MEDICAL RECORDS.

INTERNATIONAL CLASSIFICATION OF DISEASES

MANUAL
OF THE INTERNATIONAL
STATISTICAL CLASSIFICATION
OF DISEASES, INJURIES, AND
CAUSES OF DEATH

Based on the Recommendations
of the Ninth Revision Conference, 1975,
and Adopted by the Twenty-ninth World Health Assembly

Volume 2
ALPHABETICAL INDEX

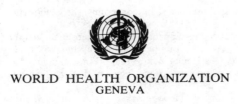

WORLD HEALTH ORGANIZATION
GENEVA

1978

First impression, 1978
Second impression, 1982

Volume 1 Introduction

List of Three-digit Categories

Tabular List of Inclusions and Four-digit Subcategories

Medical Certification and Rules for Classification

Special Lists for Tabulation

Definitions and Recommendations

Regulations

Volume 2 Alphabetical Index

ISBN 92 4 154005 2

PRINTED IN SWITZERLAND
82/5264 – Schüler SA – 10 000 (R)

CONTENTS

INTRODUCTION

INTRODUCTION

Volume 2 of the International Classification of Diseases is an alphabetical index to the Tabular List of Volume 1. Although the Index reflects the provisions of the Tabular List in regard to the notes varying the assignment of a diagnostic term when it is reported with other conditions, or under particular circumstances (e.g. certain conditions complicating pregnancy), it is not possible to express all such variations in the index terms and Volume 1 should be regarded as the primary coding tool. Reference should always be made back to the Tabular List and its notes to ensure that the code given by the Index fits the circumstances of a particular case.

The Index is, however, an essential adjunct to the Tabular List, since it contains a great number of diagnostic terms which do not appear in Volume 1. The terms included in a category of the Tabular List are not exhaustive; they serve as examples of the content of the category. The Index, on the other hand, is intended to include all diagnostic terms currently in use.

Because of its exhaustive nature, the Index inevitably includes many imprecise and undesirable terms. Since these terms are still occasionally encountered on medical records, coders need an indication of their assignment in the Classification, even if this is to a rubric for residual or ill-defined conditions. The presence of a term in this volume, therefore, should not be taken as sanction for its usage in good medical terminology.

General Arrangement of the Index

Main Sections

The Alphabetical Index consists of three sections, as follows:

Section I. – Index of diseases, syndromes, pathological conditions, injuries, signs, symptoms, problems and other reasons for contact with health services, i.e. the type of information that would be recorded by a physician. It includes all terms classifiable to categories 001–999 and V01–V82 except drugs and other chemical substances giving rise to poisoning or other adverse effects – see Section III.

Section II. – Index of external causes of injury. The terms included here are not medical diagnoses but descriptions of the circumstances under which the violence occurred (e.g. fire, explosion, fall, assault, collision, submersion). It includes all terms classifiable to E800–E999 except drugs and chemicals (Section III).

Section III. – Index of drugs and other chemical substances giving rise to poisoning or other adverse effects (referred to in Sections I and II as the Table of Drugs and Chemicals). The Table gives, for each substance, the Chapter XVII code for poisoning (960–989) and the E codes for accidental poisoning (E850–E869, E905), suicide and self-inflicted poisoning (E950–E952), and poisoning undetermined whether accidental or purposeful (E980–E982). For drugs, medicaments and biological substances, it also gives the code for these substances causing adverse effects in therapeutic use (E930–E949).

Structure

To avoid repetition, the Index is organized in the form of lead terms, which start at the extreme left of a column, and various levels of indentation, which start progressively further and further to the right. A complete index term, therefore, may be composed of several lines, sometimes quite widely separated. For example, in the entry

Erythroblastosis (fetalis) (newborn) 773.2
– due to
– – ABO
– – – antibodies 773.1
– – – incompatibility, maternal/fetal 773.1
– – – isoimmunization 773.1
– – Rh
– – – antibodies 773.0
– – – incompatibility, maternal/fetal 773.0
– – – isoimmunization 773.0

the last line stands for "Erythroblastosis due to Rh isoimmunization".

Usually, the lead term is the name of a disease or pathological condition, while the terms indented beneath it (the "modifiers") refer either to varieties of this condition, to the anatomical sites affected by it or to circumstances which affect its coding. For these, the coder should therefore first look up the disease condition as a lead term and then find the variety, anatomical site, etc., in alphabetical order below it. Thus he will find "tuberculosis of hip" under T and not under H, and stomach ulcer under U, not under S. In some diagnostic statements, the disease condition is expressed in adjectival form (e.g. "dislocated elbow") instead of the more usual noun form ("dislocation of elbow"). Sometimes the index lists both forms but often only the noun form will be found and the coder must make the necessary transformation.

Amongst the indented modifiers, it is not always feasible to include a complete listing of the various combinations of modifiers which could apply to a given term. In such instances, there are some types of modifier which tend to have priority over others. For example, under the lead term "Abscess" are indented a large number of anatomical sites and their appropriate codes. However, tuberculous abscesses are not classified to these codes but to the codes for tuberculosis of these sites. Instead of inserting an indent "tuberculous" under each anatomical site, the index uses one single indent "tuberculous" – see "Tuberculosis, abscess" under the lead term "Abscess". In general, the types of modifiers which tend to have priority over others are: in Section I, those indicating that a disease or condition was infectious or parasitic, malignant, neoplastic, psychogenic, hysterical, congenital, traumatic, complicating or affecting management of pregnancy, childbirth or the puerperium, affecting the fetus or newborn, or was reported in circumstances applicable to the supplementary "V" code. In Section II, the "priority" modifiers are those indicating transport accidents, complications of medical and surgical procedures, suicide and self-inflicted injury, homicide and assault, legal intervention, or war operations.

Section I incorporates an index of the categories in the supplementary "V" code relating to problems or circumstances rather than diseases or injuries. Some special lead terms are used for these, consisting of "key" words indicating the type of problem or circumstances, with indents indicating the codes for the complete range of appropriate categories. The main "key" words are: "Counselling", "Examination", "History (of)", "Observation (for)", "Pregnancy", "Problem (with)", "Screening (for)", "Status (post)", "Vaccination".

In both Sections I and II, this "key" word form of lead term is also used instead of, or in addition to, the standard method for certain conditions or circumstances where terminology is diverse and reported descriptions might not easily be found in the index, or where the normal method of indexing might be misleading. Such lead terms include: "Late effects of", (the only place where the code numbers of the special "Late effects" categories can be found – see Vol. 1, page 711), terms such as "Typhoid" where the implied lead term "Fever" is often omitted, "Delivery", "Pregnancy", "Puerperal", "Birth" and "Maternal condition affecting fetus or newborn", and, in Part II, "Complication", (for medical and surgical procedures), "Late effect", "Suicide", "Assault", "Legal intervention" and "War operations". Coders should remember the presence of these special lists whenever difficulty is found in locating index entries for the relevant conditions, problems or circumstances – by scrutinizing the indented terms guidance can be found as to the code numbers of all the relevant categories even if not reported in precisely the listed words.

Code numbers

The code numbers that follow the terms in the Index are those of the three-digit categories to which the terms are classified. In general, if the three-digit category is subdivided into four-digit subcategories, the appropriate fourth digit is also given in the code number. In some cases, however, the fourth digit is replaced by a dash, e.g. Burn, trunk 942.–, Arteriosclerosis, cardiorenal 404.–. This device is an indication to the coder that a fourth digit exists and should be used and that it will be found either in a note in the Index (e.g. the fourth-digit subdivision common to many sites of burns is given in a note under the lead term "Burn") or by reference to Volume 1.

Where an index term is one of the diagnostic statements for which there is a dual classification according to etiology and manifestation (see Volume 1, page XXVI), both codes are given, the first followed by a dagger (†) and the second by an asterisk (*), e.g. Pott's disease 015.0 † 730.4*.

Multiple diagnoses

The Tabular List includes a number of categories for the classification of two or more conditions jointly reported, e.g. "487.0 Influenza with pneumonia", "540.0 Acute appendicitis with generalized peritonitis". Such combinations of conditions, which are specifically classified in the Tabular List, also appear in the Index. Classification rules for certain other combinations, however, appear in the section "Medical Certification and Rules for Classification" under the heading "Notes for use in primary mortality coding" in Volume 1, e.g. "440 Atherosclerosis" excludes this condition when it is reported with conditions in "430–438 (cerebrovascular disease)". These provisions, since they are not inherent in the Classification itself, are not indexed.

Spelling

In order to avoid repetitions caused by the differences between American and English spelling, the American form has been used in the Index. This applies not only to diphthongs (e.g. anemia, anaemia; leukemia, leukaemia) but also to other variations in spelling (e.g. color, colour; labor, labour). Users familiar with the English form should remember that the first letter of diphthongs and the u in words ending in -our have been dropped, and the "re" reversed to "er" in words ending thus, etc. It is only when the initial letters of a word are affected that any great displacement in alphabetical order is caused, and in these cases, when the first two letters of a word differ in the two forms of spelling, the word is listed with the English spelling and a reference given to the American spelling, thus: "Oedema, oedematous – see Edema".

Conventions Used in the Index

Parentheses

In the Index, as in the Tabular List, parentheses have a special meaning which the coder must bear in mind. Any term which is followed by other terms in parentheses is classified to the given code number whether any of the terms in parentheses are reported or not. For example:

Abscess (infectional) (metastatic) (multiple) (pyogenic) (septic)
– adrenal (capsule) (gland) 255.8

Adrenal abscess is classified to 255.8 whether or not capsule or gland is mentioned and whether or not the abscess is described as infectional, metastatic, multiple, pyogenic, or septic.

Cross-references

Some categories, particularly those subject to notes linking them with other categories, require rather complex indexing arrangements. To avoid repeating this arrangement for each of the inclusion terms involved, a cross-reference is used. This may take a number of forms, as in the following examples:

Paralysis, paralytic
 − cerebral
 − − spastic infantile − see Palsy, cerebral

The coder is warned that the term "Cerebral spastic infantile paralysis" is to be coded in the same way as the term "Cerebral palsy". On looking up the latter term, the coder will find listed various forms of paralysis; diplegic, hemiplegic, monoplegic, etc.

Inflammation, inflamed, inflammatory (with exudation)
 − cornea (see also Keratitis) 370.9

The coder is told that if the term "Inflammation of cornea" is the only term on the medical record, the code number is 370.9, but that if any other information is present which is not found indented below he should look up "Keratitis". There he will find alternative code numbers for the condition if further or otherwise qualified as, for example, gonococcal, syphilitic, trachomatous or tuberculous.

Enlargement, enlarged − see also Hypertrophy
 − adenoids (and tonsils) 474.1
 − alveolar ridge 525.8
     etc.

If the coder does not find the site of the enlargement among the indents beneath "Enlargement," he should look among the indents beneath "Hypertrophy" where a more complete list of sites if given.

Septicemia, septicemic (generalized) (suppurative)
 − with
 − − abortion − see categories 634−639, fourth digit .0

The coder is here referred, not to another part of the Index, but to a group of categories in Volume 1, one of which will be the appropriate code number. In this case the categories 634−639 classify different types of abortion.

Bladder − see condition
Hereditary − see condition

Anatomical sites and very general adjectival modifiers are not usually used as lead terms in the Index and the coder is instructed to look up the disease or injury reported on the medical record and under that term to find the site or adjectival modifier.

Abdomen, abdominal – see also condition
– acute 789.0
– convulsive equivalent 345.5

The term "acute abdomen" is coded to 789.0 and "Abdominal convulsive equivalent" is coded to 345.5, but for other abdominal conditions, the coder should look up the disease or injury reported.

Abbreviation NEC

The letters NEC stand for "not elsewhere classified". They are added after terms classified to residual or unspecific categories and to terms in themselves ill-defined as a warning that specified forms of the conditions are classified differently and if the medical record includes more precise information the coding should be modified accordingly, e.g.

Disease, diseased – see also Syndrome
– heart (organic)
– – congenital NEC 746.9

The term "congenital heart disease" is classified to 746.9 only if no more precise description appears on the medical record. If a more precise term, e.g. interventricular septal defect, is recorded, this term should be looked up for the appropriate code.

Special signs

The following special signs will be found attached to certain code numbers or index terms:

†/*   used to designate the "etiology" code and the "manifestation" code respectively, for terms subject to dual classification. See under "Code numbers" above.

#/◊   attached to certain terms in the list of sites under "Neoplasm" to refer the coder to Notes 3 and 4 respectively at the start of that list.

SECTION I

ALPHABETICAL INDEX TO DISEASES AND NATURE OF INJURY

Section I

ALPHABETICAL INDEX TO DISEASES AND NATURE OF INJURY

A

Abasia (-astasia) 307.9
− hysterical 300.1
Abdomen, abdominal - see also condition
− acute 789.0
− convulsive equivalent 345.5
Abduction contracture, hip or other joint -
  see Contraction, joint
Aberrant (congenital) - see also
  Malposition, congenital
− adrenal gland 759.1
− breast 757.6
− endocrine gland NEC 759.2
− hepatic duct 751.6
− pancreas 751.7
− parathyroid gland 759.2
− pituitary gland 759.2
− sebaceous glands, mucous membrane,
  mouth 750.2
− spleen 759.0
− testis (descent) 752.5
− thymus (gland) 759.2
− thyroid gland 759.2
Aberration, mental (see also Disorder,
  mental, nonpsychotic) 300.9
Abetalipoproteinemia 272.5
Abiotrophy 799.8

Ablatio
− placentae - see Placenta, ablatio
− retinae (see also Detachment, retina)
  361.9
Ablation
− placenta - see Placenta, ablatio
− uterus 621.8
Ablepharia, ablepharon 743.6
Abnormal, abnormality, abnormalities - see
  also Anomaly
− acid-base balance 276.4
− − fetus - see Distress, fetal
− alveolar ridge 525.9
− amnion 658.9
− − fetus or newborn 762.9
− anatomical relationship NEC 759.9
− apertures, congenital, diaphragm 756.6
− auditory perception NEC 388.4
− autosomes NEC 758.5
− − D(1) 758.1
− − E(3) 758.2
− − G 758.0
− − 13 758.1
− − 18 758.2
− − 21 or 22 758.0
− basal metabolic rate 794.7

Abnormal - *continued*
- loss of weight 783.2
- Mantoux test 795.5
- membranes (fetal)
- - complicating pregnancy 658.8
- - fetus or newborn 762.9
- movement
- - head 781.0
- - involuntary 781.0
- - specified type NEC 333.9
- myoglobin (Aberdeen) (Annapolis) 289.9
- narrowness, eyelid 743.6
- organs or tissues of pelvis NEC
- - in pregnancy or childbirth 654.9
- - - causing obstructed labor 660.2
- - - - fetus or newborn 763.1
- - - fetus or newborn 763.8
- origin - see Malposition, congenital
- palmar creases 757.2
- Papanicolaou (smear)
- - cervix 795.0
- - other site 795.1
- parturition
- - fetus or newborn 763.9
- - mother - see Delivery, complicated
- pelvis (bony) - see Deformity, pelvis
- percussion, chest 786.7
- periods (grossly) (see also Menstruation) 626.9
- phonocardiogram 794.3
- placenta - see Placenta, abnormal
- pleural folds 748.8
- position - see also Malposition ·
- - gravid uterus 654.4
- - - causing obstructed labor 660.2
- posture 781.9
- presentation (fetus) - see Presentation, fetal, abnormal
- product of conception NEC 631
- pulmonary
- - artery 747.3
- - function, newborn 770.8
- - test results 794.2
- - ventilation, newborn 770.8
- pupillary reaction 379.4
- radiological examination 793.9
- - abdomen NEC 793.6
- - biliary tract 793.3
- - breast 793.8
- - gastrointestinal (tract) 793.4
- - genitourinary organs 793.5
- - head 793.0
- - intrathoracic organ NEC 793.2
- - lung (field) 793.1
- - musculoskeletal system 793.7
- - retroperitoneum 793.6

Abnormal - *continued*
- radiological examination - *continued*
- - skull 793.0
- red blood cell(s) 790.0
- - morphology 790.0
- - volume 790.0
- reflex NEC 796.1
- renal function test 794.4
- response to nerve stimulation 794.1
- retinal correspondence 368.3
- rhythm, heart - see also Arrhythmia
- - fetus - see Distress, fetal
- saliva 792.4
- secretion
- - gastrin 251.5
- - glucagon 251.4
- semen 792.2
- serum level (of)
- - acid phosphatase 790.5
- - alkaline phosphatase 790.5
- - amylase 790.5
- - enzymes NEC 790.5
- - lipase 790.5
- shape
- - cornea 743.4
- - gallbladder 751.6
- - gravid uterus - see Anomaly, uterus
- - organ or site, congenital NEC - see Distortion
- sinus venosus 747.4
- size
- - gallbladder 751.6
- - organ or site, congenital NEC - see Distortion
- - teeth 520.2
- skin and appendages, congenital NEC 757.9
- soft parts of pelvis - see Abnormal organs or tissues of pelvis
- spermatazoa 792.2
- sputum 786.4
- stool NEC 787.7
- - color 792.1
- - contents 792.1
- synchondrosis 756.9
- thebesian valve 746.9
- thermography - see Abnormal radiological examination
- thyroid-binding globulin 246.8
- toxicology (findings) NEC 796.0
- tracheal cartilage (congenital) 748.3
- transport protein 273.8
- ultrasound results - see Abnormal radiological examination
- umbilical cord
- - complicating delivery 663.9
- - fetus or newborn NEC 762.9

Abnormal - *continued*
- umbilical cord - *continued*
- - specified NEC 663.8
- union
- - cricoid cartilage and thyroid cartilage 748.3
- - larynx and trachea 748.3
- - thyroid cartilage and hyoid bone 748.3
- urination NEC 788.6
- urine (constituents) NEC 791.9
- uterine hemorrhage - see Hemorrhage, uterus
- vagina (acquired) (congenital) in pregnancy or childbirth 654.7
- - causing obstructed labor 660.2
- - - fetus or newborn 763.1
- visually evoked potential (VEP) 794.1
- vulva (acquired) (congenital), in pregnancy or childbirth 654.8
- - causing obstructed labor 660.2
- - - fetus or newborn 763.1
- X-ray examination - see Abnormal radiological examination
Abnormally formed uterus - see Anomaly, uterus
Abnormity (any organ or part) - see Anomaly
ABO hemolytic disease 773.1
Abolition, language 784.6
Aborter, habitual or recurrent NEC
- current abortion 634.-
- fetus or newborn 761.8
- observation in current pregnancy 646.3
- without current pregnancy 629.9
Abortion (complete) (incomplete) 637.-
- accidental - see Abortion, spontaneous
- attempted (failed) 638.-
- criminal - see Abortion, illegal
- failed (legal) 638.-
- fetus 779.6
- following threatened abortion - see Abortion, by type
- habitual or recurrent (care during pregnancy) 646.3
- - with current abortion 634.-
- - - fetus or newborn 761.8
- - without current pregnancy 629.9
- homicidal - see Abortion, illegal
- illegal 636.-
- - fetus 779.6
- induced 637.-
- - for
- - - legal indications - see Abortion, legal
- - - medical indications - see Abortion, therapeutic
- - illegal - see Abortion, illegal

Abortion - *continued*
- induced - *continued*
- - legal - see Abortion, legal
- legal 635.-
- - fetus 779.6
- missed 632
- operative - see Abortion, therapeutic
- psychiatric indication - see Abortion, therapeutic
- recurrent - see Abortion, spontaneous
- spontaneous 634.-
- - fetus 761.8
- - threatened 640.0
- - - affecting fetus or newborn 762.1
- surgical - see Abortion, therapeutic
- therapeutic 635.-
- - fetus 779.6
- threatened 640.0
- - affecting fetus or newborn 762.1
- tubal - see Pregnancy, tubal
Abrami's disease 283.9
Abrasion - see also Injury, superficial
- tooth, teeth (dentifrice) (habitual) (hard tissues) (occupational) (ritual) (traditional) (wedge defect) 521.2
Abrikossoff's tumor (M9580/0) - see also Neoplasm, connective tissue, benign
- malignant (M9580/3) - see Neoplasm, connective tissue, malignant
Abruptio placentae - see Placenta, abruptio
Abruption, placenta - see Placenta, abruptio
Abscess (infectional) (metastatic) (multiple) (pyogenic) (septic) 682.9
- with lymphangitis - code by site under Abscess
- abdomen, abdominal
- - cavity - see Abscess, peritoneum
- - wall 682.2
- abdominopelvic - see Abscess, peritoneum
- accessory sinus (chronic) (see also Sinusitis) 473.9
- adrenal (capsule) (gland) 255.8
- alveolar 522.5
- amebic 006.3
- - brain (and liver or lung abscess) 006.5
- - liver (without mention of brain or lung abscess) 006.3
- - lung (and liver) (without mention of brain abscess) 006.4
- - specified site NEC 006.8
- - spleen 006.8
- ankle 682.6
- anorectal 566
- antecubital space 682.3
- antrum (chronic) (Highmore) (see also Sinusitis, maxillary) 473.0

Abscess - *continued*
- anus 566
- apical (tooth) 522.5
- — with sinus (alveolar) 522.7
- appendix 540.1
- areola (acute) (chronic) (nonpuerperal) 611.0
- — puerperal, postpartum 675.1
- arm (any part, above wrist) 682.3
- artery (wall) 447.2
- auricle (ear) (staphylococcal) (streptococcal) 380.1
- axilla (region) 682.3
- — lymph gland or node 683
- back (any part) 682.2
- Bartholin's gland 616.3
- Bezold's 383.0
- bile, biliary, duct or tract (see also Cholecystitis) 576.8
- bladder (wall) 595.8
- bone (subperiosteal) 730.0
- — accessory sinus (chronic) (see also Sinusitis) 473.9
- — chronic or old 730.1
- — jaw (lower) (upper) 526.4
- — mastoid 383.0
- — petrous 383.2
- — spinal (tuberculous) 015.0 † 730.4*
- — — nontuberculous 730.0
- bowel 569.5
- brain (any part) 324.0
- — amebic (with abscess of any other site) 006.5
- — cystic 324.0
- — otogenic 324.0
- — tuberculous 013.8 † 324.0*
- breast (acute) (chronic) (nonpuerperal) 611.0
- — newborn 771.5
- — puerperal, postpartum 675.1
- broad ligament (see also Disease, pelvis, inflammatory) 614.4
- Brodie's (localized) (chronic) 730.1
- bronchi 519.1
- buccal cavity 528.3
- bulbo-urethral gland 597.0
- bursa (see also Bursitis) 727.8
- — pharyngeal 478.2
- buttock 682.5
- canthus 372.2
- cartilage 733.9
- cecum 540.1
- cerebellum, cerebellar 324.0
- cerebral (embolic) 324.0
- cervical (meaning neck) 682.1
- — lymph gland or node 683
- — stump (see also Cervicitis) 616.0

Abscess - *continued*
- cervix (uteri) (see also Cervicitis) 616.0
- cheek 682.0
- — inner 528.3
- chest 510.9
- — with fistula 510.0
- — wall 682.2
- chin 682.0
- choroid 363.0
- ciliary body 364.3
- cold (tuberculous) - see also Tuberculosis, abscess
- — articular - see Tuberculosis, joint
- colon (wall) 569.5
- colostomy or enterostomy 569.6
- conjunctiva 372.0
- connective tissue NEC 682.9
- cornea 370.5
- corpus
- — cavernosum 607.2
- — luteum (see also Salpingo-oophoritis) 614.2
- Cowper's gland 597.0
- cranium 324.0
- cul-de-sac (Douglas') (posterior) (see also Disease, pelvis, inflammatory) 614.4
- dental 522.5
- — with sinus (alveolar) 522.7
- dentoalveolar 522.5
- — with sinus (alveolar) 522.7
- diaphragm, diaphragmatic - see Abscess, peritoneum
- Douglas' cul-de-sac or pouch (see also Disease, pelvis, inflammatory) 614.4
- ear (middle) 382.4
- — acute 382.0
- — external 380.1
- — inner 386.3
- elbow 682.3
- entamebic - see Abscess, amebic
- epididymis 604.0
- epidural 324.9
- — brain 324.0
- — spinal cord 324.1
- epiglottis 478.7
- epiploon, epiploic - see Abscess, peritoneum
- erysipelatous (see also Erysipelas) 035
- esophagus 530.1
- ethmoid (bone) (chronic) (sinus) 473.2
- external auditory canal 380.1
- extradural 324.9
- — brain 324.0
- — spinal cord 324.1
- extraperitoneal - see Abscess, peritoneum
- eye 360.0

Abscess - *continued*
- eyelid 373.1
- face (any part, except eye) 682.0
- fallopian tube (see also
  Salpingo-oophoritis) 614.2
- fascia 728.8
- fauces 478.2
- fecal 569.5
- femoral (region) 682.6
- filaria, filarial (see also Infestation,
  filarial) 125.9
- finger (any) 681.0
- fistulous NEC 682.9
- foot (except toe) 682.7
- forearm 682.3
- forehead 682.0
- frontal (chronic) (sinus) 473.1
- gallbladder (see also Cholecystitis, acute)
  575.0
- gastric 535.0
- genital organ or tract NEC
- - female 616.9
- - - complication of
- - - - abortion - see categories 634-639,
        fourth digit .0
- - - - ectopic or molar pregnancy 639.0
- - - puerperal, postpartum, childbirth
      670
- - male 608.4
- gingival 523.3
- gland, glandular (lymph) (acute) NEC
  683
- gluteal (region) 682.5
- gonorrheal NEC (see also Gonococcus)
  098.0
- groin 682.2
- gum 523.3
- hand (except finger or thumb) 682.4
- head NEC 682.8
- heart (see also Carditis) 429.8
- heel 682.7
- hepatic 572.0
- - amebic (see also Abscess, liver,
    amebic) 006.3
- - duct (see also Cholecystitis) 576.8
- hip 682.6
- ileocecal 540.1
- ileostomy (bud) 569.6
- iliac (region) 682.2
- - fossa 540.1
- iliopsoas (tuberculous) 015.0 † 730.4*
- - nontuberculous 728.8
- infraclavicular (fossa) 682.3
- inguinal (region) 682.2
- - lymph gland or node 683
- intestine, intestinal 569.5
- - rectal 566

Abscess - *continued*
- intra-abdominal - see also Abscess,
  peritoneum
- intracranial 324.0
- intramammary - see Abscess, breast
- intra-orbital 376.0
- intraperitoneal - see Abscess, peritoneum
- intraspinal 324.1
- intratonsillar 475
- iris 364.3
- ischiorectal 566
- jaw (bone) (lower) (upper) 526.4
- joint 711.0
- - vertebral (tuberculous) 015.0 † 730.4*
- - - nontuberculous 724.8
- kidney 590.2
- - with calculus 592.0
- - complicating pregnancy or puerperium
    646.6
- - - fetus or newborn 760.1
- knee 682.6
- - joint 711.0
- labium (majus) (minus) 616.4
- - complicating pregnancy, childbirth or
    puerperium 646.6
- lacrimal
- - caruncle 375.3
- - gland 375.0
- - passages (duct) (sac) 375.3
- larynx 478.7
- leg, except foot 682.6
- lens 360.0
- lingual 529.0
- - tonsil 475
- lip 528.5
- Littre's gland 597.0
- liver 572.0
- - amebic 006.3
- - - with
- - - - brain abscess (and lung abscess)
        006.5
- - - - lung abscess 006.4
- - due to Entameba histolytica (see also
    Abscess, liver, amebic) 006.3
- - dysenteric (see also Abscess, liver,
    amebic) 006.3
- - tropical - see Abscess, liver, amebic
- loin (region) 682.2
- lumbar (tuberculous) 015.0 † 730.4*
- - nontuberculous 682.2
- lung (miliary) (putrid) 513.0
- - amebic (with liver abscess) 006.4
- - - with brain abscess 006.5
- lymph, lymphatic, gland or node (acute)
  683
- - any site, except mesenteric 683
- - mesentery 289.2

Abscess - *continued*
- malar 526.4
- mammary gland - see Abscess, breast
- marginal (anus) 566
- mastoid 383.0
- maxilla, maxillary 526.4
- - molar 522.5
- - premolar 522.5
- - sinus (chronic) 473.0
- mediastinum 513.1
- meibomian gland 373.1
- meninges (see also Meningitis) 320.9
- mesentery, mesenteric - see Abscess, peritoneum
- mesosalpinx (see also Salpingo-oophoritis) 614.2
- mons pubis 682.2
- mouth (floor) 528.3
- mural 682.2
- muscle 728.8
- myocardium 422.9
- nabothian (follicle) (see also Cervicitis) 616.0
- nail (chronic) (with lymphangitis) 681.9
- nasal (fossa) (septum) 478.1
- - sinus (chronic) (see also Sinusitis) 473.9
- nasopharyngeal 478.2
- navel 682.2
- - newborn NEC 771.4
- neck (region) 682.1
- - lymph gland or node 683
- nephritic (see also Abscess, kidney) 590.2
- nipple 611.0
- - puerperal, postpartum 675.0
- nose (septum) 478.1
- - external 682.0
- oesophagus 530.1
- omentum - see Abscess, peritoneum
- operative wound 998.5
- orbit, orbital 376.0
- ossifluent - see Abscess, bone
- ovary, ovarian (corpus luteum) (see also Salpingo-oophoritis) 614.2
- oviduct (see also Salpingo-oophoritis) 614.2
- palate (soft) 528.3
- - hard 526.4
- palmar (space) 682.4
- pancreas (duct) 577.0
- paradontal 523.3
- parametric, parametrium (see also Disease, pelvis, inflammatory) 614.4
- pararectal 566
- parasinus (see also Sinusitis) 473.9
- parauterine (see also Disease, pelvis, inflammatory) 614.4

Abscess - *continued*
- paravaginal (see also Vaginitis) 616.1
- parietal region 682.8
- parotid (duct) (gland) 527.3
- - region 528.3
- pectoral (region) 682.2
- pelvis, pelvic
- - female (see also Disease, pelvis, inflammatory) 614.4
- - male, peritoneal - see Abscess, peritoneum
- penis 607.2
- - gonococcal (acute) 098.0
- - - chronic or duration of 2 months or over 098.2
- perianal 566
- periapical 522.5
- - with sinus (alveolar) 522.7
- periappendiceal 540.1
- pericardial 420.9
- pericecal 540.1
- pericemental 523.3
- pericholecystic (see also Cholecystitis, acute) 575.0
- pericoronal 523.3
- peridental 523.3
- perigastric 535.0
- perimetric (see also Disease, pelvis, inflammatory) 614.4
- perinephric, perinephritic (see also Abscess, kidney) 590.2
- perineum, perineal (superficial) 682.2
- - deep (with urethral involvement) 597.0
- - urethra 597.0
- periodontal (parietal) 523.3
- periosteum, periosteal 730.3
- - with osteomyelitis 730.2
- - - acute or subacute 730.0
- - - chronic or old 730.1
- periproctic 566
- periprostatic 601.2
- perirectal 566
- perirenal (tissue) (see also Abscess, kidney) 590.2
- perisinus (nose) (see also Sinusitis) 473.9
- peritoneum, peritoneal (perforated) (ruptured) (see also Peritonitis) 567.2
- - with appendicitis 540.1
- - complication of
- - - abortion - see categories 634-639, fourth digit .0
- - - ectopic or molar pregnancy 639.0
- - pelvic
- - - female (see also Disease, pelvis, inflammatory) 614.4
- - - male 567.2

Abscess - *continued*
- subhepatic - see Abscess, peritoneum
- sublingual 528.3
- - gland 527.3
- submammary - see Abscess, breast
- submandibular (region) (space) (triangle) 682.0
- - gland 527.3
- submaxillary (region) 682.0
- - gland 527.3
- submental 682.0
- - gland 527.3
- subpectoral 682.2
- subperiosteal - see Abscess, bone
- subphrenic - see also Abscess, peritoneum
- - postoperative 998.5
- suburethral 597.0
- sudoriparous 705.8
- suppurative NEC 682.9
- supraclavicular (fossa) 682.3
- suprapelvic (see also Disease, pelvis, inflammatory) 614.4
- suprapubic 682.2
- suprarenal (capsule) (gland) 255.8
- sweat gland 705.8
- temple 682.0
- temporal region 682.0
- temporosphenoidal 324.0
- tendon (sheath) 727.8
- testis 604.0
- thecal 728.8
- thigh 682.6
- thorax 510.9
- - with fistula 510.0
- throat 478.2
- thumb 681.0
- thymus (gland) 254.1
- thyroid (gland) 245.0
- toe (any) 681.1
- tongue (staphylococcal) 529.0
- tonsil(s) (lingual) 475
- tonsillopharyngeal 475
- tooth, teeth (root) 522.5
- - with sinus (alveolar) 522.7
- - supporting structures NEC 523.3
- trachea 478.9
- trunk 682.2
- tubal (see also Salpingo-oophoritis) 614.2
- tuberculous - see Tuberculosis, abscess
- tubo-ovarian (see also Salpingo-oophoritis) 614.2
- tunica vaginalis 608.4
- umbilicus NEC 682.2
- - newborn 771.4
- upper respiratory 478.9
- urethra (gland) 597.0

Abscess - *continued*
- uterus, uterine (wall) (see also Endometritis) 615.9
- - ligament (see also Disease, pelvis, inflammatory) 614.4
- - neck (see also Cervicitis) 616.0
- uvula 528.3
- vagina (wall) (see also Vaginitis) 616.1
- vaginorectal (see also Vaginitis) 616.1
- vas deferens 608.4
- vermiform appendix 540.1
- vertebra (column) (tuberculous) 015.0 † 730.4*
- - nontuberculous 730.0
- vesical 595.8
- vesico-uterine pouch (see also Disease, pelvis, inflammatory) 614.4
- vitreous (humor) (pneumococcal) 360.0
- vocal cord 478.5
- von Bezold's 383.0
- vulva 616.4
- - complicating pregnancy, childbirth or puerperium 646.6
- vulvovaginal gland (see also Vaginitis) 616.3
- web space 682.4
- wrist 682.4
Absence (organ or part) (complete or partial)
- adrenal (gland) (congenital) 759.1
- - acquired 255.8
- albumin in blood 273.8
- alimentary tract (congenital) 751.8
- - lower 751.5
- - upper 750.9
- anus (congenital) 751.2
- aorta (congenital) 747.2
- appendix, congenital 751.2
- arm (acquired) 736.8
- - congenital 755.2
- artery (congenital) (peripheral) 747.6
- - brain 747.8
- - coronary 746.8
- - pulmonary 747.3
- atrial septum 745.6
- auditory canal (congenital) (external) 744.0
- auricle (ear), congenital 744.0
- bile, biliary duct, congenital 751.6
- bladder (acquired) 596.8
- - congenital 753.8
- bone, congenital NEC 756.9
- brain 740.0
- - part of 742.2
- breast(s) (acquired) 611.8
- - congenital 757.6
- broad ligament 752.1

Absence - *continued*
- bronchus (congenital) 748.3
- canaliculus lacrimalis, congenital 743.6
- cerebellum (vermis) 742.2
- cervix (acquired) 622.8
- - congenital 752.4
- chin, congenital 744.8
- cilia (congenital) 743.6
- - acquired 374.8
- clitoris (congenital) 752.4
- coccyx, congenital 756.1
- cold sense (see also Disturbance, sensation) 782.0
- congenital
- - lumen - see Atresia
- - organ or site NEC - see Agenesis
- - septum - see Imperfect closure
- corpus callosum 742.2
- diaphragm (with hernia) 756.6
- digestive organ(s) or tract, congenital 751.8
- - lower 751.5
- - upper 750.8
- ductus arteriosus 747.8
- ear (auricle) (external) (inner) (middle), congenital 744.0
- - lobe, lobule 744.2
- ejaculatory duct (congenital) 752.8
- endocrine gland NEC 759.2
- epididymis (congenital) 752.8
- - acquired 608.8
- epiglottis, congenital 748.3
- epileptic (atonic) (typical) 345.0
- esophagus (congenital) 750.3
- eustachian tube (congenital) 744.2
- extremity (acquired) 736.9
- - congenital 755.4
- - lower 736.8
- - - congenital 755.3
- - upper 736.8
- - - congenital 755.2
- eye (acquired) 360.8
- - congenital 743.0
- - muscle (congenital) 743.6
- eyelid (fold) (congenital) 743.6
- - acquired 374.8
- fallopian tube(s) (acquired) 620.8
- - congenital 752.1
- femur, congenital 755.3
- finger (acquired) 736.2
- - congenital 755.2
- foot (acquired) 736.7
- - congenital 755.3
- forearm (acquired) 736.0
- - congenital 755.2
- gallbladder (acquired) 575.8
- - congenital 751.6

Absence - *continued*
- gamma globulin in blood 279.0
- genital organs, congenital
- - female 752.8
- - - external 752.4
- - - internal NEC 752.8
- - male 752.8
- genitourinary organs, congenital NEC 752.8
- hand (acquired) 736.0
- - congenital 755.2
- heat sense (see also Disturbance, sensation) 782.0
- hymen (congenital) 752.4
- incus (acquired) 385.2
- - congenital 744.0
- internal ear (congenital) 744.0
- intestine (acquired) (small) 569.8
- - congenital 751.1
- - large 569.8
- - - congenital 751.2
- iris (congenital) 743.4
- joint, congenital NEC 755.8
- kidney(s) (acquired) 593.8
- - congenital 753.0
- labium (congenital) (majus) (minus) 752.4
- lacrimal apparatus (congenital) 743.6
- larynx (congenital) 748.3
- leg (acquired) 736.8
- - congenital 755.3
- lens (congenital) 743.3
- - acquired 379.3
- limb (acquired) 736.9
- - congenital 755.4
- - - lower 755.3
- - - upper 755.2
- liver (congenital) 751.6
- lung (fissure) (lobe) (bilateral) (unilateral) (congenital) 748.5
- - acquired (any part) 518.8
- menstruation 626.0
- muscle (congenital) (pectoral) 756.8
- - ocular 743.6
- neutrophile 288.0
- nipple (congenital) 757.6
- nose (congenital) 748.1
- - acquired 738.0
- ocular muscle (congenital) 743.6
- oesophagus (congenital) 750.3
- organ
- - of Corti (congenital) 744.0
- - or site, congenital NEC 759.8
- ovary (acquired) 620.8
- - congenital 752.0
- oviduct (acquired) 620.8
- - congenital 752.1

Absence - *continued*
- pancreas (congenital) 751.7
- – acquired 577.8
- parathyroid gland (congenital) 759.2
- parotid gland(s) (congenital) 750.2
- patella, congenital 755.6
- penis (congenital) 752.8
- – acquired 607.8
- pericardium (congenital) 746.8
- pituitary gland (congenital) 759.2
- prostate (congenital) 752.8
- – acquired 602.8
- punctum lacrimale (congenital) 743.6
- radius, congenital 755.2
- rectum (congenital) 751.2
- – acquired 569.4
- respiratory organ (congenital) NEC 748.9
- rib (acquired) 738.3
- – congenital 756.3
- roof of orbit (congenital) 742.0
- sacrum, congenital 756.1
- salivary gland(s) (congenital) 750.2
- scrotum, congenital 752.8
- seminal tract or duct (congenital) 752.8
- – acquired 608.8
- septum
- – atrial 745.6
- – between aorta and pulmonary artery 745.0
- – ventricular 745.3
- sex chromosome 758.8
- skull bone 756.0
- – with
- – – – anencephalus 740.0
- – – – encephalocele 742.0
- – – – hydrocephalus 742.3
- – – – – with spina bifida 741.0
- – – – microcephalus 742.1
- spermatic cord (congenital) 752.8
- spine, congenital 756.1
- spleen (congenital) 759.0
- – acquired 289.5
- sternum, congenital 756.3
- stomach (acquired) (partial) 564.2
- – congenital 750.7
- submaxillary gland(s) (congenital) 750.2
- superior vena cava (congenital) 747.4
- tendon (congenital) 756.8
- testis (congenital) 752.8
- – acquired 608.8
- thigh (acquired) 736.8
- thumb (acquired) 736.2
- – congenital 755.2
- thymus gland (congenital) 759.2
- thyroid (gland) (surgical) 246.8
- – cartilage, congenital 748.3

Absence - *continued*
- thyroid - *continued*
- – congenital 243
- toe (acquired) 735.8
- – congenital 755.3
- tongue 750.1
- tooth, teeth (congenital) 520.0
- – with abnormal spacing 524.3
- – acquired 525.1
- – – with malocclusion 524.3
- trachea (cartilage) (congenital) 748.3
- transverse aortic arch (congenital) 747.2
- umbilical artery (congenital) 747.5
- ureter (congenital) 753.4
- – acquired 593.8
- urethra, congenital 753.8
- uterus (acquired) 621.8
- – congenital 752.3
- uvula (congenital) 750.2
- vagina, congenital 752.4
- vas deferens (congenital) 752.8
- – acquired 608.8
- vein (congenital) (peripheral) 747.6
- – brain 747.8
- – great 747.4
- – portal 747.4
- – pulmonary 747.4
- vena cava (congenital) (inferior) (superior) 747.4
- ventricular septum 745.3
- vertebra, congenital 756.1
- vulva, congenital 752.4
Absinthemia 304.6
Absinthism 304.6
Absorbent system disease 459.8
Absorption
- chemical NEC 989.9
- – specified chemical or substance - see Table of drugs and chemicals
- – through placenta (fetus or newborn) 760.7
- – – obstetric anesthetic or analgesic drug 763.5
- – – suspected, affecting management of pregnancy 655.5
- drug NEC (see also Reaction, drug) 995.2
- – through placenta, fetus or newborn 760.7
- – – obstetric anesthetic or analgesic drug 763.5
- – – suspected, affecting management of pregnancy 655.5
- fat, disturbance 579.8
- lactose defect 271.3
- noxious substance - see Absorption, chemical

Absorption - *continued*
- protein, disturbance 579.8
- pus or septic, general - see Septicemia
- toxic substance - see Absorption, chemical
- uremic - see Uremia
Abstinence symptoms, syndrome
- alcohol 291.8
- drug 292.0
Abulia 799.8
Abuse
- alcohol (see also Alcoholism) 303
- - non-dependent 305.0
- child NEC 995.5
- drugs, non-dependent 305.9
- - amphetamine type 305.7
- - antidepressants 305.8
- - barbiturates 305.4
- - caffeine 305.9
- - cannabis 305.2
- - cocaine type 305.6
- - hallucinogens 305.3
- - hashish 305.2
- - LSD 305.3
- - marijuana 305.2
- - mixed 305.9
- - morphine type 305.5
- - specified NEC 305.9
- - tranquillizers 305.4
- tobacco 305.1
Acalculia 784.6
- developmental 315.1
Acanthocheilonemiasis 125.4
Acanthocytosis 272.5
Acantholysis 701.8
- bullosa 757.3
Acanthoma (benign) (M8070/0) - see also Neoplasm, benign
- malignant (M8070/3) - see Neoplasm, malignant
Acanthosis (acquired) (nigricans) 701.2
- benign 757.3
- congenital 757.3
- tongue 529.8
Acardia 759.8
Acardiacus amorphus 759.8
Acardius 759.8
Acariasis 133.9
Acarodermatitis 133.9
- urticarioides 133.9
Acarophobia 300.2
Acatalasemia 277.8
Acatalasia 277.8
Accelerated atrioventricular conduction 426.7
Accessory (congenital)
- adrenal gland 759.1

Accessory - *continued*
- anus 751.5
- appendix 751.5
- atrioventricular conduction 426.7
- auditory ossicles 744.0
- auricle (ear) 744.1
- autosome(s) NEC 758.5
- - 21 or 22 758.0
- biliary duct or passage 751.6
- bladder 753.8
- blood vessels NEC 747.6
- bone NEC 756.9
- breast tissue, axilla 757.6
- carpal bones 755.5
- cecum 751.5
- chromosome(s) NEC 758.9
- - autosome(s) NEC 758.5
- - D(1) 758.1
- - E(3) 758.2
- - G 758.0
- - sex 758.8
- - 13 758.1
- - 18 758.2
- - 21 or 22 758.0
- coronary artery 746.8
- cusp(s), heart valve NEC 746.8
- - pulmonary 746.0
- cystic duct 751.6
- digits 755.0
- ear (auricle) (lobe) 744.1
- endocrine gland NEC 759.2
- external os 752.8
- eye muscle 743.6
- eyelid 743.6
- face bone(s) 756.0
- fallopian tube (fimbria) (ostium) 752.1
- fingers 755.0
- foreskin 605
- frontonasal process 756.0
- gallbladder 751.6
- genital organ(s)
- - female 752.8
- - - external 752.4
- - - internal NEC 752.8
- - male 752.8
- genitourinary organs NEC 752.8
- heart 746.8
- - valve NEC 746.8
- - - pulmonary 746.0
- hepatic ducts 751.6
- hymen 752.4
- intestine (large) (small) 751.5
- kidney 753.3
- lacrimal canal 743.6
- leaflet, heart valve NEC 746.8
- - pulmonary 746.0
- ligament, broad 752.1

Accessory - *continued*
- liver (duct) 751.6
- lobule (ear) 744.1
- lung (lobe) 748.6
- muscle 756.8
- navicular of carpus 755.5
- nervous system, part NEC 742.8
- nipple 757.6
- nose 748.1
- organ or site not listed here - see
  Anomaly, specified type NEC
- ovary 752.0
- oviduct 752.1
- pancreas 751.7
- parathyroid gland 759.2
- parotid gland (and duct) 750.2
- pituitary gland 759.2

- preauricular appendage 744.1
- prepuce 605
- renal arteries (multiple) 747.6
- rib 756.3
- - cervical 756.2
- roots (teeth) 520.2
- salivary gland 750.2
- sesamoids 755.8
- sinus - see condition
- skin tags 757.3
- spleen 759.0
- sternum 756.3
- submaxillary gland 750.2
- tarsal bones 755.6
- tendon 756.8
- thumb 755.0
- thymus gland 759.2
- thyroid gland 759.2
- toes 755.0
- tongue 750.1
- tooth, teeth 520.1
- - causing crowding 524.3
- tragus 744.1
- ureter 753.4
- urethra 753.8
- urinary organ or tract NEC 753.8
- uterus 752.2
- vagina 752.4
- valve, heart NEC 746.8
- - pulmonary 746.0
- vertebra 756.1
- vocal cords 748.3
- vulva 752.4

Accident
- birth NEC 767.9
- cardiac (see also Infarct, myocardium)
  410
- cardiovascular (see also Disease,
  cardiovascular) 429.2

Accident - *continued*
- cerebral (see also Disease,
  cerebrovascular, acute) 436
- cerebrovascular (see also Disease,
  cerebrovascular, acute) 436
- coronary (see also Infarct, myocardium)
  410
- craniovascular (see also Disease,
  cerebrovascular, acute) 436
- during pregnancy, to mother
- - fetus or newborn 760.5
- vascular - see Disease, cerebrovascular,
  acute
Accidental - see condition
Accommodation
- disorder of 367.5
- insufficiency of 367.4
- paralysis of, hysterical 300.1
- spasm of 367.5
Accouchement - see Delivery
Accreta placenta (without hemorrhage)
  667.0
- with hemorrhage 666.0
Accretions, tooth, teeth 523.6
Accumulation secretion, prostate 602.8
Acephalia, acephalism, acephaly 740.0
Acephalobrachia monster 759.8
Acephalochirus monster 759.8
Acephalogaster 759.8
Acephalostomus monster 759.8
Acephalothorax 759.8
Acephalus 740.0
Acetonemia 790.6
- diabetic 250.1
Acetonuria 791.6
Achalasia 530.0
- cardia 530.0
- digestive organs, congenital NEC 751.8
- esophagus 530.0
- pylorus 750.5
- sphincteral NEC 564.8
Achard-Thiers syndrome 255.2
Ache(s) - see Pain
Achillobursitis 726.7
Achillodynia 726.7
Achlorhydria, achlorhydric 536.0
- anemia 280
- diarrhea 536.0
- neurogenic 536.0
- psychogenic 306.4
- secondary to vagotomy 564.2
Acholuric jaundice (familial)
  (splenomegalic) (see also Spherocytosis)
  282.0
- acquired 283.9
Achondroplasia 756.4
Achroma, cutis 709.0

Actinomycosis - *continued*
- specified site NEC 039.8
Actinoneuritis 357.8
Action, heart
- disorder 427.9
- irregular 427.9
- - psychogenic 306.2
Active - see condition
Activity decrease, functional 780.9
Acute - see also condition
- abdomen NEC 789.0
- gallbladder 575.0
Acystia 753.8
Adair-Dighton syndrome 756.5
Adamantinoblastoma (M9310/0) - see
  Ameloblastoma
Adamantinoma (M9310/0) - see
  Ameloblastoma
Adamantoblastoma (M9310/0) - see
  Ameloblastoma
Adams-Stokes(-Morgagni) disease or
  syndrome 426.9
Adaption reaction (see also Reaction,
  adjustment) 309.9
Addiction (see also Dependence)
- absinthe 304.6
- alcohol, alcoholic (ethyl) (methyl) (wood)
  303
- - complicating pregnancy, childbirth or
    puerperium 648.4
- - - fetus or newborn 760.8
- - suspected damage to fetus affecting
    management of pregnancy 655.4
- drug (see also Dependence) 304.9
- ethyl alcohol 303
- heroin 304.0
- methyl alcohol 303
- methylated spirit 303
- morphine(-like substances) 304.0
- nicotine 305.1
- opium 304.0
- tobacco 305.1
- wine 303
Addison's
- anemia 281.0
- disease (bronze) 255.4
- - tuberculous 017.6 † 255.4*
- keloid 701.0
Addisonian crisis or melanosis 255.4
Additional - see also Accessory
- chromosome(s) 758.9
- - autosome(s) NEC 758.5
- - sex 758.8
- - 21 758.0
Adduction contracture, hip or other joint -
  see Contraction, joint
Adenitis (see also Lymphadenitis) 289.3

Adenitis - *continued*
- acute, unspecified site 683
- axillary 289.3
- - acute 683
- - chronic or subacute 289.1
- Bartholin's gland 616.8
- bulbourethral gland (see also Urethritis)
  597.8
- cervical 289.3
- - acute 683
- - chronic or subacute 289.1
- chancroid (Ducrey's bacillus) 099.0
- chronic, unspecified site 289.1
- Cowper's gland (see also Urethritis)
  597.8
- epidemic, acute 075
- gangrenous 683
- gonorrheal NEC 098.8
- groin 289.3
- - acute 683
- - chronic or subacute 289.1
- infectious 075
- inguinal 289.3
- - acute 683
- - chronic or subacute 289.1
- lymph gland or node, except mesenteric
  289.3
- - acute 683
- - chronic or subacute 289.1
- mesenteric (acute) (chronic)
  (nonspecific) (subacute) 289.2
- - due to Pasteurella multocida (Past.
    septica) 027.2
- parotid gland (suppurative) 527.2
- salivary duct or gland (any) (recurring)
  (suppurative) 527.2
- scrofulous 017.2
- Skene's duct or gland (see also Urethritis)
  597.8
- strumous, tuberculous 017.2
- subacute, unspecified site 289.1
- sublingual gland (suppurative) 527.2
- submandibular gland (suppurative) 527.2
- submaxillary gland (suppurative) 527.2
- tuberculous - see Tuberculosis, lymph
  gland
- urethral gland (see also Urethritis) 597.8
- Wharton's duct (suppurative) 527.2
Adenoacanthoma (M8570/3) - see
  Neoplasm, malignant
Adenoameloblastoma (M9300/0) 213.1
- upper jaw (bone) 213.0
Adenocarcinoma (M8140/3) - see also
  Neoplasm, malignant

Note – The list of adjectival modifiers below is not exhaustive. A description of adenocarcinoma that does not appear in this list should be coded in the same manner as carcinoma with that description. Thus, "mixed acidophil-basophil adenocarcinoma" should be coded in the same manner as "mixed acidophil-basophil carcinoma", which appears in the list under "Carcinoma".

Except where otherwise indicated, the morphological varieties of adenocarcinoma in the list below should be coded by site as for "Neoplasm, malignant".

Adenocarcinoma - *continued*
– with
– – apocrine metaplasia (M8573/3)
– – cartilaginous (and osseous) metaplasia (M8571/3)
– – osseous (and cartilaginous) metaplasia (M8571/3)
– – spindle cell metaplasia (M8572/3)
– – squamous metaplasia (M8570/3)
– acidophil (M8280/3)
– – specified site - see Neoplasm, malignant
– – unspecified site 194.3
– acinar (M8550/3)
– acinic cell (M8550/3)
– adrenal cortical (M8370/3) 194.0
– alveolar (M8251/3)
– and
– – epidermoid carcinoma, mixed (M8560/3)
– – squamous cell carcinoma, mixed (M8560/3)
– apocrine (M8401/3)
– – breast - see Neoplasm, breast, malignant
– – specified site NEC - see Neoplasm, skin, malignant
– – unspecified site 173.9
– basophil (M8300/3)
– – specified site - see Neoplasm, malignant
– – unspecified site 194.3
– bile duct 156.1
– – type (M8160/3)
– – – liver 155.1
– – – specified site NEC - see Neoplasm, malignant
– – – unspecified site 155.1
– bronchiolar (M8250/3) - see Neoplasm, lung, malignant
– bronchioloalveolar (M8250/3) - see Neoplasm, lung, malignant
– ceruminous (M8420/3) 173.2

Adenocarcinoma - *continued*
– chromophobe (M8270/3)
– – specified site - see Neoplasm, malignant
– – unspecified site 194.3
– clear cell (mesonephroid type) (M8310/3)
– colloid (M8480/3)
– cylindroid type (M8200/3)
– diffuse type (M8145/3)
– – specified site - see Neoplasm, malignant
– – unspecified site 151.9
– duct (M8500/3)
– – infiltrating (M8500/3)
– – – with Paget's disease (M8541/3) - see Neoplasm, breast, malignant
– – – specified site - see Neoplasm, malignant
– – – unspecified site 174.9
– embryonal (M9070/3)
– endometrioid (M8380/3) - see Neoplasm, malignant
– eosinophil (M8280/3)
– – specified site - see Neoplasm, malignant
– – unspecified site 194.3
– follicular (M8330/3)
– – and papillary (M8340/3) 193
– – moderately differentiated type (M8332/3) 193
– – pure follicle type (M8331/3) 193
– – specified site - see Neoplasm, malignant
– – trabecular type (M8332/3) 193
– – unspecified site 193
– – well differentiated type (M8331/3) 193
– gelatinous (M8480/3)
– granular cell (M8320/3)
– Hurthle cell (M8290/3) 193
– in
– – adenomatous
– – – polyp (M8210/3)
– – – polyposis coli (M8220/3) 153.9
– – polypoid adenoma (M8210/3)
– – tubular adenoma (M8210/3)
– – villous adenoma (M8261/3)
– infiltrating duct (M8500/3)
– – with Paget's disease (M8541/3) - see Neoplasm, breast, malignant
– – specified site - see Neoplasm, malignant
– – unspecified site 174.9
– inflammatory (M8530/3)
– – specified site - see Neoplasm, malignant

Adenocarcinoma - *continued*
- inflammatory - *continued*
- - unspecified site 174.9
- intestinal type (M8144/3)
- - specified site - see Neoplasm,
  malignant
- - unspecified site 151.9

- intraductal (noninfiltrating) (M8500/2)
- - papillary (M8503/2)
- - - specified site - see Neoplasm, in situ
- - - unspecified site 233.0
- - specified site - see Neoplasm, in situ
- - unspecified site 233.0
- islet cell (M8150/3)
- - and exocrine, mixed (M8154/3)
- - - specified site - see Neoplasm,
  malignant
- - - unspecified site 157.9
- - pancreas 157.4
- - specified site NEC - see Neoplasm,
  malignant
- - unspecified site 157.4
- lobular (M8520/3)
- - specified site - see Neoplasm,
  malignant
- - unspecified site 174.9
- medullary (M8510/3)
- mesonephric (M9110/3)
- mixed cell (M8323/3)
- mucinous (M8480/3)
- mucin-producing (M8481/3)
- mucoid (M8480/3) - see also Neoplasm,
  malignant
- - cell (M8300/3)
- - - specified site - see Neoplasm,
  malignant
- - - unspecified site 194.3

- nonencapsulated sclerosing (M8350/3)
  193
- oncocytic (M8290/3)
- oxyphilic (M8290/3)
- papillary (M8260/3)
- - and follicular (M8340/3) 193
- - intraductal (noninfiltrating)
  (M8503/2)
- - - specified site - see Neoplasm, in situ
- - - unspecified site 233.0
- - serous (M8460/3)
- - - specified site - see Neoplasm,
  malignant
- - - unspecified site 183.0
- papillocystic (M8450/3)
- - specified site - see Neoplasm,
  malignant
- - unspecified site 183.0
- pseudomucinous (M8470/3)

Adenocarcinoma - *continued*
- pseudomucinous - *continued*
- - specified site - see Neoplasm,
  malignant
- - unspecified site 183.0
- renal cell (M8312/3) 189.0
- sebaceous (M8410/3) - see Neoplasm,
  skin, malignant
- serous (M8441/3) - see also Neoplasm,
  malignant
- - papillary (M8460/3)
- - - specified site - see Neoplasm,
  malignant
- - - unspecified site 183.0
- signet ring cell (M8490/3)
- superficial spreading (M8143/3)
- sweat gland (M8400/3) - see Neoplasm,
  skin, malignant
- trabecular (M8190/3)
- tubular (M8211/3)
- villous (M8262/3)
- water-clear cell (M8322/3) 194.1
Adenocarcinoma-in-situ (M8140/2) - see
  Neoplasm, in situ
Adenofibroma (M9013/0)
- clear cell (M8313/0) - see Neoplasm,
  benign
- endometrioid (M8381/0) 220
- - borderline malignancy (M8381/1)
  236.2
- - malignant (M8381/3) 183.0
- mucinous (M9015/0)
- - specified site - see Neoplasm, benign
- - unspecified site 220
- prostate 600
- serous (M9014/0)
- - specified site - see Neoplasm, benign
- - unspecified site 220
- specified site - see Neoplasm, benign
- unspecified site 220
Adenofibrosis
- breast 610.2
- endometroid 617.0
Adenoiditis 474.0
- acute 463
Adenoids (congenital) (of nasal fossa) 474.9
- hypertrophy 474.1
- vegetations 474.2
Adenolymphoma (M8561/0)
- specified site - see Neoplasm, benign
- unspecified site 210.2
Adenoma (sessile) (M8140/0) - see also
  Neoplasm, benign

Note – Except where otherwise indicated,
the morphological varieties of adenoma in

the list below should be coded by site as
for "Neoplasm, benign".

Adenoma - *continued*
- acidophil (M8280/0)
- - specified site - see Neoplasm, benign
- - unspecified site 227.3
- acidophil-basophil, mixed (M8281/0)
- - specified site - see Neoplasm, benign
- - unspecified site 227.3
- acinar (cell) (M8550/0)
- acinic cell (M8550/0)
- adrenal (cortex) (cortical) (functioning)
  (M8370/0) 227.0
- - clear cell type (M8373/0) 227.0
- - compact cell type (M8371/0) 227.0
- - glomerulosa cell type (M8374/0) 227.0
- - heavily pigmented variant (M8372/0)
  227.0
- - mixed cell type (M8375/0) 227.0
- alpha-cell (M8152/0)
- - pancreas 211.7
- - specified site NEC - see Neoplasm,
  benign
- - unspecified site 211.7
- alveolar (M8251/0)
- - breast 217
- - specified site NEC - see Neoplasm,
  skin, benign
- - unspecified site 216.9
- apocrine (M8401/0)
- - breast 217
- - specified site NEC - see Neoplasm,
  skin, benign
- - unspecified site 216.9
- basal cell (M8147/0)
- basophil (M8300/0)
- - specified site - see Neoplasm, benign
- - unspecified site 227.3
- beta-cell (M8151/0)
- - pancreas 211.7
- - specified site NEC - see Neoplasm,
  benign
- - unspecified site 211.7
- bile duct (M8160/0) 211.5
- black (M8372/0) 227.0
- bronchial (M8140/1) 235.7
- - carcinoid type (M8240/3) - see
  Neoplasm, lung, malignant
- - cylindroid type (M8200/3) - see
  Neoplasm, lung, malignant
- ceruminous (M8420/0) 216.2
- chief cell (M8321/0) 227.1
- chromophobe (M8270/0)
- - specified site - see Neoplasm, benign
- - unspecified site 227.3
- clear cell (M8310/0)

Adenoma - *continued*
- colloid (M8334/0)
- - specified site - see Neoplasm, benign
- - unspecified site 226
- duct (M8503/0)
- embryonal (M8191/0)
- endocrine, multiple (M8360/1)
- - single specified site - see Neoplasm,
  uncertain behavior
- - two or more specified sites 237.4
- - unspecified site 237.4

- endometrioid (M8380/0) - see also
  Neoplasm, benign
- - borderline malignancy (M8380/1) -
  see Neoplasm, uncertain behavior
- eosinophil (M8280/0)
- - specified site - see Neoplasm, benign
- - unspecified site 227.3
- fetal (M8333/0)
- - specified site - see Neoplasm, benign
- - unspecified site 226
- follicular (M8330/0)
- - specified site - see Neoplasm, benign
- - unspecified site 226
- hepatocellular (M8170/0) 211.5
- Hurthle cell (M8290/0) 226
- intracystic papillary (M8504/0)
- islet cell (functioning) (M8150/0)
- - pancreas 211.7
- - specified site NEC - see Neoplasm,
  benign
- - unspecified site 211.7
- liver cell (M8170/0) 211.5
- macrofollicular (M8334/0)
- - specified site - see Neoplasm, benign
- - unspecified site 226

- malignant, malignum (M8140/3) - see
  Neoplasm, malignant
- mesonephric (M9110/0)
- microfollicular (M8333/0)
- - specified site - see Neoplasm, benign
- - unspecified site 226
- mixed cell (M8323/0)
- monomorphic (M8146/0)
- mucinous (M8480/0)
- mucoid cell (M8300/0)
- - specified site - see Neoplasm, benign
- - unspecified site 227.3
- multiple endocrine (M8360/1)
- - single specified site - see Neoplasm,
  uncertain behavior
- - two or more specified sites 237.4
- - unspecified site 237.4
- nipple (M8506/0) 217
- oncocytic (M8290/0)
- oxyphilic (M8290/0)

Adenoma - *continued*
- papillary (M8260/0) - see also Neoplasm, benign
- - intracystic (M8504/0)
- papillotubular (M8263/0)
- Pick's tubular (M8640/0)
- - specified site - see Neoplasm, benign
- - unspecified site
- - - female 220
- - - male 222.0
- pleomorphic (M8940/0)
- polypoid (M8210/0)
- prostate 600
- rete cell 222.0

- sebaceous (gland) (senile) (M8410/0) - see Neoplasm, skin, benign
- Sertoli cell (M8640/0)
- - specified site - see Neoplasm, benign
- - unspecified site
- - - female 220
- - - male 222.0
- skin appendage (M8390/0) - see Neoplasm, skin, benign
- sudoriferous gland (M8400/0) - see Neoplasm, skin, benign
- sweat gland (M8400/0) - see Neoplasm, skin, benign
- testicular (M8640/0)
- - specified site - see Neoplasm, benign
- - unspecified site
- - - female 220
- - - male 222.0
- trabecular (M8190/0)
- tubular (M8211/0) - see also Neoplasm, benign
- - Pick's (M8640/0)
- - - specified site - see Neoplasm, benign
- - - unspecified site
- - - - female 220
- - - - male 222.0
- tubulovillous (M8263/0)
- villoglandular (M8263/0)
- villous (M8261/1) - see Neoplasm, uncertain behavior
- water-clear cell (M8322/0) 227.1
- wolffian duct (M9110/0)

Adenomatosis (M8220/0)
- endocrine (multiple) (M8360/1)
- - single specified site - see Neoplasm, uncertain behavior
- - two or more specified sites 237.4
- - unspecified site 237.4
- erosive of nipple (M8506/0) 217
- pluriendocrine - see Adenomatosis, multiple endocrine
- pulmonary (M8250/1) 235.7

Adenomatosis - *continued*
- pulmonary - *continued*
- - malignant (M8250/3) - see Neoplasm, lung, malignant
- specified site - see Neoplasm, benign
- unspecified site 211.3
Adenomatous
- goiter (nontoxic) 241.9
- - with hyperthyroidism 242.3
- - toxic 242.3
Adenomyoma (M8932/0) - see also Neoplasm, benign
- prostate 600
Adenomyosis 617.0
Adenopathy (lymph gland) 785.6
- inguinal 785.6
- mediastinal 785.6
- mesentery 785.6
- syphilitic (secondary) 091.4
- tracheobronchial 785.6
- - tuberculous 012.1
- - - primary, progressive 010.8
- tuberculous (see also Tuberculosis, lymph gland) 017.2
- - tracheobronchial 012.1
- - - primary, progressive 010.8
Adenosarcoma (M8960/3) 189.0
Adenosclerosis 289.3
Adenosis (sclerosing) breast 610.2
Adherent
- labia (minora) 624.4
- pericardium 423.1
- - rheumatic 393
- placenta (without hemorrhage) 667.0
- - with hemorrhage 666.0
- prepuce 605
- scar (skin) 709.2
- tendon in scar 709.2
Adhesions, adhesive (postinfectional) 568.0
- abdominal (wall) (see also Adhesions, peritoneum) 568.0
- amnion to fetus 658.8
- - fetus or newborn 762.8
- appendix 543
- bile duct (see also Disease, biliary) 576.8
- bladder (sphincter) 596.8
- bowel (see also Adhesions, peritoneum) 568.0
- cardiac 423.1
- - rheumatic 398.9
- cecum (see also Adhesions, peritoneum) 568.0
- cervicovaginal 622.3
- - congenital 752.4
- - postpartal 674.8
- - - old 622.3
- cervix 622.3

Adhesions - *continued*
- ciliary body 364.7
- clitoris 624.4
- colon (see also Adhesions, peritoneum) 568.0
- common duct (see also Disease, biliary) 576.8
- congenital - see also Anomaly, specified type NEC
- - fingers 755.1
- - omental, anomalous 751.4
- - peritoneal 751.4
- - toes 755.1
- - tongue (to gum or roof of mouth) 750.1
- conjunctiva (acquired) 372.6
- - congenital 743.6
- cornea 371.0
- cystic duct (see also Disease, gallbladder) 575.8
- diaphragm (see also Adhesions, peritoneum) 568.0
- due to foreign body - see Foreign body
- duodenum (see also Adhesions, peritoneum) 568.0
- epididymis 608.8
- epidural - see Adhesions, meninges
- epiglottis 478.7
- eyelid 374.4
- gallbladder (see also Disease, gallbladder) 575.8
- globe 360.8
- heart 423.1
- - rheumatic 398.9
- ileocecal (coil) (see also Adhesions, peritoneum) 568.0
- ileum (see also Adhesions, peritoneum) 568.0
- intestine (see also Adhesions, peritoneum) 568.0
- - with obstruction 560.8
- intra-abdominal (see also Adhesions, peritoneum) 568.0
- iris 364.7
- - to corneal graft 996.7
- joint 718.5

- labium (majus) (minus), congenital 752.4
- liver 572.8
- lung 511.0
- mediastinum 519.3
- meninges 349.2
- - cerebral (any) 349.2
- - - congenital 742.4
- - congenital 742.8
- - spinal (any) 349.2
- - - congenital 742.5

Adhesions - *continued*
- meninges - *continued*
- - tuberculous (cerebral) (spinal) 013.0 † 320.4*
- mesenteric (see also Adhesions, peritoneum) 568.0
- nasal (septum) (to turbinates) 478.1
- ocular muscle 378.6
- omentum (see also Adhesions, peritoneum) 568.0
- organ or site, congenital NEC - see Anomaly, specified type NEC
- ovary 614.6
- - congenital (to cecum, kidney or omentum) 752.0
- paraovarian 614.6
- pelvic (peritoneal)
- - female 614.6
- - male (see also Adhesions, peritoneum) 568.0
- - postpartal (old) 614.6
- - tuberculous 016.9
- penis to scrotum (congenital) 752.8
- periappendiceal (see also Adhesions, peritoneum) 568.0
- pericardium 423.1
- - rheumatic 393
- - tuberculous 017.8 † 420.0*
- pericholecystic (see also Disease, gallbladder) 575.8
- perigastric (see also Adhesions, peritoneum) 568.0
- periovarian 614.6
- periprostatic 602.8
- perirectal (see also Adhesions, peritoneum) 568.0
- perirenal 593.8
- peritoneum, peritoneal 568.0
- - with obstruction (intestinal) 560.8
- - congenital 751.4
- - pelvic, female 614.6
- - postpartal, pelvic 614.6
- - to uterus 614.6
- peritubal 614.6
- periureteral 593.8
- periuterine 621.5
- perivesical 596.8
- perivesicular (seminal vesicle) 608.8
- pleura, pleuritic 511.0
- - tuberculous 012.0
- pleuropericardial 511.0
- postoperative 997.4
- postpartal, old 624.4
- preputial, prepuce 605
- pulmonary 511.0
- pylorus (see also Adhesions, peritoneum) 568.0

Adhesions - *continued*
- sciatic nerve 355.0
- seminal vesicle 608.8
- shoulder (joint) 726.0
- sigmoid flexure (see also Adhesions, peritoneum) 568.0
- spermatic cord (acquired) 608.8
- - congenital 752.8
- spinal canal 349.2
- stomach (see also Adhesions, peritoneum) 568.0
- subscapular 726.2
- tendinitis 726.9
- - shoulder 726.0
- testis 608.8
- tongue, congenital (to gum or roof of mouth) 750.1
- trachea 519.1
- tubo-ovarian 614.6
- tunica vaginalis 608.8
- uterus 621.5
- - to abdominal wall 621.5
- vagina (chronic) (postoperative) (postradiation) 623.2
- vitreous 379.2
Adie's pupil or syndrome 379.4
Adie-Holmes syndrome 379.4
Adiponecrosis neonatorum 778.1
Adiposis 278.0
- cerebralis 253.8
- dolorosa 272.8
Adiposity 278.0
- heart (see also Degeneration, myocardial) 429.1
- localized 278.1
Adiposogenital dystrophy 253.8
Adjustment
- prosthesis or other device - see Fitting (of)
- reaction - see Reaction, adjustment
Administration, prophylactic
- antibiotics V07.3
- chemotherapeutic agents NEC V07.3
- gamma globulin V07.2
Admission for observation - see Observation (for)
Adnexitis (suppurative) (see also Salpingo-oophoritis) 614.2
Adolescence NEC V21.2
Adrenal (gland) - see condition
Adrenalism, tuberculous 017.6 † 255.4*
Adrenalitis, adrenitis 255.8
- meningococcal, hemorrhagic 036.3 † 255.5*
Adrenocortical syndrome 255.2
Adrenogenital syndrome (acquired) (congenital) 255.2

Adventitious bursa - see Bursitis
Adynamia episodica hereditaria 359.3
Aeration lung imperfect, newborn 770.5
Aerobullosis 993.3
Aerocele - see Embolism, air, by type
Aerodontalgia 993.2
Aero-embolism 993.3
Aero-otitis media 993.0
Aerophagy, aerophagia 306.4
- psychogenic 306.4
Aerosinusitis 993.1
Aerotitis 993.0
Affection - see also Disease
- sacroiliac (joint) NEC 724.9
- shoulder region NEC 726.2
Afibrinogenemia (see also Defect, coagulation) 286.9
- acquired 286.6
- congenital 286.3
- following childbirth 666.3
Aftercare V58.9
- following surgery NEC V58.4
- involving dialysis
- - extracorporeal V56.0
- - peritoneal V56.8
- - renal V56.0
- orthodontics V58.5
- orthopedic (see also Removal (of)) V54.9
- - specified NEC V54.8
- specified type NEC V58.8
After-cataract 366.5
Agalactia 676.4
Agammaglobulinemia 279.0
- with lymphopenia 279.2
- acquired (primary) (secondary) 279.0
- Bruton's X-linked 279.0
- congenital sex-linked 279.0
- Swiss type 279.2
Aganglionosis (bowel) (colon) 751.3
Age (old) (see also Senility) 797
Agenesis 759.8
- adrenal (gland) 759.1
- alimentary tract (complete) (partial) NEC 751.8
- - lower 751.2
- - upper 750.8
- anus, anal (canal) 751.2
- aorta 747.2
- appendix 751.2
- arm (complete) (partial) 755.2
- artery (peripheral) 747.6
- - brain 747.8
- - coronary 746.8
- - pulmonary 747.3
- - umbilical 747.5
- auditory (canal) (external) 744.0
- auricle (ear) 744.0

Agenesis - *continued*
- patella 755.6
- pelvic girdle (complete) (partial) 755.6
- penis 752.8
- pericardium 746.8
- pituitary (gland) 759.2
- prostate 752.8
- punctum lacrimale 743.6
- radioulnar 755.2
- radius 755.2
- rectum 751.2
- renal 753.0
- respiratory organ NEC 748.9
- rib 756.3
- roof of orbit 742.0
- round ligament 752.8
- sacrum 756.1
- salivary gland 750.2
- scapula 755.5
- scrotum 752.8
- seminal duct or tract 752.8
- septum
- - atrial 745.6
- - between aorta and pulmonary artery 745.0
- - ventricular 745.3
- shoulder girdle (complete) (partial) 755.5
- skull (bone) 756.0
- - with
- - - anencephalus 740.0
- - - encephalocele 742.0
- - - hydrocephalus 742.3
- - - - with spina bifida 741.0
- - - microcephalus 742.1
- spermatic cord 752.8
- spinal cord 742.5
- spine 756.1
- spleen 759.0
- sternum 756.3
- stomach 750.7
- tarsus 755.3
- tendon 756.8
- thymus (gland) 759.2
- thyroid (gland) 243
- - cartilage 748.3
- tibia 755.3
- tibiofibular 755.3
- toe (complete) (partial) 755.3
- tongue 750.1
- trachea (cartilage) 748.3
- ulna 755.2
- ureter 753.4
- urethra 753.8
- urinary tract NEC 753.8
- uterus 752.3
- uvula 750.2
- vagina 752.4

Agenesis - *continued*
- vas deferens 752.8
- vein(s) (peripheral) 747.6
- - brain 747.8
- - great 747.4
- - portal 747.4
- - pulmonary 747.4
- vena cava (inferior) (superior) 747.4
- vermis of cerebellum 742.2
- vertebra 756.1
- vulva 752.4
Ageusia (see also Disturbance, sensation) 781.1
Aggressive outburst 312.0
- in children and adolescents 313.9
Aggressiveness 301.3
Agitated - see condition
Agitation 307.9
- catatonic 295.2
Aglossia (congenital) 750.1
Agnail (with lymphangitis) 681.0
Agnosia (body image) (tactile) 784.6
- verbal 784.6
- - auditory 784.6
- - - developmental 315.3
- - - secondary to organic lesion 784.6
- - developmental 315.8
- - secondary to organic lesion 784.6
- - visual 784.6
- - - developmental 315.8
- - - secondary to organic lesion 784.6
Agoraphobia 300.2
Agrammatism 784.6
Agranulocytosis (angina) (chronic) (cyclical) (genetic) (infantile) (periodic) (pernicious) 288.0
Agraphia (absolute) 784.6
- developmental 315.3
Ague (see also Malaria) 084.6
- brass-founders' 985.8
- dumb 084.6
- tertian 084.1
Agyria 742.2
Ailment heart - see Disease, heart
Ainhum (disease) 136.0
Air
- anterior mediastinum 518.1
- compressed disease 993.3
- embolism (artery) (cerebral) (any site) 958.0
- - with abortion - see categories 634-639, fourth digit .6
- - due to implanted device 996.7
- - following infusion, perfusion or transfusion 999.1
- - in pregnancy, childbirth or puerperium 673.0

Air - *continued*
- embolism - *continued*
- - traumatic 958.0
- hunger, psychogenic 306.1
- rarefied, effects of - see Effect, adverse, high altitude
- sickness 994.6
Airplane sickness 994.6
Akureyri disease 049.8 † 323.4*
Alacrima (congenital) 743.6
Alactasia (hereditary) 271.3
Alalia 784.3
- developmental 315.3
- secondary to organic lesion 784.3
Alastrim 050.1
Albers-Schonberg disease 756.5
Albert's disease 726.7
Albinism, albino (cutaneous) (generalized) (isolated) (partial) 270.2
- ocular 270.2 † 743.8*
Albinismus 270.2
Albright(-McCune)(-Sternberg) syndrome 756.5
Albuminous - see condition
Albuminuria, albuminuric (acute) (chronic) (subacute) 791.0
- complicating pregnancy, childbirth or puerperium 646.2
- - with hypertension - see Toxemia, of pregnancy
- - fetus or newborn 760.1
- gravidarum 646.2
- - with hypertension - see Toxemia, of pregnancy
- - fetus or newborn 760.1
- orthostatic 593.6
- postural 593.6
- pre-eclamptic (mild) 642.4
- - fetus or newborn 760.0
- - severe 642.5
- - - fetus or newborn 760.0
- scarlatinal 034.1
Alcaptonuria 270.2
Alcohol, alcoholic
- addiction 303
- brain syndrome, chronic 291.2
- delirium 291.0
- - acute 291.0
- - chronic 291.1
- - tremens 291.0
- dementia NEC 291.2
- hallucinosis (acute) 291.3
- insanity 291.9
- intoxication (acute) 305.0
- - with dependence 303
- jealousy 291.5
- liver NEC 571.3

Alcohol - *continued*
- mania (acute) (chronic) 291.9
- paranoia 291.5
- paranoid (type) psychosis 291.5
- pellagra 265.2
- poisoning, accidental (acute) NEC 980.9
- - specified type of alcohol - see Table of drugs and chemicals
- psychosis (see also Psychosis, alcoholic) 291.9
Alcoholism 303
- with
- - psychosis (see also Psychosis, alcoholic) 291.9
- acute 303
- chronic 303
- - with psychosis 291.9
- complicating pregnancy, childbirth or puerperium 648.4
- - fetus or newborn 760.8
- Korsakoff's, Korsakov's, Korsakow's 291.1
- suspected damage to fetus affecting management of pregnancy 655.4
Alder's anomaly or syndrome 288.2
Aldosteronism (congenital) (primary) 255.1
Aldosteronoma (M8370/1) 237.2
Aldrich(-Wiskott) syndrome 279.1
Aleppo boil 085.1
Aleukemic - see condition
Aleukia hemorrhagica 284.9
Alexia 784.6
- developmental 315.0
- secondary to organic lesion 784.6
Algoneurodystrophy 733.7
Alibert's disease (M9700/3) 202.1
Alienation mental (see also Psychosis) 298.9
Alkalemia 276.3
Alkalosis 276.3
- metabolic 276.3
- respiratory 276.3
Alkaptonuria 270.2
Allergy, allergic (reaction) 995.3
- air-borne substance (see also Fever, hay) 477.9
- animal (dander) (epidermal) (hair) 477.8
- bee sting (anaphylactic shock) 989.5
- biological - see Allergy, drug
- dander (animal) 477.8
- dandruff 477.8
- dermatitis - see Dermatitis
- drug, medicament and biological (any) (correct medicinal substance properly administered) (external) (internal) 995.2
- - wrong substance given or taken NEC 977.9

Allergy - *continued*
- drug - *continued*
- - wrong substance given or taken NEC
  continued
- - - specified drug or substance - see
    Table of drugs and chemicals
- dust (house) (stock) 477.8
- eczema - see Eczema
- epidermal (animal) 477.8
- feathers 477.8
- food (any) (ingested) 693.1
- - in contact with skin 692.5
- gastrointestinal 558
- grass (pollen) 477.0
- - asthma 493.0
- - hay fever 477.0
- hair (animal) 477.8
- horse serum - see Allergy, serum
- inhalant (see also Fever, hay) 477.9
- kapok 477.8
- medicine - see Allergy, drug
- pollen (any) 477.0
- - asthma 493.0
- - hay fever 477.0
- ragweed (pollen) 477.0
- - asthma 493.0
- - hay fever 477.0
- rose 477.0
- Senecio jacoboea 477.0
- serum (prophylactic) (therapeutic) 999.5
- - anaphylactic shock 999.4
- shock (anaphylactic) (due to adverse
  effect of correct medicinal substance
  properly administered) 995.0
- - from serum or immunization 999.5
- - - anaphylactic 999.4
- tree (any) (hay fever) (pollen) 477.0
- - asthma 493.0
- upper respiratory (see also Fever, hay)
  477.9
- vaccine - see Allergy, serum
Allescheriosis 117.6
Alligator skin disease 757.1
Allocheiria, allochiria (see also Disturbance,
  sensation) 782.0
Almeida's disease 116.1
Alopecia (aerata) (atrophicans) (celsi)
  (cicatrisata) (circumscripta) (disseminata)
  (febrile) (hereditaria) (mucinosa)
  (postinfectional) (pregnancy) (prematura)
  (seborrheica) (senilis) (totalis) (toxica)
  (universalis) 704.0
- adnata 757.4
- congenital, congenitalis 757.4
- specific 091.8
- syphilitic (secondary) 091.8
- X-ray 704.0

Alper's disease 330.8
Alphalipoproteinemia 272.4
Alpine sickness 993.2
Alport's syndrome 759.8
Alternaria (infection) 118
Alternating - see condition
Altitude, high (effects) - see Effect, adverse,
  high altitude
Aluminosis (of lung) 503
Alvarez syndrome 435
Alveolitis
- allergic (extrinsic) 495.9
- - due to organisms (fungal, thermophilic
  actinomycete, other) growing in
  ventilation (air conditioning) systems
  495.7
- due to
- - Aspergillus clavatus 495.4
- - Cryptostroma corticale 495.6
- fibrosing (idiopathic) 516.3
- jaw 526.5
Alveolus, alveolar - see condition
Alymphocytosis 279.2
Alymphoplasia, thymic 279.2
Alzheimer's disease or sclerosis 331.0
- dementia in 290.1
Amastia (see also Absence, breast) 611.8
Amaurosis (acquired) (congenital) (see also
  Blindness) 369.0
- hysterical 300.1
- Leber's congenital 362.7
- uremic - see Uremia
Amaurotic family idiocy (infantile)
  (juvenile) (late) 330.1
Amblyopia (congenital) (partial)
  (deprivation) (strabismic) (suppression)
  368.0
- exanopsia 368.0
- hysterical 300.1
- nocturnal 368.6
- - vitamin A deficiency 264.5 † 368.6*
- tobacco 377.3
- toxic NEC 377.3
- uremic - see Uremia
Ameba, amebic (histolytica) - see
  Amebiasis
Amebiasis NEC 006.9
- with abscess - see Abscess, amebic
- acute 006.0
- - with abscess - see Abscess, amebic
- chronic 006.1
- - with abscess - see Abscess, amebic
- due to organism other than Entameba
  histolytica 007.8
- nondysenteric 006.2
- specified
- - organism NEC 007.8

Amebiasis NEC - *continued*
− specified - *continued*
− − site NEC 006.8
Ameboma 006.8
Amelia 755.4
− lower limb 755.3
− upper limb 755.2
Ameloblastoma (M9310/0) 213.1
− jaw (bone) (lower) 213.1
− − upper 213.0
− long bones (M9261/3) - see Neoplasm,
  bone, malignant
− malignant (M9310/3) 170.1
− − jaw (bone) (lower) 170.1
− − − upper 170.0
− mandible 213.1
− tibial (M9261/3) 170.7
Amelogenesis imperfecta 520.5
− nonhereditaria (segmentalis) 520.4
Amenorrhea (primary) (secondary) 626.0
− hyperhormonal 256.8
Amentia (see also Retardation, mental) 319
Ametropia 367.9
Amimia 784.6
Amino-acid deficiency 270.9
− anemia 281.4
Aminoaciduria 270.9
− imidazole 270.5
Amnesia (retrograde) 780.9
− auditory 784.6
− − developmental 315.3
− − secondary to organic lesion 784.6
− hysterical 300.1
− psychogenic 300.1
Amniocentesis screening (for) V28.2
− alphafetoprotein level, raised V28.1
− chromosomal anomalies V28.0
Amnion, amniotic - see condition
Amnionitis
− complicating pregnancy 658.4
− fetus or newborn 762.7
Amoral trends 301.7
Amotio retinae (see also Detachment,
  retina) 361.9
Ampulla
− lower esophagus 530.8
− phrenic 530.8
Amputation
− any part of fetus, to facilitate delivery
  763.8
− cervix (uteri) 622.8
− − in pregnancy or childbirth 654.6
− − − fetus or newborn 763.8
− congenital - see Deformity, reduction
− neuroma (traumatic) - see also Injury,
  nerve, by site
− − surgical complication (late) 997.6

Amputation - *continued*
− stump (surgical)
− − abnormal, painful, or with
    complication (late) 997.6
− − healed or old NEC 736.9
− traumatic (complete) (partial)

Note − The following fourth-digit subdivisions are for use with categories 885−886
and 895:
  .0 Without mention of complication
  .1 Complicated
"Complicated" includes traumatic amputation with delayed healing, delayed treatment, foreign body, or major infection.

Amputation - *continued*
− traumatic - *continued*
− − arm 887.4
− − − at or above elbow 887.2
− − − − complicated 887.3
− − − below elbow 887.0
− − − − complicated 887.1
− − − both (bilateral) (any level(s)) 887.6
− − − − complicated 887.7
− − − complicated 887.5

− − finger(s) (one or both hands) 886.-
− − − with thumb(s) 885.-
− − foot (except toe(s) only) 896.0
− − − both (bilateral) 896.2
− − − − complicated 896.3
− − − complicated 896.1
− − − toe(s) only (one or both feet) 895.-

− − genital organ(s) NEC 878.8
− − − complicated 878.9
− − hand (except finger(s) only) 887.0
− − − and other arm 887.6
− − − − complicated 887.7
− − − both (bilateral) 887.6
− − − − complicated 887.7
− − − complicated 887.1
− − − finger(s) (one or both hands) 886.-
− − − − with thumb(s) 885.-
− − − thumb(s) alone 885.-
− − head 874.9
− − leg 897.4
− − − and other foot 897.6
− − − − complicated 897.7
− − − at or above knee 897.2
− − − − complicated 897.3
− − − below knee 897.0
− − − − complicated 897.1
− − − both (bilateral) 897.6
− − − − complicated 897.7
− − − complicated 897.5

Amputation - *continued*
− traumatic - *continued*
− − lower limb(s) except toe(s) - see
Amputation, traumatic, leg
− − nose 873.2
− − − complicated 873.3
− − penis 878.0
− − − complicated 878.1
− − sites other than limbs - see Wound,
open
− − thumb(s) (with finger(s) of either
hand) 885.-
− − toe(s) (one or both feet) 895.-
− − upper limb(s) - see Amputation,
traumatic, arm
Amputee (bilateral) (old) 736.8
Amusia 784.6
− developmental 315.3
− secondary to organic lesion 784.6
Amyelencephalus 740.0
Amyelia 742.5
Amygdalitis - see Tonsillitis
Amygdalolith 474.8
Amyloid heart (disease) 277.3 † 425.7*
Amyloidosis (general) (generalized)
(inherited) (nephropathic) (neuropathic)
(Portuguese) (primary) (secondary)
(systemic) (Swiss) 277.3
− with lung involvement 277.3 † 517.8*
− familial 277.3
− genetic 277.3
− heart 277.3 † 425.7*
− pulmonary 277.3 † 517.8*
Amylopectinosis (brancher enzyme
deficiency) 271.0
Amyoplasia congenita 756.8
Amyotonia 728.2
− congenita 358.8
Amyotrophia, amyotrophy, amyotrophic
728.2
− congenita 756.8
− diabetic 250.5 † 358.1*
− lateral sclerosis 335.2
− neuralgic 353.5
− spinal progressive 335.2
Anacidity gastric 536.0
− psychogenic 306.4
Anaerosis of newborn 770.8
Analbuminemia 273.8
Analgesia (see also Anesthesia) 782.0
Analphalipoproteinemia 272.5
Anaphylactic shock or reaction - see Shock,
anaphylactic
Anaphylactoid shock or reaction - see
Shock, anaphylactic
Anaphylaxis - see Shock, anaphylactic
Anaplasia cervix 622.1

Anarthria 784.5
Anarthritic rheumatoid disease 446.5
Anasarca 782.3
− cardiac (see also Failure, heart,
congestive) 428.0
− fetus or newborn 778.0
− lung 514
− nutritional 262
− pulmonary 514
− renal (see also Nephrosis) 581.9
Anaspadias 752.6
Anastomosis
− aneurysmal - see Aneurysm
− arteriovenous, congenital 747.6
− − ruptured of brain (see also
Hemorrhage, subarachnoid) 430
− intestinal 569.8
− − complicated NEC 997.4
− − − involving urinary tract 997.5
− retinal and choroidal vessels 743.5
Anatomical narrow angle 365.0
Ancylostoma (infection) (infestation) 126.9
− americanus 126.1
− braziliense 126.2
− caninum 126.8
− ceylanicum 126.3
− duodenale 126.0
− Necator americanus 126.1
Ancylostomiasis (intestinal) 126.9
− americanus 126.1
− braziliense 126.2
− caninum 126.8
− ceylanicum 126.3
− duodenale 126.0
− Necator americanus 126.1
Andersen's glycogen storage disease 271.0
Anderson's disease 272.7
Andes disease 993.2
Androblastoma (M8630/1)
− benign (M8630/0)
− − specified site - see Neoplasm, benign
− − unspecified site
− − − female 220
− − − male 222.0
− malignant (M8630/3)
− − specified site - see Neoplasm,
malignant
− − unspecified site
− − − female 183.0
− − − male 186.9
− specified site - see Neoplasm, uncertain
behavior
− tubular (M8640/0)
− − with lipid storage (M8641/0)
− − − specified site - see Neoplasm, benign
− − − unspecified site
− − − − female 220

Anemia - *continued*
- due to - *continued*
- - loss of blood - *continued*
- - - acute 285.1
- - myxedema 244.9
- - prematurity 776.6
- - selective vitamin B12 malabsorption
  with proteinuria 281.1
- Dyke-Young type (secondary)
  (symptomatic) 283.9
- dyserythropoietic (congenital) 285.8
- dyshematopoietic (congenital) 285.8
- Egypt (see also Ancylostomiasis) 126.9
- elliptocytosis (see also Elliptocytosis)
  282.1
- enzyme-deficiency, drug induced 282.2
- epidemic (see also Ancylostomiasis)
  126.9
- erythrocytic glutathione deficiency 282.2
- essential 285.9
- eythroblastic
- - familial 282.4
- - fetus or newborn (see also Disease,
  hemolytic) 773.2
- - - late 773.5
- familial erythroblastic 282.4
- Fanconi's 284.0
- favism 282.2
- fetus or newborn
- - due to
- - - AB0
- - - - antibodies 773.1
- - - - incompatibility, maternal/fetal
  773.1
- - - - isoimmunization 773.1
- - - Rh
- - - - antibodies 773.0
- - - - incompatibility, maternal/fetal
  773.0
- - - - isoimmunization 773.0
- - following fetal blood loss 776.5
- folate (folic acid) deficiency 281.2
- general 285.9
- glucose-6-phosphate dehydrogenase
  deficiency 282.2
- glutathione-reductase deficiency 282.2
- goat's milk 281.2
- granulocytic 288.0
- Heinz-body, congenital 282.7
- hemoglobin deficiency 285.9
- hemolytic 282.9
- - acquired 283.9
- - - with hemoglobinuria NEC 283.2
- - - autoimmune 283.0
- - - infectious 283.1
- - - non-autoimmune 283.1
- - - toxic 283.1

Anemia - *continued*
- hemolytic - *continued*
- - acute 283.9
- - - due to enzyme deficiency NEC
  282.3
- - - fetus or newborn (see also Disease,
  hemolytic) 773.2
- - - - late 773.5
- - - Lederer's 283.1
- - autoimmune 283.0
- - chronic 282.9
- - - idiopathic 283.9
- - cold type (secondary) (symptomatic)
  283.0
- - congenital (spherocytic) (see also
  Spherocytosis) 282.0
- - due to
- - - cardiac conditions 283.1
- - - drugs 283.1
- - - enzyme deficiency NEC 282.3
- - - - drug induced 282.2
- - - presence of shunt or other internal
  prosthetic device 283.1
- - - thrombotic thrombocytopenic
  purpura 283.1 † 446.6*
- - familial 282.9
- - hereditary 282.9
- - - due to enzyme deficiency NEC
  282.3
- - idiopathic (chronic) 283.9
- - mechanical 283.1
- - microangiopathic 283.1
- - nonautoimmune 283.1
- - nonspherocytic
- - - congenital or hereditary NEC 282.3
- - - - glucose-6-phosphate
  dehydrogenase deficiency 282.2
- - - - pyruvate kinase deficiency 282.3
- - - - type
- - - - - I 282.2
- - - - - II 282.3
- - - type
- - - - I 282.2
- - - - II 282.3
- - secondary 283.1
- - - autoimmune 283.0
- - Stransky-Regala type (Hb E) (see also
  Hemoglobinopathy) 282.7
- - symptomatic 283.1
- - - autoimmune 283.0
- - toxic 283.1
- - warm type (secondary) (symptomatic)
  283.0
- hemorrhagic (chronic) 280
- - acute 285.1
- Herrick's (see also Disease, sickle cell)
  282.6

Anemia - *continued*
- specified type NEC 285.8
- spherocytic (hereditary) (see also Spherocytosis) 282.0
- splenic 285.8
- splenomegalic 285.8
- syphilitic 095
- target cell 282.4
- thalassemia 282.4
- thrombocytopenic (see also Thrombocytopenia) 287.5
- toxic 284.8
- tropical, macrocytic 281.2
- tuberculous 017.8
- vegan's 281.1
- vitamin
- - B12 deficiency (dietary) 281.1
- - B6-responsive 285.0
- von Jaksch's 285.8
- Witts' 280
- Zuelzer(-Ogden) (megaloblastic) 281.2
Anencephalus, anencephaly 740.0
- fetus (suspected), affecting management of pregnancy 655.0
Anergasia (see also Psychosis, organic) 294.9
- senile 290.0
Anesthesia, anesthetic 782.0
- complication or reaction NEC 995.2
- - due to
- - - correct substance properly administered 995.2
- - - overdose or wrong substance given 968.-
- - - - specified anesthetic - see Table of drugs and chemicals
- cornea 371.8
- death from
- - correct substance properly administered 995.4
- - during delivery 668.9
- - overdose or wrong substance given 968.-
- - - specified anesthetic - see Table of drugs and chemicals
- eye 371.8
- functional 300.1
- hysterical 300.1
- local skin lesion 782.0
- sexual (psychogenic) 302.7
- shock
- - correct substance properly administered 995.4
- - overdose or wrong substance given 968.-
- - - specified anesthetic - see Table of drugs and chemicals

Anesthesia - *continued*
- skin 782.0
Anetoderma (maculosum) 701.3
Aneuploidy NEC 758.5
Aneurin deficiency 265.1
Aneurysm (anastomotic) (artery) (cirsoid) (diffuse) (false) (fusiform) (multiple) (ruptured) (saccular) (varicose) 442.9
- abdominal (aorta) 441.4
- - dissecting 441.0
- - ruptured 441.3
- - syphilitic 093.0 † 441.7*
- aorta, aortic (nonsyphilitic) 441.6
- - abdominal 441.4
- - - ruptured 441.3
- - arch 441.2
- - - ruptured 441.1
- - arteriosclerotic NEC 441.6
- - - ruptured 441.5
- - ascending 441.2
- - - ruptured 441.1
- - congenital 747.2
- - descending 441.6
- - - abdominal 441.4
- - - - ruptured 441.3
- - - ruptured 441.5
- - - thoracic 441.2
- - - - ruptured 441.1
- - dissecting (any part) 441.0
- - due to coarctation (aorta) 747.1
- - ruptured 441.5
- - sinus, right 747.2
- - syphilitic 093.0 † 441.7*
- - thorax, thoracic (arch) 441.2
- - - ruptured 441.1
- - transverse 441.2
- - - ruptured 441.1
- - valve (heart) (see also Endocarditis, aortic) 424.1
- arteriosclerotic NEC 442.9
- - cerebral (see also Ischemia, cerebral) 437.3
- - - ruptured (see also Hemorrhage, subarachnoid) 430
- arteriovenous (congenital) (peripheral) 747.6
- - acquired NEC 447.0
- - - brain 437.3
- - - - ruptured (see also Hemorrhage, subarachnoid) 430
- - - pulmonary 417.0
- - brain 747.8
- - - ruptured (see also Hemorrhage, subarachnoid) 430
- - coronary 746.8
- - retina 743.5
- - specified site NEC 747.8

Aneurysm - *continued*
- arteriovenous - *continued*
- - specified site NEC - *continued*
- - - acquired 447.0
- - traumatic (complication) (early) 904.9
- basal - see Aneurysm, brain
- berry (congenital) (ruptured) (see also
  Hemorrhage, subarachnoid) 430
- brain 437.3
- - arteriosclerotic (see also Ischemia,
  cerebral) 437.3
- - - ruptured (see also Hemorrhage,
  subarachnoid) 430
- - arteriovenous 747.8
- - - acquired 437.3
- - - - ruptured (see also Hemorrhage,
  subarachnoid) 430
- - - ruptured (see also Hemorrhage,
  subarachnoid) 430
- - berry (congenital) (ruptured) (see also
  Hemorrhage, subarachnoid) 430
- - congenital 747.8
- - - ruptured (see also Hemorrhage,
  subarachnoid) 430
- - meninges 437.3
- - - ruptured (see also Hemorrhage,
  subarachnoid) 430
- - miliary (congenital) (ruptured) (see
  also Hemorrhage, subarachnoid) 430
- - mycotic 421.0
- - - ruptured (see also Hemorrhage,
  subarachnoid) 430
- - ruptured (see also Hemorrhage,
  subarachnoid) 430
- - syphilitic (hemorrhage) 094.8 † 430*
- - traumatic - see Injury, intracranial
- cardiac (false) (see also Aneurysm, heart)
  414.1
- carotid 442.8
- - internal 442.8
- - - ruptured into brain (see also
  Hemorrhage, subarachnoid) 430
- - syphilitic 093.8
- - - intracranial 094.8
- cavernous sinus (see also Aneurysm,
  brain) 437.3
- - arteriovenous 747.8
- - - ruptured (see also Hemorrhage,
  subarachnoid) 430
- - congenital 747.8
- - - ruptured (see also Hemorrhage,
  subarachnoid) 430
- central nervous system syphilitic 094.8
- cerebral - see Aneurysm, brain
- chest - see Aneurysm, thorax
- circle of Willis (see also Aneurysm, brain)
  437.3

Aneurysm - *continued*
- circle of Willis - *continued*
- - congenital 747.8
- - - ruptured (see also Hemorrhage,
  subarachnoid) 430
- - ruptured (see also Hemorrhage,
  subarachnoid) 430
- congenital (peripheral) 747.6
- - brain 747.8
- - - ruptured (see also Hemorrhage,
  subarachnoid) 430
- - coronary 746.8
- - pulmonary 747.3
- - retina 743.5
- - specified site NEC 747.8
- conjunctiva 372.7
- conus arteriosus (see also Aneurysm,
  heart) 414.1
- coronary (arteriosclerotic) (artery) (vein)
  (see also Aneurysm, heart) 414.1
- - arteriovenous 746.8
- - congenital 746.8
- - syphilitic 093.8
- cylindrical 441.6
- - ruptured 441.5
- - syphilitic 093.9
- dissecting 442.9
- - aorta (any part) 441.0
- - syphilitic 093.9
- ductus arteriosus 747.0
- femoral 442.3
- heart (infectional) (wall) (chronic or with
  a stated duration of over 8 weeks) 414.1
- - acute or with a stated duration of 8
  weeks or under 410
- - congenital 746.8
- - valve - see Endocarditis
- iliac (common) 442.2
- infective 421.0
- innominate (nonsyphilitic) 442.8
- - syphilitic 093.8
- interauricular septum (see also
  Aneurysm, heart) 414.1
- interventricular septum (see also
  Aneurysm, heart) 414.1
- intrathoracic (nonsyphilitic) 441.2
- - ruptured 441.1
- - syphilitic 093.0 † 441.7*
- jugular vein 453.8
- lower extremity 442.3
- malignant 093.9
- mediastinal (nonsyphilitic) 442.8
- - syphilitic 093.8
- miliary (congenital) (ruptured) (see also
  Hemorrhage, subarachnoid) 430
- mitral (heart) (valve) 424.0
- mural (see also Aneurysm, heart) 414.1

Aneurysm - *continued*
– mycotic, any site 421.0
– – ruptured, brain (see also Hemorrhage, subarachnoid) 430
– myocardium (see also Aneurysm, heart) 414.1
– patent ductus arteriosus 747.0
– peripheral NEC 442.8
– – congenital 747.6
– popliteal 442.3
– pulmonary 417.1
– – arteriovenous 747.3
– – – acquired 417.0
– – syphilitic 093.8
– – valve (heart) (see also Endocarditis, pulmonary) 424.3
– racemose 442.9
– – congenital 747.6
– Rasmussen's 011.2
– renal 442.1
– retina 362.1
– – congenital 743.5
– – diabetic 250.4 † 362.0*
– sinus aortic, sinuses of Valsalva 747.2
– spinal (cord) 442.8
– – congenital 747.6
– – syphilitic (hemorrhage) 094.8
– splenic 442.8
– subclavian 442.8
– – syphilitic 093.8
– syphilitic 093.9
– – central nervous system 094.8
– – congenital 090.5
– – spine, spinal 094.8
– thorax, thoracic (arch) (nonsyphilitic) 441.2
– – dissecting 441.0
– – ruptured 441.1
– – syphilitic 093.0 † 441.7*

– traumatic (complication) (early)
– – specified site - see Injury, blood vessel
– tricuspid (heart) (valve) - see Endocarditis, tricuspid
– upper extremity 442.0
– valve, valvular - see Endocarditis
– venous 456.8
– – congenital 747.6
– ventricle (see also Aneurysm, heart) 414.1

Angiectasis 459.8

Angiectopia 459.9

Angiitis 447.6
– allergic granulomatous 446.4
– hypersensitivity 446.2
– necrotizing 446.0

Angina (attack) (cardiac) (chest) (effort) (heart) (pectoris) (syndrome) (vasomotor) 413
– agranulocytic 288.0
– aphthous 074.0
– cruris 443.9
– decubitus 413
– diphtheritic, membranous 032.0
– ludovici 528.3
– Ludwig's 528.3
– membranous 472.1
– – diphtheritic 032.0
– mesenteric 557.1
– monocytic 075
– pre-infarctional 411
– pseudomembranous 101
– septic 034.0
– streptococcal 034.0
– Vincent's 101
Angioblastoma (M9161/1) - see Neoplasm, connective tissue, uncertain behavior
Angiocholecystitis (see also Cholecystitis, acute) 575.0
Angiocholitis (see also Cholecystitis, acute) 576.1
Angioedema (allergic) (any site) (with urticaria) 995.1
– hereditary 277.6
Angioendothelioma (M9130/1) - see Neoplasm, uncertain behavior
– benign (M9130/0) 228.0
– bone (M9130/3) - see Neoplasm, bone, malignant
– Ewing's (M9260/3) - see Neoplasm, bone, malignant
– nervous system (M9130/0) 228.0
Angiofibroma (M9160/0) - see also Neoplasm, benign
– juvenile (M9160/0)
– – specified site - see Neoplasm, benign
– – unspecified site 210.7
Angiohemophilia (A) (B) 286.4
Angioid streaks (choroid) (retina) 363.4
Angiokeratoma (M9141/0) - see Neoplasm, skin, benign
– corporis diffusum 272.7
Angioleiomyoma (M8894/0) - see Neoplasm, connective tissue, benign
Angioleucitis 683
Angiolipoma (M8861/0) 214
– infiltrating (M8861/1) - see Neoplasm, connective tissue, uncertain behavior
Angioma (M9120/0) 228.0
– malignant (M9120/3) - see Neoplasm, connective tissue, malignant
– placenta 656.7
– plexiform (M9131/0) 228.0

Angioma - *continued*
- senile 448.1
- serpiginosum 709.1
- spider 448.1
- stellate 448.1
Angiomatosis 757.3
- encephalocutaneous 759.6
- encephalotrigeminal 759.6
Angiomyolipoma (M8860/0)
- specified site - see Neoplasm, connective
  tissue, benign
- unspecified site 223.0
Angiomyoliposarcoma (M8860/3) - see
  Neoplasm, connective tissue, malignant
Angiomyoma (M8894/0) - see Neoplasm,
  connective tissue, benign
Angiomyosarcoma (M8894/3) - see
  Neoplasm, connective tissue, malignant
Angioneurosis 306.2
Angioneurotic edema (allergic) (any site)
  (with urticaria) 995.1
- hereditary 277.6
Angiopathia, angiopathy 459.9
- peripheral 443.9
- - diabetic 250.6 † 443.8*
- retinae syphilitica 093.8
- retinalis juvenalis 362.1
Angiosarcoma (M9120/3) - see Neoplasm,
  connective tissue, malignant
Angiosclerosis - see Arteriosclerosis
Angiospasm 443.9
- cerebral 435
- peripheral NEC 443.9
- traumatic 443.9
- - foot 443.9
- - leg 443.9
- vessel 443.9
Anguillulosis 127.2
Angulation
- cecum (see also Obstruction, intestine)
  560.9
- coccyx (acquired) 738.6
- - congenital 756.1
- femur (acquired) 736.3
- - congenital 755.6
- intestine (large) (small) (see also
  Obstruction, intestine) 560.9
- sacrum (acquired) 738.5
- - congenital 756.1
- sigmoid (flexure) (see also Obstruction,
  intestine) 560.9
- spine (see also Curvature, spine) 737.9
- tibia (acquired) 736.8
- - congenital 755.6
- ureter 593.3
- wrist (acquired) 736.0
- - congenital 755.5

Angulus infectiosus 686.8
Anhidrosis 705.0
Anhydration 276.5
Anhydremia 276.5
Anidrosis 705.0
Aniridia (congenital) 743.4
Anisakiasis (infection) (infestation) 127.1
Anisakis larva infestation 127.1
Aniseikonia 367.3
Anisocoria (pupil) 379.4
- congenital 743.4
Anisocytosis 790.0
Anisometropia (congenital) 367.3
Ankle - see condition
Ankyloblepharon (eyelid) (acquired) 374.4
- filiforme (adnatum) (congenital) 743.6
- total 743.6
Ankyloglossia 750.0
Ankylosis (fibrous) (osseous) 718.5
- ankle 718.5
- cricoarytenoid (cartilage) (joint) (larynx)
  478.7
- dental 521.6
- ear ossicles 385.2
- elbow 718.5
- finger 718.5
- hip 718.5
- incostapedial joint (infectional) 385.2
- joint, produced by surgical fusion 718.5
- - sacroiliac 724.6
- knee 718.5
- lumbosacral (joint) 724.6
- multiple sites 718.5
- postoperative (status) V45.8
- sacroiliac (joint) 724.6
- shoulder 718.5
- specified site NEC 718.5
- spine NEC 724.9
- surgical 718.5
- tooth, teeth (hard tissues) 521.6
- wrist 718.5
Ankylostoma - see Ancylostoma
Ankylostomiasis - see Ancylostomiasis
Ankylurethria (see also Stricture, urethra)
  598.9
Annular - see also condition
- organ or site, congenital NEC - see
  Distortion
- pancreas (congenital) 751.7
Anodontia (complete) (partial) (vera) 520.0
- with abnormal spacing 524.3
- acquired 525.1
- - with malocclusion 524.3
Anomaly, anomalous (congenital)
  (unspecified type) 759.9
- abdomen 759.9
- abdominal wall 756.7

Anomaly - *continued*
- acoustic nerve 742.9
- adrenal (gland) 759.1
- Alder's 288.2
- alimentary tract 751.9
- − lower 751.5
- − upper 750.9
- ankle (joint) 755.6
- anus 751.5
- aorta (arch) 747.2
- − coarctation (preductal) (postductal) 747.1
- aortic cusp or valve NEC 746.9
- − pulmonary 746.3
- aqueduct of Sylvius 742.3
- − with spina bifida 741.0
- arm 755.5
- arteriovenous 747.6
- artery NEC 747.6
- − cerebral 747.8
- − coronary 746.9
- − peripheral 747.6
- − pulmonary 747.3
- − retina 743.9
- − umbilical 747.5
- aryteno-epiglottic folds 748.3
- atrial
- − bands 746.9
- − folds 746.9
- − septa 745.5
- atrioventricular excitation 426.7
- auditory canal 744.3
- auricle
- − ear 744.3
- − − causing impairment of hearing 744.0
- − heart 746.9
- autosomes, autosomal, NEC 758.5
- back 759.9
- band
- − atrial 746.9
- − heart 746.9
- − ventricular 746.9
- Bartholin's duct 750.9
- biliary duct or passage 751.6
- bladder 753.9
- bone NEC 756.9
- − face 756.0
- − skull 756.0
- − − with
- − − − anencephalus 740.0
- − − − encephalocele 742.0
- − − − hydrocephalus 742.3
- − − − − with spina bifida 741.0
- − − − microcephalus 742.1
- brain 742.9
- − multiple 742.4
- − vessel 747.8

Anomaly - *continued*
- breast 757.9
- bronchus 748.3
- bursa 756.9
- canal of Nuck 752.9
- canthus 743.9
- capillary 747.6
- cardiac 746.9
- − septal closure 745.9
- − valve NEC 746.9
- − − pulmonary 746.0
- cardiovascular system 746.9
- carpus 755.5
- caruncle lacrimal 743.9
- cecum 751.5
- cerebral - see also Anomaly, brain
- − vessels 747.8
- cervix 752.4
- − in pregnancy or childbirth 654.6
- − − causing obstructed labor 660.2
- − − − fetus or newborn 763.1
- − − fetus or newborn 763.8
- Chediak-Higashi(-Steinbrink) 288.2
- cheek 744.9
- chest (wall) 756.3
- chin 744.9
- chordae tendineae 746.9
- choroid 743.9
- − plexus 742.9
- chromosomes, chromosomal 758.9
- − autosomes NEC (see also Abnormality, autosomes) 758.5
- − − deletion 758.3
- − − D(1) 758.1
- − − E(3) 758.2
- − − G 758.0
- − − sex 758.8
- − − − gonadal dysgenesis 758.6
- − − − Klinefelter's 758.7
- − − − Turner's 758.6
- − − 13 758.1
- − − 18 758.2
- − − 21 or 22 758.0
- cilia 743.9
- circulatory system NEC 747.9
- clavicle 755.5
- clitoris 752.4
- coccyx 756.1
- colon 751.5
- concha (ear) 744.3
- connection
- − renal vessels with kidney 747.6
- − total pulmonary venous 747.4
- cornea 743.9
- coronary artery or vein 746.8
- cranium - see Anomaly, skull
- cricoid cartilage 748.3

Anomaly - *continued*
- cystic duct 751.6
- dental arch relationship 524.2
- dentition 520.6
- dentofacial 524.9
- - functional 524.5
- - specified type NEC 524.8
- dermatoglyphic 757.2
- diaphragm (apertures) NEC 756.6
- digestive organ(s) or system NEC 751.9
- - lower 751.5
- - upper 750.9
- distribution, coronary artery 746.8
- ductus arteriosus 747.0
- duodenum 751.5
- dura (brain) 742.9
- - spinal cord 742.9
- ear NEC 744.3
- - causing impairment of hearing 744.0
- - middle (causing impairment of
    hearing) 744.0
- Ebstein's 746.2
- ectodermal 757.9
- ejaculatory duct 752.9
- elbow 755.5
- endocrine gland NEC 759.2
- epididymis 752.9
- epiglottis 748.3
- esophagus 750.9
- eustachian tube 744.3
- eye (any part) 743.9
- eyelid 743.9
- face 744.9
- fallopian tube 752.1
- fascia 756.9
- femur 755.6
- fibula 755.6
- finger 755.5
- fixation, intestine 751.4
- flexion (joint) 755.9
- - hip or thigh 754.3
- foot 755.6
- forearm 755.5
- forehead (see also Anomaly, skull) 756.0
- frontal bone (see also Anomaly, skull)
    756.0
- gallbladder 751.6
- gastrointestinal tract NEC 751.9
- genitalia, genital organ(s) or system
- - female 752.9
- - - external 752.4
- - - internal NEC 752.9
- - male 752.9
- genitourinary NEC 752.9
- globe (eye) 743.9
- granulation or granulocyte, genetic 288.2
- gum 750.9

Anomaly - *continued*
- hair 757.9
- hand 755.5
- head (see also Anomaly, skull) 756.0
- heart 746.9
- - auricle 746.9
- - bands 746.9
- - folds 746.9
- - septum 745.9
- - - auricular 745.5
- - - ventricular 745.4
- - valve NEC 746.9
- - - pulmonary 746.0
- - ventricle 746.9
- heel 755.6
- Hegglin's 288.2
- hepatic duct 751.6
- hip 755.6
- humerus 755.5
- hymen 752.4
- hypophyseal 759.2
- ileocecal (coil) (valve) 751.5
- ileum 751.5
- ilium 755.6
- integument 757.9
- intervertebral cartilage or disc 756.1
- intestine (large) (small) 751.5
- iris 743.9
- ischium 755.6
- jaw NEC 524.9
- - size (major) 524.0
- jaw-cranial base relationship 524.1
- joint 755.9
- kidney(s) (calyx) (pelvis) 753.9
- - vessel 747.6
- knee 755.6
- labium (majus) (minus) 752.4
- labyrinth, membranous 744.0
- lacrimal apparatus or duct 743.9
- larynx, laryngeal (muscle) 748.3
- - web(bed) 748.2
- leg (upper) (lower) 755.6
- lens 743.9
- leucocytes, genetic 288.2
- lid (fold) 743.9
- ligament 756.9
- - broad 752.1
- - round 752.9
- limb except reduction deformity 755.9
- - lower 755.6
- - upper 755.5
- lip 750.9
- liver (duct) 751.6
- lower extremity 755.6
- lumbosacral (joint) (region) 756.1
- lung (fissure) (lobe) NEC 748.6
- lymphatic system 759.9

Anomaly - *continued*
- May-Hegglin 288.2
- meningeal bands or folds 742.9
- - contriction of 742.8
- meninges 742.9
- - brain 742.4
- - spinal 742.5
- mesentery 751.9
- metacarpus 755.5
- metatarsus 755.6
- middle ear 744.0
- mitral (leaflets) (valve) 746.9
- mouth 750.9
- multiple NEC 759.7
- muscle 756.9
- musculoskeletal system, except limbs, NEC 756.9
- nail 757.9
- neck (any part) 744.9
- nervous system NEC 742.9
- neurological 742.9
- nipple 757.9
- nose, nasal (bones) (cartilage) (septum) (sinus) 748.1
- ocular muscle 743.9
- oesophagus 750.9
- opening, pulmonary veins 747.4
- optic nerve 742.9
- opticociliary vessels 743.9
- orbit (eye) 743.9
- organ NEC 759.9
- - of Corti 744.0
- origin
- - artery
- - - coronary 746.8
- - - innominate 747.6
- - - pulmonary 747.3
- - - subclavian 747.6
- - renal vessels 747.6
- ovary 752.0
- oviduct 752.1
- palate (hard) (soft) 750.9
- pancreas 751.7
- papillary muscles 746.9
- parathyroid gland 759.2
- paraurethral ducts 753.9
- parotid (gland) 750.9
- patella 755.6
- Pelger-Huet 288.2
- pelvic girdle 755.6
- pelvis (bony) 755.6
- penis (glans) 752.9
- pericardium 746.8
- Peter's 743.4
- pharynx 750.9
- pigmentation NEC 709.0
- - congenital 757.3

Anomaly - *continued*
- pituitary (gland) 759.2
- pleural folds 748.8
- portal vein 747.4
- position
- - tooth, teeth 524.3
- prepuce 752.9
- prostate 752.9
- pulmonary 748.6
- - artery 747.3
- - circulation 747.3
- - valve 746.0
- - vein 747.4
- - venous connection, total 747.4
- pupil 743.9
- pylorus 750.9
- radius 755.5
- rectum 751.5
- refraction 367.9
- renal 753.9
- - vessel 747.6
- respiratory system NEC 748.9
- rib 756.3
- - cervical 756.2
- Rieger's 743.4
- rotation - see also Malrotation
- - hip or thigh 754.3
- sacroiliac (joint) 755.6
- sacrum 756.1
- salivary duct or gland 750.9
- scapula 755.5
- scrotum 752.9
- sebaceous gland 757.9
- seminal duct or tract 752.9
- sense organs NEC 742.9
- sex chromosomes NEC (see also Anomaly, chromosomes) 758.8
- shoulder (girdle) (joint) 755.5
- sigmoid (flexure) 751.5
- sinus of Valsalva 747.2
- site NEC 759.9
- skeleton generalized NEC 756.5
- skin (appendage) 757.9
- skull 756.0
- - with
- - - anencephalus 740.0
- - - encephalocele 742.0
- - - hydrocephalus 742.3
- - - - with spina bifida 741.0
- - - microcephalus 742.1
- specified type NEC
- - adrenal (gland) 759.1
- - alimentary tract (complete) (part) 751.8
- - - lower 751.5
- - - upper 750.8
- - ankle 755.6

Anomaly - *continued*
- specified type NEC - *continued*
- - liver 751.6
- - lung (fissure) (lobe) 748.6
- - meatus urinarius 753.8
- - metacarpus 755.5
- - mouth 750.2
- - muscle 756.8
- - - eye 743.6
- - musculoskeletal system, except limbs 756.8
- - nail 757.5
- - neck 744.8
- - nerve 742.8
- - - acoustic 742.8
- - - optic 742.8
- - nervous system 742.8
- - nipple 757.6
- - nose 748.1
- - organ NEC 759.8
- - - of Corti 744.0
- - osseous meatus (ear) 744.0
- - ovary 752.0
- - oviduct 752.1
- - pancreas 751.7
- - parathyroid 759.2
- - patella 755.6
- - pelvic girdle 755.6
- - penis 752.8
- - pericardium 746.8
- - peripheral vascular system 747.6
- - pharynx 750.2
- - pituitary 759.2
- - prostate 752.8
- - radius 755.5
- - rectum 751.5
- - respiratory system 748.8
- - rib 756.3
- - round ligament 752.8
- - sacrum 756.1
- - salivary duct or gland 750.2
- - scapula 755.5
- - scrotum 752.8
- - seminal duct or tract 752.8
- - shoulder girdle 755.5
- - site NEC 759.8
- - skin 757.3
- - skull (bone(s)) 756.0
- - - with
- - - - anencephalus 740.0
- - - - encephalocele 742.0
- - - - hydrocephalus 742.3
- - - - - with spina bifida 741.0
- - - - microcephalus 742.1
- - specified organ or site NEC 759.8
- - spermatic cord 752.8
- - spinal cord 742.5

Anomaly - *continued*
- specified type NEC - *continued*
- - spine 756.1
- - spleen 759.0
- - sternum 756.3
- - stomach 750.7
- - tarsus 755.6
- - tendon 756.8
- - testis 752.8
- - thorax (wall) 756.3
- - thymus 759.2
- - thyroid (gland) 759.2
- - - cartilage 748.3
- - tibia 755.6
- - toe 755.6
- - tongue 750.1
- - trachea (cartilage) 748.3
- - ulna 755.5
- - urachus 753.7
- - ureter 753.4
- - - obstructive 753.2
- - urethra 753.8
- - - obstructive 753.6
- - urinary tract 753.8
- - uterus 752.3
- - uvula 750.2
- - vagina 752.4
- - vas deferens 752.8
- - vascular 747.6
- - - brain 747.8
- - vein(s) (peripheral) 747.6
- - - brain 747.8
- - - great 747.4
- - - portal 747.4
- - - pulmonary 747.4
- - vena cava (inferior) (superior) 747.4
- - vertebra 756.1
- - vulva 752.4
- spermatic cord 752.9
- spine, spinal 756.1
- - column 756.1
- - cord 742.9
- - - vessel 747.6
- - nerve root 742.9
- spleen 759.0
- sternum 756.3
- stomach 750.9
- submaxillary gland 750.9
- superior vena cava 747.4
- tarsus 755.6
- tendon 756.9
- testis 752.9
- thebesian valve 746.9
- thigh 755.6
- thorax (wall) 756.3
- throat 750.9
- thumb 755.5

Anomaly - *continued*
- thymus gland 759.2
- thyroid (gland) 759.2
- - cartilage 748.3
- tibia 755.6
- toe 755.6
- tongue 750.1
- tooth, teeth NEC 520.9
- - position 524.3
- - spacing 524.3
- tracheal cartilage 748.3
- trichromata 368.5
- trichromatopsia 368.5
- tricuspid (leaflet) (valve) 746.9
- - atresia or stenosis 746.1
- - Ebstein's 746.2
- trunk 759.9
- ulna 755.5
- umbilicus 759.9
- union trachea with larynx 748.3
- upper extremity 755.5
- urachus 753.7
- ureter 753.9
- - obstructive 753.2
- urethra (valve) 753.9
- urinary tract (any part, except urachus) 753.9
- uterus 752.3
- - with only one functioning horn 752.3
- - in pregnancy or childbirth 654.0
- - - causing obstructed labor 660.2
- - - - fetus or newborn 763.1
- - - fetus or newborn 763.8
- vagina 752.4
- valleculae 748.3
- valve (heart) NEC 746.9
- - pulmonary 746.0
- vas deferens 752.9
- vascular NEC 747.6
- - ring 747.2
- vein(s) (peripheral) NEC 747.6
- - brain 747.8
- - cerebral 747.8
- - coronary 746.9
- - great 747.4
- - portal 747.4
- - pulmonary 747.4
- - retina 743.9
- vena cava (inferior) (superior) 747.4
- venous return 747.4
- ventricular
- - bands 746.9
- - folds 746.9
- - septa 745.4
- vertebra 756.1
- vesicourethral orifice 753.9
- vessels NEC 747.6

Anomaly - *continued*
- vessels NEC - *continued*
- - optic papilla 743.9
- vitreous humor 743.9
- vulva 752.4
- wrist (joint) 755.5
Anomia 784.6
Anonychia 757.5
- acquired 703.8
Anophthalmos, anophthalmus (congenital) (globe) 743.0
- acquired 360.8
Anopsia (altitudinal) (quadrant) 368.4
Anorchia 752.8
Anorchism, anorchidism 752.8
Anorexia 783.0
- hysterical 300.1
- nervosa 307.1
Anosmia (see also Disturbance, sensation) 781.1
- hysterical 300.1
- postinfectional 478.9
- traumatic 951.8
Anosognosia 780.9
Anosteoplasia 756.5
Anovulatory cycle 628.0
Anoxemia 799.0
- newborn 770.8
Anoxia 799.0
- altitude 993.2
- cerebral 348.1
- - complicating
- - - abortion - see categories 634-639, fourth digit .8
- - - delivery (cesarean) (instrumental) 669.4
- - - ectopic or molar pregnancy 639.8
- - - obstetric anesthesia or sedation 668.2
- - during or resulting from a procedure 997.0
- - newborn - see Distress, fetal
- due to drowning 994.1
- heart - see Insufficiency, coronary
- high altitude 993.2
- intrauterine
- - fetal death (before onset of labor) 768.0
- - - during labor 768.1
- - liveborn infant - see Distress, fetal, liveborn infant
- myocardial - see Insufficiency, coronary
- newborn - see Asphyxia, newborn
- pathological 799.0
Anteflexion - see Anteversion
Antenatal
- care, normal pregnancy V22.1

Antenatal - *continued*
- care - *continued*
- - first V22.0
- screening (for) V28.9
- - based on amniocentesis V28.2
- - chromosomal anomalies V28.0
- - fetal growth retardation using
   ultrasonics V28.4
- - isoimmunization V28.5
- - malformations using ultrasonics V28.3
- - raised alphafetoprotein levels in
   amniotic fluid V28.1
- - specified NEC V28.8
Antepartum - see condition
Anterior - see condition
Anteversion
- cervix (see also Anteversion, uterus)
   621.6
- femur (neck), congenital 755.6
- uterus, uterine (cervix) (postinfectional)
   (postpartal, old) 621.6
- - congenital 752.3
- - in pregnancy or childbirth 654.4
- - - causing obstructed labor 660.2
- - - - fetus or newborn 763.1
- - - fetus or newborn 763.8
Anthracosilicosis 500
Anthracosis (lung) 500
Anthrax 022.9
- with pneumonia 022.1 † 484.5*
- cutaneous 022.0
- gastrointestinal 022.2
- pulmonary 022.1
- respiratory 022.1
- septicemia 022.3
- specified manifestation NEC 022.8
Anthropoid pelvis 755.6
- with disproportion 653.2
- - causing obstructed labor 660.1
- - fetus or newborn 763.1
Anthropophobia 300.2
Antibioma, breast 611.0
Antibodies, maternal (blood group) (see
   also Incompatibility) 656.2
- anti-D 656.1
- - fetus or newborn 773.0
Antimonial cholera 985.4
Antisocial personality 301.7
Antithrombinemia (see also Circulating
   anticoagulants) 286.5
Antithromboplastinemia (see also
   Circulating anticoagulants) 286.5
Antithromboplastinogenemia (see also
   Circulating anticoagulants) 286.5
Antitoxin complication or reaction - see
   Complications, vaccination
Antritis (chronic) 473.0

Antritis - *continued*
- acute 461.0
Antrum, antral - see condition
Anuria 788.5
- calculous (impacted) (recurrent) 592.9
- congenital 753.3
- following
- - abortion - see categories 634-639,
   fourth digit .3
- - ectopic or molar pregnancy 639.3
- newborn 753.3
- puerperal, postpartum, childbirth 669.3
- specified due to a procedure 997.5
- sulfonamide
- - correct substance properly
   administered 788.5
- - overdose or wrong substance given or
   taken 961.0
- traumatic (following crushing) 958.5
Anus, anal - see condition
Anusitis 569.4
Anxiety (neurosis) (reaction) (state) 300.0
- depression 300.4
- hysteria 300.2
- separation, abnormal 309.2
Aorta, aortic - see condition
Aortitis (nonsyphilitic) 447.6
- arteriosclerotic 440.0
- calcific 447.6
- Doehle-Heller 093.1 † 447.7*
- luetic 093.1 † 447.7*
- rheumatic (see also Endocarditis, acute,
   rheumatic) 391.1
- rheumatoid - see Arthritis, rheumatoid
- specific 093.1 † 447.7*
- syphilitic 093.1 † 447.7*
- - congenital 090.5 † 447.7*
Apepsia 536.8
- achlorhydric 536.0
- psychogenic 306.4
Apert's syndrome 755.5
Apgar (score)
- low NEC 768.9
- 0-3 at 1 minute 768.5
- 4-7 at 1 minute 768.6
Aphagia 783.0
- psychogenic 307.1
Aphakia
- acquired 379.3
- congenital 743.3
- unilateral 379.3
Aphasia (amnestic) (ataxic) (auditory)
   (Broca's) (choreatic) (expressive) (global)
   (jargon) (motor) (nominal) (rreceptive)
   (semantic) (sensory) (syntactic) (verbal)
   (visual) (Wernicke's) 784.3
- developmental 315.3

Aphasia - *continued*
- syphilis, tertiary 094.8
- uremic - see Uremia
Aphemia 784.3
Aphonia 784.4
- hysterical 300.1
- organic 784.4
- psychogenic 306.1
Aphthae, aphthous - see also condition
- Bednar's 528.2
- epizootic 078.4
- fever 078.4
- stomatitis 528.2
- thrush 112.0
- ulcer (oral) (recurrent) 528.2
- - genital organ(s) NEC
- - - female 629.8
- - - male 608.8
- - larynx 478.7
Apical - see condition
Aplasia - see also Agenesis
- alveolar process (acquired) 525.8
- - congenital 750.2
- aorta (congenital) 747.2
- aortic valve (congenital) 746.8
- axialis extracorticalis (congenita) 330.0
- bone marrow (myeloid) 284.9
- brain 740.0
- - part of 742.2
- bronchus 748.3
- cementum 520.4
- cerebellum 742.2
- corpus callosum 742.2
- extracortical axial 330.0
- eye 743.0
- fovea centralis (congenital) 743.5
- iris 743.4
- labyrinth, membranous 744.0
- limb (congenital) 755.4
- - lower 755.3
- - upper 755.2
- lung (bilateral) (congenital) (unilateral) 748.5
- nervous system NEC 742.8
- nuclear 742.8
- Pelizaeus-Merzbacher 330.0
- prostate 752.8
- red cell (acquired) (adult) (pure) 284.8
- - with thymoma 284.8
- - congenital 284.0
- - of infant 284.0
- - primary 284.0
- round ligament 752.8
- spinal cord 742.5
- testicle 752.8
- thymic, with immunodeficiency 279.2
- uterus 752.3

Aplasia - see also Agenesis - *continued*
- ventral horn cell 742.5
Apnea, apneic (spells) 786.0
- newborn 770.8
Apneumatosis newborn 770.4
Apophysitis (bone) (see also Osteochondrosis) 732.9
- calcaneus 732.5
- juvenile 732.6
Apoplectiform convulsions (see also Disease, cerebrovascular, acute) 436
Apoplexia, apoplexy, apoplectic (see also Disease, cerebrovascular, acute) 436
- adrenal 036.3 † 255.5*
- attack 436
- basilar (see also Disease, cerebrovascular, acute) 436
- brain (see also Disease, cerebrovascular, acute) 436
- bulbar (see also Disease, cerebrovascular, acute) 436
- capillary (see also Disease, cerebrovascular, acute) 436
- cardiac (see also Infarct, myocardium) 410
- cerebral (see also Disease, cerebrovascular, acute) 436
- chorea (see also Disease, cerebrovascular, acute) 436
- congestive (see also Disease, cerebrovascular, acute) 436
- embolic (see also Embolism, brain) 434.1
- fit (see also Disease, cerebrovascular, acute) 436
- heart (auricle) (ventricle) (see also Infarct, myocardium) 410
- heat 992.0
- hemorrhagic (stroke) (see also Hemorrhage, brain) 432.9
- lung - see Embolism, pulmonary
- meninges, hemorrhagic (see also Hemorrhage, subarachnoid) 430
- progressive (see also Disease, cerebrovascular, acute) 436
- pulmonary (artery) (vein) - see Embolism, pulmonary
- seizure (see also Disease, cerebrovascular, acute) 436
- stroke (see also Disease, cerebrovascular, acute) 436
- thrombotic 434.0
- uremic - see Uremia
Appendage
- intestine (epiploic) 751.5
- preauricular 744.1
- testicular (organ of Morgagni) 752.8
Appendicitis 541

Appendicitis - *continued*
– with
– – perforation, peritonitis, or rupture
  540.0
– – peritoneal abscess 540.1
– acute (catarrhal) (fulminating)
  (gangrenous) (obstructive) (retrocecal)
  (suppurative) 540.9
– – with
– – – perforation, peritonitis, or rupture
  540.0
– – – peritoneal abscess 540.1
– amebic 006.8
– chronic (recurrent) 542
– exacerbation - see Appendicitis, acute
– gangrenous - see Appendicitis, acute
– healed (obliterative) 542
– interval 542
– obstructive 542
– pneumococcal 541
– recurrent 542
– retrocecal 541
– subacute (adhesive) 542
– suppurative - see Appendicitis, acute
– tuberculous 014
Appendicopathia oxyurica 127.4
Appendix, appendicular - see also condition
– Morgagni 752.8
Appetite
– depraved 307.5
– excessive 783.6
– lack or loss (see also Anorexia) 783.0
– – nonorganic origin 307.5
– perverted 307.5
– – hysterical 300.1
Apprehension state 300.0
Apprehensiveness, abnormal 300.0
Apraxia (classic) (ideational) (ideokinetic)
  (ideomotor) (motor) 784.6
– verbal 784.6
Aptyalism 527.7
Arachnidism 989.5
Arachnitis - see Meningitis
Arachnodactyly 759.8
Arachnoiditis (acute) (adhesive) (basic)
  (brain) (cerebrospinal) (chiasmal)
  (chronic) (spinal) (see also Meningitis)
  322.9
– meningococcal (chronic) 036.0 † 320.5*
– syphilitic 094.2 † 320.7*
– tuberculous 013.0 † 320.4*
Araneism 989.5
Arboencephalitis, Australian 062.4 † 323.3*
Arborization block (heart) 426.6
Arches - see condition
Arcuatus uterus 752.3
Arcus (cornea)

Arcus - *continued*
– juvenilis 743.4
– senilis 371.4
Arc-welder's lung 503
Areola - see condition
Argentaffinoma (M8241/1) - see also
  Neoplasm, uncertain behavior
– benign (M8241/0) - see Neoplasm,
  benign
– malignant (M8241/3) - see Neoplasm,
  malignant
Argyll Robertson phenomenon, pupil or
  syndrome (syphilitic) 094.8 † 379.4*
– atypical 379.4
– nonsyphilitic 379.4
Argyria, argyriasis NEC 985.8
– from drug or medicament
– – correct substance properly
  administered 709.0
– – overdose or wrong substance given or
  taken 961.2
Arhinencephaly 742.2
Ariboflavinosis 266.0
Arizona enteritis 008.1
Arm - see condition
Arnold-Chiari disease, obstruction or
  syndrome 741.0
Arrest, arrested
– active phase of labor 661.1
– – fetus or newborn 763.7
– any plane in pelvis
– – complicating delivery 660.1
– – fetus or newborn 763.1
– cardiac 427.5
– – complicating
– – – abortion - see categories 634-639,
  fourth digit .8
– – – anesthesia
– – – – correct substance properly
  administered 427.5
– – – – obstetric 668.1
– – – – overdose or wrong substance
  given 968.-
– – – – – specified anesthetic - see Table
  of drugs and chemicals
– – – delivery (cesarean) (instrumental)
  669.4
– – – ectopic or molar pregnancy 639.8
– – – surgery (therapeutic)
  (nontherapeutic) 997.1
– – fetus or newborn 779.8
– – postoperative 997.1
– – – long term effect of cardiac surgery
  429.4
– cardio-respiratory (see also Arrest,
  cardiac) 427.5
– deep transverse 660.3

Arteritis - *continued*
- cerebral 437.4
- - syphilitic 094.8
- coronary (artery) 414.0
- - rheumatic 391.9
- - - chronic 398.9
- - syphilitic 093.8
- cranial (left) (right) 446.5
- deformans - see Arteriosclerosis
- giant cell 446.5
- necrosing or necrotizing 446.0
- nodosa 446.0
- obliterans - see Arteriosclerosis
- rheumatic - see Fever, rheumatic
- senile - see Arteriosclerosis
- suppurative 447.2
- syphilitic (general) 093.8
- - brain 094.8
- - coronary 093.8
- - spinal 094.8
- temporal 446.5
Artery, arterial - see condition
Arthralgia 719.4
- allergic 719.4
- psychogenic 307.8
Arthritis, arthritic (acute) (chronic) (subacute) 716.9
- allergic 716.2
- ankylosing (crippling) (spine) 720.0
- - sites other than spine 716.9
- atrophic 714.0
- - spine 720.9
- back (see also Arthritis, spine) 721.9
- blennorrhagic 098.5 † 711.4*
- cervical (see also Spondylosis, cervical) 721.0
- Charcot's 094.0 † 713.5*
- - diabetic 250.5 † 713.5*
- - syringomyelic 336.0 † 713.5*
- - tabetic 094.0 † 713.5*
- chylous 125.9 † 711.7*
- climacteric (any site) NEC 716.3
- coccyx 721.8
- crystal(-induced) - see Arthritis, due to crystals
- deformans 715.9
- - spine 721.9
- degenerative 715.9
- - spine 721.9
- due to or associated with
- - acromegaly 253.0 † 713.0*
- - amyloidosis 277.3 † 713.7*
- - bacterial disease NEC 040.8 † 711.4*
- - Behcet's syndrome 136.1 † 711.2*
- - coliform (escherichia coli) 711.0
- - colitis, ulcerative 556 † 713.1*
- - crystals NEC 275.4 † 712.9*

Arthritis - *continued*
- due to or associated with - *continued*
- - crystals NEC 275.4 † 712.9* - *cont.*
- - - dicalcium phosphate 275.4 † 712.1*
- - - pyrophosphate 275.4 † 712.2*
- - dermatoarthritis, lipoid 272.8 † 713.0*
- - dermatological disorder NEC 709.9 † 713.3*
- - dracontiasis 125.7 † 711.7*
- - dysentery 009.0 † 711.3*
- - endocrine disorder NEC 259.9 † 713.0*
- - enteritis NEC 009.1 † 711.3*
- - - infectious (see also Enteritis, infectious) 009.0 † 711.3*
- - - - specified organism NEC 008.8 † 711.3*
- - - regional 555.- † 713.1*
- - - specified organism NEC 008.8 † 711.3*
- - epiphyseal slip, nontraumatic (old) 716.8
- - erythema
- - - multiforme 695.1 † 713.3*
- - - nodosum 695.2 † 713.3*
- - gastrointestinal condition NEC 569.9 † 713.1*
- - gonococcus 098.5 † 711.4*
- - gout 274.0 † 712.0*
- - H. influenzae 711.0

- - helminthiasis NEC 128.9 † 711.7*
- - hematological disorder NEC 289.9 † 713.2*
- - hemochromatosis 275.0 † 713.0*
- - hemoglobinopathy NEC 282.7 † 713.2*
- - hemophilia NEC 286.0 † 713.2*
- - Henoch(-Schonlein) purpura 287.0 † 713.6*
- - hyperparathyroidism 252.0 † 713.0*
- - hypersensitivity reaction NEC 995.3 † 713.6*
- - hypogammaglobulinemia 279.0 † 713.0*
- - hypothyroidism NEC 244.9 † 713.0*
- - infection (see also Arthritis, infectious) 711.9
- - infectious disease NEC 136.9 † 711.8*
- - leprosy 030.- † 711.4*
- - leukemia NEC (M9800/3) 208.9 † 713.2*
- - lipoid dermatoarthritis 272.8 † 713.0*
- - Mediterranean fever, familial 277.3 † 713.7*
- - meningococcus 036.8 † 711.4*
- - metabolic disorder NEC 277.9 † 713.0*

Arthritis - *continued*
- transient 716.4
- traumatic (chronic) (old) (post) 716.1
- tuberculous - see Tuberculosis, arthritis
- urethritica 099.3 † 711.1*
- urica, uratic 274.0 † 712.0*
- venereal 099.3 † 711.1*
- vertebral (see also Arthritis, spine) 721.9
- villous (any site) 716.8
Arthrocele 719.0
Arthrodesis status V45.4
Arthrodynia 719.4
- psychogenic 307.8
Arthrofibrosis, joint 718.5
Arthrogryposis 728.3
- multiplex congenita 755.8
Arthrokatadysis 715.3
Arthropathy (see also Arthritis) 716.9
- Charcot's 094.0 † 713.5*
- - diabetic 250.5 † 713.5*
- - syringomyelic 336.0 † 713.5*
- - tabetic 094.0 † 713.5*
- crystal(-induced) - see Arthritis, due to crystals
- neurogenic, neuropathic (Charcot) (tabetic) 094.0 † 713.5*
- - diabetic 250.5 † 713.5*
- - nonsyphilitic NEC 349.9 † 713.5*
- - syringomyelic 336.0 † 713.5*
- postdysenteric NEC 009.0 † 711.3*
- postrheumatic, chronic 714.4
- psoriatic 696.0 † 713.3*
- pulmonary 731.2
- specified NEC 716.8
- syringomyelic 336.0 † 713.5*
- tabes dorsalis 094.0 † 713.5*
- tabetic 094.0 † 713.5*
- transient 716.4
- traumatic 716.1
Arthrophytis 719.8
Arthropyosis 711.0
Arthrosis (deformans) (degenerative) 715.9
- polyarticular 715.0
- spine 721.9
Arthus' phenomenon 995.2
- due to
- - correct substance properly administered 995.2
- - overdose or wrong substance given or taken 977.9
- - - specified drug - see Table of drugs and chemicals
- - serum 999.5
Articular - see condition
Artificial
- insemination V26.1
- vagina status V44.7

Arytenoid - see condition
Asbestosis 501
Ascariasis (intestinal) (lung) 127.0
Ascaridiasis 127.0
Ascaridosis 127.0
Ascaris 127.0
- lumbricoides (infestation) 127.0
- pneumonia 127.0
Ascending - see condition
Aschoff's bodies (see also Myocarditis, rheumatic) 398.0
Ascites 789.5
- abdominal NEC 789.5
- chylous (nonfilarial) 457.8
- - filarial (see also Infestation, filarial) 125.9
- congenital 778.0
- joint 719.0
- syphilitic 095
- tuberculous 014
Aseptic - see condition
Asocial personality or trends 301.7
Aspergillosis 117.3
- with pneumonia 117.3 † 484.6*
Aspergillus (flavus) (fumigatus) (infection) (terreus) 117.3
Aspermatogenesis 606
Aspermia (testis) 606
Asphyxia, asphyxiation (by) 799.0
- antenatal - see Distress, fetal
- bedclothes 994.7
- birth (see also Asphyxia, newborn) 768.9
- bunny bag 994.7
- carbon monoxide 986
- caul (see also Asphyxia, newborn) 768.9
- cave-in 994.7
- - crushing - see Injury, internal, intrathoracic
- constriction 994.7
- crushing - see Injury, internal, intrathoracic
- drowning 994.1
- fetal - see Asphyxia, intra-uterine
- food or foreign body (in larynx) 933.1
- - bronchioles 934.8
- - bronchus (main) 934.1
- - lung 934.8
- - nasopharynx 933.0
- - nose, nasal passages 932
- - pharynx 933.0
- - respiratory tract 934.9
- - - specified part NEC 934.8
- - throat 933.0
- - trachea 934.0
- gas, fumes, or vapor NEC 987.9
- - specified - see Table of drugs and chemicals

Asphyxia - *continued*
- gravitational changes 994.7
- hanging 994.7
- inhalation - see Inhalation
- intrauterine
- – fetal death (before onset of labor) 768.0
- – – during labor 768.1
- – – liveborn infant - see Distress fetal, liveborn infant
- local 443.0
- mechanical 994.7
- – during birth (see also Distress, fetal) 768.4
- mucus 933.1
- – bronchus (main) 934.1
- – larynx 933.1
- – lung 934.8
- – nasal passages 932
- – newborn 770.1
- – respiratory tract 934.9
- – – specified part NEC 934.8
- – trachea 934.0
- – vaginal (fetus or newborn) 770.1
- newborn 768.9
- – blue 768.6
- – livida 768.6
- – mild or moderate 768.6
- – pallida 768.5
- – severe 768.5
- – white 768.5
- pathological 799.0
- postnatal (see also Asphyxia, newborn) 768.9
- – mechanical 994.7
- pressure 994.7
- reticularis 782.6
- strangulation 994.7
- submersion 994.1
- traumatic NEC - see Injury, internal, intrathoracic
- vomiting, vomitus - see Asphyxia, food or foreign body
Aspiration
- amniotic fluid 770.1
- content of birth canal 770.1
- food, foreign body, or gasoline (with asphyxiation) - see Asphyxia, food or foreign body
- meconium 770.1
- mucus 933.1
- – into
- – – bronchus (main) 934.1
- – – lung 934.8
- – – respiratory tract 934.9
- – – – specified part NEC 934.8
- – – trachea 934.0

Aspiration - *continued*
- mucus - *continued*
- – – newborn 770.1
- – – vaginal (fetus or newborn) 770.1
- syndrome of newborn (massive) (meconium) 770.1
- vernix caseosa 770.1
Asplenia 759.0
- with mesocardia 746.8
Assam fever 085.0
Assimilation pelvis
- with disproportion 653.2
- – causing obstructed labor 660.1
- – fetus or newborn 763.1
Assmann's focus 011.0
Astasia(-abasia) 307.9
- hysterical 300.1
Asteatosis 706.8
Astereognosis 780.9
Asterixis 781.3
Asthenia, asthenic 780.7
- cardiac (see also Failure, heart) 428.9
- – psychogenic 306.2
- cardiovascular (see also Failure, heart) 428.9
- – psychogenic 306.2
- heart (see also Failure, heart) 428.9
- – psychogenic 306.2
- hysterical 300.1
- myocardial (see also Failure, heart) 428.9
- – psychogenic 306.2
- nervous 300.5
- neurocirculatory 306.2
- neurotic 300.5
- psychogenic 300.5
- psychoneurotic 300.5
- psychophysiologic 300.5
- reaction (psychophysiologic) 300.5
- senile 797
Asthenopia 368.1
- accommodative 367.4
- hysterical (muscular) 300.1
- psychogenic 306.7
Asthenospermia 792.2
Asthma, asthmatic (bronchial) (catarrh) (spasmodic) 493.9
- with
- – hay fever 493.0
- – rhinitis, allergic 493.0
- allergic 493.9
- – stated cause (external allergen) 493.0
- atopic 493.0
- cardiac (see also Failure, ventricular, left) 428.1
- cardiobronchial 428.1
- childhood 493.0
- colliers' 500

Asthma - *continued*
- croup 493.9
- due to
- - detergent 507.8
- - internal immunological process 493.1
- eosinophilic 518.3
- extrinsic 493.0
- grinders' 502
- hay 493.0
- heart 428.1
- intrinsic 493.1
- Kopp's 254.8
- late-onset 493.1
- Millar's 478.7
- millstone makers' 502
- miners' 500
- platinum 493.0
- pneumoconiotic NEC 505
- potters' 502
- pulmonary eosinophilic 518.3
- red-cedar 495.8
- Rostan's 428.1
- sandblasters' 502
- sequoiosis 495.8
- stonemasons' 502
- thymic 254.8
- tuberculous (see also Tuberculosis, pulmonary) 011.9
- wood 495.8
Astigmatism (compound) (congenital) (any type) 367.2
Astroblastoma (M9430/3)
- nose 748.1
- specified site NEC - see Neoplasm, malignant
- unspecified site 191.9
Astrocytoma (cystic) (M9400/3)
- anaplastic type (M9401/3)
- - specified site - see Neoplasm, malignant
- - unspecified site 191.9
- fibrillary (M9420/3)
- - specified site - see Neoplasm, malignant
- - unspecified site 191.9
- fibrous (M9420/3)
- - specified site - see Neoplasm, malignant
- - unspecified site 191.9
- gemistocytic (M9411/3)
- - specified site - see Neoplasm, malignant
- - unspecified site 191.9
- juvenile (M9421/3)
- - specified site - see Neoplasm, malignant
- - unspecified site 191.9

Astrocytoma - *continued*
- nose 748.1
- pilocytic (M9421/3)
- - specified site - see Neoplasm, malignant
- - unspecified site 191.9
- piloid (M9421/3)
- - specified site - see Neoplasm, malignant
- - unspecified site 191.9
- protoplasmic (M9410/3)
- - specified site - see Neoplasm, malignant
- - unspecified site 191.9
- specified site NEC - see Neoplasm, malignant
- subependymal (M9383/1) 237.5
- - giant cell (M9384/1) 237.5
- unspecified site 191.9
Astroglioma (M9400/3)
- nose 748.1
- specified site NEC - see Neoplasm, malignant
- unspecified site 191.9
Asymbolia 784.6
Asymmetry - see also Distortion
- face 754.0
- jaw 524.1
- pelvis with disproportion 653.0
- - causing obstructed labor 660.1
- - fetus or newborn 763.1
Asynergia 781.3
Asynergy 781.3
Asystole (heart) (see also Arrest, cardiac) 427.5
Ataxia, ataxy, ataxic 781.3
- acute 781.3
- brain 331.8
- cerebellar 334.3
- - hereditary (Marie's) 334.2
- - in
- - - alcoholism 303 † 334.4*
- - - myxedema NEC 244.9 † 334.4*
- - - neoplastic disease NEC 239.9 † 334.4*
- cerebral 331.8
- family, familial 334.2
- - cerebral (Marie's) 334.2
- - spinal (Friedreich's) 334.0
- Friedreich's (heredofamilial) (spinal) 334.0
- gait 781.2
- - hysterical 300.1
- general 781.3
- hereditary NEC 334.2
- - spastic 334.1
- heredofamilial, Marie's 334.2

Ataxia - *continued*
- hysterical 300.1
- locomotor (progressive) 094.0
- Marie's (cerebellar) (heredofamilial)
  334.2
- nonorganic origin 307.9
- partial 094.0
- progressive 094.0
- psychogenic 307.9
- Sanger-Brown's 334.2
- spastic 094.0
- - hereditary 334.1
- - syphilitic 094.0
- spinal
- - hereditary 334.0
- - progressive 094.0
- telangiectasia 334.8
Ataxia-telangiectasia 334.8
Atelectasis (absorption collapse) (complete)
  (compression) (massive) (partial)
  (postinfective) (pressure collapse)
  (pulmonary) (relaxation) 518.0
- fetus or newborn 770.5
- - primary 770.4
- primary 770.4
- tuberculous (see also Tuberculosis,
  pulmonary) 011.9
Atelia - see Distortion
Ateliosis 253.3
Atelocardia 746.9
Atelomyelia 742.5
Atheroma, atheromatous (see also
  Arteriosclerosis) 440.9
- aorta, aortic 440.0
- - valve (see also Endocarditis, aortic)
  424.1
- artery - see Arteriosclerosis
- basilar (artery) (see also Occlusion,
  artery, basilar) 433.0
- carotid (artery) (common) (internal) (see
  also Occlusion, artery, carotid) 433.1
- cerebral (arteries) 437.0
- coronary 414.0
- degeneration - see Arteriosclerosis
- heart, cardiac 414.0
- mitral (valve) 424.0
- myocardium, myocardial 414.0
- pulmonary valve (heart) (see also
  Endocarditis, pulmonary) 424.3
- skin 706.2
- tricuspid (heart) (valve) 424.2
- valve, valvular - see Endocarditis
- vertebral (artery) (see also Occlusion,
  artery, vertebral) 433.2
Atheromatosis - see Arteriosclerosis
Atherosclerosis - see Arteriosclerosis
Athetosis (acquired) 781.0

Athetosis - *continued*
- bilateral 333.7
- congenital (bilateral) 333.7
- double 333.7
- unilateral 781.0
Athlete's
- foot 110.4
- heart 429.3
Athyrea (acquired) (see also
  Hypothyroidism) 244.9
- congenital 243
Athyroidism (acquired) (see also
  Hypothyroidism) 244.9
- congenital 243
Atonia, atony, atonic
- abdominal wall 728.2
- bladder (sphincter) 596.4
- - neurogenic NEC 344.6
- capillary 448.9
- cecum 564.8
- - psychogenic 306.4
- colon 564.8
- - psychogenic 306.4
- congenital 779.8
- dyspepsia 536.8
- - psychogenic 306.4
- intestine 564.8
- - psychogenic 306.4
- stomach 536.8
- - neurotic or psychogenic 306.4
- uterus 661.2
- - fetus or newborn 763.7
Atransferrinemia, congenital 273.8
Atresia, atretic (congenital) 759.8
- alimentary organ or tract NEC 751.8
- - lower 751.2
- - upper 750.8
- ani, anus, anal (canal) 751.2
- aorta 747.2
- - arch 747.1
- - ring 747.2
- aortic (orifice) (valve) 746.8
- - arch 747.1
- - in hypoplastic left heart syndrome
  746.7
- aqueduct of Sylvius 742.3
- - with spina bifida 741.0
- artery NEC 747.6
- - cerebral 747.8
- - coronary 746.8
- - eye 743.5
- - pulmonary 747.3
- - umbilical 747.5
- auditory canal (external) 744.0
- bile duct 751.6
- - acquired (see also Obstruction, biliary)
  576.2

Atresia - *continued*
- bladder (neck) 753.6
- bronchus 748.3
- cecum 751.2
- cervix (acquired) 622.4
- - congenital 752.4
- - in pregnancy or childbirth 654.6
- - - causing obstructed labor 660.2
- - - - fetus or newborn 763.1
- - - fetus or newborn 763.8
- choana 748.0
- colon 751.2
- cystic duct 751.6
- - acquired (see also Obstruction, gallbladder) 575.8
- digestive organs NEC 751.8
- duodenum 751.1
- ear canal 744.0
- ejaculatory duct 752.8
- epiglottis 748.3
- esophagus 750.3
- eustachian tube 744.2
- fallopian tube (congenital) 752.1
- - acquired 628.2
- foramen of
- - Luschka 742.3
- - - with spina bifida 741.0
- - Magendie 742.3
- - - with spina bifida 741.0
- gallbladder 751.6
- genital organ
- - external
- - - female 752.4
- - - male 752.8
- - internal
- - - female 752.8
- - - male 752.8
- glottis 748.3
- gullet 750.3
- heart valve NEC 746.8
- - pulmonary 746.0
- - tricuspid 746.1
- hymen 752.4
- - acquired 623.3
- - postinfective 623.3
- ileum 751.1
- intestine (small) 751.1
- - large 751.2
- iris, filtration angle 743.2
- jejunum 751.1
- kidney 753.3
- lacrimal apparatus 743.6
- - acquired 375.5
- larynx 748.3
- lung 748.6
- meatus urinarius 753.6
- mitral valve 746.8

Atresia - *continued*
- mitral valve - *continued*
- - in hypoplastic left heart syndrome 746.7
- nares (anterior) (posterior) 748.0
- nasopharynx 748.8
- nose, nostril 748.0
- - acquired 478.1
- oesophagus 750.3
- organ or site NEC 759.8
- osseous meatus (ear) 744.0
- oviduct (congenital) 752.1
- - acquired 628.2
- parotid duct 750.2
- - acquired 527.8
- pulmonary (artery) 747.3
- - valve 746.0
- - vein 747.4
- pulmonic 746.0
- pupil 743.4
- rectum 751.2
- salivary duct or gland 750.2
- - acquired 527.8
- sublingual duct 750.2
- - acquired 527.8
- submaxillary duct or gland 750.2
- - acquired 527.8
- trachea 748.3
- tricuspid valve 746.1
- ureter 753.2
- ureteropelvic junction 753.2
- ureterovesical orifice 753.2
- urethra (valvular) 753.6
- urinary tract NEC 753.2
- uterus 752.3
- - acquired 621.8
- vagina (acquired) 623.2
- - congenital 752.4
- - postgonococcal (old) 098.2
- - postinfectional 623.2
- - senile 623.2
- vas deferens 752.8
- vascular NEC 747.6
- - cerebral 747.8
- vein NEC 747.6
- - great 747.4
- - portal 747.4
- - pulmonary 747.4
- vena cava (inferior) (superior) 747.4
- vesicourethral orifice 753.6
- vulva 752.4
- - acquired 624.8
Atrichia, atrichosis 704.0
- congenital (universal) 757.4
Atrophia - see also Atrophy
- cutis senilis 701.8
- dermatological, diffuse (idiopathic) 701.8

Atrophy - *continued*
– liver - *continued*
– – yellow - *continued*
– – – from injection, inoculation or
      transfusion (onset within 8 months
      after administration) 070.3 † 573.1*
– – – – with hepatic coma 070.2 † 573.1*
– – – post-immunization 070.3 † 573.1*
– – – – with hepatic coma 070.2 † 573.1*
– – – post-transfusion 070.3 † 573.1*
– – – – with hepatic coma 070.2 † 573.1*
– lung (senile) 518.8
– – congenital 748.6
– macular (dermatological) 701.3
– – syphilitic, skin 091.3
– – – striated 095
– muscle, muscular 728.2
– – Duchenne-Aran 335.1
– – extremity (lower) (upper) 728.2
– – general 728.2
– – idiopathic 728.2
– – myelopathic (progressive) 335.1
– – neuritic 356.1
– – neuropathic (peroneal) (progressive)
    356.1
– – peroneal 356.1
– – primary (idiopathic) 728.2
– – progressive (familial) (hereditary)
    (pure) 335.2
– – – adult (spinal) 335.1
– – – infantile (spinal) 335.0
– – – juvenile (spinal) 335.1
– – pseudohypertrophic 359.1
– – spinal (adult) (familial) (hereditary)
    (progressive) 335.1
– – – infantile 335.0
– – syphilitic 095 † 728.0*
– myocardium (see also Degeneration,
    myocardial) 429.1
– myometrium (senile) 621.8
– – cervix 622.8
– myotatic 728.2
– nail 703.8
– – congenital 757.5
– nasopharynx 472.2
– nerve - see also Disorder, nerve
– – abducens 378.5
– – cranial
– – – fourth (trochlear) 378.5
– – – second (optic) 377.1
– – – sixth (abducens) 378.5
– – – third (oculomotor) 378.5
– – oculomotor 378.5
– – trochlear 378.5
– nervous system, congenital 742.8
– neurogenic, bone
– – tabetic 094.0

Atrophy - *continued*
– nutritional 261
– old age 797
– olivopontocerebellar 333.0
– optic nerve (ascending) (descending)
    (familial) (hereditary) (infectional NEC)
    (Leber's) (nonfamilial) (papillomacular
    bundle) (postretinal) (primary)
    (secondary) (simple) 377.1
– – syphilitic 094.8 † 377.1*
– – – congenital 090.4 † 377.1*
– – – tabes dorsalis 094.0 † 377.1*
– orbit 376.4
– ovary (senile) 620.3
– oviduct (senile) 620.3
– palsy, diffuse 335.2
– pancreas (duct) (senile) 577.8
– parotid gland 527.0
– patches skin 701.3
– – senile 701.8
– penis 607.8
– pharynx 478.2
– pluriglandular 258.8
– polyarthritis 714.0
– prostate 602.2
– pseudohypertrophic 359.1
– renal (see also Sclerosis, renal) 587
– reticulata 701.8
– retina, retinal (postinfectional) 362.8
– salivary duct or gland 527.0
– scar 709.2
– sclerosis lobar (of brain) 331.0
– – dementia in 290.1
– scrotum 608.8
– seminal vesicle 608.8
– senile 797
– – degenerative, of skin (senile) 701.3
– skin (senile) 701.8
– – degenerative 701.3
– spermatic cord 608.8
– spinal (cord) 336.8
– – muscular (chronic) 335.1
– – paralysis 335.1
– – – acute 045.1 † 323.2*
– spine (column) 733.9
– spleen (senile) 289.5
– spots (skin) 701.3
– – senile 701.8
– stomach 537.8
– striate and macular 701.3
– – syphilitic 095
– subcutaneous 701.9
– sublingual gland 527.0
– submaxillary gland 527.0
– Sudeck's 733.7
– suprarenal (capsule) (gland) 255.4
– tarso-orbital fascia, congenital 743.6

Atrophy - *continued*
- testis 608.3
- thymus (fat) 254.8
- thyroid (gland) 246.8
- - with
- - - cretinism 243
- - - myxedema 244.9
- - congenital 243
- tongue (senile) 529.8
- - papillae 529.4
- trachea 519.1
- tunica vaginalis 608.8
- turbinate 733.9
- upper respiratory tract 478.9
- uterus, uterine (senile) 621.8
- - cervix 622.8
- - due to radiation (intended effect) 621.8
- vagina (senile) 627.3
- vas deferens 608.8
- vascular 459.8
- vertebra (senile) 733.9
- vulva (senile) 624.1
- yellow (acute) (liver) (subacute) 570
- - chronic 571.8
Attack
- akinetic 345.0
- angina - see Angina
- bilious (see also Vomiting) 787.0
- cataleptic 300.1
- cerebral (see also Disease, cerebrovascular, acute) 436
- coronary (see also Infarct, myocardium) 410
- cyanotic, newborn 770.8
- epileptic - see Epilepsy
- epileptiform 780.3
- heart (auricle) (ventricle) (see also Infarct, myocardium) 410
- hemiplegia (see also Disease, cerebrovascular, acute) 436
- hysterical 300.1
- jacksonian 345.5
- myocardium, myocardial (see also Infarct, myocardium) 410
- myoclonic 345.1
- panic 300.0
- paralysis (see also Disease, cerebrovascular, acute) 436
- paroxysmal 780.3
- psychomotor 345.4
- salaam 345.6
- schizophreniform 295.4
- sensory and motor 780.3
- syncope 780.2
- transient ischemic (TIA) 435
- unconsciousness 780.2

Attack - *continued*
- unconsciousness - *continued*
- - hysterical 300.1
- vasomotor 780.2
- vasovagal (paroxysmal) (idiopathic) 780.2
Attention to
- artificial
- - opening (of) V55.9
- - - digestive tract NEC V55.4
- - - specified NEC V55.8
- - - urinary tract NEC V55.6
- - vagina V55.7
- colostomy V55.3
- cystostomy V55.5
- gastrostomy V55.1
- ileostomy V55.2
- nephrostomy V55.6
- surgical dressings V58.3
- sutures V58.3
- tracheostomy V55.0
- ureterostomy V55.6
- urethrostomy V55.6
Attrition
- gum 523.2
- tooth, teeth (excessive) (hard tissues) 521.1
Atypical - see also condition
- distribution, vessel 747.6
- endometrium 621.9
Auditory - see condition
Aujeszky's disease 078.8
Aura, jacksonian 345.5
Aurantiasis, cutis 278.3
Auricle, auricular - see condition
Australian
- Q fever 083.0
- X disease 062.4 † 323.3*
Autism, autistic (childhood) (infantile) 299.0
Autodigestion 799.8
Autoerythrocyte sensitization 287.2
Autographism 708.3
Autoimmune disease NEC 279.4
Autoinfection, septic - see Septicemia
Autointoxication 799.8
Automatism 348.8
- epileptic 345.4
- paroxysmal, idiopathic 345.4
Autonomic, autonomous
- bladder 344.6
- - neurogenic 344.6
- hysteria seizure 300.1
Autosensitivity, erythrocyte 287.2
Autotopagnosia 780.9
Autotoxemia 799.8
Autumn - see condition

Avellis' syndrome 344.8
Aviators'
– disease or sickness (see also Effects, adverse, high altitude) 993.2
– ear 993.0
– effort syndrome 306.2
Avitaminosis (multiple NEC) (see also Deficiency, vitamin) 269.2
Avulsion (traumatic) 879.8
– blood vessel - see Injury, blood vessel
– cartilage - see also Dislocation, by site
– – knee, current (see also Tear, meniscus) 836.2
– – symphyseal (inner), complicating delivery 665.6
– complicated 879.9
– epiphysis of bone - see Fracture, by site
– external site other than limb - see Wound, open, by site
– eye 871.3
– head NEC (intracranial) 854.1
– – complete 874.9
– – external site NEC 873.8
– – – complicated 873.9
– internal organ or site - see Injury, internal, by site
– joint - see also Dislocation, by site
– – capsule - see Sprain

Avulsion - *continued*
– ligament - see Sprain, by site
– limb - see also Amputation, traumatic, by site
– – skin and subcutaneous tissue - see Wound, open
– muscle - see Sprain, strain, by site
– nerve (root) - see Injury, nerve, by site
– skin and subcutaneous tissue - see Wound, open
– symphyseal cartilage (inner), complicating delivery 665.6
– tendon - see also Sprain, by site
– – with open wound - see Wound, open, by site
– tooth 873.6
– – complicated 873.7
Awareness of heart beat 785.1
Ax(e)-grinders' disease 502
Axilla, axillary - see also condition
– breast 757.6
Axonotmesis - see Injury, nerve, by site
Ayala's disease 756.8
Ayerza's disease or syndrome 416.0
Azoospermia 606
Azotemia 791.9
Aztec ear 744.2
Azygos lobe, lung 748.6

B

Baastrup's syndrome 721.5
Babinski's syndrome 093.8
Babinski-Nageotte syndrome 344.8
Bacillary - see condition
Bacilluria 599.0
– tuberculous 016.9
Bacillus - see Infection, bacillus
Back - see condition
Backache (postural) 724.5
– psychogenic 307.8
– sacroiliac 724.6
Backflow (pyelovenous) (see also Disease, renal) 593.9
Bacteremia 790.7
– with
– – abortion - see categories 634-639, fourth digit .0
– – ectopic gestation 639.0
– – pneumonia 482.-
– anaerobic 038.3
– during labor 659.3
– gas gangrene 040.0
– gonococcal NEC 098.8
– gram-negative bacilli 038.4
– – anaerobic 038.3
– meningococcal 036.2
– plague 020.2
– pneumococcal 038.2
– puerperal, postpartum, childbirth 670
– specified organism NEC 038.8
– staphylococcal 038.1
– streptococcal (anaerobic) 038.0
Bacteria
– in blood - see Bacteremia
– in urine - see Bacteriuria
Bacterial - see condition
Bactericholia (see also Cholecystitis, acute) 575.0
Bacterid, bacteride (pustular) 686.8
Bacteriuria, bacteruria 599.0
– asymptomatic 599.0
– – in pregnancy or puerperium 646.5
– – – fetus or newborn 760.1
Bad
– heart - see Disease, heart
– trip 305.3
Baelz's disease 528.5
Bagassosis 495.1
Bagratuni's syndrome 446.5
Baker's cyst 727.5

Baker's cyst - *continued*
– tuberculous 015.2
Balanitis (circinata) (gangrenosa) (infectional) (vulgaris) 607.1
– amebic 006.8
– due to Ducrey's bacillus 099.0
– erosiva circinata et gangrenosa 607.1
– gonococcal (acute) 098.0
– – chronic or duration of 2 months or over 098.2
– nongonococcal 607.1
– phagedenic 607.1
– venereal 099.8
– xerotica obliterans 607.8
Balanoposthitis 607.1
– gonococcal (acute) 098.0
– – chronic or duration of 2 months or over 098.2
– ulcerative 099.8
Balanorrhagia - see Balanitis
Balantidiasis 007.0
Balantidiosis 007.0
Balbuties, balbutio 307.0
Baldness (see also Alopecia) 704.0
Balkan grippe 083.0
Balloon disease (see also Effect, adverse, high altitude) 993.2
Balo's disease or concentric sclerosis 341.1
Bamberger-Marie disease 731.2
Bancroft's filariasis 125.0
Band(s)
– adhesive (see also Adhesions, peritoneum) 568.0
– anomalous or congenital - see also Anomaly, specified type NEC
– – atrial 746.9
– – heart 746.9
– – intestine 751.4
– – omentum 751.4
– – ventricular 746.9
– cervix 622.3
– gallbladder (congenital) 751.6
– intestinal (adhesive) (see also Adhesions, peritoneum) 568.0
– obstructive (see also Obstruction, intestine) 560.8
– periappendiceal (congenital) 751.4
– peritoneal (adhesive) (see also Adhesions, peritoneum) 568.0
– uterus 621.5

Band(s) - *continued*
– vagina 623.2
Bandl's ring (contraction)
– complicating delivery 661.4
– – fetus or newborn 763.7
Bang's disease 023.1
Bannister's disease 995.1
Banti's disease or syndrome (with cirrhosis) (with portal hypertension) - see Cirrhosis, liver
Bar, prostate 600
Barcoo disease or rot (see also Ulcer, skin) 707.9
Barensprung's disease 110.3
Barlow's disease 267
Barodontalgia 993.2
Baron Munchhausen syndrome 301.5
Barosinusitis 993.1
Barotitis 993.0
Barotrauma 993.2
– odontalgia 993.2
– otitic 993.0 † 381.0*
– sinus 993.1
Barraquer(-Simons) disease 272.6
Barre-Guillain syndrome 357.0
Barrel chest 738.3
Barre-Lieou syndrome 723.2
Bartholin's gland - see condition
Bartholinitis (suppurating) 616.8
– gonococcal (acute) 098.0
Bartonellosis 088.0
Basal - see condition
Baseball finger 842.1
Basedow's disease 242.0
Basic - see condition
Basilar - see condition
Bason's (hidrotic) ectodermal dysplasia 757.3
Basophilia 289.8
Basophilism (cortico-adrenal) (Cushing's) (pituitary) (thymic) 255.0
Bassen-Kornzweig syndrome 272.5
Bat ear 744.2
Bateman's disease 078.0
Bathing cramp 994.1
Bathophobia 300.2
Batten's disease, retina 330.1 † 362.7*
Batten-Mayou disease 330.1 † 362.7*
Battered baby or child (syndrome) NEC 995.5
Battey mycobacterium infection 031.0
Battle exhaustion (see also Reaction, stress, acute) 308.9
Battledore placenta - see Placenta, abnormal
Baumgarten-Cruveilhier cirrhosis, disease or syndrome 571.5

Bauxite fibrosis (of lung) 503
Bayle's disease 094.1
Bazin's disease (primary) 017.1
Beach ear 380.1
Beaded hair (congenital) 757.4
Beard's disease 300.5
Beat elbow, hand or knee 727.2
Beats
– escaped, heart 427.6
– premature (atrium) (auricular) (nodal) (supraventricular) 427.6
Beau's lines 703.8
Bechterew's disease 720.0
Becker's
– disease 425.2
– dystrophy 359.1
Beckwith(-Wiedemann) syndrome 759.8
Bedclothes, asphyxiation or suffocation by 994.7
Bednar's aphthae 528.2
Bedsore 707.0
Bedwetting (see also Enuresis) 788.3
Bee sting (with allergic or anaphylactic shock) 989.5
Behavior disorder, disturbance - see Disturbance, conduct
Behcet's syndrome 136.1
Behr's disease 362.5
Beigel's disease or morbus 111.2
Bejel 104.0
Belching (see also Eructation) 787.3
Bell's
– disease 296.0
– mania 296.0
– palsy, paralysis 351.0
– – newborn 767.5
– – syphilitic 094.8
– spasm 351.1
Bence-Jones albuminuria, albumosuria or proteinuria NEC 791.0
Bends 993.3
Benedikt's paralysis or syndrome 344.8
Bennett's fracture - see Fracture, metacarpal
Benson's disease 379.2
Bent
– back (hysterical) 300.1
– nose 738.0
– – congenital 754.0
Berger's paresthesia 782.0
Bergeron's disease 300.1
Beriberi 265.0
– heart (disease) 265.0 † 425.7*
– leprosy 030.1
– neuritis 265.0 † 357.4*
Berlin's disease or edema (traumatic) 921.3
Berloque's dermatitis 692.7

Bernard-Horner syndrome 337.9
Bernard-Soulier disease or thrombopathia
  287.1
Bernhardt's disease or paresthesia 355.1
Bernhardt-Roth disease or syndrome 355.1
Bernheim's syndrome (see also Failure,
  heart, congestive) 428.0
Bertielliasis 123.8
Bertolotti's syndrome 756.1
Berylliosis (lung) 503
Besnier's
– lupus pernio 135
– prurigo 691.8
Besnier-Boeck(-Schaumann) disease 135
Best's disease 362.7
Bestiality 302.1
Beta-amino-isobutyricaciduria 277.2
Beurmann's disease 117.1
Bezoar 938
– intestine 936
– stomach 935.2
Bezold's abscess 383.0
Bianchi's syndrome 784.6
Bicornate or bicornis uterus 752.3
– in pregnancy or childbirth 654.0
– – fetus or newborn 763.8
Bicuspid aortic valve 746.4
Biedl-Bardet syndrome 759.8
Bielschowsky(-Jansky)
– amaurotic familial idiocy 330.1
– disease 330.1
Biemond's syndrome 759.8
Biermer's anemia or disease 281.0
Biett's disease 695.4
Bifid (congenital) - see also Imperfect,
  closure
– apex, heart 746.8
– clitoris 752.4
– kidney 753.3
– nose 748.1
– patella 755.6
– scrotum 752.8
– toe 755.6
– tongue 750.1
– ureter 753.4
– uterus 752.3
– uvula 749.0
– – with cleft lip 749.2
Biforis uterus (suprasimplex) 752.3
Bifurcation (congenital) - see also
  Imperfect, closure
– gallbladder 751.6
– kidney pelvis 753.3
– renal pelvis 753.3
– rib 756.3
– tongue 750.1
– trachea 748.3

Bifurcation - *continued*
– ureter 753.4
– urethra 753.8
– uvula 749.0
– – with cleft lip 749.2
– vertebra 756.1
Bigeminal pulse 427.8
Bilateral - see condition
Bile
– duct - see condition
– pigments in urine 791.4
Bilharziasis (see also Schistosomiasis) 120.9
– chyluria 120.0
– galacturia 120.0
– hematochyluria 120.0
– intestinal 120.1
– lipemia 120.9
– lipuria 120.0
– oriental 120.2
– piarhemia 120.9
– pulmonary 120.2
– tropical hematuria 120.0
– vesical 120.0
Biliary - see condition
Bilious (attack) (see also Vomiting) 787.0
Biliuria 791.4
Billroth's disease - see Disease, Billroth's
Bilocular stomach 536.8
Bing-Horton's syndrome 346.2
Biparta, bipartite - see also Imperfect,
  closure
– carpal scaphoid 755.5
– patella 755.6
– vagina 752.4
Bird
– face 756.0
– fanciers' lung or disease 495.2
Birth
– abnormal, fetus or newborn NEC 763.9
– complications in mother - see Delivery,
  complicated
– compression during NEC 767.9
– defect - see Anomaly
– delayed, fetus 763.9
– difficult nec, affecting fetus or newborn
  763.9
– dry, affecting fetus or newborn 761.1
– forced, nec, affecting fetus or newborn
  763.8
– forceps, affecting fetus or newborn 763.2
– immature 765.1
– – extremely 765.0
– inattention, after or at 995.5
– induced, affecting fetus or newborn 763.8
– injury NEC 767.9
– – basal ganglia 767.0
– – brachial plexus 767.6

Birth - *continued*
- injury NEC - *continued*
- - brain (compression) (pressure) 767.0
- - cerebellum 767.0
- - cerebral hemorrhage 767.0
- - eye 767.8
- - fracture
- - - bone, any except clavicle or spine 767.3
- - - clavicle 767.2
- - - femur 767.3
- - - humerus 767.3
- - - long bone 767.3
- - - radius and ulna 767.3
- - - skeleton NEC 767.3
- - - skull 767.3
- - - spine 767.4
- - - tibia and fibula 767.3
- - hematoma of sternomastoid 767.8
- - intracranial 767.0
- - laceration
- - - brain 767.0
- - - by scalpel 767.8
- - - peripheral nerve 767.7
- - liver 767.8
- - meninges
- - - brain 767.0
- - - spinal cord 767.4
- - nerve (cranial) (peripheral) 767.7
- - - brachial plexus 767.6
- - - facial 767.5
- - scalp 767.1
- - scalpel wound 767.8
- - spinal cord 767.4
- - spleen 767.8
- - subdural hemorrhage 767.0
- - tentorial tear 767.0
- - testes 767.8
- - vulva 767.8
- instrumental, nec, affecting fetus or newborn 763.2
- lack of care, after or at 995.5
- multiple 761.5
- neglect, after or at 995.5
- palsy or paralysis, newborn, NEC 767.7
- precipitate, fetus or newborn 763.6
- premature (infant) 765.1
- prolonged, affecting fetus or newborn 763.9
- retarded, fetus or newborn 763.9
- shock, newborn 779.8
- trauma NEC 767.9
- twin 761.5
- ventouse, affecting fetus or newborn 763.3
Birthmark 757.3
Bisalbuminemia 273.8

Biskra's button 085.1
Bite(s)   •
- with intact skin surface - see Contusion
- animal - see also Wound, open
- - intact skin surface - see Contusion
- centipede 989.5
- chigger 133.8
- flea - see Injury, superficial
- human (open wound) - see also Wound, open
- - intact skin surface - see Contusion
- insect (nonvenomous) - see also Injury, superficial
- - venomous 989.5
- mad dog, death from 071
- poisonous 989.5
- reptile 989.5
- - nonvenomous - see Wound, open
- snake 989.5
- - nonvenomous - see Wound, open
- spider (venomous) 989.5
- - nonvenomous - see Injury, superficial
- venomous 989.5
Biting, cheek or lip 528.9
Black
- death 020.9
- hairy tongue 529.3
Blackfan-Diamond anemia or syndrome 284.0
Blackhead 706.1
Blackout 780.2
Bladder - see condition
Blast
- blindness 921.3
- concussion - see Blast injury
- injury 869.-
- - abdomen or thorax - see Injury, internal, by site
- - brain 850
- - - with skull fracture - see Fracture, skull
- - ear (acoustic nerve trauma) 951.5
- - - with perforation, tympanic membrane - see Wound, open, ear
Blastomycosis, blastomycotic (chronic) (cutaneous) (disseminated) (lung) (pulmonary) (systemic) 116.0
- Brazilian 116.1
- European 117.5
- keloidal 116.2
- North American 116.0
- primary pulmonary 116.0
- South American 116.1
Bleb(s) 709.8
- emphysematous (lung) 492
- lung (ruptured) 492
- - congenital 770.5

Bleeder (familial) (hereditary) (see also
  Defect, coagulation) 286.9
– nonfamilial 286.9
Bleeding (see also Hemorrhage) 459.0
– atonic, following delivery 666.1
– capillary 448.9
– due to subinvolution 621.1
– – puerperal 666.2
– familial (see also Defect, coagulation)
  286.9
– following intercourse 626.7
– hemorroids (see also Hemorrhoids) 455.8
– intermenstrual
– – irregular 626.6
– – regular 626.5
– irregular NEC 626.4
– menopausal 627.0
– ovulation 626.5
– postclimacteric 627.1
– postcoital 626.7
– postmenopausal 627.1
– postoperative 998.1
– preclimacteric 627.0
– puberty 626.3
– – excessive, with onset of menstrual
     periods 626.3
– rectum, rectal 569.3
– tendencies (see also Defect, coagulation)
  286.9
– umbilical stump 772.3
– uterus, uterine 626.9
– – climacteric 627.0
– – dysfunctional 626.8
– – functional 626.8
– – unrelated to menstrual cycle 626.6
– vagina, vaginal 623.8
– – functional 626.8
– vicarious 625.8
Blennorrhagia, blennorrhagic - see
  Blennorrhea
Blennorrhea (acute) 098.0
– adultorum 098.4 † 372.0*
– alveolaris 523.4
– chronic or duration of 2 months or over
  098.2
– gonococcal (neonatorum) 098.4 † 372.0*
– inclusion (newborn) (neonatal) 771.6
Blepharelosis 374.0
Blepharitis (angularis) (ciliaris) (eyelid)
  (marginal) (nonulcerative) (squamous)
  (ulcerative) 373.0
Blepharochalasis 374.3
– congenital 743.6
Blepharoclonus 374.4
Blepharoconjunctivitis (see also
  Conjunctivitis) 372.2
Blepharophimosis (eyelid) 374.4

Blepharophimosis - *continued*
– congenital 743.6
Blepharoptosis 374.3
– congenital 743.6
Blepharopyorrhea 098.4 † 372.0*
Blepharospasm 333.8
Blighted ovum 631
Blind - see also Blindness
– bronchus (congenital) 748.3
– loop syndrome 579.2
– sac, fallopian tube (congenital) 752.1
– spot, enlarged 368.4
– tract or tube, congenital NEC - see
  Atresia
Blindness (acquired) (congenital) (both
  eyes) 369.0
– blast 921.3
– – with nerve injury - see Injury, optic
– Bright's - see Uremia
– color 368.5
– concussion - see Injury, optic
– day 368.1
– due to injury - see Injury, optic
– eclipse (total) 363.3
– emotional 300.1
– hysterical 300.1
– mind 784.6
– night 368.6
– – vitamin A deficiency 264.5 † 368.6*
– one eye (other eye normal) 369.6
– – low vision, other eye 369.1
– psychic 784.6
– river 125.3 † 360.1*
– snow 370.2
– sun 363.3
– traumatic - see Injury, optic
– word (developmental) 315.0
– – acquired 784.6
– – secondary to organic lesion 784.6
Blister - see also Injury, superficial
– beetle dermatitis 692.8
– due to burn - see Burn
– fever 054.9
– multiple, skin, nontraumatic 709.8
Bloating 787.3
Bloch-Sulzberger disease or syndrome
  757.3
Block
– alveolocapillary 516.3
– arborization (heart) 426.6
– arrhythmic 426.9
– atrioventricular (incomplete) (partial)
  426.1
– – complete 426.0
– auriculoventricular (incomplete) (partial)
  426.1
– – complete 426.0

Block - *continued*
- bundle branch (complete) (false) (incomplete) 426.5
- - left 426.3
- - - hemiblock 426.2
- - right 426.4
- - Wilson's type 426.4
- cardiac 426.9
- conduction 426.9
- foramen Magendie (acquired) 331.3
- - congenital 742.3
- - - with spina bifida 741.0
- heart 426.9
- - congenital 746.8
- - specified type NEC 426.6
- hepatic vein 453.0
- intraventricular 426.6
- kidney (see also Disease, renal) 593.9
- - postcystoscopic 997.5
- myocardial (see also Block, heart) 426.9
- nodal 426.1
- organ or site, congenital NEC - see Atresia
- portal (vein) 452
- sinoatrial 426.6
- sinoauricular 426.6
- tubal 628.2
- vein NEC 453.9
Blocq's disease 307.9
Blood
- constituents, abnormal NEC 790.6
- disease 289.9
- dyscrasia 289.9
- - complicating
- - - abortion - see categories 634-639, fourth digit .1
- - - ectopic or molar pregnancy 639.1
- - fetus or newborn NEC 776.9
- - puerperal, postpartum 666.3
- flukes NEC (see also Infestation, schistosoma) 120.9
- in
- - feces (see also Melena) 578.1
- - urine (see also Hematuria) 599.7
- mole 631
- poisoning - see Septicemia
- pressure
- - decreased, due to shock following injury 958.4
- - fluctuating 459.8
- - high (see also Hypertension) 401.9
- - - incidental reading, without diagnosis of hypertension 796.2
- - low (see also Hypotension) 458.9
- - - incidental reading, without diagnosis of hypotension 796.3
- spitting (see also Hemoptysis) 786.3

Blood - *continued*
- staining cornea 371.1
- tranfusion
- - reaction or complication - see Complications, transfusion
- - without reported diagnosis V58.2
- tumor - see Hematoma
- vessel rupture - see Hemorrhage
- vomiting (see also Hematemesis) 578.0
Blood-forming organs, disease 289.9
Bloodgood's disease 610.1
Bloom(-Machacek)(-Torre) syndrome 757.3
Blotch palpebral 372.5
Blount's disease 732.4
Blue
- baby 746.9
- disease 746.9
- dome cyst 610.0
- sclera 743.4
- - with fragility of bone and deafness 756.5
Blueness (see also Cyanosis) 782.5
Blushing (abnormal) (excessive) 782.6
Boarder, hospital V65.0
Bockhart's impetigo 704.8
Body, bodies
- Aschoff's (see also Myocarditis, rheumatic) 398.0
- asteroid, vitreous 379.2
- cytoid (retina) 362.8
- drusen (retina) 362.5
- - optic nerve 377.2
- foreign - see Foreign body
- loose
- - joint 718.1
- - - knee 717.6
- - sheath, tendon 727.8
- Mallory's 034.1
- Mooser's 081.0
- Negri 071
- rice 718.1
- - knee 717.6
Boeck's
- disease 135
- lupoid (miliary) 135
- sarcoid 135
Boggy
- cervix 622.8
- uterus 621.8
Boil - see also Carbuncle
- Aleppo 085.1
- Baghdad 085.1
- Delhi 085.1
- eyelid 373.1
- Gafsa 085.1
- lacrimal

Boil - see also Carbuncle - *continued*
− lacrimal - *continued*
− − gland 375.0
− − passages (duct) (sac) 375.3
− Natal 085.1
− orbit, orbital 376.0
− tropical 085.1
Bold hives (see also Urticaria) 708.9
Bombe, iris 364.7
Bone - see condition
Bonnevie-Ullrich syndrome 758.6
Bonnier's syndrome 386.1
Bony block of joint 718.8
Borderline pelvis 653.1
− with obstruction during labor 660.1
− − fetus or newborn 763.1
Borna disease 062.9 † 323.3*
Bornholm disease 074.1
Borrelia vincenti (mouth) (pharynx)
  (tonsils) 101
Boston exanthem 048
Botulism 005.1
Bouba (see also Yaws) 102.9
Bouffee delirante 298.3
Bouillaud's disease or syndrome 391.9
Bourneville's disease 759.5
Boutonniere hand (intrinsic) 736.2
Bouveret's syndrome 427.2
Bovine heart - see Hypertrophy, cardiac
Bowel - see condition
Bowen's
− dermatosis (precancerous) (M8081/2) -
  see Neoplasm, skin, in situ
− disease (M8081/2) - see Neoplasm, skin,
  in situ
− epithelioma (M8081/2) - see Neoplasm,
  skin, in situ
− type
− − epidermoid carcinoma-in-situ
  (M8081/2) - see Neoplasm, skin, in
  situ
− − intraepidermal squamous cell
  carcinoma (M8081/2) - see Neoplasm,
  skin, in situ
Bowing
− femur 736.8
− − congenital 754.4
− fibula 736.8
− − congenital 754.4
− forearm 736.0
− leg(s), long bones, congenital 754.4
− radius 736.0
Bowleg(s) 736.4
− congenital 754.4
− rachitic 268.1
Boyd's dysentery 004.2
Brachial - see condition

Brachycardia 427.8
Bradycardia (any type) (sinoatrial) (sinus)
  (vagal) 427.8
− fetal - see Distress, fetal
Bradypnea 786.0
Brailsford's disease 732.3
− radial head 732.3
− tarsal scaphoid 732.5
Brain - see also condition
− syndrome - see Syndrome, brain
Branched chain amino acid disease 270.3
Branchial - see condition
Brash (water) 787.1
Brass-founders' ague 985.8
Bravais-jacksonian epilepsy 345.5
Braxton-Hicks contractures 644.0
Braziers' disease 985.8
Breakdown
− device, implant or graft - see
  Complications, mechanical chanical
− nervous (see also Disorder, mental,
  nonpsychotic) 300.9
− perineum 674.2
Breast - see condition
Breath
− foul 784.9
− holder, child 312.8
− holding spell 786.9
− shortness 786.0
Breathing
− exercises V57.0
− labored 786.0
− mouth 784.9
− periodic 786.0
Breathlessness 786.0
− exercises V57.0
Breda's disease (see also Yaws) 102.9
Breech
− delivery, affecting fetus or newborn 763.0
− extraction, affecting fetus or newborn
  763.0
− presentation 652.2
− − with successful version 652.1
− − before labor, affecting fetus or
    newborn 761.7
− − causing obstructed labor 660.0
− − during labor, affecting fetus or
    newborn 763.0
Breisky's disease 624.0
Brenneman's syndrome 289.2
Brenner
− tumor (benign) (M9000/0) 220
− − borderline malignancy (M9000/1)
    236.2
− − malignant (M9000/3) 183.0
− − proliferating (M9000/1) 236.2
Bretonneau's disease 032.0

Breus' mole 631
Brevicollis 756.1
Bricklayers' itch 692.8
Bright's
— blindness - see Uremia
— disease (see also Nephritis) 583.9
— — arteriosclerotic (see also Hypertension, kidney) 403.9
Brill's disease (flea or louse borne) 081.1
Brill-Symmer's disease (M9690/3) 202.0
Brill-Zinsser disease 081.1
Briquet's disorder or syndrome 300.8
Brissaud's infantilism 244.9
Brittle
— bones 756.5
— nails 703.8
— — congenital 757.5
Broad ligament - see also condition
— laceration syndrome 620.6
Brock's syndrome 518.0
Brocq's disease 691.8
Brodie's abscess or disease (joint) 730.1
Broken
— arches 734
— — congenital 755.6
— back - see Fracture, vertebra
— bone - see Fracture
— compensation - see Disease, heart
— implant or internal device - see Complications, mechanical
— neck - see Fracture, vertebra, cervical
— nose 802.0
— — open 802.1
— tooth, teeth 873.6
— — complicated 873.7
Bromhidrosis 705.8
Bromidism, bromism
— acute
— — correct substance properly administered 349.8
— — overdose or wrong substance given or taken 967.3
— chronic 304.1
Bromidrosiphobia 300.2
Bromidrosis 705.8
Bronchi, bronchial - see condition
Bronchiectasis (cylindrical) (diffuse) (fusiform) (localized) (moniliform) (postinfectional) (recurrent) (saccular) 494
— congenital 748.6
— tuberculous 011.5
Bronchiolectasis - see Bronchiectasis
Bronchiolitis (acute) (infectional) (subacute) 466.1
— with
— — bronchospasm or obstruction 466.1
— — influenza, flu or grippe 487.1

Bronchiolitis - *continued*
— chemical 506.0
— — chronic 506.4
— chronic (obliterative) 491.8
— due to external agent - see Bronchitis, acute, due to
— influenzal 487.1
— obliterative (chronic) (subacute) 491.8
Bronchitis (diffuse) (hypostatic) (infectional) (inflammatory) (with tracheitis) 490
— with
— — influenza, flu or grippe 487.1
— — obstruction (airway) (lung) 491.2
— — tracheitis 490
— — — acute or subacute 466.0
— — — chronic 491.8
— acute or subacute 466.0
— — with
— — — bronchospasm or obstruction 466.0
— — — tracheitis 466.0
— — chemical (due to fumes or vapors) 506.0
— — due to
— — — radiation 508.8
— allergic (acute) (see also Asthma) 493.9
— arachidic 934.1
— asthmatic (see also Asthma) 493.9
— — chronic 491.2
— capillary 466.1
— — with bronchospasm or obstruction 466.1
— — chronic 491.8
— caseous 011.3
— Castellani's 104.8
— catarrhal 490
— — acute - see Bronchitis, acute
— — chronic 491.0
— chemical (acute) (subacute) 506.0
— — chronic 506.4
— chronic 491.9
— — with
— — — airways obstruction 491.2
— — — tracheitis (chronic) 491.8
— — asthmatic 491.2
— — chemical (due to fumes or vapors) 506.4
— — due to
— — — fumes or vapors (chemical) (inhalation) 506.4
— — — radiation 508.8
— — emphysematous 491.2
— — mucopurulent 491.1
— — obstructive 491.2
— — purulent 491.1
— — simple 491.0
— croupous 466.0

Bronchitis - *continued*
- emphysematous 491.2
- exudative 466.0
- fetid 491.1
- fibrinous, acute or subacute 466.0
- grippal 487.1
- influenzal 487.1
- membranous, acute or subacute 466.0
- moulders' 502
- mucopurulent (chronic) (recurrent) 491.1
- - acute or subacute 466.0
- obliterans 491.8
- obstructive (chronic) (diffuse) 491.2
- plastic 466.0
- pneumococcal, acute or subacute 466.0
- pseudomembranous 466.0
- purulent (chronic) (recurrent) 491.1
- - acute or subacute 466.0
- senile 491.9
- septic, acute or subacute 466.0
- smokers' 491.0
- spirochetal 104.8
- suffocative, acute or subacute 466.0
- summer (see also Asthma) 493.9
- suppurative (chronic) 491.1
- - acute or subacute 466.0
- tuberculous 011.3
- ulcerative 491.8
- - Vincent's 101
- Vincent's 101
- viral, acute or subacute 466.0
Broncho-alveolitis 485
Bronchoaspergillosis 117.3
Bronchocele 240.9
Bronchohemisporosis 117.9
Broncholithiasis 518.8
- tuberculous 011.3
Bronchomoniliasis 112.8
Bronchomycosis 112.8
Bronchonocardiosis 039.1

Bronchopleuropneumonia - see Pneumonia,
  broncho
Bronchopneumonia - see Pneumonia,
  broncho
Bronchopneumonitis - see Pneumonia,
  broncho
Bronchopulmonary - see condition
Bronchopulmonitis - see Pneumonia,
  broncho
Bronchorrhagia 786.3
- newborn 770.3
- tuberculous 011.3

Bronchorrhea (chronic) (purulent) 491.0
- acute 466.0
Bronchospasm 519.1
- with

Bronchospasm - *continued*
- with - *continued*
- - bronchiolitis, acute (conditions in
    466.1) 466.1
- - bronchitis, acute (conditions in 466.0)
    466.0
- due to external agent - see condition,
  respiratory, acute, due to
Bronchospirochetosis 104.8
Bronchostenosis 519.1
Bronchus - see condition
Brooke's tumor (M8100/0) - see Neoplasm,
  skin, benign
Brown's sheath syndrome 378.6
Brown-Sequard disease, paralysis or
  syndrome 344.8
Brucella, brucellosis (infection) 023.9
- abortus 023.1
- canis 023.3
- dermatitis, skin 023.9
- melitensis 023.0
- mixed 023.8
- suis 023.2
Bruck's disease 733.9
Bruck-Lange disease 759.8
Brugsch's syndrome 757.3
Bruhl's disease 285.8
Bruise (skin surface intact) - see also
  Contusion
- with
- - fracture - see Fracture
- - open wound - see Wound, open
- internal organ (abdomen, chest or pelvis)
  - see Injury, internal
- umbilical cord 663.6
- - affecting fetus or newborn 762.6
Bruit 785.9
Brushburn - see Injury, superficial, by site
Bruton's X-linked agammaglobulinemia
  279.0
Bruxism 306.8
Bubbly lung syndrome 770.7
Bubo 289.3
- blennorrhagic 098.8
- chancroidal 099.0
- climatic 099.1
- due to Hemophilus ducreyi 099.0
- gonococcal 098.8
- indolent 099.8
- inguinal 099.8
- - chancroidal 099.0
- - climatic 099.1
- - due to H. ducreyi 099.0
- - infective 099.8
- - venereal 099.8
- phagedenic 099.8
- scrofulous 017.2

Bubo - *continued*
– soft chancre 099.0
– suppurating 683
– syphilitic 091.0
– – congenital 090.0
– tropical 099.1
– venereal 099.8
– virulent 099.0
Bubonocele - see Hernia, inguinal
Buccal - see condition

Buchanan's disease or osteochondrosis
732.1
Buchman's disease or osteochondrosis
732.1
Bucket handle fracture (semilunar cartilage)
- see Tear, meniscus
Budd-Chiari syndrome 453.0
Budgerigar fanciers' disease or lung 495.2
Budinger-Ludloff-Laewen disease 717.8
Buerger's disease 443.1
Bulbar - see condition

Bulbus cordis (left ventricle) (persistent)
745.8
Bulimia 783.6
Bulky uterus 621.2
Bulla(e) 709.8
– lung 492
Bullet wound - see also Wound, open
– fracture - code as Fracture, open
– internal organ (abdomen, chest, or pelvis)
- see Injury, internal, by site, with open
wound
– intracranial 851.1
Bundle
– branch block (complete) (false)
(incomplete) 426.5
– – left 426.3
– – – hemiblock 426.2
– – right 426.4
– of His - see condition
Bungpagga 040.8 † 728.0*
Bunion 727.1

Buphthalmia, buphthalmos (congenital)
743.2
Burger-Grutz disease 272.3
Buried roots 525.3
Burkitt's
– tumor (M9750/3) 200.2
– type malignant lymphoma, lymphoblastic
or undifferentiated (M9750/3) 200.2

Burn (acid) (cathode ray) (caustic)
(chemical) (electric heating appliance)
(electricity) (fire) (flame) (hot liquid or
object) (irradiation) (lime) (radiation)
(steam) (thermal) (x-ray) 949.-

Note – The following fourth-digit subdivisions are for use with categories 941–946 and 949:
.0 *Unspecified degree*
.1 *Erythema*
 First degree
.2 *Blisters, epidermal loss*
 Second degree
.3 *Full-thickness skin loss*
 Subcutaneous
 Third degree
.4 *Deep necrosis of underlying tissue*
 Deep third degree.

Burn - *continued*
– abdomen, abdominal (muscle) (wall) -
see Burn, trunk
– ankle - see Burn, leg
– anus - see Burn, trunk
– arm(s) 943.-
– – with specified sites classifiable to more
than one category in 940-945 946.-
– auditory canal (external) - see Burn, head
– auricle (ear) - see Burn, head
– axilla - see Burn, arm
– back - see Burn, trunk
– biceps
– – brachii - see Burn, arm
– – femoris - see Burn, leg
– breast(s) - see Burn, trunk
– brow - see Burn, head
– buttock(s) - see Burn, trunk
– canthus (eye) 940.1
– – chemical 940.0
– cervix 947.4
– cheek (cutaneous) - see Burn, head
– chest wall - see Burn, trunk
– chin - see Burn, head
– clitoris - see Burn, trunk
– colon 947.3
– conjunctiva (and cornea) 940.4
– – chemical NEC 940.4
– – – acid 940.3
– – – alkaline 940.2
– cornea (and conjunctiva) 940.4
– – chemical NEC 940.4
– – – acid 940.3
– – – alkaline 940.2
– costal region - see Burn, trunk
– due to ingested chemical agent - see
Burn, internal organs
– ear (auricle) (external) (drum) (canal) -
see Burn, head
– elbow - see Burn, arm
– electricity, electric current - see Burn, by
site
– entire body 946.-

Burn - *continued*
- scrotum - see Burn, trunk
- septum, nasal - see Burn, head
- shoulder(s) - see Burn, arm
- skin NEC 949.-
- skull - see Burn, head
- sternal region - see Burn, trunk
- stomach 947.3
- subconjunctival - see Burn, conjunctiva
- submaxillary region - see Burn, head
- submental region - see Burn, head
- supraclavicular fossa - see Burn, head
- supra-orbital - see Burn, head
- temple - see Burn, head
- temporal region - see Burn, head
- testis - see Burn, trunk
- thigh - see Burn, leg
- thorax (external) - see Burn, trunk
- throat 947.0
- thumb(s) - see Burn, hand
- toe(nail) (subungual) - see Burn, leg
- tongue 947.0
- tonsil 947.0
- trachea 947.1
- trunk 942.-
- - with specified sites classifiable to more
  than one category in 940-945 946.-
- tunica vaginalis - see Burn, trunk
- tympanic membrane - see Burn, head
- tympanum - see Burn, head
- unspecified site with extent of body
  surface involved specified
- - less than 10 per cent 948.0
- - 10-19 per cent 948.1
- - 20-29 per cent 948.2
- - 30-39 per cent 948.3
- - 40-49 per cent 948.4
- - 50-59 per cent 948.5
- - 60-69 per cent 948.6
- - 70-79 per cent 948.7
- - 80-89 per cent 948.8
- - 90 per cent or more 948.9
- uterus 947.4
- uvula 947.0
- vagina 947.4
- vulva - see Burn, trunk
- wrist(s) - see Burn, hand
Burnett's syndrome 999.9
Burning
- feet syndrome 266.2
- sensation (see also Disturbance,
  sensation) 782.0
- tongue 529.6

Burns's disease or osteochondrosis 732.3
Bursa - see also condition
- pharynx 478.2
Bursitis NEC 727.3
- Achilles 726.7
- adhesive 726.9
- - shoulder 726.0
- ankle 726.7
- calcaneal 726.7
- Duplay's 726.2
- elbow 726.3
- finger 726.8
- foot 726.7
- gonococcal 098.5 † 727.3*
- hand 726.4
- hip 726.5
- knee 726.6
- occupational NEC 726.2
- olecranon 726.3
- pharyngeal 478.2
- popliteal 726.6
- prepatellar 726.6
- radiohumeral 727.3
- scapulohumeral 726.1
- - adhesive 726.0
- shoulder 726.1
- - adhesive 726.0
- subacromial 726.1
- - adhesive 726.0
- subcoracoid 726.1
- subdeltoid 726.1
- - adhesive 726.0
- syphilitic 095 † 727.3*
- Thornwaldt, Tornwaldt 478.2
- toe 726.7
- trochanteric (area) 726.5
- wrist 726.4
Burst stitches or sutures (complication of
  surgery) 998.3
Buruli ulcer 031.1
Bury's disease 695.8
Buschke's scleredema 710.1
Busse-Buschke disease 117.5
Buttock - see condition
Button
- Biskra 085.1
- Delhi 085.1
- oriental 085.1
Buttonhole hand (intrinsic) 736.2
Bwamba fever 066.3
Byssinosis 504
Bywater syndrome 958.5

C

Calcification - *continued*
- pleura 511.0
- - postinfectional 518.8
- - tuberculous 012.0
- pulp (dental) (nodular) 522.2
- riders' bone 733.9
- sclera 379.1
- semilunar cartilage 717.8
- spleen 289.5
- subcutaneous 709.3
- suprarenal (capsule) (gland) 255.4
- tendon (sheath) 727.8
- - with bursitis, synovitis or tenosynovitis 727.8
- trachea 519.1
- ureter 593.8
- uterus 621.8
- vitreous 379.2
Calcified - see Calcification
Calcinosis (interstitial) (tumoral) (universalis) 275.4
- circumscripta 709.3
- cutis 709.3
Calcium
- blood
- - high 275.4
- - low (see also Hypocalcemia) 275.4
- deposits - see also Calcification, by site
- - bursa 727.8
- - tendon (sheath) 727.8
- salts or soaps in vitreous 379.2
Calciuria 791.9
Calculi - see Calculus
Calculosis, intrahepatic (see also Choledocholithiasis) 574.5
Calculus, calculi, calculous 592.9
- ampulla of Vater (see also Choledocholithiasis) 574.5
- appendix 543
- bile duct (any) (see also Choledocholithiasis) 574.5
- biliary (see also Cholelithiasis) 574.2
- bilirubin, multiple (see also Cholelithiasis) 574.2
- bladder (encysted) (impacted) (urinary) 594.1
- - diverticulum 594.0
- bronchus 519.1
- calyx (kidney) (renal) 592.0
- - congenital 753.3
- cholesterol (pure) (solitary) (see also Cholelithiasis) 574.2
- common duct (bile) (see also Choledocholithiasis) 574.5
- conjunctiva 372.5
- cystic 594.1
- - duct (see also Cholelithiasis) 574.2

Calculus - *continued*
- dental 523.6
- - subgingival 523.6
- - supragingival 523.6
- epididymis 608.8
- gallbladder (see also Cholelithiasis) 574.2
- - congenital 751.6
- hepatic (duct) (see also Choledocholithiasis) 574.5
- intestinal (impaction) (obstruction) 560.3
- kidney (impacted) (multiple) (pelvis) (recurrent) (staghorn) 592.0
- - congenital 753.3
- lacrimal passages 375.5
- liver (impacted) (see also Choledocholithiasis) 574.5
- lung 518.8
- nephritic (impacted) (recurrent) 592.0
- nose 478.1
- pancreas (duct) 577.8
- parotid gland 527.5
- pelvis, encysted 592.0
- prostate 602.0
- pulmonary 518.8
- pyelitis (impacted) (recurrent) 592.9
- pyelonephritis (impacted) (recurrent) 592.9
- pyonephrosis (impacted) (recurrent) 592.9
- renal (impacted) (recurrent) 592.0
- - congenital 753.3
- salivary (duct) (gland) 527.5
- seminal vesicle 608.8
- staghorn 592.0
- Stensen's duct 527.5
- sublingual duct or gland 527.5
- - congenital 750.2
- submaxillary duct, gland or region 527.5
- suburethral 594.8
- tonsil 474.8
- tooth, teeth 523.6
- tunica vaginalis 608.8
- ureter (impacted) (recurrent) 592.1
- urethra (impacted) 594.2
- urinary (duct) (impacted) (passage) 592.9
- - lower tract NEC 594.9
- vagina 623.8
- vesical (impacted) 594.1
- Wharton's duct 527.5
Caliectasis 593.8
Caligo cornea 371.0
Callositas, callosity (infected) 700
Callus (infected) 700
- excessive, following fracture - code as Late effect of fracture 905.5
- - current - see Fracture
Calve(-Perthes) disease 732.1

Calvities (see also Alopecia) 704.0
Cameroon fever (see also Malaria) 084.6
Camptocormia 300.1
Camurati-Engelmann disease 756.5
Canal - see condition
Canaliculitis (lacrimal) (acute) (subacute) 375.3
— actinomyces 039.8
— chronic 375.4
Canavan's disease 330.0
Cancer (M8000/3) - see also Neoplasm, malignant

Note – The term "cancer" when modified by an adjective or adjectival phrase indicating a morphological type should be coded in the same manner as "carcinoma" with that adjective or phrase. Thus, "squamous-cell cancer" should be coded in the same manner as "squamous-cell carcinoma", which appears in the list under "Carcinoma".

Cancer - *continued*
— bile duct type (M8160/3), liver 155.1
— hepatocellular (M8170/3) 155.0
Cancerous (M8000/3) - see Neoplasm, malignant
Cancerphobia 300.2
Cancrum oris 528.1
Candidiasis, candidal 112.9
— congenital 771.7
— disseminated 112.5
— endocarditis 112.8 † 421.1*
— intertrigo 112.3
— lung 112.4 † 484.7*
— meningitis 112.8 † 321.0*
— mouth 112.0
— nails 112.3
— onychia 112.3
— paronychia 112.3
— perionyxis 112.3
— pneumonia 112.4 † 484.7*
— skin 112.3
— specified site NEC 112.8
— systemic 112.5
— urogenital site NEC 112.2
— vagina 112.1 † 616.1*
— vulva 112.1 † 616.1*
— vulvovaginitis 112.1 † 616.1*
Candidiosis - see Candidiasis
Candiru infection or infestation 136.8
Canities (premature) 704.3
— congenital 757.4
Canker (sore) (mouth) 528.2
Cannabinosis 504

Canton fever 081.9
Capillariasis 127.5
Capillary - see condition
Caplan syndrome 714.8 † 517.0*
Capsule - see condition
Capsulitis (joint) 726.9
— adhesive (shoulder) 726.0
— thyroid 245.9
Caput
— crepitus 756.0
— medusae 456.8
— succedaneum 767.1
Car sickness 994.6
Carapata's disease 087.1
Carate - see Pinta
Carboxyhemoglobinemia 986
Carbuncle 680.9
— abdominal wall 680.2
— ankle 680.6
— anus 680.5
— arm (any part, above wrist) 680.3
— axilla 680.3
— back (any part) 680.2
— breast 680.2
— buttock 680.5
— chest wall 680.2
— corpus cavernosum 607.2
— ear (any part) (external) 680.0
— eyelid 373.1
— face (any part, except eye) 680.0
— finger (any) 680.4
— foot (any part) 680.7
— forearm 680.3
— gluteal (region) 680.5
— groin 680.2
— hand (any part) 680.4
— head (any part, except face) 680.8
— heel 680.7
— hip 680.6
— kidney (see also Abscess, kidney) 590.2
— knee 680.6
— labia 616.4
— lacrimal
— — gland 375.0
— — passages (duct) (sac) 375.3
— leg, any part except foot 680.6
— lower extremity, any part except foot 680.6
— malignant 022.0
— multiple sites, so stated 680.9
— neck 680.1
— nose (septum) 680.0
— orbit, orbital 376.0
— partes posteriores 680.5
— penis 607.2
— perineum 680.2
— scalp (any part) 680.8

Carbuncle - *continued*
- scrotum 608.4
- shoulder 680.3
- skin NEC 680.9
- specified site NEC 680.8
- temple (region) 680.0
- thigh 680.6
- thumb 680.4
- toe (any) 680.7
- trunk 680.2
- umbilicus 680.2
- upper arm 680.3
- urethra 597.0
- vulva 616.4
- wrist 680.4
Carbunculus (see also Carbuncle) 680.9
Carcinoid (tumor) (M8240/1) - see also
  Neoplasm, uncertain behavior
- and struma ovarii (M9091/1) 236.2
- argentaffin (M8241/1) - see Neoplasm,
  uncertain behavior
- - malignant (M8241/3) - see Neoplasm,
  malignant
- benign (M9091/0) 220
- composite (M8244/3) - see Neoplasm,
  malignant
- goblet cell (M8243/3) - see Neoplasm,
  malignant
- malignant (M8240/3) - see Neoplasm,
  malignant
- nonargentaffin (M8242/1) - see
  Neoplasm, uncertain behavior
- - malignant (M8242/3) - see Neoplasm,
  malignant
- strumal (M9091/1) 236.2
- syndrome 259.2
- type bronchial adenoma (M8240/3) - see
  Neoplasm, lung, malignant
Carcinoma (M8010/3) - see also Neoplasm,
  malignant

Note – Except where otherwise indicated,
the morphological varieties of carcinoma
in the list below should be coded by site as
for "Neoplasm, malignant".

Carcinoma - *continued*
- with
- - apocrine metaplasia (M8573/3)
- - cartilaginous (and osseous) metaplasia
  (M8571/3)
- - osseous (and cartilaginous) metaplasia
  (M8571/3)
- - productive fibrosis (M8141/3)
- - spindle cell metaplasia (M8572/3)
- - squamous metaplasia (M8570/3)

Carcinoma - *continued*
- acidophil (M8280/3)
- - specified site - see Neoplasm,
  malignant
- - unspecified site 194.3
- acidophil-basophil, mixed (M8281/3)
- - specified site - see Neoplasm,
  malignant
- - unspecified site 194.3
- acinar (cell) (M8550/3)
- acinic cell (M8550/3)
- adenocystic (M8200/3)
- adenoid
- - cystic (M8200/3)
- - squamous cell (M8075/3)
- adenosquamous (M8560/3)
- adnexal (skin) (M8390/3) - see
  Neoplasm, skin, malignant
- adrenal cortical (M8370/3) 194.0
- alveolar (M8251/3)
- - cell (M8250/3) - see Neoplasm, lung,
  malignant
- anaplastic type (M8021/3)
- apocrine (M8401/3)
- - breast - see Neoplasm, breast,
  malignant
- - specified site NEC - see Neoplasm,
  skin, malignant
- - unspecified site 173.9
- basal cell (pigmented) (M8090/3) - see
  also Neoplasm, skin, malignant
- - fibro-epithelial type (M8093/3) - see
  Neoplasm, skin, malignant
- - morphea type (M8092/3) - see
  Neoplasm, skin, malignant
- - multicentric (M8091/3) - see
  Neoplasm, skin, malignant
- basaloid (M8123/3)
- basal-squamous cell, mixed (M8094/3) -
  see Neoplasm, skin, malignant
- basophil (M8300/3)
- - specified site - see Neoplasm,
  malignant
- - unspecified site 194.3
- basophil-acidophil, mixed (M8281/3)
- - specified site - see Neoplasm,
  malignant
- - unspecified site 194.3
- basosquamous (M8094/3) - see
  Neoplasm, skin, malignant
- bile duct type (M8160/3)
- - and hepatocellular, mixed (M8180/3)
  155.0
- - liver 155.1
- - specified site NEC - see Neoplasm,
  malignant
- - unspecified site 155.1

Carcinoma - *continued*
- branchial or branchiogenic 146.8
- bronchial or bronchogenic - see
  Neoplasm, lung, malignant
- bronchiolar (terminal) (M8250/3) - see
  Neoplasm, lung, malignant
- bronchioloalveolar (M8250/3) - see
  Neoplasm, lung, malignant
- C cell
- - specified site - see Neoplasm,
  malignant
- - unspecified site 193
- ceruminous (M8420/3) 173.2
- chorionic (M9100/3)
- - specified site - see Neoplasm,
  malignant
- - unspecified site
- - - female 181
- - - male 186.9
- chromophobe (M8270/3)
- - specified site - see Neoplasm,
  malignant
- - unspecified site 194.3
- clear cell (mesonephroid type)
  (M8310/3)
- cloacogenic (M8124/3)
- - specified site - see Neoplasm,
  malignant
- - unspecified site 154.8
- colloid (M8480/3)
- cribriform (M8201/3)
- cylindroid type (M8200/3)
- diffuse type (M8145/3)
- - specified site - see Neoplasm,
  malignant
- - unspecified site 151.9
- duct (cell) (M8500/3)
- - with Paget's disease (M8541/3) - see
  Neoplasm, breast, malignant
- - infiltrating (M8500/3)
- - - specified site - see Neoplasm,
  malignant
- - - unspecified site 174.9
- ductal (M8500/3)
- ductular, infiltrating (M8521/3)
- embryonal (M9070/3)
- - and teratoma, mixed (M9081/3)
- - combined with choriocarcinoma
  (M9101/3)
- - infantile type (M9071/3)
- - liver 155.0
- - polyembryonal type (M9072/3)
- endometrioid (M8380/3)
- eosinophil (M8280/3)
- - specified site - see Neoplasm,
  malignant
- - unspecified site 194.3

Carcinoma - *continued*
- epidermoid (M8070/3) - see also
  Carcinoma, squamous cell
- - and adenocarcinoma, mixed
  (M8560/3)
- - in situ, Bowen's type (M8081/2) - see
  Neoplasm, skin, in situ
- fibroepithelial type basal cell (M8093/3) -
  see Neoplasm, skin, malignant
- follicular (M8330/3)
- - and papillary (mixed) (M8340/3) 193
- - moderately differentiated type
  (M8332/3) 193
- - pure follicle type (M8331/3) 193
- - specified site - see Neoplasm,
  malignant
- - trabecular type (M8332/3) 193
- - unspecified site 193
- - well differentiated type (M8331/3)
  193
- gelatinous (M8480/3)
- giant cell (M8031/3)
- - and spindle cell (M8030/3)
- granular cell (M8320/3)
- granulosa cell (M8620/3) 183.0
- hepatic cell (M8170/3) 155.0
- hepatocellular (M8170/3) 155.0
- - and bile duct, mixed (M8180/3) 155.0
- hepatocholangiolitic (M8180/3) 155.0
- Hurthle cell (M8290/3) 193
- hypernephroid (M8311/3)
- in
- - adenomatous
- - - polyp (M8210/3)
- - - polyposis coli (M8220/3) 153.9
- - pleomorphic adenoma (M8940/3)
- - polypoid adenoma (M8210/3)
- - situ (M8010/2) - see
  Carcinoma-in-situ
- - tubular adenoma (M8210/3)
- - villous adenoma (M8261/3)
- infiltrating duct (M8500/3)
- - with Paget's disease (M8541/3) - see
  Neoplasm, breast, malignant
- - specified site - see Neoplasm,
  malignant
- - unspecified site 174.9
- inflammatory (M8530/3)
- - specified site - see Neoplasm,
  malignant
- - unspecified site 174.9
- intestinal type (M8144/3)
- - specified site - see Neoplasm,
  malignant
- - unspecified site 151.9
- intraductal (noninfiltrating) (M8500/2)
- - papillary (M8503/2)

Carcinoma - *continued*
- intraductal - *continued*
- - papillary - *continued*
- - - specified site - see Neoplasm, in situ
- - - unspecified site 233.0
- - specified site - see Neoplasm, in situ
- - unspecified site 233.0
- intraepidermal (M8070/2) - see Neoplasm, in situ
- - squamous cell, Bowen's type (M8081/2) - see Neoplasm, skin, in situ
- intraepithelial (M8010/2) - see Neoplasm, in situ
- - squamous cell (M8070/2) - see Neoplasm, in situ
- intraosseous (M9270/3) 170.1
- - upper jaw (bone) 170.0
- islet cell (M8150/3)
- - and exocrine, mixed (M8154/3)
- - - specified site - see Neoplasm, malignant
- - - unspecified site 157.9
- - pancreas 157.4
- - specified site NEC - see Neoplasm, malignant
- - unspecified site 157.4
- juvenile, breast (M8502/3) - see Neoplasm, breast, malignant
- large cell (M8012/3)
- - squamous cell, nonkeratinizing type (M8072/3)
- Leydig cell (testis) (M8650/3)
- - specified site - see Neoplasm, malignant
- - unspecified site
- - - female 183.0
- - - male 186.9
- liver cell (M8170/3) 155.0
- lobular (infiltrating) (M8520/3)
- - noninfiltrating (M8520/2)
- - - specified site - see Neoplasm, in situ
- - - unspecified site 233.0
- - specified site - see Neoplasm, malignant
- - unspecified site 174.9
- lymphoepithelial (M8082/3)
- medullary (M8510/3)
- - with
- - - amyloid stroma (M8511/3)
- - - - specified site - see Neoplasm, malignant
- - - - unspecified site 193
- - - lymphoid stroma (M8512/3)
- - - - specified site - see Neoplasm, malignant
- - - - unspecified site 174.9

Carcinoma - *continued*
- mesometanephric (M9110/3)
- mesonephric (M9110/3)
- metastatic (M8010/6) - see Secondary neoplasm
- metatypical (M8095/3) - see Neoplasm, skin, malignant
- morphea type basal cell (M8092/3) - see Neoplasm, skin, malignant
- mucinous (M8480/3)
- mucin-producing (M8481/3)
- mucin-secreting (M8481/3)
- mucoepidermoid (M8430/3)
- mucoid (M8480/3)
- - cell (M8300/3)
- - - specified site - see Neoplasm, malignant
- - - unspecified site 194.3
- mucous (M8480/3)
- nonencapsulated sclerosing (M8350/3) 193
- noninfiltrating
- - intracystic (M8504/2) - see Neoplasm, in situ
- - intraductal (M8500/2)
- - - papillary (M8503/2)
- - - - specified site - see Neoplasm, in situ
- - - - unspecified site 233.0
- - - specified site - see Neoplasm, in situ
- - - unspecified site 233.0
- - lobular (M8520/2)
- - - specified site - see Neoplasm, in situ
- - - unspecified site 233.0
- oat cell (M8042/3)
- - specified site - see Neoplasm, malignant
- - unspecified site 162.9
- odontogenic (M9270/3) 170.1
- - upper jaw (bone) 170.0
- oncocytic (M8290/3)
- oxyphilic (M8290/3)
- papillary (M8050/3)
- - and follicular (mixed) (M8340/3) 193
- - epidermoid (M8052/3)
- - intraductal (noninfiltrating) (M8503/2)
- - - specified site - see Neoplasm, in situ
- - - unspecified site 233.0
- - serous (M8460/3)
- - - specified site - see Neoplasm, malignant
- - - surface (M8461/3)
- - - - specified site - see Neoplasm, malignant
- - - - unspecified site 183.0
- - - unspecified site 183.0

Carcinoma - *continued*
- papillary - *continued*
- - squamous cell (M8052/3)
- - transitional cell (M8130/3)
- papillocystic (M8450/3)
- - specified site - see Neoplasm, malignant
- - unspecified site 183.0
- parafollicular cell (M8510/3)
- - specified site - see Neoplasm, malignant
- - unspecified site 193
- pleomorphic (M8022/3)
- polygonal cell (M8034/3)
- prickle cell (M8070/3)
- pseudoglandular, squamous cell (M8075/3)
- pseudomucinous (M8470/3)
- - specified site - see Neoplasm, malignant
- - unspecified site 183.0
- pseudosarcomatous (M8033/3)
- Regaud type (M8082/3) - see Neoplasm, nasopharynx, malignant
- renal cell (M8312/3) 189.0
- reserve cell (M8041/3)
- round cell (M8041/3)
- Schminke (M8082/3) - see Neoplasm, nasopharynx, malignant
- Schneiderian (M8121/3)
- - specified site - see Neoplasm, malignant
- - unspecified site 160.0
- scirrhous (M8141/3)
- sebaceous (M8410/3) - see Neoplasm, skin, malignant
- secondary (M8010/6) - see Secondary neoplasm
- secretory, breast (M8502/3) - see Neoplasm, breast, malignant
- serous (M8441/3)
- - papillary (M8460/3)
- - - specified site - see Neoplasm, malignant
- - - unspecified site 183.0
- - surface, papillary (M8461/3)
- - - specified site - see Neoplasm, malignant
- - - unspecified site 183.0
- Sertoli cell (M8640/3)
- - specified site - see Neoplasm, malignant
- - unspecified site 186.9
- signet ring cell (M8490/3)
- - metastatic (M8490/6) - see Secondary neoplasm
- simplex (M8231/3)

Carcinoma - *continued*
- skin appendage (M8390/3) - see Neoplasm, skin, malignant
- small cell (M8041/3)
- - fusiform cell type (M8043/3)
- - squamous cell, nonkeratinizing type (M8073/3)
- solid (M8230/3)
- - with amyloid stroma (M8511/3)
- - - specified site - see Neoplasm, malignant
- - - unspecified site 193
- spheroidal cell (M8035/3)
- spindle cell (M8032/3)
- - and giant cell (M8030/3)
- spinous cell (M8070/3)
- squamous (cell) (M8070/3)
- - adenoid type (M8075/3)
- - and adenocarcinoma, mixed (M8560/3)
- - keratinizing type (large cell) (M8071/3)
- - large cell, nonkeratinizing type (M8072/3)
- - microinvasive (M8076/3)
- - - specified site - see Neoplasm, malignant
- - - unspecified site 180.9
- - nonkeratinizing type (M8072/3)
- - papillary (M8052/3)
- - pseudoglandular (M8075/3)
- - small cell, nonkeratinizing type (M8073/3)
- - spindle cell type (M8074/3)
- - verrucous (M8051/3)
- superficial spreading (M8143/3)
- sweat gland (M8400/3) - see Neoplasm, skin, malignant
- theca cell (M8600/3) 183.0
- thymic (M8580/3) 164.0
- trabecular (M8190/3)
- transitional (cell) (M8120/3)
- - papillary (M8130/3)
- - spindle cell type (M8122/3)
- tubular (M8211/3)
- undifferentiated type (M8020/3)
- urothelial (M8120/3)
- ventriculi 151.9
- verrucous (epidermoid)(squamous cell) (M8051/3)
- villous (M8262/3)
- water-clear cell (M8322/3) 194.1
- wolffian duct (M9110/3)
Carcinoma-in-situ (M8010/2) - see also Neoplasm, in situ
- epidermoid (M8070/2) - see also Neoplasm, in situ

Carcinoma-in-situ - *continued*
− epidermoid - *continued*
− − with questionable stromal invasion
  (M8076/2)
− − − specified site - see Neoplasm, in situ
− − − unspecified site 233.1
− − Bowen's type (M8081/2) - see
  Neoplasm, skin, in situ
− intraduct (M8500/2)
− − specified site - see Neoplasm, in situ
− − unspecified site 233.0
− lobular (M8520/2)
− − specified site - see Neoplasm, in situ
− − unspecified site 233.0
− papillary (M8050/2) - see Neoplasm, in
  situ
− squamous cell (M8070/2) - see also
  Neoplasm, in situ
− − with questionable stromal invasion
  (M8076/2)
− − − specified site - see Neoplasm, in situ
− − − unspecified site 233.1
− transitional cell (M8120/2) - see
  Neoplasm, in situ
Carcinomaphobia 300.2
Carcinomatosis
− peritonei (M8010/6) 197.6
− specified site NEC (M8010/3) - see
  Neoplasm, malignant
− unspecified site (M8010/6) 199.0
Carcinosarcoma (M8980/3) - see
  Neoplasm, malignant
− embryonal type (M8981/3) - see
  Neoplasm, malignant
Cardia, cardial - see condition
Cardiac - see also condition
− death - see Disease, heart
− pacemaker
− − fitting or adjustment V53.3
− − in situ V45.0
− tamponade 423.9
Cardialgia (see also Pain, precordial) 786.5
Cardiectasis - see Hypertrophy, cardiac
Cardiochalasia 530.0
Cardiomalacia (see also Degeneration,
  myocardial) 429.1
Cardiomegalia glycogenica diffusa 271.0
Cardiomegaly (see also Hypertrophy,
  cardiac) 429.3
− congenital 746.8
− glycogen 271.0
− idiopathic 425.4
Cardiomyopathy (congestive) (constrictive)
  (familial) (idiopathic) (obstructive) 425.4
− alcoholic 425.5
− amyloid 277.3 † 425.7*
− beriberi 265.0 † 425.7*

Cardiomyopathy - *continued*
− congenital 425.3
− hypertrophic
− − nonobstructive 425.4
− − obstructive 425.1
− − − congenital 746.8
− in
− − Chagas's disease 086.0 † 425.6*
− − sarcoidosis 135 † 425.8*
− metabolic 277.9 † 425.7*
− nutritional 269.9 † 425.7*
− obscure of Africa 425.2
− postpartum 674.8
− secondary 425.9
− thyrotoxic 242.- † 425.7*
− tuberculous 017.8 † 425.8*
Cardionephritis 404.9
Cardionephropathy 404.9
Cardionephrosis 404.9
Cardiopathy (see also Disease, heart) 429.9
− idiopathic 425.4
− mucopolysaccharidosis 277.5 † 425.7*

Cardiopericarditis (see also Pericarditis)
  423.9
Cardiophobia 300.2
Cardiorenal - see condition
Cardiorrhexis (see also Infarct,
  myocardium) 410
Cardiosclerosis 414.0
Cardiosis - see Disease, heart
Cardiospasm (esophagus) (reflex)
  (stomach) 530.0
− congenital 750.7
Cardiostenosis - see Disease, heart
Cardiovascular - see condition

Carditis (acute) (bacterial) (chronic)
  (subacute) 429.8
− meningococcal 036.4 † 429.8*
− rheumatic - see Disease, heart, rheumatic
− rheumatoid 714.2
Care (of)
− family member (handicapped) (sick)
− − creating problem for family V61.4
− holiday relief V60.5
− improper 995.5
− lack of (at or after birth) (infant) 995.5
− postpartum
− − immediately after delivery V24.0
− − routine follow-up V24.2
− unavailable, due to
− − absence of person rendering care
  V60.4
− − inability (any reason) of person
  rendering care V60.4
Caries (bone) 015.9 † 730.6*
− cementum 521.0

Caries - *continued*
- cerebrospinal (tuberculous) 015.0 †
730.4*
- dental (acute) (chronic) (incipient)
(infected) (with pulp exposure) 521.0
- dentin (acute) (chronic) 521.0
- enamel (acute) (chronic, incipient) 521.0
- external meatus 380.8
- hip 015.1 † 730.5*
- knee 015.2 † 730.5*
- labyrinth 386.8
- limb NEC 015.7 † 730.6*
- mastoid process (chronic) 383.1
- middle ear 385.8
- nose 015.7 † 730.6*
- orbit 015.7 † 730.6*
- ossicle 385.2
- petrous bone 383.2
- sacrum (tuberculous) 015.0 † 730.4*
- spine, spinal (column) (tuberculous)
015.0 † 730.4*
- syphilitic 095 † 730.8*
- - congenital 090.0 † 730.8*
- tooth, teeth 521.0
- vertebra (column) (tuberculous) 015.0 †
730.4*
Carious teeth 521.0
Carneous mole 631
Carotid body or sinus syndrome 337.0
Carotidynia 337.0
Carotinemia (dietary) 278.3
Carotinosis (cutis) (skin) 278.3
Carpal tunnel syndrome 354.0
Carpenter's syndrome 759.8
Carpopedal spasm (see also Tetany) 781.7
Carrier (suspected) of
- amebiasis V02.2
- bacterial disease NEC V02.5
- cholera V02.0
- diphtheria V02.4
- gastrointestinal pathogens NEC V02.3
- gonorrhea V02.7
- hepatitis
- - Australia-antigen (HAA) V02.6
- - viral V02.6
- infectious organism NEC V02.9
- typhoid V02.1
- venereal disease NEC V02.8
Carrion's disease 088.0
Carter's relapsing fever (Asiatic) 087.0
Cartilage - see condition
Caruncle (inflamed)
- conjunctiva 372.0
- eyelid 372.2
- labium (majus) (minus) 616.8
- lacrimal 375.3
- urethra (benign) 599.3

Caruncle - *continued*
- vagina (wall) 616.8
Caseation lymphatic gland 017.2
Castellani's bronchitis 104.8
Castration, traumatic 878.2
- complicated 878.3
Casts in urine 791.7
Cat's ear 744.2
Catalepsy 300.1
- catatonic (acute) 295.2
- hysterical 300.1
- schizophrenic 295.2
Cataplexy (idiopathic) 347
Cataract (anterior cortical) (anterior polar)
(black) (capsular) (central) (cortical)
(hypermature) (immature) (incipient)
(mature) (nuclear) (sunflower) 366.9
- anterior
- - and posterior axial embryonal 743.3
- - pyramidal 743.3
- blue dot 743.3
- cerulean 743.3
- complicated 366.3
- congenital 743.3
- coronary 743.3
- diabetic 250.4 † 366.4*
- drug-induced 366.4
- due to
- - infection 366.4
- - radiation 366.4
- electric 366.4
- glass blowers' 366.4
- heat ray 366.4
- heterochromic 366.3
- in eye disease 366.3
- infantile 366.0
- irradiational 366.4
- juvenile 366.0
- lamellar 743.3
- morgagnian 366.1
- myxedema 244.9 † 366.4*
- posterior, polar (capsular) 743.3
- presenile 366.0
- punctate 743.3
- secondary (membrane) 366.5
- senile 366.1
- toxic 366.4
- traumatic 366.2
- zonular (perinuclear) 743.3
Cataracta 366.1
- brunescens 366.1
- cerulea 743.3
- complicata 366.3
- congenita 743.3
- coralliformis 743.3
- coronaria 743.3
- membranacea

Cataracta - *continued*
− membranacea - *continued*
− − accreta 366.5
− − congenita 743.3
Catarrh, catarrhal (inflammation) (see also
 Condition) 460
− acute 460
− bowel - see Enteritis
− bronchial (see also Bronchitis) 490
− chest (see also Bronchitis) 490
− chronic 472.0
− congestion 472.0
− due to syphilis 095
− − congenital 090.0
− enteric - see Enteritis
− epidemic 487.1
− eustachian 381.5
− eye (acute) (vernal) 372.0
− fauces (see also Pharyngitis) 462
− febrile 460
− fibrinous, acute 466.0
− gastroenteric - see Enteritis
− gastrointestinal - see Enteritis
− hay (see also Fever, hay) 477.9
− infectious 460
− intestinal - see Enteritis
− larynx (see also Laryngitis, chronic) 476.0
− lung (see also Bronchitis) 490
− middle ear, chronic 381.1
− nasal (chronic) (see also Rhinitis) 472.0
− − acute 460
− nasobronchial 472.2
− nasopharyngeal (chronic) 472.2
− − acute 460
− nose - see Catarrh, nasal
− pneumococcal, acute 466.0
− pulmonary (see also Bronchitis) 490
− spring (eye) 372.1
− suffocating NEC 493.9
− summer (hay) (see also Fever, hay) 477.9
− throat 472.1
− tubotympanal 381.4
− − acute 381.0
− − chronic 381.1
− vasomotor (see also Fever, hay) 477.9
Catarrhus aestivus (see also Fever, hay)
 477.9
Catastrophe, cerebral (see also Disease,
 cerebrovascular, acute) 436
Catatonia, catatonic (acute) 295.2
− agitation 295.2
− dementia (praecox) 295.2
− excitation 295.2
− schizophrenia 295.2
− stupor 295.2
Cat-scratch - see also Injury, superficial
− disease or fever 078.3

Cauda equina - see condition
Caul over face 768.9
Cauliflower ear 738.7
Causalgia 354.4
Cause
− external, general effects NEC 994.9
− not stated 799.9
− unknown 799.9
Caustic burn - see also Burn
− from swallowing caustic or corrosive
 substance - see Burn, internal organs
Cavare's disease 359.3
Cave-in, injury
− crushing (severe) 869.1
− suffocation 994.7
Cavernitis (penis) 607.2
Cavernositis 607.2
Cavernous - see condition
Cavitation of lung 011.2
− nontuberculous 518.8
− primary, progressive 010.8
Cavity
− lung - see Cavitation of lung
− optic papilla 743.5
− pulmonary - see Cavitation of lung
Cavus foot (congenital) 754.7
− acquired 736.7
Cazenave's
− disease NEC 694.4
− lupus 695.4
Cecitis (see also Appendicitis) 541
− with perforation, peritonitis, or rupture
 540.0
− acute 540.9
− − with perforation, peritonitis or rupture
 540.0
Cecum - see condition
Celiac infantilism 579.0
Cell, cellular - see also condition
− anterior chamber (eye) (positive aqueous
 ray) 364.0
Cellulitis (diffuse) (with lymphangitis) (see
 also Abscess) 682.9
− abdominal wall 682.2
− anaerobic (see also Gas gangrene) 040.0
− ankle 682.6
− anus 566
− arm (any part, above wrist) 682.3
− axilla 682.3
− back (any part) 682.2
− buttock 682.5
− cervical (meaning neck) 682.1
− cervix (uteri) (see also Cervicitis) 616.0
− chest wall 682.2
− chronic NEC 682.9
− corpus cavernosum 607.2
− drainage site (following operation) 998.5

Cellulitis - *continued*
- ear (external) 380.1
- erysipelar (see also Erysipelas) 035
- eyelid 373.1
- face (any part, except eye) 682.0
- finger (intrathecal) (periosteal)
  (subcutaneous) (subcuticular) 681.0
- foot (except toe) 682.7
- gangrenous (see also Gangrene) 785.4
- genital organ NEC
- - female - see Abscess, genital organ,
  female
- - male 608.4
- gluteal (region) 682.5
- gonococcal NEC 098.0
- groin 682.2
- hand (except finger or thumb) 682.4
- head NEC 682.8
- heel 682.7
- hip 682.6
- jaw (region) 682.0
- knee 682.6
- labium (majus) (minus) (see also
  Vulvitis) 616.1
- larynx 478.7
- leg, except foot 682.6
- lip 528.5
- mouth (floor) 528.3
- multiple sites, so stated 682.9
- nasopharynx 478.2
- navel 682.2
- - newborn NEC 771.4
- neck (region) 682.1
- nose 478.1
- - external 682.0
- orbit, orbital 376.0
- palate (soft) 528.3
- pectoral (region) 682.2
- pelvis, pelvic (chronic)
- - female (see also Disease, pelvis,
  inflammatory) 614.4
- - following
- - - abortion - see categories 634-639,
  fourth digit .o
- - - ectopic gestation 639.0
- - male (see also Abscess, peritoneum)
  567.2
- - puerperal, postpartum, childbirth 670
- penis 607.2
- perineal, perineum 682.2
- perirectal 566
- peritonsillar 475
- periurethral 597.0
- periuterine (see also Disease, pelvis,
  inflammatory) 614.4
- pharynx 478.2
- rectum 566

Cellulitis - *continued*
- retroperitoneal (see also Peritonitis)
  567.2
- scalp (any part) 682.8
- scrotum 608.4
- septic NEC 682.9
- shoulder 682.3
- specified sites NEC 682.8
- suppurative NEC 682.9
- thigh 682.6
- thumb (intrathecal) (periosteal)
  (subcutaneous) (subcuticular) 681.0
- toe (intrathecal) (periosteal)
  (subcutaneous) (subcuticular) 681.1
- tonsil 475
- trunk 682.2
- tuberculous (primary) 017.0
- umbilicus 682.2
- - newborn NEC 771.4
- vaccinal 999.3
- vocal cords 478.5
- vulva (see also Vulvitis) 616.1
- wrist 682.4
Cementoblastoma, benign (M9273/0) 213.1
- upper jaw (bone) 213.0
Cementoma (M9272/0) 213.1
- gigantiform (M9275/0) 213.1
- - upper jaw (bone) 213.0
- upper jaw (bone) 213.0
Cementoperiostitis 523.4
Cephalematocele, cephalhematocele
- birth injury 767.0
- fetus or newborn 767.0
- traumatic 920
Cephalematoma, cephalhematoma
  (calcified)
- birth injury 767.1
- fetus or newborn 767.1
- traumatic 920
Cephalgia, cephalalgia (see also Headache)
  784.0
- nonorganic origin 307.8
Cephalic - see condition
Cephalitis - see Encephalitis
Cephalocele 742.0
Cephalomenia 625.8
Cephalopelvic - see condition
Cerebellitis - see Encephalitis
Cerebellum, cerebellar - see condition
Cerebral - see condition
Cerebritis - see Encephalitis
Cerebromacular degeneration 330.1
Cerebromalacia (see also Softening, brain)
  434.9
Cerebrosidosis 272.7
Cerebrospasticity - see Palsy, cerebral
Cerebrospinal - see condition

Cerebrum - see condition
Cerumen (accumulation) (impacted) 380.4
Cervical - see also condition
- auricle 744.4
- rib 756.2
Cervicalgia 723.1
Cervicitis (acute) (chronic) (nonvenereal)
  (subacute) 616.0
- with ulceration 616.0
- complicating pregnancy or puerperium
  646.6
- - fetus or newborn 760.8
- gonococcal 098.1 † 616.0*
- - chronic or duration of 2 months or over
  098.3
- senile (atrophic) 616.0
- syphilitic 095
- trichomonal 131.0 † 616.0*
- tuberculous 016.4
Cervicocolpitis (emphysematosa) (see also
  Cervicitis) 616.0
Cervix - see condition
Cesarean operation or section NEC 669.7
- affecting fetus or newborn 763.4
- post mortem, affecting fetus or newborn
  761.6
- previous, affecting management of
  pregnancy 654.2
Cestan's syndrome 344.8
Cestan-Chenais paralysis 344.8
Cestode infestation NEC 123.9
- specified type NEC 123.8
Cestodiasis 123.9
Chabert's disease 022.9
Chafing 709.8
Chagas' disease (see also Trypanosomiasis,
  American) 086.2
Chagres fever 084.0
Chalasia (cardiac sphincter) 530.0
Chalazion 373.2
Chalazoderma 757.3
Chalcosis 360.2
- cornea 371.1
- crystalline lens 366.3
- retina 360.2
Chalicosis (pulmonum) 502
Chancre (any genital site) (hard)
  (indurated) (infecting) (primary)
  (recurrent) 091.0
- congenital 090.0
- conjunctiva 091.2
- Ducrey's 099.0
- extragenital 091.2
- eyelid 091.2
- hunterian 091.0
- lip (syphilis) 091.2
- mixed 099.8

Chancre - *continued*
- nipple 091.2
- Nisbet's 099.0
- of
- - carate 103.0
- - pinta 103.0
- - yaws 102.0
- palate soft 091.2
- phagedenic 099.0
- Ricord's 091.0
- Rollet's (syphilitic) 091.0
- seronegative 091.0
- seropositive 091.0
- simple 099.0
- soft 099.0
- - bubo 099.0
- urethra 091.0
- yaws 102.0
Chancroid 099.0
- anus 099.0
- penis (Ducrey's bacillus) 099.0
- perineum 099.0
- rectum 099.0
- scrotum 099.0
- urethra 099.0
- vulva 099.0
Change(s) (of) - see also Removal of
- arteriosclerotic - see Arteriosclerosis
- bone 733.9
- - diabetic 250.7 † 731.8*
- cardiorenal (vascular) 404.9
- cardiovascular - see Disease,
  cardiovascular
- circulatory 459.9
- cognitive (nonpsychotic) NEC 310.1
- color, tooth, teeth
- - during formation 520.8
- - posteruptive 521.7
- contraceptive device V25.4
- coronary (see also Ischemia, heart) 414.9
- degenerative, spine or vertebra 721.9
- dental pulp, regressive 522.2
- dressing V58.3
- fixation device V54.8
- - external V54.8
- - internal V54.0
- heart - see Disease, heart
- hip joint 718.9
- hyperplastic larynx 478.7
- hypertrophic
- - nasal sinus (see also Sinusitis) 473.9
- - upper respiratory tract 478.9
- inflammatory - see Inflammation
- joint 718.9
- - sacroiliac 724.6
- Kirschner wire V54.8
- knee 717.9

Change(s) - *continued*
- malignant (M----/3) - code as Primary malignant neoplasm of the site of the lesion 199.1

Note – For malignant change occuring in a neoplasm, use the appropriate M code with behavior digit /3 e.g. malignant change in uterine fibroid – M8890/3. For malignant change occuring in a non-neoplastic condition (e.g. gastric ulcer) use the M code M8000/3.

Change(s) - *continued*
- mental NEC 300.9
- myocardium, myocardial - see Degeneration, myocardial
- of life (see also Menopause) 627.2
- personality (nonpsychotic) NEC 310.1
- plaster cast V54.8
- retina, myopic 360.2
- sacroiliac joint 724.6
- senile (see also Senility) 797
- sensory (see also Disturbance, sensation) 782.0
- skin texture 782.8
- spinal cord 336.9
- splint, external V54.8
- suture V58.3
- traction device V54.8
- vascular 459.9
- vasomotor 443.9
- voice 784.4
- - psychogenic 306.1
Chapping skin 709.8
Charcot's
- arthropathy 094.0 † 713.5*
- cirrhosis - see Cirrhosis, biliary
- disease, spinal cord 094.0
- fever (biliary) (hepatic) (intermittent) (see also Choledocholithiasis) 574.5
- joint (disease) 094.0 † 713.5*
- - diabetic 250.5 † 713.5*
- syndrome 443.9
Charcot-Marie-Tooth disease, paralysis or syndrome 356.1
Charley-horse (quadriceps) 843.8
- muscle, except quadriceps - see Sprain, strain
Chauffeur's fracture 813.4
- open 813.5
Cheadle's disease 267
Checking (of)
- device
- - contraceptive V25.4
- - fixation V54.8

Checking - *continued*
- device - *continued*
- - fixation - *continued*
- - - external V54.8
- - - internal V54.0
- - traction V54.8
- Kirschner wire V54.8
- plaster cast V54.8
- splint, external V54.8
Checkup, health V70.0
Chediak-Higashi(-Steinbrink) anomaly, disease or syndrome 288.2
Cheek - see condition
Cheese itch 133.8
Cheese-washers' lung 495.8
Cheilitis 528.5
- actinic (due to sun) 692.7
- - other than from sun 692.8
Cheilodynia 528.5
Cheiloschisis 749.1
- with cleft palate 749.2
Cheilosis 528.5
- with pellagra 265.2
- angular 528.5
- due to
- - dietary deficiency 266.0
- - vitamin deficiency 266.0
Cheiromegaly 729.8
Cheiropompholyx 705.8
Cheloid (see also Keloid) 701.4
Chemical burn - see also Burn
- from swallowing chemical - see Burn, internal organs
Chemodectoma (M8693/1) - see Paraganglioma, nonchromaffin
Chemoprophylaxis V07.3
Chemosis, conjunctiva 372.7
Chemotherapy
- maintenance V58.1
- prophylactic NEC V07.3
Cherubism 526.8
Chest - see condition
Cheyne-Stokes respiration 786.0
Chiari's
- disease or syndrome 453.0
- network 746.8
Chiari-Frommel syndrome 676.6
Chicago disease 116.0
Chickenpox 052
Chiclero ulcer 085.4
Chiggers 133.8
Chignon 111.2
- fetus or newborn (from vacuum extraction) 767.1
Chilblains 991.5
Child behavior causing concern V61.2
Childbirth - see also Delivery

Childbirth - see also Delivery - *continued*
- puerperal complications - see Puerperal
Childhood, period of rapid growth V21.0
Chill(s) 780.9
- with fever 780.6
- in malarial regions 084.6
- septic - see Septicemia
- urethral 599.8
Chilomastigiasis 007.8
Chin - see condition
Chloasma 709.0
- cachecticorum 709.0
- eyelid 374.5
- - congenital 757.3
- - hyperthyroid 242.0
- idiopathic 709.0
- skin 709.0
- symptomatic 709.0
Chloroma (M9930/3) 205.3
Chlorosis 280
- Egyptian (see also Ancylostomiasis)
  126.9
- miners' (see also Ancylostomiasis) 126.9
Chocolate cyst (ovary) 617.1
Choked
- disc or disk 377.0
- on food, phlegm, or vomitus NEC (see
  also Asphyxia, food) 933.1
- while vomiting NEC (see also Asphyxia,
  food) 933.1
Chokes (resulting from bends) 993.3
Choking sensation 784.9
Cholangiectasis (see also Disease,
  gallbladder) 575.8
Cholangiocarcinoma (M8160/3)
- and hepatocellular carcinoma, combined
  (M8180/3) 155.0
- liver 155.1
- specified site NEC - see Neoplasm,
  malignant
- unspecified site 155.1
Cholangiohepatoma (M8180/3) 155.0
Cholangiolitis (acute) (chronic)
  (extrahepatic) (gangrenous) 576.1
- intrahepatic 575.8
Cholangioma (M8160/0) 211.5
- malignant (M8160/3) - see
  Cholangiocarcinoma
Cholangitis (ascending) (catarrhal)
  (chronic) (infective) (malignant) (primary)
  (recurrent) (sclerosing) (secondary)
  (stenosing) (suppurative) 576.1
- chronic nonsuppurative destructive 571.6
Cholecystdocholithiasis (see also
  Choledocholithiasis) 574.5
Cholecystitis (chronic) 575.1
- with

Cholecystitis - *continued*
- with - *continued*
- - calculus, stones in
- - - bile duct (common) (hepatic) 574.4
- - - gallbladder 574.1
- - choledocholithiasis 574.4
- - cholelithiasis 574.1
- acute 575.0
- - with
- - - calculus, stones in
- - - - bile duct (common) (hepatic)
      574.3
- - - - gallbladder 574.0
- - - choledocholithiasis 574.3
- - - cholelithiasis 574.0
- emphysematous - see Cholecystitis, acute
- gangrenous - see Cholecystitis, acute
- suppurative - see Cholecystitis, acute
Choledochitis (suppurative) 576.1
Choledocholith (see also
  Choledocholithiasis) 574.5
Choledocholithiasis 574.5
- with cholecystitis (chronic) 574.4
- - acute 574.3
Cholelithiasis (impacted) (multiple) 574.2
- with cholecystitis (chronic) 574.1
- - acute 574.0
Cholemia (see also Jaundice) 782.4
- familial 277.4
- Gilbert's 277.4
Cholemic gallstone (see also Cholelithiasis)
  574.2
Choleperitoneum, choleperitonitis (see also
  Disease, gallbladder) 567.8
Cholera (algid) (Asiatic) (asphyctic)
  (epidemic) (gravis) (Indian) (malignant)
  (morbus) (pestilential) (spasmodic) 001.9
- antimonial 985.4
- classical 001.0
- due to Vibrio cholerae (Inaba, Ogawa,
  Hikojima serotypes) 001.0
- - El Tor 001.1
- El Tor 001.1
Cholerine (see also Cholera) 001.9
Cholestasis (see also Disease, gallbladder)
  575.8
Cholesteatoma (ear (middle)) (mastoid)
  (with reaction) 385.3
- external ear (canal) 380.2
Cholesteremia 272.0
Cholesterin in vitreous 379.2
Cholesterol
- deposit
- - retina 362.8
- - vitreous 379.2
- imbibition of gallbladder (see also
  Disease, gallbladder) 575.6

Cholesterolemia 272.0
- essential 272.0
- familial 272.0
- hereditary 272.0
Cholesterolosis (gallbladder) 575.6
Cholesterosis (gallbladder) 575.6
Cholocolic fistula (see also Fistula,
  gallbladder) 575.5
Choluria 791.4
Chondritis (purulent) 733.9
- costal 730.9
- - Tietze's 733.6
- tuberculous (see also Tuberculosis, bone)
  015.9
- - intervertebral 015.0 † 730.4*
Chondroblastoma (M9230/0) - see also
  Neoplasm, bone, benign
- malignant (M9230/3) - see Neoplasm,
  bone, malignant
Chondrocalcinosis 275.4 † 712.3*
- due to
- - dicalcium phosphate crystals 275.4 †
  712.1*
- - pyrophosphate crystals 275.4 † 712.2*
Chondrodermatitis nodularis helicis or
  anthelicis 380.0
Chondrodysplasia 756.4
- angiomatose 756.4
- calcificans congenita 756.5
- hereditary deforming 756.4
Chondrodystrophia (fetalis) 756.4
- calcarea 756.4
- calcificans congenita 756.5
- punctata 756.5
- tarda 277.5
Chondrodystrophy (familial) (hypoplastic)
  756.4
Chondroectodermal dysplasia 756.5

Chondroma (M9220/0) - see also
  Neoplasm, cartilage, benign
- juxtacortical (M9221/0) - see Neoplasm,
  bone, benign
- periosteal (M9221/0) - see Neoplasm,
  bone, benign
Chondromalacia 733.9
- epiglottis 748.3
- larynx 748.3
- patella, patellae 717.7
- systemic 733.9
Chondromatosis (M9220/1) - see also
  Neoplasm, cartilage, uncertain behavior
Chondromyxosarcoma (M9220/3) - see
  Neoplasm, cartilage, malignant
Chondro-osteodysplasia 277.5
- Morquio-Brailsford type 277.5
Chondro-osteodystrophy 277.5

Chondro-osteoma (M9210/0) - see
  Neoplasm, bone, benign
Chondropathia tuberosa 733.9
Chondrosarcoma (M9220/3) - see
  Neoplasm, cartilage, malignant
- juxtacortical (M9221/3) - see Neoplasm,
  bone, malignant
- mesenchymal (M9240/3) - see Neoplasm,
  connective tissue, malignant
Chordee (nonvenereal) 607.8
- congenital 752.6
- gonococcal 098.2
Chorditis (fibrinous) (nodosa) (tuberosa)
  478.5
Chordoma (M9370/3) - see also Neoplasm,
  malignant
Chorea (gravis) (minor) (spasmodic) 333.5
- with
- - heart involvement - see Chorea, with
    rheumatic heart disease
- - rheumatic heart disease (chronic,
    inactive, or quiescent) (conditions in
    393-398) - code to rheumatic heart
    condition involved 398.9
- - - active or acute (conditions in 391)
      392.0
- apoplectic (see also Disease,
  cerebrovascular, acute) 436
- chronic 333.4
- gravidarum - see Eclampsia, pregnancy
- habit 307.2
- hereditary 333.4
- Huntington's 333.4
- posthemiplegic 344.8
- pregnancy - see Eclampsia, pregnancy
- progressive 333.4
- - chronic 333.4
- - hereditary 333.4
- rheumatic (chronic) 392.9
- - with heart involvement - see Chorea,
    with rheumatic heart disease
- senile 333.5
- Sydenham's 392.9
- - with heart involvement - see Chorea,
    with rheumatic heart disease
- - nonrheumatic 333.5
Choreoathetosis (paroxysmal) 333.5
Chorioadenoma (destruens) (M9100/1)
  236.1
Chorioamnionitis 658.4
- fetus or newborn 762.7
Chorioangioma (M9120/0) 219.8
Choriocarcinoma (M9100/3)
- combined with
- - embryonal carcinoma (M9101/3) - see
    Neoplasm, malignant

Choriocarcinoma - *continued*
– combined with - *continued*
– – teratoma (M9101/3) - see Neoplasm,
   malignant
– specified site - see Neoplasm, malignant
– unspecified site
– – female 181
– – male 186.9
Chorio-encephalitis, lymphocytic (acute)
   (serous) 049.0 † 321.6*
Chorioepithelioma (M9100/3) - see
   Choriocarcinoma
Choriomeningitis (acute) (benign)
   (lymphocytic) (serous) 049.0 † 321.6*
Chorionepithelioma (M9100/3) - see
   Choriocarcinoma
Chorionitis (see also Scleroderma) 710.1
Chorioretinitis 363.2
– disseminated 363.1
– – in neurosyphilis 094.8 † 363.1*
– due to
– – histoplasmosis 115.- † 363.0*
– – toxoplasmosis (acquired) 130 † 363.0*
– – – congenital (active) 771.2 † 363.0*
– focal (acute) (chronic) (central)
   (exudative) (Jensen's) 363.0
– histoplasmic 115.- † 363.0*
– juxtapapillaris 363.0
– juxtapapillary 363.0
– progressive myopia (degeneration) 360.2
– syphilitic (secondary) 091.5 † 363.1*
– – congenital (early) 090.0 † 363.1*
– – – late 090.5 † 363.1*
– – late 095 † 363.1*
– tuberculous 017.3 † 363.1*
Chorioretinopathy, central serous 362.4
Choroid - see condition
Choroideremia, choroidermia 363.5
Choroiditis (see also Chorioretinitis) 363.2
– leprous 030.- † 363.1*
– syphilitic (secondary) 091.5 † 363.1*
– – congenital (early) 090.0 † 363.1*
– – – late 090.5 † 363.1*
– – late 095 † 363.1*
– tuberculous 017.3 † 363.1*
Choroidopathy NEC 363.9
– degenerative 363.4
– hereditary 363.5
Choroidoretinitis - see Chorioretinitis
Choroidosis, central serous 362.4
Choroidretinopathy, serous 362.4
Christian-Weber disease 729.3
Christmas disease 286.1
Chromaffinoma (M8700/0) - see also
   Neoplasm, benign
– malignant (M8700/3) - see Neoplasm,
   malignant

Chromatopsia 368.8
Chromhidrosis 705.8
Chromidrosis 705.8
Chromoblastomycosis 117.2
Chromomycosis 117.2
Chromophytosis 111.0
Chromotrichomycosis 111.8
Chronic - see condition
Chyle cyst, mesentery 457.8
Chylocele (nonfilarial) 457.8
– filarial (see also Infestation, filarial)
   125.9
– tunica vaginalis 608.8
– – filarial (see also Infestation, filarial)
   125.9
Chylothorax (nonfilarial) 457.8
– filarial (see also Infestation, filarial)
   125.9
Chylous - see condition
Chyluria 791.1
– bilharziasis 120.0
– due to
– – Brugia (malayi) 125.1
– – Wuchereria (bancrofti) 125.0
– – – malayi 125.1
– filarial (see also Infestation, filarial)
   125.9
– nonfilarial 791.1
Cicatricial (deformity) - see Cicatrix
Cicatrix (adherent) (contracted) (painful)
   (vicious) 709.2
– adenoid 474.8
– alveolar process 525.8
– anus 569.4
– auricle 380.8
– bile duct (see also Disease, biliary) 576.8
– bladder 596.8
– bone 733.9
– brain 348.8
– cervix (postoperative) (postpartal) 622.3
– common duct (see also Disease, biliary)
   576.8
– cornea 371.0
– – tuberculous 017.3 † 371.0*
– duodenum (bulb) 537.3
– eyelid 374.4
– hypopharynx 478.2
– lacrimal apparatus 375.5
– larynx 478.7
– lung 518.8
– middle ear 385.8
– mouth 528.9
– muscle 728.8
– nasopharynx 478.2
– palate (soft) 528.9
– penis 607.8
– prostate 602.8

Cicatrix - *continued*
- rectum 569.4
- retina 363.3
- semilunar cartilage - see Derangement, meniscus
- seminal vesicle 608.8
- skin 709.2
- - infected 686.8
- - postinfectional 709.2
- - tuberculous 017.0
- throat 478.2
- tongue 529.8
- tonsil (and adenoid) 474.8
- trachea 478.9
- tuberculous NEC 011.9
- ureter 593.8
- urethra 599.8
- uterus 621.8
- vagina 623.4
- vocal cord 478.5
- wrist, constricting (annular) 709.2
Cinchonism
- correct substance properly administered 386.9
- overdose or wrong substance given or taken 961.4
Circle of Willis - see condition
Circular - see also condition
- hymen 752.4
Circulating anticoagulants 286.5
- following childbirth 666.3
Circulation
- collateral (venous), any site 459.8
- defective 459.9
- - congenital 747.9
- - lower extremity 459.8
- embryonic 747.9
- failure (peripheral) 785.5
- - fetus or newborn 779.8
- fetal, persistence 747.9
- heart, incomplete 747.9

Circulatory system - see condition

Circulus senilis 371.4

Circumcision
- in absence of medical indication V50.2
- ritual V50.2
- routine V50.2

Circumscribed - see condition

Circumvallata placenta - see Placenta, abnormal

Cirrhosis, cirrhotic 571.5
- alcoholic (liver) 571.2
- atrophic (of liver) - see Cirrhosis, portal
- Baumgarten-Cruveilhier 571.5

Cirrhosis - *continued*
- biliary (cholangiolitic) (cholangitic) (cholostatic) (extrahepatic) (hypertrophic) (intrahepatic) (nonobstructive) (obstructive) (posthepatitic) (pericholangiolitic) (primary) (secondary) 571.6
- - due to
- - - clonorchiasis 121.1
- - - flukes 121.3
- brain 331.9
- capsular - see Cirrhosis, portal
- cardiac 571.5
- - alcoholic 571.2
- central (liver) - see Cirrhosis, liver
- Charcot's 571.6
- cholangiolitic - see Cirrhosis, biliary
- cholangitic - see Cirrhosis, biliary
- cholostatic - see Cirrhosis, biliary
- clitoris (hypertrophic) 624.2
- congestive (liver) - see Cirrhosis, cardiac
- Cruveilhier-Baumgarten 571.5
- cryptogenic (of liver) 571.5
- - alcoholic 571.2
- dietary (see also Cirrhosis, portal) 571.5
- due to
- - bronzed diabetes 275.0
- - cystic fibrosis 277.0
- - hemachromatosis 275.0
- - hepatolenticular degeneration 275.1
- - Wilson's disease 275.1
- - xanthomatosis 272.2
- extrahepatic (obstructive) - see Cirrhosis, biliary
- fatty 571.8
- - alcoholic 571.0
- Glisson's 571.5
- Hanot's (hypertropic) 571.6
- hepatic - see Cirrhosis, liver
- hepatolienal - see Cirrhosis, liver
- hobnail - see Cirrhosis, portal
- hypertrophic - see Cirrhosis, liver
- infectious NEC - see Cirrhosis, portal
- insular - see Cirrhosis, portal
- intrahepatic - see Cirrhosis, biliary
- juvenile (see also Cirrhosis, portal) 571.5
- kidney (see also Sclerosis, renal) 587
- Laennec's (of liver) 571.2
- - nonalcoholic 571.5
- liver (chronic) (hepatolienal) (hypertrophic) (nodular) (splenomegalic) (unilobar) 571.5
- - alcoholic 571.2
- - congenital (due to failure of obliteration of umbilical vein) 777.8
- - pigmentary 275.0
- - syphilitic 095 † 573.2*

Cirrhosis - *continued*
- lung (chronic) (see also Fibrosis, lung) 515
- macronodular (of liver) 571.5
- - alcoholic 571.2
- malarial 084.9
- metabolic NEC 571.5
- micronodular (of liver) 571.5
- - alcoholic 571.2
- monolobular - see Cirrhosis, portal
- multilobular - see Cirrhosis, portal
- nodular - see Cirrhosis, liver
- nutritional (fatty) 571.5
- obstructive (biliary) (extrahepatic) (intrahepatic) - see Cirrhosis, biliary
- ovarian 620.8
- paludal 084.9
- pancreas (duct) 577.8
- periportal - see Cirrhosis, portal
- pigment, pigmentary (of liver) 275.0
- portal (of liver) 571.5
- - alcoholic 571.2
- posthepatitic (see also Cirrhosis, postnecrotic) 571.5
- postnecrotic (of liver) 571.5
- - alcoholic 571.2
- primary (intrahepatic) - see Cirrhosis, biliary
- pulmonary (see also Fibrosis, lung) 515
- renal (see also Sclerosis, renal) 587
- septal (see also Cirrhosis, postnecrotic) 571.5
- spleen 289.5
- splenomegalic (of liver) - see Cirrhosis, liver
- stomach 535.4
- Todd's 571.6
- toxic (nodular) - see Cirrhosis, postnecrotic
- trabecular - see Cirrhosis, postnecrotic
- unilobar - see Cirrhosis, liver
- vascular (of liver) - see Cirrhosis, liver
- xanthomatous (biliary) 571.6
- - due to xanthomatosis (familial) (metabolic) (primary) 272.2
Citrullinemia 270.6
Citrullinuria 270.6
Civatte's disease or poikiloderma 709.0
Clap - see Gonorrhea
Clark's paralysis 343.9
Clastothrix 704.2
Claude Bernard-Horner syndrome 337.9
Claude's syndrome 352.6
Claudication, intermittent 443.9
- cerebral (artery) 435
- spinal cord (arteriosclerotic) 435
- - syphilitic 094.8

Claustrophobia 300.2
Clavus (infected) 700
Clawfoot (congenital) 754.7
- acquired 736.7
Clawhand (acquired) 736.0
- congenital 755.5
Clawtoe (congenital) 754.7
- acquired 735.5
Cleansing of artificial opening - see Attention to artificial opening
Cleft (congenital) - see also Imperfect closure
- alveolar process 525.8
- branchial (cyst) (persistent) 744.4
- cricoid cartilage, posterior 748.3
- facial 749.1
- - with cleft palate 749.2
- lip 749.1
- - with cleft palate 749.2
- nose 748.1
- palate (complete) (incomplete) 749.0
- - with cleft lip 749.2
- penis 752.8
- scrotum 752.8
- thyroid cartilage 748.3
- uvula 749.0
- - with cleft lip 749.2
Cleidocranial dysostosis 755.5
Cleidotomy 763.8
Cleptomania 312.2
Climacteric (see also Menopause) 627.2
- arthritis (any site) NEC 716.3
- depression 296.1
- disease 627.2
- male (symptoms) (syndrome) NEC 608.8
- melancholia 296.1
- paranoid state 297.2
- paraphrenia 297.2
- polyarthritis NEC 716.3
- symptoms (female) 627.2
Clitoris - see condition
Cloaca persistent 751.5
Clonorchiasis 121.1
Clonorchiosis 121.1
Clonorchis infection, liver 121.1
Clonus 781.0
Closure
- congenital, nose 748.0
- cranial sutures, premature 756.0
- defective or imperfect NEC - see Imperfect closure
- fistula, delayed - see Fistula
- foramen ovale, imperfect 745.5
- hymen 623.3
- interauricular septum, defective 745.5
- interventricular septum, defective 745.4
- lacrimal duct 375.5

Closure - *continued*
- lacrimal duct 375.5 - *continued*
- - congenital 743.6
- of artificial opening - see Attention to artificial opening
- vagina 623.2
- valve - see Endocarditis
- vulva 624.8
Clot (blood)
- artery (obstruction) (occlusion) (see also Embolism) 444.9
- bladder 596.7
- brain (intradural or extradural) (see also Thrombosis, brain) 434.0
- circulation 444.9
- heart (see also Infarct, myocardium) 410
- vein (see also Thrombosis) 453.9
Clouded state 780.0
- epileptic 345.9
- paroxysmal (idiopathic) 345.9
Cloudy antrum, antra 473.0
Clouston's (hidrotic) ectodermal dysplasia 757.3
Clubbing of fingers 781.5
Clubfinger 781.5
- congenital 754.8
Clubfoot (congenital) 754.7
- acquired 736.7
- paralytic 736.7
Clubhand (congenital) 754.8
- acquired 736.0
Clubnail 703.8
- congenital 757.5
Clump, kidney 753.3
Clumsiness syndrome 315.4
Cluttering 307.0
Clutton's joints 090.5
Coagulation, intravascular (diffuse) (disseminated) (see also Defibrination syndrome) 286.6
- newborn 776.2
Coagulopathy (see also Defect, coagulation) 286.9
- consumption 286.6
Coal miner's
- elbow 727.2
- lung 500
Coalition, calcaneo-scaphoid 755.6
Coalworkers' lung or pneumoconiosis 500
Coarctation of aorta (preductal) (postductal) 747.1
Coated tongue 529.3
Coats' disease 362.1
Cocainism 304.2
Coccidioidomycosis 114
- lung 114 † 484.7*
- meninges 114 † 321.0*

Coccidioidomycosis - *continued*
- prostate 114
Coccidioidosis 114
- lung 114 † 484.7*
- meninges 114 † 321.0*
Coccidiosis 007.2
Coccydynia 724.7
Coccygodynia 724.7
Coccyx - see condition
Cock's peculiar tumor 706.2
Cockayne's syndrome 759.8
Cocked up toe 735.2
Codman's tumor (M9230/0) - see Neoplasm, bone, benign
Coffee workers' lung 495.8
Cogan's syndrome 370.5
Coitus, painful (female) 625.0
- male 608.8
- psychogenic 302.7
Cold 460
- with influenza, flu, or grippe 487.1
- agglutinin disease or hemoglobinuria 283.0
- allergic (see also Fever, hay) 477.9
- bronchi or chest - see Bronchitis
- - with grippe or influenza 487.1
- common (head) 460
- deep 464.1
- effects of 991.9
- - specified effect NEC 991.8
- excessive 991.9
- - specified effect NEC 991.8
- exhaustion from 991.8
- exposure to 991.9
- - specified effect NEC 991.8
- head 460
- injury syndrome (newborn) 778.2
- on lung - see Bronchitis
- rose 477.0
- sensitivity, auto-immune 283.0
- virus 460
Coldsore (see also Herpes simplex) 054.9
Colibacillosis 041.8
- generalized 038.4
Colic (recurrent) 789.0
- abdomen 789.0
- - psychogenic 306.4
- appendicular 543
- appendix 543
- bile duct (see also Choledocholithiasis) 574.5
- biliary (see also Cholelithiasis) 574.2
- bilious (see also Cholelithiasis) 574.2
- common duct (see also Choledocholithiasis) 574.5
- Devonshire NEC 984.9
- flatulent 787.3

Colic - *continued*
- gallbladder or gallstone (see also Cholelithiasis) 574.2
- hepatic (duct) (see also Choledocholithiasis) 574.5
- hysterical 300.1
- infantile 789.0
- intestinal 789.0
- kidney 788.0
- lead NEC 984.9
- - specified type of lead - see Table of drugs and chemicals
- liver (duct) (see also Choledocholithiasis) 574.5
- mucous 564.1
- nephritic 788.0
- painters' NEC 984.9
- pancreas 577.8
- psychogenic 306.4
- renal 788.0
- saturnine NEC 984.9
- spasmodic 789.0
- ureter 788.0
- urethral 599.8
- - due to calculus 594.2
- uterus 625.8
- - menstrual 625.4
- worm NEC 128.9
Colicystitis (see also Cystitis) 595.9
Colitis (acute) (catarrhal) (croupous) (exudative) (gravis) (hemorrhagic) (phlegmonous) (presumed infectious) (see also Enteritis and note at category 009.3) 009.1
- allergic 558
- amebic (see also Amebiasis) 006.9
- - nondysenteric 006.2
- anthrax 022.2
- bacillary (see also Infection, Shigella) 004.9
- balantidial 007.0
- chronic 558
- coccidial 007.2
- dietetic 558
- giardial 007.1
- granulomatous 555.1
- infectious (see also Enteritis, infectious) 009.0
- ischaemic 557.9
- - acute 557.0
- - chronic 557.1
- membranous 564.1
- mucous 564.1
- noninfectious 558
- protozoal NEC 007.8
- pseudomucinous 564.1
- regional 555.1

Colitis - *continued*
- septic (see also Enteritis, infectious) 009.0
- spastic 564.1
- thromboulcerative (chronic) 557.0
- toxic 558
- trichomonal 007.3
- tuberculous (ulcerative) 014
- ulcerative (chronic) 556
Collagen disease NEC 710.9
- nonvascular 710.9
- vascular (allergic) 446.2

Collagenosis (see also Collagen disease) 710.9
- cardiovascular 425.4

Collapse 780.2
- adrenal 255.8
- cardiorenal 404.9
- cardiorespiratory 785.5
- - fetus or newborn 779.8
- cardiovascular (see also Disease, heart) 785.5
- circulatory (peripheral) 785.5
- - complicating
- - - abortion - see categories 634-639, fourth digit .5
- - - ectopic or molar pregnancy 639.5
- - during or after labor and delivery 669.1
- - fetus or newborn 779.8
- during or after labor and delivery 669.1
- - fetus or newborn 779.8
- external ear canal 380.5
- general 780.2
- heart - see Disease, heart
- heat 992.1
- hysterical 300.1
- labyrinth, membranous (congenital) 744.0
- lung (massive) (see also Atelectasis) 518.0
- - pressure, during labor 668.0
- myocardial - see Disease, heart
- nervous (see also Disorder, mental, nonpsychotic) 300.9
- neurocirculatory 306.2
- nose 738.0
- postoperative (cardiovascular) 998.0
- pulmonary (see also Atelectasis) 518.0
- thorax 512
- trachea 519.1
- valvular - see Endocarditis
- vascular (peripheral) 785.5
- - cerebral (see also Disease, cerebrovascular, acute) 436
- - complication of

Collapse - *continued*
- vascular - *continued*
- - complication of - *continued*
- - - abortion - see categories 634-639,
  fourth digit .5
- - - ectopic or molar pregnancy 639.5
- - during or after labor and delivery
  669.1
- - fetus or newborn 779.8
- vertebra 733.1
Colles' fracture 813.4
- open 813.5
Collet's syndrome 352.6
Collet-Sicard syndrome 352.6
Colliers'
- asthma 500
- lung 500
- phthisis 011.4
Colloid milium 709.3
Coloboma (iris) 743.4
- fundus 743.5
- optic disc 743.5
Coloenteritis - see Enteritis
Colon - see condition
Coloptosis 569.8
Color blindness 368.5
Colostomy
- attention to V55.3
- fitting or ajustment V53.5
- malfunctioning 569.6
- status V44.3
Colpitis (see also Vaginitis) 616.1
Colpocele 618.6
Colpocystitis (see also Vaginitis) 616.1

Column, spinal, vertebral - see condition
Coma 780.0
- apoplectic (see also Disease,
  cerebrovascular, acute) 436
- diabetic (with ketoacidosis) 250.2
- - hyperosmolar 250.2
- eclamptic (see also Eclampsia) 780.3
- epileptic 345.3
- hepatic 572.2
- hyperglycemic 250.2
- hyperosmolar (diabetic) 250.2
- hypoglycemic 251.0
- - diabetic 250.2
- insulin 251.0
- Kussmaul's 250.2
- newborn 779.2
- prediabetic 250.2
- uremic - see Uremia

Combat fatigue (see also Reaction, stress,
  acute) 308.9
Combined - see condition
Comedo 706.1

Comedocarcinoma (M8501/3) - see also
  Neoplasm, breast, malignant
- noninfiltrating (M8501/2)
- - specified site - see Neoplasm, in situ
- - unspecified site 233.0
Comedomastitis 610.4
Comedones 706.1
- lanugo 757.4
Comminuted fracture - code as Fracture,
  closed
Common
- atrioventricular canal 745.6
- atrium 745.6
- truncus (arteriosus) 745.0
- ventricle 745.3
Commotio, commotion (current)
- brain 850
- - with skull fracture - see Fracture, skull
- cerebri 850
- - with skull fracture - see Fracture, skull
- retinae 921.3
- spinal cord - see Injury, spinal, by region
- spinalis - see Injury, spinal, by region
Communication
- abnormal - see also Fistula
- - between
- - - base of aorta and pulmonary artery
    745.0
- - - left ventricle and right atrium 745.4
- - - pericardial sac and pleural sac 748.8
- - - pulmonary artery and pulmonary
    vein 747.3
- - congenital between uterus and
- - - anterior abdominal wall 752.3
- - - bladder 752.3
- - - intestine 752.3
- - - rectum 752.3
Compensation
- broken - see Disease, heart
- failure - see Disease, heart
- neurosis, psychoneurosis 300.1
Complaint - see also Disease
- bowel, functional 564.9
- - psychogenic 306.4
- intestine, functional 564.9
- - psychogenic 306.4
- kidney (see also Disease, renal) 593.9
- miners' 500
Complete - see condition
Complex
- cardiorenal 404.9
- Costen's 524.6
- Eisenmenger 745.4
- homosexual 302.0
- hypersexual 302.8
- jumped process
- - spine - see Dislocation, vertebra

Complex - *continued*
- primary, tuberculous 010.0
- Taussig-Bing 745.1

Complications
- abortion NEC - see categories 634-639, fourth digit .9
- accidental puncture or laceration during procedure 998.2
- amputation stump (surgical) (late) 997.6
- anastomosis (and bypass) NEC 996.7
- - infection 996.6
- - inflammation 996.6
- - intestinal (internal) NEC 997.4
- - - involving urinary tract 997.5
- - mechanical - see Complications, mechanical
- - urinary tract (involving intestinal tract) 997.5
- anesthesia, anesthetic NEC (see also Anesthesia, complication) 995.2
- - in labor and delivery 668.9
- - - cardiac 668.1
- - - central nervous system 668.2
- - - fetus or newborn 763.5
- - - pulmonary 668.0
- arthroplasty 996.4
- bile duct implant (prosthetic) NEC 996.7
- - infection or inflammation 996.6
- - mechanical 996.5
- breast implant (prosthetic) NEC 996.7
- - infection or inflammation 996.6
- - mechanical 996.5
- bypass - see Complications, anastomosis
- cardiac (see also Disease, heart) 429.9
- - device, implant or graft NEC 996.7
- - - infection or inflammation 996.6
- - - long-term effect 429.4
- - - mechanical 996.1
- - postoperative NEC 997.1
- - - long-term effect 429.4
- cardiorenal 404.9
- catheter device NEC 996.7
- - infection 996.6
- - inflammation 996.6
- - mechanical - see Complications, mechanical, catheter
- cesarean section wound 674.3
- chin implant (prosthetic) NEC 996.7
- - infection or inflammation 996.6
- - mechanical 996.5
- contraceptive device, intrauterine NEC 996.7
- - infection 996.6
- - inflammation 996.6
- - mechanical 996.3
- cord (umbilical) - see Complications, umbilical cord

Complications - *continued*
- delivery 669.9
- - procedure (instrumental) (manual) (surgical) 669.4
- - specified NEC 669.8
- dialysis (hemodialysis) (peritoneal) (renal) NEC 999.9
- - catheter NEC 996.7
- - - infection 996.6
- - - inflammation 996.6
- - - mechanical 996.1
- due to (presence of) any device, implant or graft classified to 996.0 - 996.5 NEC 996.7
- - infection 996.6
- - inflammation 996.6
- - mechanical - see Complications, mechanical
- during dialysis NEC 999.9
- ectopic or molar pregnancy NEC 639.9
- electroshock therapy NEC 999.9
- extracorporeal circulation NEC 999.9
- eye implant (prosthetic) NEC 996.7
- - infection or inflammation 996.6
- - mechanical 996.5
- gastrointestinal, postoperative NEC 997.4
- genitourinary device, implant or graft NEC 996.7
- - infection or inflammation 996.6
- - mechanical 996.3
- graft (bypass) (patch) NEC 996.7
- - bone marrow NEC 999.8
- - infection 996.6
- - inflammation 996.6
- - mechanical - see Complications, mechanical, graft
- - organ (immune or nonimmune cause) (partial) (total) 996.8
- - skin NEC 996.7
- - - infection 996.6
- - - rejection 996.5
- heart - see Disease, heart
- hyperalimentation therapy NEC 999.9
- immunization (procedure) - see Complications, vaccination
- implant NEC 996.7
- - infection 996.6
- - inflammation 996.6
- - mechanical - see Complications, mechanical
- infusion (procedure) NEC 999.9
- - blood - see Complications, transfusion
- - infection NEC 999.3
- - sepsis NEC 999.3
- inhalation therapy NEC 999.9
- injection (procedure NEC) 999.9

Complications - *continued*
- injection - *continued*
- - drug reaction (see also Reaction, drug) 995.2
- - infection NEC 999.3
- - sepsis NEC 999.3
- - serum (prophylactic) (therapeutic) - see Complications, vaccination
- - vaccine (any) - see Complications, vaccination
- inoculation (any) - see Complications, vaccination
- internal device (catheter) (electronic) (fixation) (prosthetic) NEC 996.7
- - infection 996.6
- - inflammation 996.6
- - mechanical - see Complications, mechanical
- labor 669.9
- - specified NEC 669.8
- lumbar puncture 349.0
- mechanical 996.-
- - anastomosis - see Complications, mechanical, graft
- - bypass - see Complications, mechanical, graft
- - catheter NEC 996.5
- - - cardiac 996.0
- - - cystostomy 996.3
- - - dialysis 996.1
- - - during a procedure 998.2
- - - urethral, indwelling 996.3
- - device NEC 996.5
- - - balloon (counterpulsation), intra-aortic 996.1
- - - cardiac 996.0
- - - - long-term effect 429.4
- - - contraceptive, intrauterine 996.3
- - - counterpulsation, intra-aortic 996.1
- - - fixation, internal (nail, rod, plate) 996.4
- - - genitourinary 996.3
- - - nervous system 996.2
- - - orthopedic, internal 996.4
- - - prosthetic NEC 996.5
- - - umbrella, vena cava 996.1
- - - vascular 996.1
- - dorsal column stimulator 996.2
- - electrode NEC 996.5
- - - brain 996.2
- - - cardiac 996.0
- - - spinal column 996.2
- - fistula, arteriovenous, surgically created 996.1
- - graft NEC 996.5
- - - aortic (bifurcation) 996.1
- - - blood vessel NEC 996.1

Complications - *continued*
- mechanical - *continued*
- - graft NEC - *continued*
- - - bone 996.4
- - - cardiac 996.0
- - - carotid artery bypass 996.1
- - - cartilage 996.4
- - - coronary bypass 996.0
- - - genitourinary 996.3
- - - muscle 996.4
- - - nervous system 996.2
- - - organ (immune or nonimmune cause) 996.8
- - - orthopedic, internal 996.4
- - - peripheral nerve 996.2
- - - prosthetic NEC 996.5
- - - skin 996.5
- - - specified NEC 996.5
- - - tendon 996.4
- - - tooth 996.5
- - - ureter, without mention of resection 996.3
- - - vascular 996.1
- - heart valve prosthesis 996.0
- - - long-term effect 429.4
- - implant NEC 996.5
- - - cardiac 996.0
- - - - long-term effect 429.4
- - - electrode NEC 996.5
- - - - brain 996.2
- - - - cardiac 996.0
- - - - spinal column 996.2
- - - nervous system 996.2
- - - orthopedic, internal 996.4
- - - prosthetic 996.5
- - - - in
- - - - - bile duct 996.5
- - - - - breast 996.5
- - - - - chin 996.5
- - - - - orbit of eye 996.5
- - - vascular 996.1
- - nonabsorbable surgical material 996.5
- - pacemaker NEC 996.5
- - - brain 996.2
- - - cardiac 996.0
- - - nerve (phrenic) 996.2
- - patch - see Complications, mechanical, graft
- - prosthesis NEC 996.5
- - - reconstruction, vas deferens 996.3
- - reimplant NEC 996.5
- - - extremity 996.9
- - - organ 996.8
- - repair - see Complications, mechanical, graft
- - shunt NEC 996.5

Complications - *continued*
- mechanical - *continued*
- - shunt NEC - *continued*
- - - arteriovenous, surgically created 996.1
- - - ventricular (communicating) 996.2
- medical care NEC 999.9
- - cardiac NEC 997.1
- - gastrointestinal 997.4
- - nervous system NEC 997.0
- - peripheral vascular NEC 997.2
- - respiratory NEC 997.3
- - urinary NEC 997.5
- nervous system
- - device, implant or graft NEC 349.1
- - - mechanical 996.2
- - postoperative NEC 997.0
- obstetric 669.9
- - procedure (instrumental) (manual) (surgical) 669.4
- - specified NEC 669.8
- - surgical wound 674.3
- orthopedic device, implant or graft
- - internal (fixation) (nail) (plate) (rod) NEC 996.7
- - - infection 996.6
- - - inflammation 996.6
- - - mechanical 996.4
- perfusion NEC 999.9
- perineal repair (obstetrical) 674.3
- - disruption 674.2
- phototherapy 999.9
- postmastoidectomy 383.3
- postoperative - see Complications, surgical procedures
- pregnancy NEC 646.9
- prosthetic device, internal NEC 996.7
- - infection 996.6
- - inflammation 996.6
- - mechanical NEC 996.5
- puerperium - see Puerperal
- puncture, spinal 349.0
- - headache or reaction 349.0
- radiation 990
- radiotherapy NEC 990
- reattached extremity (infection) (rejection) 996.9
- reimplant NEC 996.7
- - extremity 996.9
- - - due to infection 996.9
- - infection 996.6
- - mechanical - see Complications, mechanical, graft
- - organ (immune or nonimmune cause) (partial) (total) 996.8
- - prosthetic device NEC 996.7
- - - infection or inflammation 996.6

Complications - *continued*
- reimplant NEC - *continued*
- - prosthetic device NEC - *continued*
- - - mechanical - see Complications, mechanical
- respiratory 519.9
- - device, implant or graft NEC 996.7
- - - infection or inflammation 996.6
- - - mechanical 996.5
- - postoperative NEC 997.3
- - therapy NEC 999.9
- sedation during labor and delivery 668.9
- - cardiac 668.1
- - central nervous system 668.2
- - fetus or newborn 763.5
- - pulmonary 668.0
- shunt NEC 996.7
- - infection or inflammation 996.6
- - mechanical - see Complications, mechanical, shunt
- specified body system NEC
- - device, implant or graft NEC 996.7
- - - infection or inflammation 996.6
- - - mechanical 996.5
- - postoperative NEC 997.9
- spinal puncture or tap 349.0
- stoma, external
- - gastrointestinal tract NEC 997.4
- - urinary tract 997.5
- surgical procedures 998.9
- - accidental puncture or laceration 998.2
- - amputation stump (late) 997.6
- - burst stitches or sutures 998.3
- - cardiac 997.1
- - - long term effect following cardiac surgery 429.4
- - catheter device - see Complications, catheter device
- - colostomy malfunction 569.6
- - dehiscence (of incision) 998.3
- - dialysis NEC (see also Complications, dialysis) 999.9
- - disruption of wound 998.3
- - dumping syndrome (postgastrectomy) 564.2
- - elephantiasis or lymphedema 997.9
- - - postmastectomy 457.0
- - emphysema (surgical) 998.8
- - enterostomy malfunction 569.6
- - evisceration 998.3
- - fistula (peristent postoperative) 998.6
- - foreign body inadvertently left in wound (sponge) (suture) (swab) 998.4
- - gastrointestinal NEC 997.4
- - hemorrhage or hematoma 998.1
- - internal prosthetic device NEC 996.7
- - - hemolytic anemia 283.1

Complications - *continued*
- surgical procedures - *continued*

- - - internal prosthetic device NEC - *cont.*
- - - - infection 996.6
- - - - malfunction - see Complications, mechanical
- - - - mechanical complication - see Complications, mechanical
- - - - thrombus 996.7
- - - malfunction of colostomy or enterostomy 569.6
- - - nervous system NEC 997.0
- - - other body system NEC 997.9
- - - peripheral vascular NEC 997.2
- - - postcardiotomy syndrome 429.4
- - - postcholecystectomy syndrome 576.0
- - - postcommissurotomy syndrome 429.4
- - - postgastrectomy dumping syndrome 564.2
- - - postmastectomy lymphedema syndrome 457.0
- - - postvagotomy syndrome 564.2
- - - postvalvulotomy syndrome 429.4
- - - reattached extremity (infection) (rejection) 996.9
- - - respiratory NEC 997.3
- - - shock (endotoxic) (hypovolemic) (septic) 998.0
- - - shunt, prosthetic (hemolytic anemia) (thrombus) 996.7
- - - - infection or inflammation 996.6
- - - - malfunction or other mechanical complication - see Complications, mechanical, shunt
- - - specified NEC 998.8
- - - stitch abscess 998.5
- - - transplant - see Complications, graft
- - - urinary NEC 997.5
- - - wound infection 998.5

- transfusion (blood) (bone marrow) (lymphocytes) (plasma) 999.8
- - atrophy, liver, yellow, subacute (within 8 months of administration) 070.3 † 573.1*
- - - with hepatic coma 070.2 † 573.1*
- - embolism
- - - air 999.1
- - hemolysis 999.8
- - hepatitis (serum) (type B) (within 8 months of administration) 070.3 † 573.1*
- - - with hepatic coma 070.2 † 573.1*
- - incompatibility reaction (ABO) (blood group) 999.6
- - - Rh (factor) 999.7
- - infection 999.3

Complications - *continued*
- transfusion - *continued*

- - jaundice (serum) (within 8 months of administration) 070.3 † 573.1*
- - - with hepatic coma 070.2 † 573.1*
- - sepsis 999.3
- - shock or reaction NEC 999.8
- - thromboembolism 999.2
- - thrombus 999.2
- transplant NEC (see also Complications, graft) 996.7
- - organ (immune or nonimmune cause) (partial) (total) 996.8
- trauma NEC (early) 958.8
- ultrasound therapy NEC 999.9
- umbilical cord
- - complicating delivery 663.9
- - - specified NEC 663.8
- - fetus or newborn NEC 762.6
- urethral catheter NEC 996.7
- - infection 996.6
- - mechanical 996.3
- urinary, postoperative NEC 997.5
- vaccination 999.9
- - anaphylaxis NEC 999.4
- - cellulitis 999.3
- - encephalitis or encephalomyelitis 323.5
- - hepatitis (serum) (type B) (within 8 months of administration) 070.3 † 573.1*
- - - with hepatic coma 070.2 † 573.1*
- - infection (general) (local) NEC 999.3
- - jaundice (serum) (within 8 months of administration) 070.3 † 573.1*
- - - with hepatic coma 070.2 † 573.1*
- - meningitis 997.0 † 321.8*
- - myelitis 323.5
- - protein sickness 999.5
- - reaction (allergic) 999.9
- - - Herxheimer's 995.0
- - - serum 999.5
- - sepsis 999.3
- - serum intoxication, sickness, rash, or other serum reaction NEC 999.5
- - shock (allergic) (anaphylactic) 999.4
- - subacute yellow atrophy of liver (within 8 months of administration) 070.3 † 573.1*
- - - with hepatic coma 070.2 † 573.1*
- - vaccinia (generalized) 999.0
- - - localized 999.3
- vascular
- - device, implant or graft NEC 996.7
- - - infection or inflammation 996.6
- - - mechanical NEC 996.1
- - - - cardiac 996.0

Complications - *continued*
- vascular - *continued*
- - following infusion, perfusion or transfusion 999.2
- - postoperative NEC 997.2
- ventilation therapy NEC 999.9
Compressed air disease 993.3
Compression
- with injury - code by nature of injury
- artery 447.1
- - coeliac, syndrome 447.4
- brachial plexus 353.0
- brain (stem) 348.4
- - due to
- - - injury NEC (see also Hemorrhage, brain, traumatic) 853.0
- - - laceration or contusion, brain (see also Laceration, cerebral) 851.0
- bronchus 519.1
- by cicatrix - see Cicatrix
- cauda equina 344.6
- cerebral - see Compression, brain
- cord (umbilical) - see Compression, umbilical cord
- divers' squeeze 993.3
- during birth 767.9
- esophagus 530.3
- eustachian tube 381.6
- facies 754.0
- fracture - see Fracture
- heart - see Disease, heart
- intestine (see also Obstruction, intestine) 560.9
- laryngeal nerve, recurrent 478.7
- lumbosacral plexus 353.1
- lung 518.8
- lymphatic vessel 457.1
- medulla - see Compression, brain
- nerve NEC - see also Disorder, nerve
- - due to displacement of intervertebral disc 722.2
- - - with myelopathy (any site) 722.7 † 336.3*
- - - cervical 722.0
- - - lumbar, lumbosacral 722.1
- - - thoracic, thoracolumbar 722.1
- - median (in carpal tunnel) 354.0
- - optic 377.4
- - posterior tibial (in tarsal tunnel) 355.5
- - root NEC 724.9
- - sciatic (acute) 355.0
- - sympathetic 337.9
- - traumatic - see Injury, nerve
- oesophagus 530.3
- spinal (cord) 336.9
- - by displacement of intervertebral disc - see Displacement, intervertebral disc

Compression - *continued*
- spinal - *continued*
- - nerve
- - - root NEC 724.9
- - - - traumatic - see Injury, nerve, spinal
- - - traumatic - see Injury, nerve, spinal
- - spondylogenic 721.9 † 336.3*
- - - cervical 721.1 † 336.3*
- - - lumbar, lumbosacral 721.4 † 336.3*
- - - thoracic 721.4 † 336.3*
- - traumatic - see also Injury, spinal, by region
- - - with fracture, vertebra - code by region under Fracture, vertebra, with spinal cord lesion
- spondylogenic - see Compression, spinal cord, spondylogenic
- sympathetic nerve NEC 337.9
- syndrome 958.5
- thorax 512
- trachea 519.1
- umbilical cord
- - complicating delivery 663.2
- - - cord
- - - - around neck 663.1
- - - - - prolapsed 663.0
- - fetus or newborn 762.5
- - - cord prolapsed 762.4
- vein 459.2
- vena cava (inferior) (superior) 459.2
- vertebral NEC - see Compression, spinal (cord)
Compulsion, compulsive
- neurosis (obsessive) 300.3
- personality 301.4
- states (mixed) 300.3
- swearing 300.3
- - in Gilles de la Tourette's syndrome 307.2
- tics and spasms 307.2
Concato's disease
- peritoneal 568.8
- pleural - see Pleurisy
Concavity chest wall 738.3
Concealed penis 752.8
Concrescence (teeth) 520.2
Concretio cordis 423.2
Concretion - see also Calculus
- appendicular 543
- canaliculus 375.5
- clitoris 624.8
- conjunctiva 372.5
- eyelid 374.5
- intestinal (impaction) (obstruction) 560.3
- lacrimal apparatus 375.5
- prepuce (male) 605

Concretion - see also Calculus - *continued*
- salivary gland (any) 527.5
- seminal vesicle 608.8
- stomach 537.8
- tonsil 474.8
Concussion (current) 850
- blast (air) (hydraulic) (immersion)
    (underwater)
- - abdomen or thorax - see Injury,
    internal, by site
- - brain - see Concussion, brain
- - ear (acoustic nerve trauma) 951.5
- - - with perforation, tympanic
    membrane 872.6
- - - - complicated 872.7
- brain 850
- - with skull fracture - see Fracture, skull
- cauda equina 952.4
- cerebral 850
- - with skull fracture - see Fracture, skull
- conus medullaris 952.4
- hydraulic - see Concussion, blast
- internal organ(s) - see Injury, internal, by
    site
- labyrinth (see also Injury, intracranial)
    854.0
- ocular 921.3
- - osseous labyrinth (see also Injury,
    intracranial) 854.0
- spinal (cord) - see also Injury, spinal, by
    region
- - due to
- - - broken
- - - - back - code by region under
    Fracture, vertebra, with spinal
    cord lesion
- - - - neck (closed) 806.0
- - - - - open 806.1
- - - fracture, vertebra - code by region
    under Fracture, vertebra, with spinal
    cord lesion 806.8
- syndrome 310.2
- underwater blast - see Concussion, blast
Condition - see also Disease
- psychiatric 298.9
- respiratory NEC
- - acute or subacute NEC 519.9
- - - due to
- - - - external agent 508.9
- - - - - specified NEC 508.8
- - - - fumes or vapors (chemical)
    (inhalation) 506.3
- - - - radiation 508.8
- - chronic NEC
- - - due to
- - - - external agent 508.9
- - - - - specified NEC 508.8

Condition - see also Disease - *continued*
- respiratory NEC - *continued*
- - chronic NEC - *continued*
- - - due to - *continued*
- - - - fumes or vapors (chemical)
    (inhalation) 506.4
- - - - radiation 508.8
- - due to
- - - external agent 508.9
- - - - specified NEC 508.8
- - - fumes or vapors (chemical)
    (inhalation) 506.9
Conduct disturbance 312.9
- adjustment reaction 309.3
- hyperkinetic 314.2
Condyloma 091.3
- acuminatum 078.1
- gonorrheal 098.0
- latum 091.3
- syphilitic 091.3
- - congenital 090.0
- venereal, syphilitic 091.3
Confinement - see also Delivery
Conflagration - see also Burn
- asphyxia (by inhalation of smoke, gases,
    fumes or vapors) 987.9
- - specified agent - see Table of drugs and
    chemicals
Confluent - see condition

Confusion, confused (mental) (state) 298.9
- epileptic 293.0
- psychogenic 298.2
- reactive (from emotional stress,
    psychological trauma) 298.2
Congelation 991.9
Congenital - see also condition
- aortic septum 747.2
- intrinsic factor deficiency 281.0
- malformation - see Anomaly

Congestion (chronic) (passive)
- bladder 596.8
- bowel 569.8
- brain (see also Disease, cerebrovascular
    NEC) 437.8
- - malarial 084.9
- breast 611.7
- bronchi 519.1
- bronchial tube 519.1
- cerebral - see Congestion, brain
- cerebrospinal - see Congestion, brain
- chest 514
- circulatory NEC 459.9
- duodenum 537.3
- eye 372.7
- general 799.8
- glottis 476.0

Congestion - *continued*
- heart (see also Failure, heart, congestive) 428.0
- hepatic 573.0
- hypostatic (lung) 514
- intestine 569.8
- intracranial - see Congestion, brain
- kidney 593.8
- labyrinth 386.5
- larynx 476.0
- liver 573.0
- lung 514
- - active or acute (see also Pneumonia) 486
- - - congenital 770.0
- - hypostatic 514
- malaria, malarial (brain) (fever) (see also Malaria) 084.6
- medulla - see Congestion, brain
- orbit, orbital 376.8
- - inflammatory (chronic) 376.1
- - - acute 376.0
- ovary 620.8
- pancreas 577.8
- pelvic, female 625.5
- pleural 511.0
- prostate (active) 602.1
- pulmonary - see Congestion, lung
- renal 593.8
- retina 362.8
- seminal vesicle 608.8
- spinal cord 336.1
- spleen 289.5
- stomach 537.8
- trachea 464.1
- urethra 599.8
- uterus 625.5
- viscera 799.8
Congestive - see Congestion
Conical
- cervix 622.6
- cornea 371.6
- teeth 520.2

Conjoined twins 759.4
Conjugal maladjustment V61.1
Conjunctiva - see condition

Conjunctivitis NEC 372.3
- acute (actinic) (allergic) (anaphylactic) (atopic) (catarrhal) (follicular) (infectious) (influenzal) (membranous) (mucopurulent) (pneumococcal) (pseudomembranous) (purulent) (pustular) (serous) (simple) (staphylococcal) (streptococcal) 372.0
- adenoviral (acute) NEC 077.3 † 372.0*
- Apollo 077.4 † 372.0*

Conjunctivitis NEC - *continued*
- blennorrhagic (neonatorum) 098.4 † 372.0*
- chlamydial 077.9 † 372.0*
- - specified NEC 077.8 † 372.0*
- chronic (nodosa) (petrificans) (phlyctenular) (vernal) 372.1
- diphtheritic 032.8 † 372.0*
- due to
- - enterovirus type 70 077.4 † 372.0*
- - syphilis 095 † 372.1*
- epidemic 077.1 † 370.4*
- - hemorrhagic 077.4 † 372.0*
- gonococcal (neonatorum) 098.4 † 372.0*
- granular (trachomatous) 076.1 † 372.0*
- hemorrhagic (acute) (epidemic) 077.4 † 372.0*
- inclusion 077.0 † 372.0*
- Koch-Week's 372.0
- meningococcic 036.8 † 372.0*
- Morax-Axenfeld 372.0
- neonatal 771.6
- - gonococcal 098.4 † 372.0*
- Newcastle's 077.8 † 372.0*
- of Beal 077.3 † 372.0*
- Parinaud's 372.0
- Reiter's 099.3 † 372.3*
- rosacea 695.3 † 372.3*
- swimming pool 077.0 † 372.0*
- trachomatous 076.1 † 372.0*
- tuberculous 017.3 † 370.3*
- tularemic 021 † 372.0*
- tularensis 021 † 372.0*
- viral 077.9 † 372.0*
- - specified NEC 077.8 † 372.0*
Conn's syndrome 255.1
Connective tissue - see condition
Conradi(-Hunermann) disease 756.5
Consanguinity V19.7
Consecutive - see condition
Consolidation lung (base) - see Pneumonia, lobar
Constipation (atonic) (simple) (spastic) 564.0
- drug induced
- - correct substance properly administered 564.0
- - overdose or wrong substance given or taken 977.9
- - - specified drug - see Table of drugs and chemicals
- neurogenic 564.0
- psychogenic 306.4
Constitutional - see also condition
- state, developmental V21.9
- - specified NEC V21.8
Constitutionally substandard 301.6

Constriction
- anomalous, meningeal bands or folds 742.8
- asphyxiation or suffocation by 994.7
- bronchi 519.1
- canal, ear 380.5
- duodenum 537.3
- gallbladder (see also Obstruction, gallbladder) 575.2
- intestine (see also Obstruction, intestine) 560.9
- larynx 478.7
- - congenital 748.3
- organ or site, congenital NEC - see Atresia
- prepuce (congenital) 605
- pylorus 537.0
- - adult hypertrophic 537.0
- - congenital or infantile 750.5
- ring (uterus) 661.4
- - fetus or newborn 763.7
- spastic - see also Spasm
- - ureter 593.3
- - urethra 599.8
- stomach 537.8
- ureter 593.3
- visual field (peripheral) (functional) 368.4
Constrictive - see condition
Consultation
- medical - see Counselling, medical
- without complaint or sickness V65.9
Consumption - see Tuberculosis
Contact
- with
- - cholera V01.0
- - communicable disease V01.9
- - - specified NEC V01.8
- - - viral NEC V01.7
- - German measles V01.4
- - poliomyelitis V01.2
- - rabies V01.5
- - rubella V01.4
- - smallpox V01.3
- - tuberculosis V01.1
- - venereal disease V01.6
- - viral disease NEC V01.7
- dermatitis - see Dermatitis
Contamination, food (see also Poisoning, food) 005.9
Contraception, contraceptive
- advice V25.0
- counselling V25.0
- device (intrauterine) (in situ) V45.5
- - causing menorrhagia 996.7
- - checking V25.4
- - complications 996.3

Contraception - *continued*
- device - *continued*
- - in place V45.5
- - insertion V25.1
- - reinsertion V25.4
- - removal V25.4
- maintenance V25.4
- - examination V25.4
- management NEC V25.9
- prescription V25.0
- - repeat V25.4
- surveillance V25.4

Contraction, contracture, contracted
- Achilles tendon (see also Short, tendon, Achilles) 727.8
- anus 564.8
- axilla 729.9
- bile duct (see also Disease, biliary) 576.8
- bladder 596.8
- - neck or sphincter 596.0
- bowel, cecum, colon or intestine, any part (see also Obstruction, intestine) 560.9
- bronchi 519.1
- burn (old) - see Cicatrix
- cervix (see also Stricture, cervix) 622.4
- - congenital 752.4
- cicatricial - see Cicatrix
- conjunctiva trachomatous, active 076.1 † 372.0*
- Dupuytren's 728.6
- eyelid 374.4
- face 729.9
- fascia (lata) (postural) 728.8
- finger NEC 736.2
- - congenital 755.5
- - joint (see also Contraction, joint) 718.4
- flaccid - see Contraction, paralytic
- gallbladder or gall duct (see also Disease, gallbladder) 575.2
- hamstring 728.8
- heart valve - see Endocarditis
- hip (see also Contraction, joint) 718.4
- hourglass
- - bladder 596.8
- - - congenital 753.8
- - gallbladder (see also Disease, gallbladder) 575.2
- - - congenital 751.6
- - stomach 536.8
- - - congenital 750.7
- - - psychogenic 306.4
- - uterus 661.4
- - - fetus or newborn 763.7
- hysterical 300.1
- infantile 345.6

Contraction - *continued*
- internal os (see also Stricture, cervix)
622.4
- joint (abduction) (acquired) (adduction)
(flexion) (rotation) 718.4
- - congenital NEC 755.8
- - - generalized or multiple 755.8
- - - - lower limb joints 754.8
- - - hip 754.3
- - - lower limb (including pelvic girdle)
not involving hip 754.8
- - - upper limb (including shoulder
girdle) 755.5
- - hysterical 300.1
- kidney (granular) (secondary) (see also
Sclerosis, renal) 587
- - congenital 753.3
- - hydronephritic 591
- - pyelonephritic (see also Pyelitis,
chronic) 590.0
- - tuberculous 016.0
- ligament 728.8
- - congenital 756.8
- muscle (postinfectional) (postural) NEC
728.8
- - congenital 756.8
- - extraocular 378.6
- - eye (extrinsic) (see also Strabismus)
378.9
- - - paralytic 378.5
- - hysterical 300.1
- - ischemic (Volkmann's) 958.6
- - psychogenic 306.0
- - - specified as conversion reaction
300.1
- neck (see also Torticollis) 723.5
- - psychogenic 306.0
- ocular muscle (see also Strabismus) 378.9
- - paralytic 378.5
- organ or site, congenital NEC - see
Atresia
- outlet (pelvis) - see Contraction, pelvis
- palmar fascia 728.6
- paralytic
- - joint (see also Contraction, joint)
718.4
- - muscle 728.8
- - - ocular (see also Strabismus) 378.5
- pelvis (acquired) (general) 738.6
- - in pregnancy or childbirth NEC 653.1
- - - causing obstructed labor 660.1
- - - fetus or newborn 763.1
- - - inlet 653.2
- - - outlet 653.3
- plantar fascia 728.7
- premature
- - auricular 427.6

Contraction - *continued*
- premature - *continued*
- - auriculoventricular 427.6
- - heart (atrial) (auricular)
(auriculoventricular) (junctional)
(nodal) (ventricular) 427.6
- - junctional 427.6
- - ventricular 427.6
- prostate 602.8
- pylorus (see also Pylorospasm) 537.8
- rectum, rectal (sphincter) 564.8
- - psychogenic 306.4
- ring (Bandl's) 661.4
- - fetus or newborn 763.7
- scar - see Cicatrix
- socket, eye 372.6
- spine 737.9
- sternocleidomastoid (muscle) 754.1
- stomach 536.8
- - hourglass 536.8
- - - congenital 750.7
- - - psychogenic 306.4
- - psychogenic 306.4
- tendon (sheath) (see also Short, tendon)
727.8
- toe 735.8
- ureterovesical orifice (postinfectional)
593.3
- urethra 599.8
- uterus 621.8
- - abnormal NEC 661.9
- - - fetus or newborn (any abnormality)
763.7
- - clonic 661.4
- - dyscoordinate 661.4
- - hourglass 661.4
- - hypotonic NEC 661.2
- - incoordinate 661.4
- - irregular 661.2
- - tetanic 661.4
- vagina (outlet) 623.2
- vesical 596.8
- - neck or urethral orifice 596.0
- visual field 368.4
- Volkmann's (ischemic) 958.6
Contusion (skin surface intact) 924.9
- with
- - crush injury - see Crush
- - dislocation - see Dislocation
- - fracture - see Fracture
- - internal injury - see Injury, internal
- - nerve injury - see Injury, nerve
- - open wound - see Wound, open
- abdomen, abdominal (muscle) (wall)
922.2
- - organs NEC 868.-
- adnexa, eye NEC 921.9

Contusion - *continued*
- ankle (and foot) 924.2
- arm 923.9
- - lower (and elbow) 923.1
- - upper (and shoulder) 923.0
- auditory canal (external) (meatus) (and other part(s) of neck, scalp, or face except eye) 920
- auricle, ear (and other part(s) of neck, scalp, or face except eye) 920
- axilla (and shoulder) (and upper arm) 923.0
- back 922.3
- bone NEC 924.9
- brain (any part) (with hemorrhage) 851.0
- - with
- - - open intracranial wound 851.1
- - - skull fracture - see Fracture, skull
- breast 922.0
- brow (and other part(s) of neck, scalp, or face except eye) 920
- buttock 922.3
- canthus 921.1
- cerebellum (see also Contusion, brain) 851.0
- cerebral (see also Contusion, brain) 851.0
- cheek(s) (and other part(s) of neck, scalp, or face except eye) 920
- chest (wall) 922.1
- chin (and other part(s) of neck, scalp, or face except eye) 920
- clitoris 922.4
- conjunctiva 921.2
- cornea 921.3
- corpus cavernosum 922.4
- cortex (brain) (cerebral) (see also Contusion, brain) 851.0
- costal region 922.1
- elbow (and forearm) 923.1
- epididymis 922.4
- epigastric region 922.2
- eye NEC 921.9
- eyeball 921.3
- eyelid(s) (and periocular area) 921.1
- face (any part, except eye(s), and neck or scalp) 920
- femoral triangle 922.2
- fetus or newborn 772.6
- finger(s) (nail) (subungual) 923.3
- flank 922.2
- foot (excluding toe(s)) 924.2
- forearm (and elbow) 923.1
- forehead (and other part(s) of neck, scalp, or face except eye) 920
- genital organs, external 922.4
- globe (eye) 921.3
- groin 922.2

Contusion - *continued*
- gum(s) (and other part(s) of neck, scalp, or face except eye) 920
- hand(s) (except fingers alone) 923.2
- head (any part, except eye) (and face) (and neck) 920
- heel 924.2
- hip (and thigh) 924.0
- iliac region 922.2
- inguinal region 922.2
- internal organs (abdomen, chest or pelvis) - see Injury, internal, by site
- interscapular region 922.3
- iris (eye) 921.3
- knee (and lower leg) 924.1
- labius (majus) (minus) 922.4
- lacrimal apparatus, gland or sac 921.1
- larynx (and other parts of neck, scalp or face, except eye) 920
- leg 924.5
- - lower 924.1
- lens 921.3
- lingual (and other parts of neck, scalp or face, except eye) 920
- lip(s) (and other part(s) of neck, scalp, or face except eye) 920
- lower extremity 924.5
- - multiple sites 924.4
- lumbar region 922.3
- malar region (and other part(s) of neck, scalp, or face except eye) 920
- mandibular joint (and other part(s) of neck, scalp, or face except eye) 920
- mastoid region (and other part(s) of neck, scalp, or face except eye) 920
- membrane, brain (see also Contusion, brain) 851.0
- midthoracic region 922.1
- mouth (and other part(s) of neck, scalp, or face except eye) 920
- multiple sites (not classifiable to same three-digit category) 924.8
- - lower limb 924.4
- - trunk 922.8
- - upper limb 923.8
- muscle NEC 924.9
- nasal (septum) (and other part(s) of neck, scalp, or face except eye) 920
- neck (and scalp, or face any part except eye) 920
- nerve - see Injury, nerve, by site
- nose (and other part(s) of neck, scalp, or face except eye) 920
- occipital region (scalp) (and neck or face, except eye) 920
- - lobe (see also Contusion, brain) 851.0
- orbit (region) (tissues) 921.2

Contusion - *continued*
- palate (soft) (and other part(s) of neck, scalp, or face except eye) 920
- parietal region (scalp) (and neck or face, except eye) 920
- – lobe (see also Contusion, brain) 851.0
- penis 922.4
- perineum 922.4
- periocular area 921.1
- pharynx (and other part(s) of neck, scalp, or face except eye) 920
- popliteal space (and lower leg) 924.1
- prepuce 922.4
- pubic region 922.4
- pudenda 922.4
- quadriceps femoris 924.0
- rib cage 922.1
- sacral region 922.3
- salivary ducts or glands (and other part(s) of neck, scalp, or face except eye) 920
- scalp (and neck, or face any part except eye) 920
- scapular region 923.0
- sclera (eye) 921.3
- scrotum 922.4
- shoulder (and upper arm) 923.0
- skin NEC 924.9
- spermatic cord 922.4
- spinal cord - see also Injury, spinal, by region
- – cauda equina 952.4
- – conus medullaris 952.4
- sternal region 922.1
- stomach 863.0
- – with open wound into cavity 863.1
- subconjunctival 921.2
- subcutaneous NEC 924.9
- submaxillary region (and other part(s) of neck, scalp, or face except eye) 920
- submental region (and other part(s) of neck, scalp, or face except eye) 920
- subperiosteal NEC 924.9
- supraclavicular fossa (and other parts of neck, scalp, or face except eye) 920
- supra-orbital (and other part(s) of neck, scalp, or face except eye) 920
- temple (region) (and other part(s) of neck, scalp, or face except eye) 920
- testis 922.4
- thigh (and hip) 924.0
- thorax 922.1
- – organ - see Injury, internal, intrathoracic
- throat (and other part(s) of neck, scalp, or face except eye) 920
- thumb(s) (nail) (subungual) 923.3
- toe(s) (nail) (subungual) 924.3

Contusion - *continued*
- tongue (and other part(s) of neck, scalp, or face except eye) 920
- trunk 922.9
- – multiple sites 922.8
- – specified site - code by site under Contusion
- tunica vaginalis 922.4
- tympanum (membrane) (and other part(s) of neck, scalp, or face except eye) 920
- upper extremity 923.9
- – multiple sites 923.8
- uvula (and other part(s) of neck, scalp, or face except eye) 920
- vagina 922.4
- vocal cord(s) (and other parts of neck, scalp, or face except eye) 920
- vulva 922.4
- wrist 923.2
Conus (congenital) (any type) 743.5
- acquired 371.6
- medullaris syndrome 336.8
Convalescence (following) V66.9
- chemotherapy V66.2
- psychotherapy V66.3
- radiotherapy V66.1
- surgery NEC V66.0
- treatment (for) NEC V66.5
- – combined V66.6
- – fracture V66.4
- – mental disorder NEC V66.3
- – specified disorder NEC V66.5
Conversion
- hysteria, hysterical, any type 300.1
- neurosis, any 300.1
- reaction, any 300.1
Convulsions (idiopathic) 780.3
- apoplectiform (see also Disease, cerebrovascular, acute) 436
- due to trauma NEC - see Injury, intracranial
- epileptic (see also Epilepsy) 345.9
- epileptiform (see also Seizure, epileptiform) 780.3
- epileptoid (see also Seizure, epileptiform) 780.3
- ether
- – anesthetic
- – – correct substance properly administered 780.3
- – – overdose or wrong substance given 968.2
- – other specified type - see Table of drugs and chemicals
- febrile 780.3
- generalized 780.3

Convulsions - *continued*
- hysterical 300.1
- infantile 780.3
- - epilepsy - see Epilepsy
- jacksonian 345.5
- myoclonic 333.2
- newborn 779.0
- paretic 094.1
- pregnancy (nephritic) (uremic) - see Eclampsia, pregnancy
- psychomotor 345.4
- puerperal, postpartum - see Eclampsia, pregnancy
- reflex 781.0
- scarlatinal 034.1
- tetanus, tetanic (see also Tetanus) 037
- thymic 254.8
- uremic 586
Convulsive - see also Convulsions
- equivalent, abdominal 345.5
Cooley's anemia 282.4
Cooper's
- disease 610.1
- hernia - see Hernia, abdominal
Copra itch 133.8
Coprolith 560.3
Coprostasis 560.3
Cor
- biloculare 745.7
- bovinum - see Hypertrophy, cardiac
- bovis - see Hypertrophy, cardiac
- pulmonale (chronic) 416.9
- - acute 415.0
- triatriatum, triatrium 746.8
- triloculare 746.8
- - biatriatum 745.3
- - biventriculare 745.6
Corbus' disease 607.1
Cord - see also condition
- around neck (tightly) (with compression)
- - affecting fetus or newborn 762.5
- - complicating delivery 663.2
- bladder 344.6
- - tabetic 094.0
Cordis ectopia 746.8
Corditis (spermatic) 608.4
Corectopia 743.4
Cori type glycogen storage disease - see Disease, glycogen storage
Corkhandlers' disease or lung 495.3
Corkscrew esophagus 530.5
Corlett's pyosis 684
Corn (infected) 700
Cornea - see also condition
- guttata (dystrophy) 371.5
- plana 743.4
Cornu cutaneum 702

Cornual gestation or pregnancy - see Pregnancy, cornual
Coronary (artery) - see condition
Corpora - see also condition
- amylacea, prostate 602.8
- cavernosa - see condition
Corpulence (see also Obesity) 278.0
Corpus - see condition
Corrosive burn - see Burn
Corsican fever (see also Malaria) 084.6
Cortical - see condition
Cortico-adrenal - see condition
Coryza (acute) 460
- with grippe or influenza 487.1
- syphilitic 095
- - congenital (chronic) 090.0
Costen's syndrome or complex 524.6
Costiveness (see also Constipation) 564.0
Cough 786.2
- with hemorrhage (see also Hemoptysis) 786.3
- bronchial 786.2
- - with grippe or influenza 487.1
- chronic 786.2
- epidemic 786.2
- functional 306.1
- hysterical 300.1
- laryngeal, spasmodic 786.2
- nervous 786.2
- psychogenic 306.1
- smokers' 491.0
- tea tasters' 112.8
Counselling NEC V65.9
- dietary V65.3
- for non-attending third party V65.1
- genetic V26.3
- health (advice) (education) (instruction) (see also Counselling, medical) V65.4
- medical (for) V65.9
- - boarding school resident V60.6
- - condition not demonstrated V65.5
- - feared complaint and no disease found V65.5
- - institutional resident V60.1
- - on behalf of another V65.1
- - person living alone V60.3
- procreative V26.4
- sex V65.4
- specified NEC V65.4
Coupled rhythm 427.8
Couvelaire uterus (complicating delivery) - see Placenta, separation
Cowper's gland - see condition
Cowperitis (see also Urethritis) 597.8
Cowpox 051.0
- eyelid 051.0 † 373.5*
Coxa

Coxa - *continued*
- plana 732.1
- valga or vara (acquired) 736.3
- - congenital 755.6
- - late effects of rickets 268.1
Coxae malum senilis 715.2
Coxalgia (nontuberculous) 719.4
- tuberculous 015.1 † 730.5*
Coxalgic pelvis 736.3
Coxitis 716.6
Coxsackie (virus) (infection) 079.2
- carditis 074.2 † 422.0*
- central nervous system NEC 048
- endocarditis 074.2 † 421.1*
- enteritis 008.6
- meningitis (aseptic) 047.0 † 321.1*
- myocarditis 074.2 † 422.0*
- pericarditis 074.2 † 420.0*
- pharyngitis 074.0
- pleurodynia 074.1
- specific disease NEC 074.8
Crabs, meaning pubic lice 132.2
Cracked nipple 611.2
- puerperal, postpartum 676.1
Craft neurosis 300.8
Craigiasis 007.8
Cramp(s) 729.8
- abdominal 789.0
- bathing 994.1
- colic 789.0
- - psychogenic 306.4
- extremity (lower) (upper) NEC 729.8
- fireman 992.2
- heat 992.2
- immersion 994.1
- intestinal 789.0
- - psychogenic 306.4
- linotypist's 300.8
- - organic 333.8
- muscle (extremity) (general) 729.8
- - due to immersion 994.1
- - hysterical 300.1
- occupational (hand) 300.8
- - organic 333.8
- salt-depletion 276.1
- stoker 992.2
- telegrapher's 300.8
- - organic 333.8
- typist's 300.8
- - organic 333.8
- uterus 625.8
- - menstrual 625.3
- writer's 300.8
- - organic 333.8
Cranial - see condition
Cranioclasis 763.8
Craniocleidodysostosis 755.5

Craniofenestria (skull) 756.0
Craniolacunia (skull) 756.0
Craniopagus 759.4
Craniopathy, metabolic 733.3
Craniopharyngeal - see condition
Craniopharyngioma (M9350/1) 237.0
Craniorachischisis (totalis) 740.1
Cranioschisis 756.0
Craniostenosis 756.0
Craniosynostosis 756.0

Craniotabes (cause unknown) 733.3
- rachitic 268.1
- syphilitic 090.5
Craniotomy, fetal 763.8
Cranium - see condition
Craw-craw 125.3
Creaking joint 719.6
Creeping palsy or paralysis 335.2
Crenated tongue 529.8
Creotoxism 005.9
Crepitus
- caput 756.0
- joint 719.6
Crescent or conus choroid, congenital 743.5
Cretin 243
- pelvis 243
- - with disproportion 653.0
- - - causing obstructed labor 660.1
- - - fetus or newborn 763.1
Cretinism (congenital) (endemic)
   (nongoitrous) (sporadic) 243
- pituitary 253.3
Cretinoid degeneration 243

Creutzfeldt-Jakob syndrome 046.1 † 331.5*
- with dementia 290.1
Crib death 798.0
Cribriform hymen 752.4
Crigler-Najjar disease or syndrome 277.4
Criminalism 301.7
Crisis
- abdomen 789.0
- addisonian 255.4
- adrenal (cortical) 255.4
- brain, cerebral (see also Disease,
   cerebrovascular, acute) 436
- emotional NEC 309.2
- - acute reaction to stress 308.0
- - adjustment reaction 309.9
- - specific to childhood and adolescence
   313.9
- gastric (tabetic) 094.0
- glaucomatocyclitic 364.2
- heart (see also Failure, heart) 428.9
- nitritoid
- - correct substance properly
   administered 458.9

Crisis - *continued*
- nitritoid - *continued*
- − overdose or wrong substance given or taken 961.1
- oculogyric 378.8
- − psychogenic 306.7
- Pel's 094.0
- rectum 094.0
- renal 593.8
- stomach (tabetic) 094.0
- tabetic 094.0
- thyroid (see also Hyperthyroidism) 242.9
- thyrotoxic (see also Thyrotoxicosis) 242.9
- vascular - see Disease, cerebrovascular, acute
Crohn's disease - see Disease, Crohn's
Crooked septum, nasal 470
Cross eye 378.0
Crossbite (anterior) (posterior) 524.2
Crossed ectopia of kidney 753.3
Croup, croupous (angina) (catarrhal) (infectious) (inflammatory) (laryngeal) (membranous) (nondiphtheritic) (pseudomembranous) 464.4
- asthmatic 493.9
- bronchial 466.0
- diphtheritic 032.3
- false 478.7
- spasmodic 478.7
- − diphtheritic 032.3
- stridulous 478.7
- − diphtheritic 032.3
Crouzon's disease 756.0
Crowding, tooth, teeth 524.3
Cruchet's disease 049.8 † 323.4*
Cruelty in children - see Disturbance, conduct
Crush, crushed, crushing 929.9
- with fracture - see Fracture
- ankle (and foot, excluding toe(s) alone) 928.2
- arm 927.9
- − lower (and elbow) 927.1
- − upper (and shoulder) 927.0
- axilla 927.0
- back 926.1
- breast 926.1
- buttock 926.1
- cheek 925
- chest - see Injury, internal, chest
- ear 925
- elbow (and forearm) 927.1
- face 925
- finger(s) (and thumb(s)) 927.3
- − with hand(s) (and wrist(s)) 927.2
- foot, excluding toe(s) alone (and ankle) 928.2

Crush - *continued*
- forearm (and elbow) 927.1
- genitalia, external (male) (female) 926.0
- hand, except finger(s) alone (and wrist) 927.2
- head - see Fracture, skull
- heel 928.2
- hip (and thigh) 928.0
- internal organ (abdomen, chest, or pelvis) - see Injury, internal, by site
- knee (and leg, lower) 928.1
- labium (majus) (minus) 926.0
- larynx 925
- leg 928.9
- − lower (and knee) 928.1
- − upper (and hip) 928.0
- limb
- − lower 928.9
- − − multiple sites (classifiable to more than one subcategory in 928.0-928.3) 928.8
- − upper 927.9
- − − multiple sites (classifiable to more than one subcategory in 927.0-927.3) 927.8
- multiple sites NEC 929.0
- neck 925
- nerve - see Injury, nerve, by site
- nose 802.0
- − open 802.1
- penis 926.0
- pharynx 925
- scalp 925
- scapular region 927.0
- scrotum 926.0
- severe, unspecified site 869.1
- shoulder (and upper arm) 927.0
- skull or cranium - see Fracture, skull
- spinal cord - see Injury, spinal, by region
- syndrome (complication of trauma) 958.5
- testis 926.0
- thigh (and hip) 928.0
- throat 925
- thumb(s) (and finger(s)) 927.3
- toe(s) 928.3
- − with foot (and ankle) 928.2
- trunk 926.9
- − internal organ - see Injury, internal, by site
- − multiple sites 926.8
- − specified site NEC 926.1
- vulva 926.0
- wrist (and hand, except finger(s) alone) 927.2
Crusta lactea 691.8
Crutch paralysis 953.4
Cruveilhier's disease 335.2

Cruveilhier-Baumgarten cirrhosis, disease
or syndrome 571.5
Cryoglobulinemia (mixed) 273.2
Crypt, anal 569.4
Cryptitis (anal) (rectal) 569.4
Cryptococcosis (European) (pulmonary)
(systemic) 117.5
Cryptococcus
— epidermicus 117.5
— neoformans, infection by 117.5
Cryptopapillitis (anus) 569.4
Cryptophthalmos 743.0
Cryptorchid, cryptorchism, cryptorchidism
752.5
Crystalluria 791.9
Cuban itch 050.1
Cubitus valgus or varus (acquired) 736.0
— congenital 755.5
— late effects of rickets 268.1
Cultural deprivation or shock V62.4
Curling's ulcer - see Ulcer, duodenum
Curvature
— organ or site, congenital NEC - see
Distortion
— penis (lateral) 752.8
— Pott's (spinal) 015.0 † 737.4*
— radius, idiopathic, progressive
(congenital) 755.5
— spine (acquired) (angular) (idiopathic)
(incorrect) (postural) 737.9
— — congenital 754.2
— — due to or associated with
— — — Charcot-Marie-Tooth disease
356.1 † 737.4*
— — — osteitis
— — — — deformans 731.0 † 737.4*
— — — — fibrosa cystica 252.0 † 737.4*
— — — tuberculosis (Pott's curvature)
015.0 † 737.4*
— — late effects of rickets 268.1 † 737.4*
— — tuberculous 015.0 † 737.4*
Cushing's
— basophilism, disease or syndrome
(iatrogenic) (idiopathic)
(pituitary-dependent) 255.0
— ulcer - see Ulcer, peptic
Cushingoid due to steroid therapy
— correct substance properly administered
255.0
— overdose or wrong substance given or
taken 962.0
Cut (external) - see Wound, open
Cutis - see also condition
— hyperelastic 757.3
— — acquired 701.8
— laxa - see also Dermatolysis
— — senilis 701.8

Cutis - see also condition - *continued*
— marmorata 782.6
— osteosis 709.3
— pendula - see Dermatolysis
— rhomboidalis nuchae 701.8
— verticis gyrata 757.3
— — acquired 701.8
Cyanosis 782.5
— congenital 770.8
— conjunctiva 372.7
— enterogenous 289.7
— fetus or newborn 770.8
— paroxysmal digital 443.0
— retina, retinal 362.1
Cycle
— anovulatory 628.0
— menstrual, irregular 626.4
Cyclencephaly 759.8
Cyclical vomiting 536.2
— psychogenic 306.4
Cyclitic membrane 364.7
Cyclitis (see also Iridocyclitis) 364.3
— Fuch's heterochromic 364.2
— posterior 363.2
Cyclophoria 378.4
Cyclopia, cyclops 759.8
Cycloplegia 367.5
Cyclospasm 367.5
Cyclothymia 296.5
— currently
— — depressed 296.3
— — manic 296.2
— mixed 296.4
Cyclothymic personality 301.1
Cyclotropia 378.3
Cylindroma (M8200/3) - see also
Neoplasm, malignant
— eccrine dermal (M8200/0) - see
Neoplasm, skin, benign
— skin (M8200/0) - see Neoplasm, skin,
benign
Cylindruria 791.7
Cyllosoma 759.8
Cynanche
— diphtheritic 032.3
— tonsillaris 475
Cyphosis - see Kyphosis
Cyst (colloid) (epidermoid) (epithelial)
(mucous) (retention) (serous) (simple)
(solitary)

Note — In general, cysts are not neoplastic
and are classified to the appropriate category
for disease of the specified anatomical site.
This generalization does not apply to certain
types of cysts which are neoplastic in nature,
for example, dermoid, nor does it apply to

cysts of certain structures, for example, branchial cleft, which are classified as developmental anomalies.

The following listing includes some of the most frequently reported sites of cysts as well as qualifiers which indicate the type of cyst. The latter qualifiers usually are not repeated under the anatomical sites. Since the code assignment for a given site may vary depending upon the type of cyst, the coder should refer to the listings under the specified type of cyst before consideration is given to the site.

Cyst - *continued*
- cornea 371.2
- corpora quadrigemina 348.0
- corpus
- - albicans 620.2
- - luteum (ruptured) 620.1
- Cowper's gland (benign) (infected) 599.8
- cranial meninges 348.0
- craniobuccal pouch 253.8
- craniopharyngeal pouch 253.8
- cystic duct (see also Disease, gallbladder) 575.8
- cysticercus 123.1
- Dandy-Walker 742.3
- - with spina bifida 741.0
- dental 522.8
- - developmental 526.0
- - eruption 526.0
- - lateral periodontal 526.0
- - primordial 526.0
- - root 522.8
- dentigerous 526.0
- - mandible 526.0
- - maxilla 526.0
- dermoid (M9084/0) - see also Neoplasm, benign
- - with malignant transformation (M9084/3) 183.0
- - implantation
- - - external area or site (skin) NEC 709.8
- - - iris 364.6
- - - vagina 623.8
- - - vulva 624.8
- - mouth 528.4
- - oral soft tissue 528.4
- developmental of ovary, ovarian 752.0
- dura (cerebral) 348.0
- - spinal 349.2
- ear (external) 706.2
- echinococcal (see also Echinococcus) 122.9
- endometrial 621.8
- - ectopic 617.9
- endometrium (uterus) 621.8
- enteric 751.5
- enterogenous 751.5
- epidermal (inclusion) (see also Cyst, skin) 706.2
- epidermoid (inclusion) (see also Cyst, skin) 706.2
- - mouth 528.4
- - oral soft tissue 528.4
- epididymis 608.8
- epiglottis 478.7
- epiphysis cerebri 259.8

Cyst - *continued*
- epithelial (inclusion) (see also Cyst, skin) 706.2
- epoophoron 752.1
- eruption 526.0
- esophagus 530.8
- ethmoid sinus 478.1
- eye 379.8
- - congenital 743.0
- eyebrow 706.2
- eyelid (sebaceous) 373.3
- - infected 373.1
- falciform ligament (inflammatory) 573.8
- fallopian tube 620.8
- female genital organs NEC 624.8
- fimbrial 752.1
- fissural (oral region) 526.1
- follicle (graafian) 620.0
- - nabothian 616.0
- follicular (atretic) (ovarian) 620.0
- - dentigerous 526.0
- frontal sinus 478.1
- gallbladder or duct 575.8
- ganglion 727.4
- Gartner's duct 752.1
- gingiva 523.8
- gland of Moll 374.8
- globulo-maxillary 526.1
- graafian follicle 620.0
- granulosa lutein 620.2
- hemangiomatous (M9121/0) 228.0
- hydatid (see also Echinococcus) 122.9
- - liver NEC 122.8
- - lung NEC 122.9
- - Morgagni 752.8
- - specified site NEC 122.9
- hymen 623.8
- - embryonal 752.4
- hypopharynx 478.2
- hypophysis, hypophyseal (duct) (recurrent) 253.8
- - cerebri 253.8
- implantation (dermoid)
- - external area or site (skin) NEC 709.8
- - iris 364.6
- - vagina 623.8
- - vulva 624.8
- incisor canal 526.1
- inclusion (epidermal) (epithelial) (epidermoid) (squamous) (see also Cyst, skin) 706.2
- - not of skin - code by site under Cyst
- intestine (large) (small) 569.8
- intracranial - see Cyst, brain
- intraligamentous 728.8
- - knee 717.8
- intrasellar 253.8

Cyst - *continued*
- iris (exudative) (implantation) 364.6
- jaw (bone) (aneurysmal) (hemorrhagic) (traumatic) 526.2
- - developmental (odontogenic) 526.0
- - fissural 526.1
- kidney (congenital) (multiple) 753.1
- - acquired 593.2
- - calyceal (see also Hydronephrosis) 591
- - pyelogenic (see also Hydronephrosis) 591
- - solitary (not congenital) 593.2
- labium (majus) (minus) 624.8
- - sebaceous 624.8
- lacrimal apparatus or sac 375.4
- larynx 478.7
- lens 379.3
- - congenital 743.3
- lip (gland) 528.5
- liver 573.8
- - congenital 751.6
- - hydatid 122.8
- - - granulosus 122.0
- - - multilocularis 122.5
- lung 518.8
- - congenital 748.4
- - giant bullous 492
- lutein 620.1
- lymphangiomatous (M9173/0) 228.1
- lymphoepithelial
- - oral soft tissue 528.4
- malignant (M8000/3) - see Neoplasm, malignant
- mammary gland - see Cyst, breast
- mandible 526.2
- - dentigerous 526.0
- - radicular 522.8
- maxilla 526.2
- - dentigerous 526.0
- - radicular 522.8
- median palatal 526.1
- meibomian (gland) 373.2
- - infected 373.1
- membrane brain 348.0
- meninges (cerebral) 348.0
- - spinal 349.2
- meniscus knee 717.5
- mesentery, mesenteric 568.8
- - chyle 457.8
- - gas 568.8
- mesonephric duct 752.8
- milk 611.5
- Morgagni (hydatid) 752.8
- mouth 528.4
- muellerian duct 752.1
- multilocular (ovary) (M8000/1) 239.5
- myometrium 621.8

Cyst - *continued*
- nabothian (follicle) (ruptured) 616.0
- nasoalveolar 528.4
- nasolabial 528.4
- nasopalatine (duct) 526.1
- nasopharynx 478.2
- neoplastic (M8000/1) - see also Neoplasm, unspecified nature
- - benign (M8000/0) - see Neoplasm, benign
- nervous system - see Cyst, brain
- neuroenteric 742.5
- nipple 610.0
- nose 478.1
- - skin of 706.2
- odontogenic, developmental 526.0
- oesophagus 530.8
- omentum (lesser) 568.8
- - congenital 751.8
- ora serrata 361.1
- oral soft tissue (dermoid) (epidermoid) (lymphoepithelial) 528.4
- orbit 376.8
- ovary, ovarian (twisted) 620.2
- - adherent 620.2
- - chocolate 617.1
- - corpus
- - - albicans 620.2
- - - luteum 620.1
- - dermoid (M9084/0) 220
- - developmental 752.0
- - due to failure or involution NEC 620.2
- - follicular (graafian) (hemorrhagic) 620.0
- - hemorrhagic 620.2
- - in pregnancy or childbirth 654.4
- - - with obstructed labor 660.2
- - - - fetus or newborn 763.1
- - - fetus or newborn 763.8
- - multilocular (M8000/1) 239.5
- - pseudomucinous (M8470/0) 220
- - retention 620.2
- - serous 620.2
- - theca lutein 620.2
- - tuberculous 016.4
- - unspecified 620.2
- oviduct 620.8
- palatal papilla (jaw) 526.1
- palate 526.1
- - fissural 526.1
- - median (fissural) 526.1
- pancreas, pancreatic 577.2
- - congenital 751.7
- - false 577.2
- - hemorrhagic 577.2
- - true 577.2
- paraovarian 752.1

Cyst - *continued*
- paraphysis, cerebri 742.4
- parasitic NEC 136.9
- parathyroid (gland) 252.8
- paratubal 620.8
- paraurethral duct 599.8
- paroophoron 752.1
- parotid gland 527.6
- - mucous extravasation or retention 527.6
- parovarian 752.1
- pelvis, female
- - in pregnancy or childbirth 654.4
- - - causing obstructed labor 660.2
- - - - fetus or newborn 763.1
- - - - fetus or newborn 763.8
- penis 607.8
- - sebaceous 607.8
- periapical 522.8
- pericardial (congenital) 746.8
- pericoronal 526.0
- periodontal 522.8
- - lateral 526.0
- peripancreatic 577.2
- peritoneum 568.8
- - chylous 457.8
- pharynx (wall) 478.2
- pilonidal (infected) (rectum) 685.1
- - with abscess 685.0
- - malignant (M9084/3) 173.5
- pituitary (duct) (gland) 253.8
- placenta (amniotic) - see Placenta, abnormal
- pleura 519.8
- popliteal 757.5
- porencephalic 742.4
- - acquired 348.0
- postanal (infected) 685.1
- - with abscess 685.0
- postmastoidectomy cavity 383.3
- preauricular 744.4
- prepuce 607.8
- - congenital 752.8
- primordial (jaw) 526.0
- prostate 600
- pseudomucinous (ovary) (M8470/0) 220
- pupillary, miotic 364.5
- radicular (residual) 522.8
- ranular 527.6
- Rathke's pouch 253.8
- rectum (epithelium) (mucous) 569.4
- renal - see Cyst, kidney
- residual (radicular) 522.8
- retention (ovary) 620.2
- retina 361.1
- retroperitoneal 568.8
- salivary gland or duct 527.6

Cyst - *continued*
- salivary gland or duct - *continued*
- - mucous extravasation or retention 527.6
- Sampson's 617.1
- sclera 379.1
- scrotum 706.2
- - sebaceous 706.2
- sebaceous (duct) (gland) 706.2
- - breast 610.8
- - eyelid 373.3
- - genital organ NEC
- - - female 629.8
- - - male 608.8
- - scrotum 706.2
- semilunar cartilage (knee) (multiple) 717.5
- seminal vesicle 608.8
- serous (ovary) 620.2
- sinus (nasal) 478.1
- Skene's gland 599.8
- skin (epidermal) (epithelial) (epidermoid, inclusion) (inclusion) (sebaceous) 706.2
- - breast 610.8
- - eyelid 373.3
- - genital organ NEC
- - - female 629.8
- - - male 608.8
- - scrotum 706.2
- - sweat gland or duct 705.8
- solitary
- - bone 733.2
- - kidney 593.2
- spermatic cord 608.8
- sphenoid sinus 478.1
- spinal meninges 349.2
- spine 733.2
- spleen NEC 289.5
- - hydatid (see also Echinococcus) 122.9
- spring water (pericardium) 746.8
- subdural 348.0
- - spinal cord 349.2
- sublingual gland 527.6
- - mucous extravasation or retention 527.6
- submaxillary gland 527.6
- - mucous extravasation or retention 527.6
- suburethral 599.8
- suprarenal gland 255.8
- suprasellar - see Cyst, brain
- sweat gland or duct 705.8
- synovial 727.4
- tarsal 373.2
- tendon (sheath) 727.4
- testis 608.8
- Thornwaldt's 478.2

Cystadenoma - *continued*
- mucinous (M8470/0)
- - borderline malignancy (M8470/1)
- - - specified site - see Neoplasm,
     uncertain behavior
- - - unspecified site 236.2
- - papillary (M8471/0)
- - - borderline malignancy (M8471/1)
- - - - specified site - see Neoplasm,
       uncertain behavior
- - - - unspecified site 236.2
- - - specified site - see Neoplasm, benign
- - - unspecified site 220
- - specified site - see Neoplasm, benign
- - unspecified site 220
- papillary (M8450/0)
- - borderline malignancy (M8450/1)
- - - specified site - see Neoplasm,
     uncertain behavior
- - - unspecified site 236.2
- - lymphomatosum (M8561/0) 210.2
- - mucinous (M8471/0)
- - - borderline malignancy (M8471/1)
- - - - specified site - see Neoplasm,
       uncertain behavior
- - - - unspecified site 236.2
- - - specified site - see Neoplasm, benign
- - - unspecified site 220
- - pseudomucinous (M8471/0)
- - - borderline malignancy (M8471/1)
- - - - specified site - see Neoplasm,
       uncertain behavior
- - - - unspecified site 236.2
- - - specified site - see Neoplasm, benign
- - - unspecified site 220
- - serous (M8460/0)
- - - borderline malignancy (M8460/1)
- - - - specified site - see Neoplasm,
       uncertain behavior
- - - - unspecified site 236.2
- - - specified site - see Neoplasm, benign
- - - unspecified site 220
- - specified site - see Neoplasm, benign
- - unspecified site 220
- pseudomucinous (M8470/0)
- - borderline malignancy (M8470/1)
- - - specified site - see Neoplasm,
     uncertain behavior
- - - unspecified site 236.2
- - papillary (M8471/0)
- - - borderline malignancy (M8471/1)
- - - - specified site - see Neoplasm,
       uncertain behavior
- - - - unspecified site 236.2
- - - specified site - see Neoplasm, benign
- - - unspecified site 220
- - specified site - see Neoplasm, benign

Cystadenoma - *continued*
- pseudomucinous - *continued*
- - unspecified site 220
- serous (M8441/0)
- - borderline malignancy (M8441/1)
- - - specified site - see Neoplasm,
     uncertain behavior
- - - unspecified site 236.2
- - papillary (M8460/0)
- - - borderline malignancy (M8460/1)
- - - - specified site - see Neoplasm,
       uncertain behavior
- - - - unspecified site 236.2
- - - specified site - see Neoplasm, benign
- - - unspecified site 220
- - specified site - see Neoplasm, benign
- - unspecified site 220
Cystathioninemia 270.4
Cystathioninuria 270.4
Cystic - see also condition
- breast, chronic 610.1
- corpora lutea 620.1
- duct - see condition
- kidney, congenital 753.1
- liver, congenital 751.6
- lung 518.8
- - congenital 748.4
- ovary 620.2
- pancreas, congenital 751.7
Cysticerciasis 123.1
Cysticercosis (mammary) (subretinal) 123.1
Cysticercus 123.1
- cellulosae infestation 123.1
Cystinosis (malignant) 270.0
Cystinuria 270.0
Cystitis (bacillary) (colli) (diffuse)
  (exudative) (hemorrhagic) (malignant)
  (purulent) (recurrent) (septic)
  (suppurative) (ulcerative) 595.9
- acute 595.0
- allergic 595.8
- amebic 006.8
- blennorrhagic 098.1 † 595.4*
- - chronic or duration of 2 months or over
     098.3 † 595.4*
- bullous 595.8
- calculous 594.1
- chronic 595.2
- - interstitial 595.1
- complicating pregnancy, childbirth or
  puerperium 646.6
- - fetus or newborn 760.1
- cystic(a) 595.8
- diphtheritic 032.8 † 595.4*
- emphysematous 595.8
- encysted 595.8
- gangrenous 595.8

D

Da Costa's syndrome 306.2
Dabney's grip 074.1
Dacryoadenitis, dacryadenitis (acute)
  (chronic) 375.0
Dacryocystitis (acute) (phlegmonous) 375.3
– chronic 375.4
– neonatal 771.6
– syphilitic 095 † 375.4*
– – congenital 090.0 † 375.4*
– trachomatous, active 076.1 † 375.4*
Dacryocystoblenorrhea 375.3
Dacryocystocele 375.4
Dacryolith 375.5
Dacryolithiasis 375.5
Dacryoma 375.4
Dacryopericystitis (acute) (subacute) 375.3
– chronic 375.4
Dacryops 375.1
Dacryosialadenopathy, atrophic 710.2
Dacryostenosis 375.5
– congenital 743.6
Dactylitis 686.9
– bone (see also Osteomyelitis) 730.2
– syphilitic 095
– tuberculous 015.7 † 730.5*
Dactylolysis spontanea 136.0
Dactylosymphysis 755.1
Damage
– arteriosclerotic - see Arteriosclerosis
– brain 348.9
– – anoxic, hypoxic 348.1
– – – during or resulting from a procedure
      997.0
– – child NEC 343.9
– – due to birth injury 767.0
– – newborn 767.0
– cardiorenal (vascular) 404.-
– cerebral NEC - see Damage, brain
– coccyx, complicating delivery 665.6
– coronary (see also Ischemia, heart) 414.9
– eye, birth injury 767.8
– heart - see also Disease, heart
– – valve - see Endocarditis
– liver 571.9
– – alcoholic 571.3
– myocardium (see also Degeneration,
  myocardial) 429.1
– pelvic
– – joint or ligament, during delivery 665.6
– – organ NEC

Damage - continued
– pelvic - continued
– – organ NEC - continued
– – – complication of
– – – – abortion - see categories 634-639,
          fourth digit .2
– – – – ectopic or molar pregnancy 639.2
– – – during delivery 665.5
– renal (see also Disease, renal) 593.9
– subendocardium, subendocardial (see
  also Degeneration, myocardial) 429.1
– vascular 459.9
Dana-Putnam syndrome - see
  Degeneration, combined
Dandruff 690
Dandy-Walker syndrome 742.3
– with spina bifida 741.0
Dangle foot 736.7
Danlos' syndrome 756.8
Darier's
– disease (congenital) 757.3
– – meaning erythema annulare
    centrifugum 695.0
– – vitamin A deficiency 264.8 † 701.1*
Darier-Roussy sarcoid 135
Darling's
– disease (congenital) 115.0
– histoplasmosis 115.0
Dartre 054.9
Darwin's tubercle 744.2
Dawson's encephalitis 046.2 † 323.1*

De Beurmann-Gougerot disease 117.1
De Lange's syndrome 759.8
De Morgan's spots 448.1
De Quervain's
– disease 727.0
– thyroiditis 245.1
De Toni-Fanconi(-Debre) syndrome 270.0
Dead
– fetus, retained 656.4
– – early pregnancy 632
– labyrinth 386.5
– ovum, retained 631
Deaf and dumb NEC 389.7

Deafmutism (acquired) (congenital) NEC
  389.7
– endemic 243
– hysterical 300.1
– syphilitic congenital 090.0

Deafness (acquired) (congenital)
(hereditary) (bilateral) (complete)
(partial) 389.9
— with blue sclera and fragility of bone
756.5
— auditory fatigue 389.9
— aviation 993.0
— boilermaker's 951.5
— central - see Deafness, sensorineural
— conductive 389.0
— — and sensorineural, mixed 389.2
— emotional (complete) 300.1
— functional (complete) 300.1
— high frequency 389.8
— hysterical (complete) 300.1
— injury 951.5
— low frequency 389.8
— mental 784.6
— mixed conductive and sensorineural
389.2
— nerve - see Deafness, sensorineural
— neural - see Deafness, sensorineural
— noise-induced 388.1
— — nerve injury 951.5
— nonspeaking 389.7

— perceptive - see Deafness, sensorineural
— psychogenic (complete) 306.7
— sensorineural 389.1
— — and conductive mixed 389.2
— sensory - see Deafness, sensorineural
— specified type NEC 389.8
— sudden NEC 388.2
— syphilitic 094.8
— transient ischemic 388.0
— traumatic 951.5
— word (secondary to organic lesion) 784.6
— — developmental 315.3

Death
— after delivery (cause not stated) (sudden)
674.9
— anesthetic
— — due to
— — — correct substance properly
administered 995.4
— — — overdose or wrong substance given
968.-
— — — — specified anesthetic - see Table of
drugs and chemicals
— — during delivery 668.9
— cardiac - see Disease, heart
— cause unknown 798.2
— cot 798.0
— crib 798.0
— fetus, fetal (cause not stated)
(intrauterine) 779.9
— — early, with retention 632

Death - *continued*
— fetus - *continued*
— — late, affecting management of
pregnancy 656.4
— from pregnancy NEC 646.9
— instantaneous 798.1
— intrauterine complicating pregnancy
656.4
— maternal, affecting fetus or newborn
761.6
— neonatal NEC 779.9
— sudden (cause unknown) 798.1
— — during delivery 669.9
— — — under anesthesia NEC 668.9
— — infant 798.0
— — puerperal, during puerperium 674.9
— unattended (cause unknown) 798.9
— under anesthesia NEC
— — due to
— — — correct substance properly
administered 995.4
— — — overdose or wrong substance given
968.-
— — — — specified anesthetic - see Table of
drugs and chemicals
— — during delivery 668.9
Debility (general) (infantile)
(postinfectional) 799.3
— congenital or neonatal NEC 779.9
— nervous 300.5
— old age 797
— senile 797
Decalcification
— bone 733.0
— teeth 521.8
Decapitation 874.9
— fetal (to facilitate delivery) 763.8

Decapsulation, kidney 593.8
Decay
— dental 521.0
— senile 797
— tooth, teeth 521.0
Deciduitis (acute)
— with
— — abortion - see categories 634-639,
fourth digit .0
— — ectopic gestation 639.0
— fetus or newborn 760.8
— in pregnancy 646.6
— puerperal, postpartum, childbirth 670
Deciduoma malignum (M9100/3) 181

Decline (general) (see also Debility) 799.3
Decompensation
— cardiac (acute) (chronic) (see also
Disease, heart) 429.9
— cardiorenal 404.9

Decompensation - *continued*
- cardiovascular (see also Disease, cardiovascular) 429.2
- heart (see also Disease, heart) 429.9
- hepatic 572.2
- myocardial (acute) (chronic) (see also Disease, heart) 429.9
- respiratory 519.9
Decompression sickness 993.3
Decrease(d)
- blood
- - platelets (see also Thrombocytopenia) 287.5
- - pressure, due to shock following injury 958.4
- estrogen 256.3
- fragility of erythrocytes 289.8
- function
- - adrenal medulla 255.5
- - ovary in hypopituitarism 253.4
- - parenchyma of pancreas 577.8
- - pituitary (gland) (anterior) (lobe) 253.2
- - - posterior (lobe) 253.2
- functional activity 780.9
- respiration, due to shock following injury 958.4
- tear secretion NEC 375.1
- tolerance
- - fat 579.8
- - glucose 790.2
Decubiti 707.0
Decubitus (ulcer) 707.0
Deepening acetabulum 718.8
Defect, defective 759.9
- abdominal wall, congenital 756.7
- aortic septal 745.0
- aorticopulmonary septum 745.0
- atrial septal (ostium secundum type) 745.5
- - ostium primum type 745.6
- atrioventricular
- - canal 745.6
- - septum 745.4
- auricular septal 745.5
- bilirubin excretion 277.4
- biosynthesis, testicular androgen 257.2
- bulbar septum 745.0
- circulation 459.9
- - congenital 747.9
- - newborn 747.9
- coagulation (factor) (see also Deficiency, factor) 286.9
- - with
- - - abortion - see categories 634-639, fourth digit .1
- - - ectopic gestation 639.1

Defect - *continued*
- coagulation - *continued*
- - antepartum or intrapartum 641.3
- - - fetus or newborn 762.1
- - newborn, transient 776.3
- - postpartum 666.3
- conduction 426.9
- - bone - see Deafness, conductive
- congenital, organ or site not listed - see Anomaly
- cushion, endocardial 745.6
- Descemet's membrane, congenital 743.4
- developmental - see also Anomaly
- - cauda equina 742.5
- diaphragm
- - with elevation, eventration or hernia - see Hernia, diaphragm
- - congenital 756.6
- - - with elevation, eventration, or hernia 756.6
- - - gross (with elevation, eventration or hernia) 756.6
- ectodermal, congenital 757.9
- Eisenmenger's 745.4
- esophagus, congenital 750.9
- extensor retinacular 728.9
- filling
- - bladder 793.5
- - kidney 793.5
- - ureter 793.5
- Gerbode's 745.4
- Hageman (factor) 286.3
- hearing (see also Deafness) 389.9
- high grade 317
- interatrial septal 745.5
- interauricular septal 745.5
- interventricular septal 745.4
- - in tetralogy of Fallot 745.2
- learning, specific 315.2
- mental - see Retardation, mental
- ostium
- - primum 745.6
- - secundum 745.5
- pericardium 746.8
- placental blood supply - see Placenta, insufficiency
- platelets, qualitative 287.1
- postural, spine 737.9
- pulmonic cusps, congenital 746.0
- renal pelvis 753.9
- - obstructive 753.2
- respiratory system, congenital 748.9
- septal (heart) NEC 745.9
- speech NEC 784.5
- - developmental 315.3
- - secondary to organic lesion 784.5
- vascular (local) 459.9

Defect - *continued*
- vascular - *continued*
- - congenital 747.6
- ventricular septal 745.4
- - atrioventricular canal type 745.6
- - between infundibulum and anterior
    portion 745.4
- - in tetralogy of Fallot 745.2
- - isolated anterior 745.4
- vision NEC 369.9
- visual field 368.4
- voice 784.4
- wedge (abrasion) 521.2
- 11 hydroxylase 255.2
- 21 hydroxylase 255.2
- 3B hydroxysteroid dehydrogenase 255.2
Deferentitis 608.4
- gonorrheal (acute) 098.1
- - chronic or duration of 2 months or over
    098.3
Defibrination (syndrome) 286.6
- with
- - abortion - see categories 634-639,
    fourth digit .1
- - ectopic gestation 639.1
- antepartum or intrapartum 641.3
- - fetus or newborn 762.1
- neonatal NEC 776.3
- postpartum 666.3
Deficiency, deficient
- abdominal muscle syndrome 756.8
- AC globulin (congenital) 286.3
- - acquired 286.7
- aldolase (hereditary) 271.2
- alpha 1-antitrypsin 277.6
- amino-acids 270.9
- anemia - see Anemia
- aneurin 265.1
- anti-hemophilic globulin NEC 286.0
- ascorbic acid 267
- biotin 266.2
- brancher enzyme (amylopectinosis) 271.0
- calciferol 268.9
- - with
- - - osteomalacia 268.2
- - - rickets (see also Rickets) 268.0
- calcium 275.4
- - dietary 269.3
- calorie, severe 261
- cardiac (see also Insufficiency,
    myocardial) 428.0
- carotene 264.9
- central nervous system 349.9
- ceruloplasmin 275.1
- cevitamic acid 267
- choline 266.2
- citrin 269.1

Deficiency - *continued*
- clotting (blood) (see also Deficiency,
    coagulation factor) 286.9
- coagulation factor NEC 286.9
- - with
- - - abortion - see categories 634-639,
    fourth digit .1
- - - ectopic gestation 639.1
- - acquired (any) 286.7
- - antepartum or intrapartum 641.3
- - - fetus or newborn 762.1
- - due to
- - - liver disease 286.7
- - - vitamin K deficiency 286.7
- - newborn, transient 776.3
- - postpartum 666.3
- - specified NEC 286.3
- corticoadrenal 255.4
- craniofacial axis 756.0
- cyanocobalamine 266.2
- debrancher enzyme (limit dextrinosis)
    271.0
- diet 269.9
- disaccharidase 271.3
- edema 262
- endocrine 259.9
- enzymes, circulating NEC 277.6
- ergosterol 268.9
- - with
- - - osteomalacia 268.2
- - - rickets (see also Rickets) 268.0
- factor - see also Deficiency, coagulation
    factor
- - Hageman 286.3
- - I (congenital) 286.3
- - II (congenital) 286.3
- - IX (congenital) (functional) 286.1
- - multiple (congenital) 286.9
- - - acquired 286.7
- - V (congenital) 286.3
- - VII (congenital) 286.3
- - VIII (congenital) (functional) 286.0
- - - with vascular defect 286.4
- - X (congenital) 286.3
- - XI (congenital) 286.2
- - XII (congenital) 286.3
- - XIII (congenital) 286.3
- fibrin stabilizing factor (congenital) (see
    also Defect, coagulation) 286.3
- - acquired 286.7
- fibrinogen (congenital) (see also Defect,
    coagulation) 286.3
- - acquired 286.6
- folic acid 266.2
- fructokinase 271.2
- galactose-1-phosphate uridyl transferase
    271.1

Deficiency - *continued*
- gammaglobulin in blood 279.0
- glucose-6-phosphatase 271.0
- glucose-6-phosphate dehydrogenase anemia 282.2
- glycogen synthetase 271.0
- Hageman factor (see also Defect, coagulation) 286.3
- hemoglobin 285.9
- hepatophosphorylase 271.0
- homogentisic acid oxidase 270.2
- hormone
- - anterior pituitary (isolated) (partial) NEC 253.4
- - - growth 253.3
- - growth (isolated) 253.3
- - testicular 257.2
- hypoxanthine-guanine-phosphoribosyl-transferase (HG-PRT) 277.2
- immunity 279.3
- - cell-mediated 279.1
- - combined 279.2
- - humoral 279.0
- inositol 266.2
- intrinsic factor (congenital) 281.0
- iodine 269.3
- labile factor (congenital) (see also Defect, coagulation) 286.3
- - acquired 286.7
- lacrimal fluid (acquired) 375.1
- - congenital 743.6
- lecithin cholesterol acyltransferase 272.5
- lipocaic 577.8
- lipoprotein, familial (high density) 272.5
- mental (familial) (hereditary) - see Retardation, mental
- mineral NEC 269.3
- moral 301.7
- myocardial (see also Insufficiency, myocardial) 428.0
- myophosphorylase 271.0
- NADH diaphorase or reductase (congenital) 289.7
- NADH-methemoglobin-reductase (congenital) 289.7
- niacin(amide)(-tryptophan) 265.2
- nicotinamide 265.2
- nicotinic acid 265.2
- number of teeth (see also Anodontia) 520.0
- nutrition, nutritional 269.9
- ornithine transcarbamylase 270.6
- oxygen (see also Anoxia) 799.0
- pantothenic acid 266.2
- parathyroid (gland) 252.1
- phenylalanine hydroxylase 270.1

Deficiency - *continued*
- placenta - see Placenta, insufficiency
- plasma thromboplastin
- - antecedent (PTA) 286.2
- - component (PTC) 286.1
- polyglandular 258.9
- potassium (K) 276.8
- proaccelerin (congenital) 286.3
- - acquired 286.7
- proconvertin factor (congenital) (see also Defect,coagulation) 286.3
- - acquired 286.7
- protein 260
- prothrombin (congenital) (see also Defect, coagulation) 286.3
- - acquired 286.7
- pseudocholinesterase 289.8
- psychobiological 301.6
- PTA 286.2
- PTC 286.1
- pyracin (alpha) (beta) 266.1
- pyridoxamine, pyridoxal 266.1
- pyridoxine (derivatives) 266.1
- riboflavin 266.0
- salt 276.1
- secretion
- - ovary 256.3
- - salivary gland (any) 527.7
- - urine 788.5
- serum
- - antitripsin, familial 277.6
- - protein 273.8
- sodium (Na) 276.1
- SPCA (see also Defect, coagulation) 286.3
- stable factor (congenital) (see also Defect, coagulation) 286.3
- - acquired 286.7
- Stuart-Prower (see also Defect, coagulation) 286.3
- syndrome, multiple 260
- thiamine, thiaminic (chloride) 265.1
- thyroid (gland) 244.9
- tocopherol 269.1
- tooth bud 520.0
- vascular 459.9
- viosterol (see also Deficiency, calciferol) 268.9
- vitamin (multiple) NEC 269.2
- - A 264.9
- - - with
- - - - Bitot's spot 264.1 † 372.5*
- - - - - corneal 264.2 † 371.4*
- - - - - - with corneal ulceration 264.3 † 370.0*
- - - - keratomalacia 264.4 † 371.4*
- - - - night blindness 264.5 † 368.6*

Deformity - *continued*
- capillary - *continued*
- – congenital 747.6
- cardiac - see Deformity, heart
- cardiovascular system (congenital) 746.9
- caruncle lacrimal (congenital) 743.9
- – acquired 375.6
- cecum (congenital) 751.5
- – acquired 569.8
- cerebral (congenital) 742.9
- – acquired 348.8
- cervix (uterus) (acquired) 622.8
- – congenital 752.4
- cheek (acquired) 738.1
- – congenital 744.9
- chest (acquired) (wall) 738.3
- – congenital 754.8
- – late effects of rickets 268.1
- chin (acquired) 738.1
- – congenital 744.9
- choroid (congenital) 743.9
- – acquired 363.8
- – plexus 742.9
- cicatricial - see Cicatrix
- cilia (congenital) 743.9
- – acquired 374.4

- circulatory system (congenital) 747.9
- clavicle (acquired) 738.8
- – congenital 755.5
- clitoris (congenital) 752.4
- – acquired 624.8
- clubfoot - see Clubfoot
- coccyx (acquired) 738.6
- – congenital 756.1
- colon (congenital) 751.5
- – acquired 569.8

- concha (ear) (congenital) (see also Deformity, ear) 744.3
- – acquired 380.3
- congenital, organ or site not listed (see also Anomaly) 759.9
- cornea (congenital) 743.9
- – acquired 371.7
- coronary artery (congenital) 746.9
- – acquired (see also Ischemia, heart) 414.9
- cranium (acquired) 738.1
- – congenital (see also Deformity, skull, congenital) 756.0
- cricoid cartilage (congenital) 748.3
- – acquired 478.7
- cystic duct (congenital) 751.6
- – acquired (see also Disease, gallbladder) 575.8
- diaphragm (congenital) 756.6
- – acquired 738.8

Deformity - *continued*
- digestive organ(s) or system (congenital) NEC 751.9
- ductus arteriosus 747.9
- duodenal bulb 537.8
- duodenum (congenital) 751.5
- – acquired 537.8
- dura (congenital) 742.9
- – brain 742.9
- – – acquired 349.2
- – spinal 742.5
- – – acquired 349.2
- ear (auricle) (external) (lobule) (congenital) 744.3
- – acquired 380.3
- – causing impairment of hearing 744.0
- – internal 744.0
- – middle 744.0
- ectodermal (congenital) NEC 757.9
- ejaculatory duct (congenital) 752.9
- – acquired 608.8
- elbow (joint) (acquired) (see also Deformity, joint) 736.0
- – congenital 755.5
- endocrine gland NEC 759.2
- epididymis (congenital) 752.9
- – acquired 608.8
- epiglottis (congenital) 748.3
- – acquired 478.7
- esophagus (congenital) 750.9
- – acquired 530.8
- eustachian tube (congenital) NEC 744.3
- extremity (acquired) 736.9
- – congenital, except reduction deformity 755.9
- – – lower 755.6
- – – upper 755.5
- eye (congenital) 743.9
- – muscle 743.9
- eyelid (congenital) 743.9
- – acquired 374.4
- face (acquired) 738.1
- – congenital 744.9
- fallopian tube (congenital) 752.1
- – acquired 620.8
- femur (acquired) 736.8
- – congenital 755.6
- fetal
- – with fetopelvic disproportion 653.7
- – causing obstructed labor 660.1
- – – affecting fetus or newborn 763.1
- – known or suspected, affecting management of pregnancy 655.9
- finger (acquired) 736.2
- – congenital 755.5
- flexion (joint) (acquired) 736.9
- – congenital NEC 755.9

Deformity - *continued*
- flexion - *continued*
- − − hip or thigh (acquired) 736.3
- − − − congenital 754.3
- − foot (acquired) 736.7
- − − congenital NEC 754.7
- − − valgus (congenital) 754.6
- − − − acquired 736.7
- − − varus (congenital) 754.5
- − − − acquired 736.7
- − forearm (acquired) 736.0
- − − congenital 755.5
- − forehead (acquired) 738.1
- − − congenital (see also Deformity, skull,
   congenital) 756.0
- − frontal bone (acquired) 738.1
- − − congenital (see also Deformity, skull,
   congenital) 756.0
- − gallbladder (congenital) 751.6
- − − acquired (see also Disease,
   gallbladder) 575.8
- − gastro-intestinal tract (congenital) NEC
   751.9
- − − acquired 569.8
- − genitalia, genital organ(s) or system NEC
- − female (congenital) 752.9
- − − − acquired 629.8
- − − − external 752.4
- − − − internal 752.9
- − − male (congenital) 752.9
- − − − acquired 608.8
- − globe (eye) (congenital) 743.9
- − − acquired 360.4
- − gum (congenital) 750.9
- − − acquired 523.9
- − gunstock 738.8
- − hand (claw) (intrinsic) (minus) (pill
   roller) (plus) (swan neck) (acquired)
   736.0
- − − congenital 755.5
- − head (acquired) 738.1
- − − congenital (see also Deformity, skull,
   congenital) 756.0
- − heart (congenital) 746.9
- − − auricle (congenital) 746.9
- − − septum 745.9
- − − − auricular 745.5
- − − − ventricular 745.4
- − − valve (congenital) NEC 746.9
- − − − acquired - see Endocarditis
- − − − pulmonary 746.0
- − − ventricle (congenital) 746.9
- − heel (acquired) 736.7
- − − congenital 755.6
- − hepatic duct (congenital) 751.6
- − − acquired (see also Disease, biliary)
   576.8

Deformity - *continued*
- − hip (joint) (acquired) 736.3
- − − congenital 755.6
- − hourglass - see Contraction, hourglass
- − humerus (acquired) 736.8
- − − congenital 755.5
- − hymen (congenital) 752.4
- − hypophyseal (congenital) 759.2
- − ileocecal (coil) (valve) (congenital) 751.5
- − − acquired 569.8
- − ileum (congenital) 751.5
- − − acquired 569.8
- − ilium (acquired) 738.6
- − − congenital 755.6
- − integument (congenital) 757.9
- − intervertebral cartilage or disc (acquired)
   - see Displacement, intervertebral disc
- − − congenital 756.1
- − intestine (large) (small) (congenital)
   751.5
- − − acquired 569.8
- − iris (acquired) 364.7
- − − congenital 743.9
- − ischium (acquired) 738.6
- − − congenital 755.6
- − jaw (acquired) (congenital) NEC 524.9
- − joint (acquired) NEC 738.8
- − − congenital 755.9
- − kidney(s) (calyx) (pelvis) (congenital)
   753.9
- − − acquired 593.8
- − − vessel (congenital) 747.6
- − − − acquired 459.9
- − Klippel-Feil 756.1
- − knee (acquired) NEC 736.6
- − − congenital 755.6
- − labium (majus) (minus) (congenital)
   752.4
- − − acquired 624.8
- − lacrimal apparatus or duct (congenital)
   743.9
- − − acquired 375.6
- − larynx (muscle) (congenital) 748.3
- − − acquired 478.7
- − − web (glottic) (sub-glottic) 748.2
- − leg (upper) (lower) (acquired) NEC
   736.8
- − − congenital 755.6
- − lens (congenital) 743.9
- − − acquired 379.3
- − lid (fold) (congenital) 743.9
- − − acquired 374.4
- − ligament (acquired) 728.9
- − − congenital 756.9
- − limb (acquired) 736.9
- − − congenital, except reduction deformity
   755.9

Deformity - *continued*
- limb - *continued*
- - congenital - *continued*
- - - lower 755.6
- - - upper 755.5
- - specified NEC 736.8
- lip (congenital) NEC 750.9
- - acquired 528.5
- liver (congenital) 751.6
- - acquired 573.8
- - duct (congenital) 751.6
- - - acquired (see also Disease, biliary) 576.8
- lumbosacral (congenital) (joint) (region) 756.1
- - acquired 738.5
- lung (congenital) 748.6
- - acquired 518.8
- lymphatic system, congenital 759.9
- Madelung's (radius) 755.5
- maxilla (acquired) 524.9
- - congenital 524.9
- meninges or membrane (congenital) 742.9
- - brain 742.9
- - - acquired 349.2
- - spinal (cord) 742.5
- - - acquired 349.2
- mesentery (congenital) 751.9
- - acquired 568.8
- metacarpus (acquired) 736.0
- - congenital 755.5
- metatarsus (acquired) 736.7
- - congenital 754.7
- middle ear (congenital) 744.0
- mitral (congenital) (leaflets) (valve) 746.9
- - acquired - see Endocarditis, mitral
- - Ebstein's 746.8
- - stenosis, congenital 746.5
- mouth
- - acquired 528.9
- - congenital NEC 750.9
- multiple, congenital NEC 759.7
- muscle (acquired) 728.9
- - congenital 756.9
- musculoskeletal system, congenital NEC 756.9
- nail (acquired) 703.9
- - congenital 757.9
- nasal - see Deformity, nose
- neck (acquired) NEC 738.2
- - congenital 744.9
- - - sternocleidomastoid 754.1
- nervous system (congenital) 742.9
- nipple (congenital) 757.9
- - acquired 611.8

Deformity - *continued*
- nose (acquired) (cartilage) 738.0
- - bone (turbinate) 738.0
- - congenital 748.1
- - - bent 754.0
- - - squashed 754.0
- - septum 470
- - - congenital 748.1
- - sinus (wall) (congenital) 748.1
- - syphilitic (congenital) 090.5
- - - late 095
- ocular muscle (congenital) 743.9
- - acquired 378.6
- oesophagus (congenital) 750.9
- - acquired 530.8
- opticociliary vessels (congenital) 743.9
- orbit (eye) (congenital) 743.9
- - acquired 376.4
- organ of Corti (congenital) 744.0
- ovary (congenital) 752.0
- - acquired 620.8
- oviduct (congenital) 752.1
- - acquired 620.8
- palate (congenital) 750.9
- - acquired 526.8
- - cleft (congenital) 749.0
- - - with cleft lip 749.2
- - soft, acquired 528.9
- pancreas (congenital) 751.7
- - acquired 577.8
- parathyroid (gland) 759.2
- parotid (gland) (congenital) 750.9
- - acquired 527.8
- patella (acquired) 736.6
- - congenital 755.6
- pelvis, pelvic (acquired) (bony) 738.6
- - with disproportion 653.0
- - - causing obstructed labor 660.1
- - - fetus or newborn 763.1
- - congenital 755.6
- - rachitic (late effect) 268.1
- penis (glans) (congenital) 752.9
- - acquired 607.8
- pericardium (congenital) 746.9
- - acquired - see Pericarditis
- pharynx (congenital) 750.9
- - acquired 478.2
- Pierre Robin (congenital) 756.0
- pinna, acquired 380.3
- pituitary (congenital) 759.2
- pleural fold (congenital) 748.9
- portal vein (congenital) 747.4
- posture - see Curvature, spine
- prepuce (congenital) 752.9
- - acquired 607.8
- prostate (congenital) 752.9
- - acquired 602.8

Deformity - *continued*
- pupil (congenital) 743.9
- - acquired 364.7
- pylorus (congenital) 750.9
- - acquired 537.8
- rachitic (acquired), old or healed 268.1
- radius (acquired) 736.0
- - congenital 755.5
- rectum (congenital) 751.5
- - acquired 569.4
- reduction (extremity) (limb) 755.4
- - brain 742.2
- - lower 755.3
- - upper 755.2
- renal - see Deformity, kidney
- respiratory system (congenital) 748.9
- rib (acquired) 738.3
- - congenital 756.3
- - - cervical 756.2
- rotation (joint) (acquired) 736.9
- - congenital 755.9
- - hip or thigh 736.3
- - - congenital 754.3
- sacro-iliac joint (congenital) 755.6
- - acquired 738.5
- sacrum (acquired) 738.5
- - congenital 756.1
- saddle
- - back 737.8
- - nose 738.0
- - - syphilitic 090.5
- salivary gland or duct (congenital) 750.9
- - acquired 527.8
- scapula (acquired) 736.8
- - congenital 755.5
- scrotum (congenital) 752.9
- - acquired 608.8
- sebaceous gland, acquired 706.8
- seminal tract or duct (congenital) 752.9
- - acquired 608.8
- shoulder (joint) (acquired) 736.8
- - congenital 755.5
- sigmoid (flexure) (congenital) 751.5
- - acquired 569.8
- sinus of Valsalva 747.2
- skin (congenital) 757.9
- skull (acquired) 738.1
- - congenital 756.0
- - - with
- - - - anencephalus 740.0
- - - - encephalocele 742.0
- - - - hydrocephalus 742.3
- - - - - with spina bifida 741.0
- - - - microphalus 742.1
- soft parts, organs or tissues (of pelvis)
- - in pregnancy or childbirth NEC 654.9
- - - causing obstructed labor 660.2

Deformity - *continued*
- soft parts - *continued*
- - in pregnancy or childbirth NEC - *cont.*
- - - causing obstructed labor - *continued*
- - - - fetus or newborn 763.1
- - - fetus or newborn 763.8
- spermatic cord (congenital) 752.9
- - acquired 608.8
- spinal
- - column (acquired) - see Deformity, spine
- - cord (congenital) 742.9
- - - acquired 336.8
- - - vessel (congenital) 747.6
- - nerve root (congenital) 742.9
- - - acquired 724.9
- spine (acquired) NEC 738.5
- - congenital 756.1
- - rachitic 268.1
- spleen
- - acquired 289.5
- - congenital 759.0
- Sprengel's (congenital) 755.5
- sternum (acquired) 738.3
- - congenital 756.3
- stomach (congenital) 750.9
- - acquired 537.8
- submaxillary gland (congenital) 750.9
- - acquired 527.8
- talipes - see Talipes
- testis (congenital) 752.9
- - acquired 608.8
- thigh (acquired) 736.8
- - congenital 755.6
- thorax (acquired) (wall) 738.3
- - congenital 754.8
- - late effects of rickets 268.1
- thumb (acquired) 736.2
- - congenital 755.5
- thymus (tissue) (congenital) 759.2
- thyroid (gland) (congenital) 759.2
- - cartilage 748.3
- - - acquired 478.7
- tibia (acquired) 736.8
- - congenital 755.6
- - saber 090.5
- toe (acquired) 735.9
- - congenital 755.6
- tongue (congenital) 750.1
- - acquired 529.8
- tooth, teeth NEC 520.9
- trachea (rings) (congenital) 748.3
- - acquired 519.1
- transverse aortic arch (congenital) 747.2
- tricuspid (congenital) (leaflets) (valve) 746.9
- - acquired - see Endocarditis, tricuspid

Deformity - *continued*
- tricuspid - *continued*
- - atresia or stenosis 746.1
- trunk (acquired) 738.3
- - congenital 759.9
- ulna (acquired) 736.0
- - congenital 755.5
- urachus (congenital) 753.7
- ureter (opening) (congenital) 753.9
- - acquired 593.8
- urethra (congenital) 753.9
- - acquired 599.8
- urinary tract (congenital) 753.9
- uterus (congenital) 752.3
- - acquired 621.8
- uvula (congenital) 750.9
- - acquired 528.9
- vagina (congenital) 752.4
- - acquired 623.8
- valve, valvular (congenital) (heart) 746.9
- - acquired - see Endocarditis
- - pulmonary 746.0
- vas deferens (congenital) 752.9
- - acquired 608.8
- vascular (congenital) NEC 747.6
- - acquired 459.9
- vein (congenital) NEC 747.6
- - brain 747.8
- - coronary 746.9
- - great 747.4
- vena cava (inferior) (superior) (congenital) 747.4
- vertebra - see Deformity, spine
- vesicourethral orifice (acquired) 596.8
- - congenital NEC 753.9
- vessels of optic papilla (congenital) 743.9
- visual field (contraction) 368.4
- vitreous humor (congenital) 743.9
- - acquired 379.2
- vulva (congenital) 752.4
- - acquired 624.8
- wrist (joint) (acquired) 736.0
- - congenital 755.5
Degeneration, degenerative
- adrenal (capsule) (gland) 255.8
- - fatty 255.8
- - hyaline 255.8
- - infectional 255.8
- amyloid (any site) (general) 277.3
- anterior cornua, spinal cord 336.8
- aorta, aortic 440.0
- - fatty 447.8
- aortic valve (heart) (see also Endocarditis, aortic) 424.1
- arteriovascular - see Arteriosclerosis
- artery, arterial (atheromatous) (calcareous) - see also Arteriosclerosis

Degeneration - *continued*
- artery - *continued*
- - amyloid 277.3
- - medial 440.2
- articular cartilage NEC 718.0
- - elbow 718.0
- - knee 717.5
- - shoulder 718.0
- atheromatous - see Arteriosclerosis
- basal nuclei or ganglia NEC 333.0
- bone 733.9
- brain (cortical) (progressive) 331.9
- - arteriosclerotic 437.0
- - childhood 330.9
- - - specified NEC 330.8
- - cystic 348.0
- - - congenital 742.4
- - in
- - - alcoholism 303 † 331.7*
- - - beriberi 265.0 † 331.7*
- - - cerebrovascular disease 437.9 † 331.7*
- - - congenital hydrocephalus 742.3 † 331.7*
- - - - with spina bifida 741.0 † 331.7*
- - - Fabry's disease 272.7 † 330.2*
- - - Gaucher's disease 272.7 † 330.2*
- - - Hunter's disease or syndrome 277.5 † 330.3*
- - - lipidosis
- - - - cerebral 330.1
- - - - generalized 272.7 † 330.2*
- - - mucopolysaccharidosis 277.5 † 330.3*
- - - myxedema NEC 244.9 † 331.7*
- - - neoplastic disease NEC (M8000/1) 239.9 † 331.7*
- - - Niemann-Pick disease 272.7 † 330.2*
- - - sphingolipidosis 272.7 † 330.2*
- - - vitamin B12 deficiency 266.2 † 331.7*
- - senile 331.2
- breast - see Disease, breast
- Bruch's membrane 363.4
- calcareous NEC 275.4
- capillaries 448.9
- - amyloid 277.3
- - fatty 448.9
- cardiac (see also Degeneration, myocardial) 429.1
- - valve, valvular - see Endocarditis
- cardiorenal 404.9
- cardiovascular (see also Disease, cardiovascular) 429.2
- - renal 404.9
- cerebellar NEC 334.9

Degeneration - *continued*
- cerebellar NEC - *continued*
- - primary (hereditary) (sporadic) 334.2
- cerebral - see Degeneration, brain
- cerebromacular 330.1
- cerebrovascular 437.1
- cervix 622.8
- - due to radiation (intended effect) 622.8
- - - adverse effect or misadventure 622.8
- changes, spine or vertebra 721.9
- chorioretinal 363.4
- - hereditary 363.5
- choroid (colloid) (drusen) 363.4
- - hereditary 363.5
- cochlear 386.8
- combined (spinal cord) (subacute) 266.2 † 336.2*
- - with anemia (pernicious) 281.0 † 336.2*
- - - due to dietary deficiency 281.1 † 336.2*
- - due to vitamin B12 deficiency anemia (dietary) 281.1 † 336.2*
- cornea 371.4
- - familial, hereditary 371.5
- - hyaline (of old scars) 371.4
- - senile 371.4
- cortical (cerebellar) (parenchymatous) 334.2
- - alcoholic 303 † 334.4*
- - diffuse, due to arteriopathy 437.0
- corticostriatal-spinal 334.8
- cretinoid 243
- cutis 709.3
- - amyloid 277.3
- dental pulp 522.2
- disc disease - see Degeneration, intervertebral disc
- dorsolateral (spinal cord) - see Degeneration, combined
- extrapyramidal NEC 333.9
- eye, macular 362.5
- - congenital or hereditary 362.7
- fatty
- - liver 571.8
- - - alcoholic 571.0
- - placenta - see Placenta, abnormal
- grey matter 330.8
- heart (see also Degeneration, myocardial) 429.1
- - amyloid 277.3 † 425.7*
- - atheromatous 414.0
- - gouty 274.8 † 425.7*
- hepatolenticular (Wilson's) 275.1
- hepatorenal 572.4

Degeneration - *continued*
- hyaline (diffuse) (generalized) 728.8
- - localized - see also Degeneration, by site
- - - keratitis (see also Keratitis) 371.4
- internal semilunar cartilage 717.3
- intervertebral disc 722.6
- - with myelopathy (any site) 722.7 † 336.3*
- - cervical, cervicothoracic 722.4
- - - with myelopathy 722.7 † 336.3*
- - lumbar, lumbosacral 722.5
- - - with myelopathy 722.7 † 336.3*
- - thoracic, thoracolumbar 722.5
- - - with myelopathy 722.7 † 336.3*
- intestine 569.8
- - amyloid 277.3
- iris (pigmentary) 364.5
- ischemic - see Ischemia
- joint disease 715.9
- - multiple 715.0
- - spine 721.9
- kidney (see also Sclerosis, renal) 587
- - amyloid 277.3
- - cystic, congenital 753.1
- - fatty 593.8
- - fibrocystic (congenital) 753.1
- - polycystic (congenital) 753.1
- lens 366.9
- lenticular (familial) (progressive) (Wilson's) (with cirrhosis of liver) 275.1
- - striate artery 437.0
- liver (diffuse) 572.8
- - amyloid 277.3
- - cystic 572.8
- - - congenital 751.6
- - fatty 571.8
- - - alcoholic 571.0
- - hypertrophic 572.8
- - parenchymatous, acute or subacute (see also Necrosis, liver) 570
- - pigmentary 572.8
- - toxic (acute) 573.8
- lung 518.8
- lymph gland 289.3
- - hyaline 289.3
- macula, macular (acquired) (atrophic) (exsudative) (senile) 362.5
- - congenital or hereditary 362.7
- membranous labyrinth, congenital (causing impairment of hearing) 744.0
- mitral - see Insufficiency, mitral
- Monckeberg's 440.2
- moral 301.7
- mural (see also Degeneration, myocardial) 429.1

Degeneration - *continued*
- mural - *continued*
- – heart, cardiac (see also Degeneration, myocardial) 429.1
- – myocardium, myocardial (see also Degeneration, myocardial) 429.1
- muscle 728.9
- – fatty 728.9
- – fibrous 728.9
- – heart (see also Degeneration, myocardial) 429.1
- – hyaline 728.9
- muscular progressive 728.2
- myelin, central nervous system NEC 341.9
- myocardium, myocardial (with arteriosclerosis) (brown) (calcareous) (fatty) (fibrous) (hyaline) (mural) (muscular) (pigmentary) (senile) 429.1
- – with
- – – rheumatic fever (conditions in 390) 398.0
- – – – active, acute or subacute 391.2
- – – – – with chorea 392.0
- – – – inactive or quiescent (with chorea) 398.0
- – congenital 746.8
- – fetus or newborn 779.8
- – gouty 274.8 † 425.7*
- – hypertensive (see also Hypertension, heart) 402.9
- – rheumatic - see Degeneration, myocardium, with rheumatic fever
- – syphilitic 093.8
- nerve - see Disorder, nerve
- nervous system 349.8
- – amyloid 277.3
- – fatty 349.8
- – peripheral autonomic NEC 337.9
- nipple 611.9
- olivopontocerebellar (hereditary) (familial) 333.0
- osseous labyrinth 386.8
- ovary 620.8
- – cystic 620.2
- – microcystic 620.2
- pallidal pigmentary (progressive) 333.0
- pancreas 577.8
- – tuberculous 017.8
- penis 607.8
- peritoneum 568.8
- pigmentary (diffuse) (general)
- – localized - see Degeneration by site
- – pallidal (progressive) 333.0
- pineal gland 259.8
- pituitary (gland) 253.8
- placenta - see Placenta, abnormal

Degeneration - *continued*
- posterolateral (spinal cord) - see Degeneration, combined
- pulmonary valve (heart) (see also Endocarditis, pulmonary) 424.3
- pupillary margin 364.5
- renal (see also Sclerosis, renal) 587
- – fibrocystic 753.1
- – polycystic 753.1
- retina (lattice) (microcystoid) (palisade) (paving stone) (peripheral) (reticular) (senile) 362.6
- – hereditary (cerebroretinal) (congenital) (juvenile) (macula) (peripheral) (pigmentary) 362.7
- – Kuhnt-Junius 362.5
- – macula (cystic) (exudative) (hole) (nonexudative) (pseudohole) (senile) (toxic) 362.5
- – pigmentary (primary) 362.7
- – posterior pole 362.5
- saccule, congenital (causing impairment of hearing) 744.0
- senile 797
- – brain 331.2
- – cardiac, heart or myocardium 429.1
- – vascular - see Arteriosclerosis
- sinus (cystic) (see also Sinusitis) 473.9
- – polypoid 471.1
- skin 709.3
- – amyloid 277.3
- – colloid 709.3
- spinal (cord) 336.8
- – amyloid 277.3
- – column 733.9
- – combined (subacute) - see Degeneration, combined
- – dorsolateral - see Degeneration, combined
- – familial NEC 336.8
- – fatty 336.8
- – funicular - see Degeneration, combined
- – posterolateral - see Degeneration, combined
- – subacute combined - see Degeneration, combined
- – tuberculous 013.8 † 323.4*
- spine 733.9
- spleen 289.5
- – amyloid 277.3
- stomach 537.8
- strionigral 333.0
- sudoriparous (cystic) 705.8
- suprarenal (capsule) (gland) 255.8
- sweat gland 705.8
- synovial membrane (pulpy) 727.9

Delivery - *continued*
- cesarean - *continued*
- - chin presentation 652.4
- - cicatrix of cervix 654.6
- - contracted pelvis (general) 653.1
- - - inlet 653.2
- - - outlet 653.3
- - cord presentation or prolapse 663.0
- - cystocele 654.4
- - deformity (acquired) (congenital)
- - - pelvic organs or tissues NEC 654.9
- - - pelvis (bony) NEC 653.0
- - displacement, uterus NEC 654.4
- - disproportion NEC 653.9
- - distress
- - - fetal 656.3
- - - maternal 669.0
- - eclampsia 642.6
- - face presentation 652.4
- - failed
- - - forceps 660.7
- - - trial of labour NEC 660.6
- - - vacuum extraction 660.7
- - - ventouse 660.7
- - fetal-maternal hemorrhage 656.0
- - fetus, fetal
- - - deformity 653.7
- - - distress 656.3
- - - prematurity 656.8
- - fibroid (tumor) (uterus) 654.1
- - hemorrhage (antepartum)
  (intrapartum) NEC 641.9
- - hydrocephalic fetus 653.6
- - incarceration of uterus 654.3
- - incoordinate uterine action 661.4
- - inertia, uterus 661.2
- - - primary 661.0
- - - secondary 661.1
- - lateroversion, uterus or cervix 654.4
- - mal lie 652.9
- - malposition
- - - fetus 652.9
- - - - in multiple gestation 652.6
- - - pelvic organs or tissues NEC 654.9
- - - uterus NEC or cervix 654.4
- - malpresentation NEC 652.9
- - - in multiple gestation 652.6
- - maternal
- - - diabetes mellitus 648.0
- - - heart disease NEC 648.6
- - meconium in liquor 656.3
- - oblique presentation 652.3
- - oversize fetus 653.5
- - pelvic tumor NEC 654.9
- - placenta previa 641.0
- - - with hemorrhage 641.1
- - placental insufficiency 656.5

Delivery - *continued*
- cesarean - *continued*
- - poor dilatation, cervix 661.0
- - pre-eclampsia 642.4
- - - severe 642.5
- - previous
- - - cesarean section 654.2
- - - surgery (to)
- - - - cervix 654.6
- - - - gynecological NEC 654.9
- - - - uterus 654.2
- - - - vagina 654.7
- - prolapse
- - - arm or hand 652.7
- - - uterus 654.4
- - prolonged labor 662.1
- - rectocele 654.4
- - retroversion, uterus or cervix 654.3
- - rigid
- - - cervix 654.6
- - - pelvic floor 654.4
- - - perineum 654.8
- - - vagina 654.7
- - - vulva 654.8
- - sacculation, pregnant uterus 654.4
- - scar(s)
- - - cervix 654.6
- - - cesarean section 654.2
- - - uterus 654.2
- - shirodkar suture in situ 654.5
- - shoulder presentation 652.8
- - stenosis or stricture, cervix 654.6
- - transverse presentation or lie 652.3
- - tumor, pelvic organs or tissues NEC
  654.4
- - umbilical cord presentation or prolapse
  663.0
- completely normal case (see also Note at
  category 650) 650
- complicated 669.9
- - by
- - - abnormal, abnormality of
- - - - cervix 660.2
- - - - forces of labor 661.9
- - - - pelvic organs or tissues 660.2
- - - - pelvis (bony) (major) NEC 660.1
- - - - presentation or position 660.0
- - - - size, fetus 660.1
- - - - soft parts (of pelvis) 660.2
- - - - uterine contractions NEC 661.9
- - - - uterus 660.2
- - - - vagina 660.2
- - - acromion presentation 660.0
- - - adherent placenta 667.0
- - - - with hemorrhage 666.0
- - - amnionitis 658.4
- - - anesthetic death 668.9

Delivery - *continued*
- complicated - *continued*
- – by - *continued*
- – – hemorrhage - *continued*
- – – – due to - *continued*
- – – – – retained placenta 666.0
- – – – – trauma 641.8
- – – – – uterine leiomyoma 641.8
- – – – – placenta NEC 641.9
- – – – – postpartum (atonic) (immediate) 666.1
- – – – – with retained or trapped placenta 666.0
- – – – – delayed 666.2
- – – – – secondary 666.2
- – – – – third stage 666.0
- – – – hourglass contraction, uterus 661.4
- – – – hydramnios 657
- – – – hydrocephalic fetus 660.1
- – – – hypertension - see Hypertension, complicating pregnancy
- – – – impacted shoulders 660.4
- – – – incarceration of uterus 660.2
- – – – incomplete dilatation (cervix) 661.0
- – – – incoordinate uterus 661.4
- – – – inertia uterus 661.2
- – – – – primary 661.0
- – – – – secondary 661.1
- – – – infantile
- – – – – genitalia 654.4
- – – – – uterus 654.4
- – – – injury (to mother) NEC 665.9
- – – – inversion uterus 665.2
- – – – laceration 664.9
- – – – – anus (sphincter) 664.2
- – – – – – with mucosa 664.3
- – – – – bladder (urinary) 665.5
- – – – – bowel 665.5
- – – – – central 664.4
- – – – – cervix (uteri) 665.3
- – – – – fourchette 664.0
- – – – – hymen 664.0
- – – – – labia 664.0
- – – – – pelvic
- – – – – – floor 664.1
- – – – – – organ NEC 665.5
- – – – – perineum, perineal 664.4
- – – – – – first degree 664.0
- – – – – – fourth degree 664.3
- – – – – – muscles 664.1
- – – – – – second degree 664.1
- – – – – – skin 664.0
- – – – – – slight 664.0
- – – – – – third degree 664.2
- – – – – peritoneum 665.5
- – – – – rectovaginal (septum) (without perineal laceration) 665.4

Delivery - *continued*
- complicated - *continued*
- – by - *continued*
- – – laceration - *continued*
- – – – rectovaginal - *continued*
- – – – – with perineum 664.2
- – – – – – with anal mucosa 664.3
- – – – – specified NEC 664.8
- – – – – sphincter ani 664.2
- – – – – – with mucosa 664.3
- – – – – urethra 665.5
- – – – – uterus 665.1
- – – – – – before labour 665.0
- – – – – vagina, vaginal (deep) (high) (without perineal laceration) 665.4
- – – – – – with perineum 664.0
- – – – – – muscles, with perineum 664.1
- – – – – vulva 664.0
- – – – lateroversion, uterus or cervix 660.2
- – – – mal lie 660.0
- – – – malposition
- – – – – fetus NEC 660.0
- – – – – pelvic organs or tissues NEC 660.2
- – – – – placenta 641.1
- – – – – – without hemorrhage 641.0
- – – – – uterus NEC or cervix 660.2
- – – – malpresentation NEC 660.0
- – – – marginal sinus (bleeding) (rupture) 641.2
- – – – meconium in liquor 656.3
- – – – metrorrhexis - see Delivery, complicated by, rupture, uterus
- – – – multiparity (grand) 659.4
- – – – nonengagement of fetal head 660.1
- – – – oblique presentation 660.0
- – – – obstetric trauma NEC 665.9
- – – – obstructed labor 660.9
- – – – – due to
- – – – – – conditions in 652- 660.0
- – – – – – conditions in 654- 660.2
- – – – – – deep transverse arrest 660.3
- – – – – – impacted shoulders 660.4
- – – – – – locked twins 660.5
- – – – – – persistent occipito posterior 660.3
- – – – oversize fetus 660.1
- – – – pathological retraction ring, uterus 661.4
- – – – pelvic tumor NEC 660.2
- – – – penetration, pregnant uterus by instrument 665.1
- – – – perforation - see Delivery complicated by laceration
- – – – persistent occiput anterior or posterior 660.3

Delivery - *continued*
- delayed NEC - *continued*
- - following rupture of membranes
  (spontaneous) 658.2
- - - artificial 658.3
- - second twin, triplet, etc. 662.3
- difficult NEC 669.9
- - previous, affecting management of
  pregnancy, childbirth V23.4
- early onset (spontaneous) 644.1
- forceps NEC 669.5
- - affecting fetus or newborn 763.2
- missed (at or near term) 656.4
- normal - see category 650
- precipitate 661.3
- - fetus or newborn 763.6
- premature NEC 644.1
- - previous, affecting management of
  pregnancy V23.4
- term pregnancy NEC - see category 650
- threatened premature 644.1
- uncomplicated - see category 650
- vacuum extractor NEC 669.5
- - affecting fetus or newborn 763.3
- ventouse NEC 669.5
- - affecting fetus or newborn 763.3
Delusions (paranoid) 297.9
- systematized 297.1
Dementia (see also Psychosis) 298.9
- alcoholic NEC 291.2
- Alzheimer's 290.1
- arteriosclerotic 290.4
- catatonic (acute) 295.2
- congenital (see also Retardation, mental)
  319
- developmental (see also Schizophrenia)
  295.9
- due to or associated with conditions
  classified elsewhere 294.1
- hebephrenic (acute) 295.1
- in
- - Alzheimer's disease 290.1
- - arteriosclerotic brain disease 290.4
- - cerebral lipidoses 294.1
- - epilepsy 294.1
- - general paralysis of the insane 294.1
- - hepatolenticular degeneration 294.1
- - Huntington's chorea 294.1
- - Jakob-Creutzfeldt d disease 290.1
- - multiple sclerosis 294.1
- - Pick's disease 290.1
- - polyarteritis nodosa 294.1
- old age 290.0
- paralytica, paralytic 094.1
- - juvenilis 090.4
- - syphilitic 094.1
- - - congenital 090.4

Dementia - *continued*
- paralytica - *continued*
- - tabetic form 094.1
- paranoid 295.3
- paraphrenic 295.3
- paretic 094.1
- praecox (see also Schizophrenia) 295.9
- presenile 290.1
- primary (acute) 295.0
- progressive, syphilitic 094.1
- schizophrenic (see also Schizophrenia)
  295.9
- senile 290.0
- - with acute confusional state 290.3
- - depressed or paranoid type 290.2
- - exhaustion 290.0
- simple type (acute) 295.0
- simplex (acute) 295.0
- uremic - see Uremia
Demineralization, ankle 733.0
Demodex folliculorum (infestation) 133.8
Demyelination, demyelinization
- central nervous system 341.9
- - specified NEC 341.8
- global 340
Dengue (fever) 061
- sandfly 061
Dens
- evaginatus 520.2
- in dente 520.2
- invaginatus 520.2
Density
- increased, bone (disseminated)
  (generalized) (spotted) 733.9
- lung (nodular) 518.8
Dental - see condition
Dentia praecox 520.6
Denticles (pulp) 522.2
Dentigerous cyst 526.0
Dentin
- irregular (in pulp) 522.3
- secondary (in pulp) 522.3
- sensitive 521.8
Dentinogenesis imperfecta 520.5
Dentinoma (M9271/0) 213.1
- upper jaw (bone) 213.0
Dentition 520.7
- abnormal 520.6
- anomaly 520.6
- delayed 520.6
- difficult 520.7
- disorder of 520.6
- precocious 520.6
- retarded 520.6
Denture sore mouth 528.9
Dependence
- absinthe 304.6

Dependence - *continued*
- amobarbital 304.1
- amphetamine(s) (type) (drugs classifiable to 969.7) 304.4
- amytal (sodium) 304.1
- analgesic NEC 304.6
- anesthetic (agent) (gas) (general) (local) NEC 304.6
- barbital(s) 304.1
- barbiturate(s) (compounds) (drugs classifiable to 967.-) 304.1
- benzedrine 304.4
- bhang 304.3
- bromide(s) NEC 304.1
- caffeine 304.4
- cannabis (sativa) (indica) (resin) (derivatives) (type) 304.3
- chloral (betaine) (hydrate) 304.1
- chlordiazepoxide 304.1
- coca (leaf) (and derivatives) 304.2
- cocaine 304.2
- codeine 304.0
- combinations of drugs - see Dependence, drug, combinations
- dagga 304.3
- demerol 304.0
- dexamphetamine 304.4
- dexedrine 304.4
- dextromethorphan 304.0
- dextromoramide 304.0
- dextro-nor-pseudo-ephedrine 304.4
- dextrorphan 304.0
- diazepam 304.1
- dilaudid 304.0
- D-lysergic acid diethylamide 304.5
- drug NEC 304.9
- - analgesic NEC 304.6
- - combinations NEC 304.8
- - - excluding morphine(-type) 304.8
- - - morphine(-type) with any other 304.7
- - complicating pregnancy, childbirth or puerperium 648.3
- - - fetus or newborn 779.5
- - hallucinogenic 304.5
- - hypnotic NEC 304.1
- - narcotic NEC 304.9
- - psychostimulant NEC 304.4
- - sedative 304.1
- - soporific NEC 304.1
- - specified NEC 304.6
- - suspected damage to fetus affecting management of pregnancy 655.5
- - synthetic, with morphine-like effect 304.0
- - tranquilizing 304.1
- ethyl

Dependence - *continued*
- ethyl - *continued*
- - alcohol 303
- - bromide 304.6
- - carbamate 304.6
- - chloride 304.6
- - morphine 304.0
- ganja 304.3
- glue (airplane) (sniffing) 304.6
- glutethimide 304.1
- hallucinogenics 304.5
- hashish 304.3
- hemp 304.3
- heroin (salt) (any) 304.0
- hypnotic NEC 304.1
- Indian hemp 304.3
- khat 304.4
- laudanum 304.0
- LSD(-25) (and derivatives) 304.5
- luminal 304.1
- lysergic acid 304.5
- maconha 304.3
- marihuana 304.3
- meprobamate 304.1
- mescaline 304.5
- methadone 304.0
- methamphetamine(s) 304.4
- methaqualone 304.1
- methyl
- - alcohol 303
- - bromide 304.6
- - morphine 304.0
- - sulfonal 304.1
- methylphenidate 304.4
- morphine (sulfate) (sulfite) (type) (drugs classifiable to 965.0) 304.0
- morphine-type drug (drugs classifiable to 965.0) with any other drug 304.7
- narcotic (drug) NEC 304.9
- nembutal 304.1
- neraval 304.1
- neravan 304.1
- neurobarb 304.1
- nicotine 305.1
- nitrous oxide 304.6
- nonbarbiturate sedatives and tranquilizers with similar effect 304.1
- on
- - aspirator V46.0
- - machine (enabling) V46.9
- - - specified type NEC V46.8
- - respirator V46.1
- opiate 304.0
- opioids 304.0
- opium (alkaloids) (derivatives) (tincture) 304.0
- paraldehyde 304.1

Dependence - *continued*
- paregoric 304.0
- pentobarbital 304.1
- pentobarbitone (sodium) 304.1
- pentothal 304.1
- peyote 304.5
- phenmetrazine 304.4
- phenobarbital 304.1
- psilocibin 304.5
- psilocin 304.5
- psilocybin 304.5
- psilocyline 304.5
- psilocyn 304.5
- psycho-stimulant NEC 304.4
- secobarbital 304.1
- seconal 304.1
- sedative NEC 304.1
- − nonbarbiturate with barbiturate effect 304.1
- specified drug NEC 304.6
- tobacco 305.1
- tranquilizer NEC 304.1
- − nonbarbiturate with barbiturate effect 304.1

Dependency
- passive 301.6
- reactions 301.6

Depersonalization (episode in neurotic state) (neurotic) (syndrome) 300.6

Depletion
- potassium 276.8
- salt or sodium 276.1
- − causing heat exhaustion or prostration 992.4
- volume 276.5
- − extracellular fluid 276.5
- − plasma 276.5

Deposit
- bone in Boeck's sarcoid 135
- calcareous, calcium - see Calcification
- cholesterol
- − retina 362.8
- − vitreous (humor) 379.2
- cornea 371.1
- crystallin, vitreous (humor) 379.2
- hemosiderin in old scars of cornea 371.1
- metallic in lens 366.4
- skin 709.3
- tooth, teeth (betel) (black) (green) (materia alba) (orange) (tobacco) (soft) 523.6
- urate, kidney (see also Disease, renal) 593.9

Depraved appetite 307.5

Depression 311
- acute 296.1
- agitated 296.1

Depression - *continued*
- anxiety 300.4
- arches 734
- − congenital 755.6
- basal metabolic rate 794.7
- bone marrow 289.9
- cerebral 331.9
- − newborn 779.2
- cerebrovascular 437.8
- chest wall 738.3
- endogenous 296.1
- functional activity 780.9
- hysterical 300.1
- involutional, climacteric, or menopausal 296.1
- manic (see also Psychosis, manic-depressive) 296.6
- medullary 348.8
- − newborn 779.2
- mental 300.4
- metatarsal heads - see Depression, arches
- metatarsus - see Depression, arches
- monopolar 296.1
- nervous 300.4
- neurotic 300.4
- nose 738.0
- psychogenic 300.4
- − reactive 298.0
- psychoneurotic 300.4
- psychotic 296.1
- reactive 300.4
- − neurotic 300.4
- − psychogenic 298.0
- − psychoneurotic 300.4
- − psychotic 298.0
- recurrent 296.1
- respiratory center 348.8
- − newborn 770.8
- senile 290.2
- skull 754.0
- sternum 738.3
- visual field 368.4

Depressive reaction - see Reaction, depressive

Deprivation
- cultural V62.4
- emotional V62.8
- − affecting infant or child 995.5
- food 994.2
- protein (familial) 260
- social V62.4
- − affecting infant or child 995.5
- symptoms, syndrome, drug (narcotic) (see also Dependence) 304.9
- vitamins (see also Deficiency, vitamin) 269.2
- water 994.3

Derangement
- cartilage (articular) NEC 718.0
- - knee 717.9
- - - recurrent 718.3
- - recurrent 718.3
- elbow (internal) 718.9
- - current injury (see also Dislocation,
    elbow) 832.-
- - recurrent 718.3
- gastro-intestinal 536.9
- joint (internal) 718.9
- - current injury - see also Dislocation
- - - knee, meniscus or cartilage (see also
      Tear, meniscus) 836.2
- - elbow 718.9
- - knee 717.9
- - - recurrent 718.3
- - recurrent 718.3
- - shoulder 718.9
- - temporomandibular 524.6
- knee NEC 717.9
- - current injury (see also Tear,
    meniscus) 836.2
- - recurrent 718.3
- low back NEC 724.9
- meniscus NEC 717.5
- - lateral 717.4
- - medial 717.3
- - - anterior horn 717.1
- - - posterior horn 717.2
- - recurrent 718.3
- mental (see also Psychosis) 298.9
- semilunar cartilage (knee) 717.5
- - current injury 836.2
- - - lateral 836.1
- - - medial 836.0
- - recurrent 718.3
- shoulder (internal) 718.9
- - current injury (see also Dislocation,
    shoulder) 831.-
- - recurrent 718.3
Dercum's disease 272.8
Derealization (neurotic) 300.6
Dermal - see condition
Dermaphytid - see Dermatophytosis
Dermatergosis - see Dermatitis
Dermatitis (allergic) (contact)
  (occupational) (venenata) 692.9
- ab igne 692.8
- acneiform 692.9
- actinic (due to sun) 692.7
- - other than from sun 692.8
- ambustionis
- - due to
- - - burn or scald - see Burn
- - - sunburn 692.7
- amebic 006.6

Dermatitis - *continued*
- anaphylactoid NEC 692.9
- arsenical 692.4
- artefacta 698.4
- atopic 691.8
- atrophicans 701.8
- - diffusa 701.8
- - maculosa 701.3
- berlock 692.7
- berloque 692.7
- blastomycetic 116.0
- blister beetle 692.8
- brucella NEC 023.9
- bullosa 694.9
- - striata pratensis 692.6
- bullous
- - mucosynechial, atrophic 694.6
- - seasonal 694.8
- calorica
- - due to
- - - burn or scald - see Burn
- - - cold 692.8
- - - sunburn 692.7
- caterpillar 692.8
- cercarial 120.3
- combustionis
- - due to
- - - burn or scald - see Burn
- - - sunburn 692.7
- congelationis 991.5
- contusiformis 695.2
- diabetic 250.7 † 709.8*
- diaper 691.0
- diphtheritica 032.8
- due to
- - acetone 692.2
- - acids 692.4
- - adhesive plaster 692.4
- - alcohol (skin contact) (substances in
    980.-) 692.4
- - - taken internally 693.8
- - alkalis 692.4
- - arsenic 692.4
- - - taken internally 693.8
- - carbon disulphide 692.2
- - caustics 692.4
- - chemical(s) NEC 692.4
- - - internal 693.8
- - - irritant NEC 692.4
- - - taken internally 693.8
- - cold weather 692.8
- - cosmetics 692.8
- - detergents 692.0
- - dichromate 692.4
- - drugs and medicaments (correct
    substance properly administered)
    (internal use) 693.0

Dermatitis - *continued*
– due to - *continued*
– – drugs and medicaments - *continued*
– – – external (in contact with skin) 692.3
– – – – wrong substance given or taken 976.-
– – – – – specified substance - see Table of drugs and chemicals
– – – in contact with skin 692.3
– – – wrong substance given or taken 977.9
– – – – specified substance - see Table of drugs and chemicals
– – dyes 692.8
– – epidermophytosis - see Dermatophytosis
– – external irritant NEC 692.9
– – food (ingested) 693.1
– – – in contact with skin 692.5
– – furs 692.8
– – greases NEC 692.1
– – hot
– – – objects and materials - see Burn
– – – weather or places 692.8
– – infrared rays, except from sun 692.8
– – – solar 692.7
– – ingested substance 693.9
– – – drugs and medicaments (see also Dermatitis, due to drugs and medicaments) 693.0
– – – food 693.1
– – – specified NEC 693.8
– – ingestion or injection of
– – – chemical 693.8
– – – drug (correct substance properly administered) 693.0
– – – – wrong substance given or taken 977.9
– – – – – specified substance - see Table of drugs and chemicals
– – insecticide 692.4
– – internal agent 693.9
– – – drugs and medicaments (see also Dermatitis, due to drugs and medicaments) 693.0
– – – food 693.1
– – irradiation 692.8
– – lacquer tree 692.6
– – light (sun) 692.7
– – – other 692.8
– – low temperature 692.8
– – nylon 692.4
– – oils NEC 692.1
– – paint solvent 692.2
– – petroleum products (substances in 981) 692.4
– – plants NEC 692.6

Dermatitis - *continued*
– due to - *continued*
– – plasters, medicated (any) 692.3
– – plastic 692.4
– – poison
– – – ivy 692.6
– – – oak 692.6
– – – plant or vine 692.6
– – – sumac 692.6
– – preservatives 692.8
– – primrose 692.6
– – primula 692.6
– – radiation 692.8
– – – sun 692.7
– – radioactive substance 692.8
– – radium 692.8
– – ragweed 692.6
– – Rhus 692.6
– – – diversiloba 692.6
– – – radicans 692.6
– – – toxicodendron 692.6
– – – venenata 692.6
– – – verniciflua 692.6
– – rubber 692.4
– – Senecio jacobaea 692.6
– – solvents (substances in 982.-) 692.2
– – – chlorocompound group 692.2
– – – cyclohexane group 692.2
– – – ester group 692.2
– – – glycol group 692.2
– – – hydrocarbon group 692.2
– – – ketone group 692.2
– – – paint 692.2
– – specified agent NEC 692.8
– – sunburn 692.7
– – sunshine 692.7
– – tetrachlorethylene 692.2
– – toluene 692.2
– – turpentine 692.2
– – ultraviolet rays, except from sun 692.8
– – – sun 692.7
– – vaccine or vaccination (correct substance properly administered) 693.0
– – – wrong substance given or taken
– – – – bacterial vaccine 978.-
– – – – – specified - see Table of drugs and chemicals
– – – – other vaccines NEC 979.-
– – – – – specified - see Table of drugs and chemicals
– – varicose veins - see Varicose vein, inflamed or infected
– – X-rays 692.8
– dysmenorrheica 625.8
– eczematoid NEC 692.9
– eczematous NEC 692.9

Dermatitis - *continued*
- epidemica 695.8
- escharotica - see Burn
- exfoliativa, exfoliative 695.8
- - generalized 695.8
- eyelid 373.3
- - herpes (zoster) 053.2 † 373.5*
- - - simplex 054.4 † 373.5*
- facta, factitia 698.4
- ficta 698.4
- flexural 691.8
- follicularis 704.8
- friction 709.8
- fungus 111.9
- - specified type NEC 111.8
- gangrenosa, gangrenous (see also Gangrene) 785.4
- - infantum 785.4
- gestationis 646.8
- harvest mite 133.8
- heat 692.8
- herpetiformis (bullous) (erythematous) (pustular) (vesicular) 694.0
- - juvenile 694.2
- - senile 694.5
- hiemalis 692.8
- hypostatic, hypostatica 454.1
- - with ulcer 454.2
- infectiosa eczematoides 690
- infective eczematoid 690
- Jacquet's 691.0
- leptus 133.8
- lichenified NEC 692.9
- medicamentosa (correct substance properly administered) (internal use) (see also Dermatitis, due to drug) 693.0
- - due to contact with skin 692.3
- mite 133.8
- multiformis 694.0
- napkin 691.0
- nummular NEC 692.9
- papillaris capillitii 706.1
- pellagrous 265.2
- perioral 695.3
- perstans 696.1
- pruritic NEC 692.9
- purulent 686.0
- pustular contagious 051.2
- pyococcal 686.0
- pyogenica 686.0
- repens 696.1
- Schamberg's 709.0
- schistosome 120.3
- seasonal bullous 694.8
- seborrheic 690
- - infantile 691.8
- sensitization NEC 692.9

Dermatitis - *continued*
- septic 686.0
- solare 692.7
- statis - see Varix, with stasis dermatitis
- suppurative 686.0
- traumatic NEC 709.8
- ultraviolet, except from sun 692.8
- - due to sun 692.7
- varicose 454.1
- - with ulcer 454.2
- vegetans 686.8
- verrucosa 117.2
Dermatoarthritis, lipoid 272.8 † 713.0*
Dermatofibroma (lenticulare) (M8832/0) - see also Neoplasm, skin, benign
- protuberans (M8832/1) - see Neoplasm, skin, uncertain behavior
Dermatofibrosarcoma (protuberans) (M8832/3) - see Neoplasm, skin, malignant
Dermatographia 708.3
Dermatolysis (exfoliativa) (congenital) 757.3
- acquired 701.8
- eyelids 374.5
- palpebrarum 374.5
- senile 701.8
Dermatomegaly NEC 701.8
Dermatomucosomyositis 710.3
Dermatomycosis 111.9
- furfuracea 111.0
- specified type NEC 111.8
Dermatomyositis (acute) (chronic) 710.3
Dermatoneuritis of children 985.0
Dermatophiliasis 134.1
Dermatophytide - see Dermatophytosis
Dermatophytosis (epidermophyton) (infection) (Microsporum) (tinea) (Trichophyton) 110.9
- beard 110.0
- body 110.5
- deep seated 110.6
- foot 110.4
- groin 110.3
- hand 110.2
- nail 110.1
- perianal (area) 110.3
- scalp 110.0
- scrotal 110.8
- specified site NEC 110.8
Dermatopolyneuritis 985.0
Dermatorrhexis 757.3
- acquired 701.8
Dermatosclerosis (see also Scleroderma) 710.1
- localized 701.0
Dermatosis 709.9

Dermatosis - *continued*
- Bowen's (M8081/2) - see Neoplasm, skin, in situ
- bullous NEC 694.9
- exfoliativa 695.8
- factitial 698.4
- gonococcal 098.8
- herpetiformis 694.0
- hysterical 300.1
- menstrual NEC 709.8
- occupational (see also Dermatitis) 692.9
- papulosa nigra 709.8
- pigmentary NEC 709.0
- - progressive 709.0
- - Schamberg's 709.0
- pustular, subcorneal 694.1
- senile NEC 709.3
Dermographia 708.3
Dermographism 708.3
Dermoid (cyst) (M9084/0) - see Neoplasm, benign
- with malignant transformation (M9084/3) 183.0
Dermopathy, senile NEC 709.3
Dermophytosis - see Dermatophytosis
Descemet's membrane - see condition
Descemetocele 371.7
Descending - see condition
Descensus uteri (incomplete) (partial) 618.1
Desensitization to allergens V07.1
Desert
- rheumatism 114
- sore (see also Ulcer, skin) 707.9
Desertion (newborn) 995.5
- Desmoid (extra-abdominal) (tumor) (M8821/1) - see Neoplasm, connective tissue, uncertain behavior
- abdominal (M8822/1) - see Neoplasm, connective tissue, uncertain behavior
Despondency 300.4
Destruction
- articular facet 718.9
- - vertebra 724.9
- bone 733.9
- - syphilitic 095 † 730.8*
- joint 718.9
- - sacroiliac 724.6
- kidney 593.8
- live fetus to facilitate delivery 763.8
- rectal sphincter 569.4
- septum (nasal) 478.1
- tuberculous NEG (see also Tuberculosis) 011.9
- tympanic membrane 384.8
- tympanum 385.8
- vertebral disc - see Degeneration, intervertebral disc

Destructiveness (see also Disturbance, conduct) 312.9
- adjustment reaction 309.3
Detachment
- cartilage - see also Sprain, strain
- - knee - see Tear, meniscus
- cervix annular 622.8
- - complicating delivery 665.3
- choroid (old) (postinfectional) (simple) (spontaneous) 363.7
- knee, medial meniscus (old) 717.5
- - current injury 836.0
- ligament - see Sprain, strain
- placenta (premature) - see Placenta, separation
- retina 361.9
- - with
- - - giant tear of retina 361.0
- - - retinal defect 361.0
- - pigment epithelium 362.4
- - rhegmatogenous 361.0
- - serous 361.2
- - traction 361.8
- - without retinal defect 361.2
- vitreous humor 379.2
Deterioration
- epileptic 294.1
- heart, cardiac (see also Degeneration, myocardial) 429.1
- mental (see also Psychosis) 298.9
- myocardium, myocardial (see also Degeneration, myocardial) 429.1
- senile (simple) 797
Deuteranomaly 368.5
Deuteranopia (anomalous trichromat) (complete) (incomplete) 368.5
Deutschlander's disease - see Fracture, foot
Development
- abnormal, bone 756.9
- arrested 783.4
- - bone 733.9
- - child 783.4
- - due to malnutrition 263.2
- - fetus 764.9
- - - affecting management of pregnancy 656.5
- - tracheal rings (congenital) 748.3
- defective, congenital - see also Anomaly
- - cauda equina 742.5
- - left ventricle 746.9
- - - in hypoplastic left heart syndrome 746.7
- delayed (see also Delay, development) 783.4
- - arithmetical skills 315.1
- - language (skills) 315.3
- - learning skill, specified NEC 315.2

Development - *continued*
- delayed - *continued*
- - mixed skills 315.5
- - motor coordination 315.4
- - reading 315.0
- - specified learning skill NEC 315.8
- - speech 315.3
- - - associated with hyperkinesis 314.1
- - spelling 315.0
- imperfect, congenital - see also Anomaly
- - heart 746.9
- - lungs 748.6
- incomplete (fetus) 764.9
- - affecting management of pregnancy
  656.5
- - bronchial tree 748.3
- - organ or site not listed - see Hypoplasia
- - respiratory system 748.9
- tardy, mental (see also Retardation,
  mental) 319
Developmental - see condition

Devergie's disease 696.4
Deviation
- conjugate (eye) (spastic) 378.8
- esophagus 530.8
- eye, skew 378.8
- midline (jaw) (teeth) 524.2
- - specified site NEC - see Malposition
- oesophagus 530.8
- organ or site, congenital NEC - see
  Malposition, congenital
- septum (nasal) (acquired) 470
- - congenital 754.0
- sexual 302.9
- - bestiality 302.1
- - erotomania 302.8
- - exhibitionism 302.4
- - fetishism 302.8
- - homosexuality 302.0
- - lesbianism 302.0
- - masochism 302.8
- - narcissism 302.8
- - necrophilia 302.8
- - nymphomania 302.8
- - pederosis 302.2
- - pedophilia 302.2
- - sadism 302.8
- - satyriasis 302.8
- - specified type NEC 302.8
- - transvestism 302.3
- - voyeurism 302.8
- teeth, midline 524.2
- trachea 519.1
- ureter (congenital) 753.4

Devic's disease 341.0
Device

Device - *continued*
- cerebral ventricle (communicating) in situ
  V45.2
- contraceptive - see Contraceptive, device
- drainage, cerebrospinal fluid, in situ
  V45.2
Devitalized tooth 522.9
Devonshire colic 984.-
- specified type of lead - see Table of drugs
  and chemicals
Dextra transposition, aorta 745.1
Dextraposition, aorta 747.2
- in tetralogy of Fallot 745.2
Dextrinosis, limit (debrancher enzyme
  deficiency) 271.0
Dextrocardia (true) 746.8
- with
- - complete transposition of viscera 759.3
- - situs inversus 759.3
Dhobie itch 110.3
Di George's syndrome 279.1
Di Guglielmo's disease (M9841/3) 207.0
Diabetes, diabetic (mellitus) (congenital)
  (controlled) (familial) (severe) (slight)
  250.0
- acetonemia 250.1
- acidosis 250.1
- bone change 250.7 † 731.8*
- bronze, bronzed 275.0
- cataract 250.4 † 366.4*
- chemical 790.2
- coma 250.2
- - hyperglycemic 250.2
- - hyperosmolar 250.2
- complicating pregnancy, childbirth or
  puerperium (maternal) 648.0
- - affecting fetus or newborn 775.0
- complication NEC 250.9
- gangrene 250.6 † 785.4*
- hemochromatosis 275.0
- insipidus 253.5
- - nephrogenic 588.1
- - pituitary 253.5
- - vasopressin resistant 588.1
- intercapillary glomerulosclerosis 250.3 †
  581.8*
- iritis 250.4 † 364.8*
- ketosis, ketoacidosis 250.1
- Lancereaux's 250.7 † 261*
- latent 790.2
- neonatal, transient 775.1
- nephropathy 250.3 † 583.8*
- nephrosis 250.3 † 581.8*
- neuralgia 250.5 † 357.2*
- neuritis 250.5 † 357.2*
- neuropathy 250.5 † 357.2*
- phosphate 275.3

Diabetes - *continued*
- renal 271.4
- - true 271.4
- retinal hemorrhage 250.4 † 362.0*
- retinitis 250.4 † 362.0*
- retinopathy 250.4 † 362.0*
- steroid induced
- - correct substance properly
  administered 251.8
- - overdose or wrong substance given or
  taken 962.0
- sugar 250.0
Diacyclothrombopathia 287.1
Diagnosis deferred 799.9
Dialysis (intermittent) (preparation)
  (treatment)
- anterior retinal 361.0
- extracorporeal V56.0
- peritoneal V56.8
- renal V56.0
- specified type NEC V56.8
Diaphragm - see condition
Diaphragmitis 519.4
Diaphysial aclasis 756.4
Diaphysitis 733.9
Diarrhea, diarrheal (autumn) (bilious)
  (bloody) (catarrhal) (choleraic) (disease)
  (endemic) (gravis) (green) (infantile)
  (lienteric) (parenteral) (presumed
  infectious) (putrefactive) (sporadic)
  (summer) (thermic) (zymotic) (see also
  Note at category 009.3) 009.3
- achlorhydric 536.0
- allergic 558
- amebic (see also Amebiasis) 006.9
- - with abscess - see Abscess, amebic
- - acute 006.0
- - chronic 006.1
- - nondysenteric 006.2
- bacillary - see Dysentery, bacillary
- bacterial NEC 008.5
- balantidial 007.0
- cachectic NEC 558
- Chilomastix 007.8
- choleriformis 001.1
- chronic 558
- - ulcerative 556
- coccidial 007.2
- Cochin-China 579.1
- - anguilluliasis 127.2
- - psilosis 579.1
- Dientameba 007.8
- dietetic 558
- due to
- - Aerobacter aerogenes 008.2
- - Bacillus coli 008.0
- - bacteria 008.5

Diarrhea - *continued*
- due to - *continued*
- - bacteria - *continued*
- - - specified type NEC 008.4
- - Clostridium perfringens (C) (F) 008.4
- - enterococci 008.4
- - Escherichia coli 008.0
- - irritating foods 558
- - Paracolobactrum Arizona 008.1
- - Paracolon bacillus NEC 008.4
- - - Arizona 008.1
- - Proteus (bacillus) (mirabilis)
  (morganii) 008.3
- - Pseudomonas aeruginosa 008.4
- - specified organism NEC 008.8
- - - bacterial 008.4
- - - viral 008.6
- - Staphylococcus 008.4
- - virus (see also Enteritis, viral) 008.8
- dysenteric 009.2
- - due to specified organism NEC 008.8
- dyspeptic 558
- epidemic 009.2
- - due to specified organism NEC 008.8
- fermentative 558
- flagellate 007.9
- Flexner's (ulcerative) 004.1
- functional 564.5
- - following gastrointestinal surgery
  564.4
- - psychogenic 306.4
- Giardia lamblia 007.1
- giardial 007.1
- hill 579.1
- hyperperistalsis (nervous) 306.4
- infectious 009.2
- - due to specified organism NEC 008.8
- inflammatory 009.3
- - due to specified organism NEC 008.8
- malarial (see also Malaria) 084.6
- mite 133.8
- mycotic 117.9
- nervous 306.4
- neurogenic 564.5
- noninfectious 558
- protozoal NEC 007.9
- psychogenic 306.4
- septic (see also Enteritis) 009.2
- specified
- - bacteria NEC 008.4
- - organism, nonbacterial NEC 008.8
- - virus NEC 008.6
- Staphylococcus 008.4
- Streptococcus 008.4
- toxic 558
- trichomonal 007.3
- tropical 579.1

Diarrhea - *continued*
- tuberculous 014
- ulcerative (chronic) 556
- viral (see also Enteritis, viral) 008.8
Diastasis
- cranial bones 733.9
- - congenital 756.0
- joint (traumatic) - see Dislocation
- muscle 728.8
- - congenital 756.8
- recti (abdomen) 728.8
- - complicating delivery 665.8
- - congenital 756.7
Diastema, tooth, teeth 524.3
Diastematomyelia 742.5
Diataxia, cerebral, infantile 343.0
Diathesis
- cystine (familial) 270.0
- gouty 274.9
- hemorrhagic (familial) 287.9
- - newborn NEC 776.0
- scrofulous 017.2
- uric acid 274.9
Diaz's disease or osteochondrosis 732.5
Dibothriocephaliasis 123.4
- larval 123.5
Dibothriocephalus (latus) (infection)
   (infestation) 123.4
- larval 123.5
Dicephalus 759.4
Dichotomy teeth 520.2
Dichromat (congenital) 368.5
Dichromatopsia (congenital) 368.5
Dichuchwa 104.0
Dicroceliasis 121.8
Didelphys, didelphic (see also Double
   uterus) 752.2
Didymytis (see also Orchitis) 604.9
Died - see also Death
- without
- - medical attention (cause unknown)
     798.9
- - sign of disease 798.2
Dietary
- inadequacy or deficiency 269.9
- surveillance and counselling V65.3
Dieulafoy's ulcer - see Ulcer, stomach
Difficult
- birth, affecting fetus or newborn 763.9
- delivery NEC 669.9
Difficulty
- feeding 783.3
- - newborn 779.3
- - nonorganic (infant) 307.5
- mechanical, gastroduodenal stoma 537.8
- reading 315.0
- specific, spelling 315.0

Difficulty - *continued*
- swallowing (see also Dysphagia) 787.2
- walking 719.7
Diffuse - see condition

Diffused ganglion 727.4
Digestive - see condition
Diktyoma (M9501/3) - see Neoplasm,
   malignant
Dilaceration, tooth 520.4

Dilatation
- anus 564.8
- - venule - see Hemorrhoids
- aorta (focal) (general) (see also
   Aneurysm, aorta) 441.6
- - congenital 747.2
- - infectional 093.0 † 441.7*
- - ruptured 441.5
- - syphilitic 093.0 † 441.7*
- artery 447.8
- bladder (sphincter) 596.8
- - congenital 753.8
- blood vessel 459.8
- bronchi 494
- calyx (due to obstruction) 593.8
- capillaries 448.9
- cardiac (acute) (chronic) (see also
   Hypertrophy, cardiac) 429.3
- - congenital 746.8
- - - valve NEC 746.8
- - - - pulmonary 746.0
- cavum septi pellucidi 742.5
- cecum 564.8
- - psychogenic 306.4
- cervix (uteri) - see also Incompetency,
   cervix
- - incomplete, poor, slow
- - - complicating delivery 661.0
- - - fetus or newborn 763.7
- colon 564.7
- - congenital 751.3
- - psychogenic 306.4
- common duct 751.6
- - acquired (see also Disease, biliary)
     576.8
- cystic duct 751.6
- - acquired (any bile duct) 575.8
- duodenum 564.8
- esophagus 530.8
- - congenital 750.4
- eustachian tube, congenital 744.2
- fontanel 756.0
- gallbladder (see also Disease,
   gallbladder) 575.8
- gastric 536.8
- - acute 536.1
- - psychogenic 306.4

Dilatation - *continued*
- heart (acute) (chronic) (see also Hypertrophy, cardiac) 429.3
- - congenital 746.8
- - valve - see Endocarditis
- - - congenital 746.8
- ileum 564.8
- - psychogenic 306.4
- inguinal rings 550.9
- jejunum 564.8
- - psychogenic 306.4
- kidney (calyx) (collecting structures) (cystic) (parenchyma) (pelvis) 593.8
- lacrimal apparatus or duct 375.6
- lymphatic vessel 457.1
- mammary duct 610.4
- Meckel's diverticulum (congenital) 751.0
- meningeal vessels, congenital 742.8
- myocardium (acute) (chronic) (see also Hypertrophy, cardiac) 429.3
- oesophagus 530.8
- - congenital 750.4
- organ or site, congenital NEC - see Distortion
- pancreatic duct 577.8
- pericardium - see Pericarditis
- pharynx 478.2
- prostate 602.8
- pulmonary
- - artery (idiopathic) 417.8
- - valve, congenital 746.0
- pupil 379.4
- rectum 564.8
- saccule, congenital 744.0
- sphincter ani 564.8
- stomach 536.8
- - acute 536.1
- - psychogenic 306.4
- submaxillary duct 527.8
- trachea, congenital 748.3
- ureter (idiopathic) 593.8
- - congenital 753.2
- urethra (acquired) 599.8
- vasomotor 443.9
- vein 459.8
- ventricular, ventricle (acute) (chronic) (see also Hypertrophy, cardiac) 429.3
- - cerebral, congenital 742.4
- venule 459.8
- vesical orifice 596.8
Dilated, dilation - see Dilatation
Diminished hearing (acuity) (see also Deafness) 389.9
Diminution, sense or sensation (cold) (heat) (tactile) (vibratory) (see also Disturbance, sensation) 782.0
Dimitri-Sturge-Weber disease 759.6

Dimple
- parasacral 685.1
- - with abscess 685.0
- pilonidal 685.1
- - with abscess 685.0
- postanal 685.1
- - with abscess 685.0
Dioctophyma renale (infection) (infestation) 128.8
Dipetalonemiasis 125.4
Diphallus 752.8
Diphtheria, diphtheritic (gangrenous) (hemorrhagic) 032.9
- cutaneous 032.8
- faucial 032.0
- infection of wound 032.8
- laryngeal 032.3
- myocarditis 032.8 † 422.0*
- nasal anterior 032.2
- nasopharyngeal 032.1
- neurological complication 032.8
- specified site NEC 032.8
Diphyllobothriasis (intestine) 123.4
- larval 123.5
Diplacusis 388.4
Diplegia (upper limbs) 344.2
- brain or cerebral 437.8
- infantile or congenital (cerebral) (spastic) (spinal) 343.0
- lower limbs 344.1
Diplococcus, diplococcal - see condition
Diplopia 368.2
Dipsomania 303
- with psychosis (see also Psychosis, alcoholic) 291.9
Dipylidiasis 123.8
- intestine 123.8
Direction, teeth abnormal 524.3
Dirt-eating child 307.5
Disability
- heart - see Disease, heart
- special spelling 315.0
Disarticulation 718.9
- meaning
- - dislocation, traumatic or congenital - see Dislocation
- - traumatic amputation - see Amputation, traumatic
Disaster, cerebrovascular (see also Disease, cerebrovascular, acute) 436
Discharge
- breast (female) (male) 611.7
- diencephalic autonomic idiopathic 345.5
- ear 388.6
- excessive urine 788.4
- nipple 611.7
- postnasal - see Sinusitis

Discharge - *continued*
- sinus from mediastinum 510.0
- urethral 788.7
- vaginal 623.5
Discoid
- meniscus, congenital 717.5
- semilunar cartilage 717.5
Discoloration, nails 703.8
Discomycosis - see Actinomycosis
Discrepancy leg length (acquired) 736.8
- congenital 755.3
Discrimination
- political V62.4
- racial V62.4
- religious V62.4
- sex V62.4
Disease, diseased - see also Syndrome
- Abrami's 283.9
- absorbent system 459.8
- Acosta's 993.2
- Adams-Stokes(-Morgagni) 426.9
- Addison's (bronze) 255.4
- - tuberculous 017.6 † 255.4*
- adenoids (and tonsils) 474.9
- adrenal (capsule) (gland) 255.9
- - cortex 255.9
- ainhum 136.0
- Akureyri 049.8 † 323.4*
- Albers-Schonberg 756.5
- Albert's 726.7
- Alibert's (M9700/3) 202.1
- alimentary canal 569.9
- alligator-skin 757.1
- - acquired 701.1
- Almeida's 116.1
- Alper's 330.8
- alveoli, teeth 525.9
- Alzheimer's 331.0
- - dementia in 290.1
- amyloid (any site) 277.3
- anarthritic rheumatoid 446.5
- Anderson's 272.7
- Andes 993.2
- angiospastic 443.9
- - cerebral 435
- - vein 459.8
- anterior
- - chamber 364.9
- - horn cell 335.9
- - - specified NEC 335.8
- anus NEC 569.4
- aorta (nonsyphilitic) 447.9
- - syphilitic NEC 093.8
- aortic (heart) (valve) (see also Endocarditis, aortic) 424.1
- Apollo 077.4 † 372.0*
- aponeuroses 726.9

Disease - *continued*
- appendix 543
- aqueous (chamber) 364.9
- Arnold-Chiari 741.0
- arterial 447.9
- - occlusive 447.1
- arteriocardiorenal 404.9
- arteriolar (obliterative) (generalized) 447.9
- arteriorenal - see Hypertension, kidney
- arteriosclerotic - see also Arteriosclerosis
- - coronary 414.0
- - heart 414.0
- - vascular - see Arteriosclerosis
- artery 447.9
- - cerebral 437.9
- arthropod-borne NEC 088.9
- - specified type NEC 088.8
- atticoantral, chronic 382.2
- auditory canal, ear 380.9
- Aujeszky's 078.8
- auricle, ear NEC 380.3
- Australian X 062.4 † 323.3*
- autoimmune NEC 279.4
- - hemolytic (cold type) (warm type) 283.0
- aviators' (see also Effect, adverse, high altitude) 993.2
- ax(e)-grinders' 502
- Ayala's 756.8
- Ayerza's 416.0
- back bone NEC 733.9
- bacterial NEC 040.8
- - zoonotic NEC 027.9
- - - specified type NEC 027.8
- balloon (see also Effect, adverse, high altitude) 993.2
- Balo's 341.1
- Bamberger-Marie 731.2
- Bang's 023.1
- Bannister's 995.1
- Banti's (with cirrhosis) (with portal hypertension) - see Cirrhosis, liver
- Barcoo (see also Ulcer, skin) 707.9
- Barensprung's 110.3
- Barlow's 267
- Barraquer(-Simons) 272.6
- basal ganglia 333.9
- - degenerative NEC 333.0
- - specified NEC 333.8
- Basedow's 242.0
- Bateman's 078.0
- Batten-Mayou (retina) 330.1 † 362.7*
- Battey 031.0
- Baumgarten-Cruveilhier 571.5
- Bayle's 094.1
- Bazin's 017.1

Disease - *continued*
- Beard's 300.5
- Bechterew's 720.0
- Becker's 425.2
- Behr's 362.5
- Beigel's 111.2
- Bell's 296.0
- Benson's 379.2
- Bergeron's 300.1
- Bernard-Soulier's 287.1
- Bernhardt(-Roth) 355.1
- Besnier-Boeck(-Schaumann) 135
- Best's 362.7
- Beurmann's 117.1
- Bielschowsky(-Jansky) 330.1
- Biermer's 281.0
- Biett's 695.4
- bile duct (see also Disease, biliary) 576.9
- biliary (duct) (tract) 576.9
- - with calculus, choledocholithiasis or stones 574.5
- Billroth's 741.9
- - with hydrocephalus 741.0
- bird fanciers' 495.2
- bladder 596.9
- - specified NEC 596.8
- Bloch-Sulzberger 757.3
- Blocq's 307.9
- blood 289.9
- - forming organs 289.9
- - vessel 459.9
- Bloodgood's 610.1
- Blount's 732.4
- blue 746.9
- Boeck's 135
- bone 733.9
- - fibrocystic NEC 733.2
- - - jaw 526.2
- - Paget's 731.0
- bone-marrow 289.9
- Borna 062.9 † 323.3*
- Bornholm 074.1
- Bouillaud's 391.9
- Bourneville's 759.5
- bowel 569.9
- - functional 564.9
- - - psychogenic 306.4
- Bowen's (M8081/2) - see Neoplasm, skin, in situ
- Brailsford's 732.3
- - radius, head 732.3
- - tarsal, scaphoid 732.5
- brain 348.9
- - arterial, artery 437.9
- - arteriosclerotic 437.0
- - congenital 742.9
- - degenerative - see Degeneration, brain

Disease - *continued*
- brain - *continued*
- - inflammatory - see Encephalitis
- - organic 348.9
- - - arteriosclerotic 437.0
- - parasitic NEC 123.9
- - Pick's 331.1
- - - dementia in 290.1
- - senile 331.2
- brazier's 985.8
- breast 611.9
- - cystic (chronic) 610.1
- - fibrocystic 610.1
- - Paget's 174.0
- - puerperal, postpartum NEC 676.3
- - specified NEC 611.8
- Breda's (see also Yaws) 102.9
- Bretonneau's 032.0
- Bright's (see also Nephritis) 583.9
- - arteriosclerotic (see also Hypertension, kidney) 403.9
- Brill's 081.1
- - flea borne 081.0
- - louse borne 081.1
- Brill-Symmers's (M9690/3) 202.0
- Brill-Zinsser 081.1
- broad ligament, noninflammatory 620.9
- - specified NEC 620.8
- Brocq's 691.8
- - meaning
- - - dermatitis, herpetiformis 694.0
- - - parapsoriasis 696.2
- Brodie's (joint) 730.1
- bronchi 519.1
- bronchopulmonary 519.1
- bronze (Addison's) 255.4
- - tuberculous 017.6 † 255.4*
- Brown-Sequard 344.8
- Bruck's 733.9
- Bruck-Lange 759.8
- Bruhl's 285.8
- buccal cavity 528.9
- Buchanan's 732.1
- Buchman's 732.1
- budgerigar fanciers' 495.2
- Budinger-Ludloff-Laewen 718.2
- Buerger's 443.1
- Burger-Grutz 272.3
- Burn's 732.3
- bursa 727.9
- Bury's 695.8
- Busse-Buschke 117.5
- Caffey's 756.5
- caisson 993.3
- California 114
- Calve(-Perthes) 732.1
- Camurati-Engelmann 756.5

Disease - *continued*
- Canavan's 330.0
- capillaries 448.9
- Carapata 087.1
- cardiac - see Disease, heart
- cardiopulmonary, chronic 416.9
- cardiorenal (hepatic) (hypertensive) (vascular) 404.9
- cardiovascular (arteriosclerosis) 429.2
- - congenital 746.9
- - hypertensive - see Hypertension, heart
- - renal (hypertensive) 404.9
- - syphilitic (asymptomatic) 093.9
- Carrion's 088.0
- cartilage NEC 733.9
- cat scratch 078.3
- Cavare's 359.3
- Cazenave's 694.4
- cecum 569.9
- celiac (adult) 579.0
- - infantile 579.0
- cellular tissue NEC 709.9
- central core 359.0
- cerebellar, cerebellum - see Disease, brain
- cerebral (see also Disease, brain) 348.9
- - degenerative - see Degeneration, brain
- cerebrospinal 349.9
- cerebrovascular NEC 437.9
- - acute 436
- - - embolic - see Embolism, brain
- - - puerperal, postpartum, childbirth 674.0
- - - thrombotic - see Thrombosis, brain
- - arteriosclerotic 437.0
- - embolic - see Embolism, brain
- - occlusive 437.1
- - puerperal, postpartum, childbirth 674.0
- - thrombotic - see Thrombosis, brain
- cervix (uteri)
- - inflammatory 616.9
- - - specified NEC 616.8
- - noninflammatory 622.9
- - - specified NEC 622.8
- Chabert's 022.9
- Chagas' (see also Trypanosomiasis, American) 086.2
- Charcot's (joint) (spinal (cord)) 094.0
- Charcot-Marie-Tooth 356.1
- Cheadle's 267
- Chediak-Higashi(-Steinbrink) 288.2
- cheek, inner 528.9
- chest 519.9
- Chiari's 453.0
- Chicago 116.0
- chigo 134.1

Disease - *continued*
- chigoe 134.1
- chlamydial NEC 078.8
- cholecystic (see also Disease, gallbladder) 575.1
- choroid 362.9
- Christian-Weber 729.3
- Christmas 286.1
- ciliary body 364.9
- circulatory (system) NEC 459.9
- - chronic, maternal, affecting fetus or newborn 760.3
- - syphilitic 093.9
- - - congenital 090.5
- Civatte's 709.0
- climacteric (female) 627.2
- - male 608.8
- coagulation factor deficiency (congenital) (see also Defect, coagulation) 286.9
- Coat's 362.1
- coccidioidal pulmonary (primary) (residual) 114
- cold
- - agglutinin 283.0
- - - or hemoglobinuria 283.0
- - - - paroxysmal (cold) (nocturnal) 283.2
- - hemagglutinin (chronic) 283.0
- collagen NEC 710.9
- - nonvascular 710.9
- - specified NEC 710.8
- - vascular (allergic) 446.2
- colon 569.9
- - functional 564.9
- - - congenital 751.3
- combined system - see Degeneration, combined
- compressed air 993.3
- Concato's
- - peritoneal 568.8
- - pleural - see Pleurisy
- conjunctiva 372.9
- - chlamydial 077.9 † 372.0*
- - - specified NEC 077.8 † 372.0*
- - viral 077.9 † 372.0*
- - - specified NEC 077.8 † 372.0*
- connective tissue, diffuse - see Disease, collagen
- Conradi(-Hunermann) 756.5
- Cooper's 610.1
- Corbus' 607.1
- corkhandlers' 495.3
- cornea 371.9
- coronary (see also Ischemia, heart) 414.9
- - congenital 746.8
- - ostial, syphilitic 093.2 † 424.9*
- - - aortic 093.2 † 424.1*

Disease - *continued*
- coronary - *continued*
- – ostial - *continued*
- – – mitral 093.2 † 424.0*
- – – pulmonary 093.2 † 424.3*
- Coxsackie (virus) NEC 074.8
- Crigler-Najjer 277.4
- Crohn's 555.9
- – intestine 555.9
- – – large (bowel, colon or rectum) 555.1
- – – small (duodenum, ileum or jejunum) 555.0
- – – – with large intestine 555.2
- Crouzon's 756.0
- Cruchet's 049.8 † 323.4*
- Cruveilhier's 335.2
- Cushing's 255.0
- cystic
- – breast (chronic) 610.1
- – kidney, congenital 753.1
- – liver, congenital 751.6
- – lung 518.8
- – – congenital 748.8
- – pancreas, congenital 751.7
- – semilunar cartilage 717.5
- cystine storage (with renal sclerosis) 270.0
- cytomegalic inclusion (generalized) 078.5
- – with pneumonia 078.5 † 484.1*
- Darier's (congenital) 757.3
- – meaning erythema annulare centrifugum 695.0
- – vitamin a deficiency 264.8 † 701.1*
- Darling's 115.0
- de Beurmann-Gougerot 117.1
- de Quervain's 727.0
- deficiency 269.9
- Degos' 447.8
- Dejerine-Sottas 356.0
- Deleage's 359.8
- demyelinating, demyelinizating (nervous system) 341.9
- – specified NEC 341.8
- Dercum's 272.8
- Deutschlander's - see Fracture, foot
- Devergie's 696.4
- Devic's 341.0
- di Guglielmo's (M9841/3) 207.0
- diaphorase deficiency 289.7
- diaphragm 519.4
- Diaz's 732.5
- digestive system 569.9
- Dimitri-Sturge-Weber 759.6
- disc, degenerative - see Degeneration, intervertebral disc
- discogenic 722.9
- – with myelopthy 722.7 † 336.3*

Disease - *continued*
- diverticular - see Diverticula
- Dubois' (thymus gland) 090.5
- Duchenne's 094.0
- – locomotor ataxia 094.0
- – muscular dystrophy 359.1
- – paralysis 335.2
- Duchenne-Griesinger 359.1
- ductless glands 259.9
- Duhring's 694.0
- Dukes(-Filatow) 057.8
- Duplay's 726.2
- Dupuytren's 728.6
- Durand-Nicolas-Favre 099.1
- Duroziez's 746.5
- Dutton's 086.9
- Eales' 362.1
- ear (chronic) (inner) NEC 388.9
- Eberth's 002.0
- Ebstein's
- – heart 746.2
- – meaning diabetes 250.3 † 581.8*
- echinococcus (see also Echinococcus) 122.9
- echo virus NEC 078.8
- Economo's 049.8 † 323.4*
- Eddowes' 756.5
- Edsall's 992.2
- Eichstedt's 111.0
- endocrine glands or system NEC 259.9
- Engelmann's 756.5
- Engman's 690
- enteroviral, enterovirus NEC 078.8
- – central nervous system NEC 048
- epidemic NEC 136.9
- epididymis 608.9
- epigastric, functional 536.9
- – psychogenic 306.4
- Erb's 359.1
- Erb-Goldflam 358.0
- Erichsen's 300.1
- esophagus 530.9
- – psychogenic 306.4
- Eulenburg's 359.2
- eustachian tube 381.8
- external auditory canal 380.9
- extrapyramidal NEC 333.9
- eye 379.9
- – anterior chamber 364.9
- – inflammatory NEC 364.3
- – muscle 378.9
- eyeball 360.9
- eyelid 374.9
- eyeworm of Africa 125.2
- Fabry's 272.7
- facial nerve (seventh) 351.9
- – newborn 767.5

Disease - *continued*
- Hallopeau's 701.0
- hand, foot and mouth 074.3
- Hand-Schuller-Christian 277.8
- Hanot's - see Cirrhosis, biliary

- Hansen's 030.9
-   - benign form 030.1
-   - malignant form 030.0
- Harley's 283.2
- Hart's 270.0
- Hartnup 270.0
- Hashimoto's 245.2
- Hass's 732.3
- Hb - see Disease, hemoglobin

- heart (organic) 429.9
- - with
- - - acute pulmonary edema (see also
  Failure, ventricular, left) 428.1
- - - rheumatic fever (conditions in 390)
- - - - active 391.9
- - - - inactive or quiescent (with
  chorea) 398.9
- - amyloid 277.3 † 425.7*
- - aortic (valve) (see also Endocarditis,
  aortic) 424.1
- - arteriosclerotic or sclerotic (senile)
  414.0
- - artery, arterial 414.0
- - beriberi 265.0 † 425.7*
- - black 416.0
- - congenital NEC 746.9
- - - cyanotic 746.9
- - - maternal, affecting fetus or newborn
  760.3
- - congestive (see also Failure, heart,
  congestive) 428.0
- - coronary 414.0
- - cryptogenic 429.9
- - fetal 746.9
- - - inflammatory 746.8
- - fibroid (see also Myocarditis) 429.0
- - functional 427.9
- - - psychogenic 306.2
- - glycogen storage 271.0 † 425.7*
- - gonococcal 098.8 † 429.9*
- - hypertensive (see also Hypertension,
  heart) 402.9
- - hyperthyroid (see also
  Hyperthyroidism) 242.9 † 425.7*
- - ischemic (see also Ischemia, heart)
  414.9
- - - asymptomatic 412
- - - diagnosed on ecg or other special
  investigation, but currently
  presenting no symptoms 412
- - kyphoscoliotic 416.1

Disease - *continued*
- heart - *continued*
- - mitral (see also Endocarditis, mitral)
  394.9
- - muscular (see also Degeneration,
  myocardial) 429.1
- - psychogenic (functional) 306.2
- - pulmonary (chronic) 416.9
- - - acute 415.0
- - - specified NEC 416.8
- - rheumatic (chronic) (inactive) (old)
  (quiescent) (with chorea) 398.9
- - - active or acute 391.9
- - - - with chorea (acute) (rheumatic)
  (Sydenham's) 392.0
- - - maternal, affecting fetus or newborn
  760.3
- - rheumatoid - see Arthritis, rheumatoid
- - senile (see also Myocarditis) 429.0
- - syphilitic 093.8
- - - aortic 093.1 † 447.7*
- - - - aneurism 093.0 † 441.7*
- - - asymptomatic 093.8
- - - congenital 090.5
- - thyroid (gland) (see also
  Hyperthyroidism) 242.9 † 425.7*
- - thyrotoxic (see also Thyrotoxicosis)
  242.9 † 425.7*
- - valve, valvular (obstructive)
  (regurgitant) - see also Endocarditis
- - - congenital NEC 746.9
- - - - pulmonary 746.0
- - vascular - see Disease, cardiovascular
- heavy chain 273.2
- Heberden's 715.0
- Hebra's
- - meaning
- - - dermatitis exfoliativa 695.8
- - - erythema multiforme exudativum
  695.1
- - - pityriasis rubra 695.8
- - - prurigo 698.2
- Heerfordt's 135
- Heidenhain's 290.1
- - with dementia 290.1
- Heilmeyer-Schoner (M9842/3) 207.1
- Heine-Medin 045.9 † 323.2*
- Heller's 299.1
- hematopoietic organs 289.9
- hemoglobin or Hb
- - abnormal (mixed) NEC 282.7
- - - with thalassemia 282.4
- - C (Hb G) (high fetal gene) 282.7
- - - with other abnormal hemoglobin
  NEC 282.7
- - - elliptocytosis 282.7
- - - Hb S 282.6

Disease - *continued*
- hemoglobin or Hb - *continued*
- - C - *continued*
- - - sickle cell 282.6
- - - thalassemia 282.4
- - D 282.7
- - - with other abnormal hemoglobin
  NEC 282.7
- - - Hb S 282.6
- - - sickle cell 282.6
- - - thalassemia 282.4
- - E 282.7
- - - with other abnormal hemoglobin
  NEC 282.7
- - - Hb S 282.6
- - - sickle cell 282.6
- - - thalassemia 282.4
- - elliptocytosis 282.7
- - H 282.7
- - - with other abnormal hemoglobin
  NEC 282.7
- - - thalassemia 282.4
- - I thalassemia 282.4
- - M 289.7
- - S - see Disease, sickle cell
- - spherocytosis 282.7
- - unstable, hemolytic 282.7
- hemolytic (fetus) (newborn) 773.2
- - autoimmune (cold type) (warm type)
  283.0
- - due to or with
- - - incompatibility
- - - - ABO (blood group) 773.1
- - - - blood (group) (Duffy) (K(ell))
  (Kidd) (Lewis) (M) (S) NEC
  773.2
- - - - Rh (blood group) (factor) 773.0
- - - Rh negative mother 773.0
- hemorrhagic 287.9
- - newborn 776.0
- Henoch(-Schonlein) 287.0
- hepatic - see Disease, liver
- Hers' 271.0
- Heubner's 094.8
- high fetal gene or hemoglobin
  thalassemia 282.4
- Hildenbrand's 081.9
- hip (joint) NEC 719.9
- - congenital 755.6
- - suppurative 711.0
- - tuberculous 015.1 † 730.5*
- Hippel's 759.6
- Hirschsprung's 751.3
- His-Werner 083.1
- Hodgkin's (M9650/3) 201.9
- - lymphocytic
- - - depletion (M9653/3) 201.7

Disease - *continued*
- Hodgkin's - *continued*
- - lymphocytic - *continued*
- - - depletion - *continued*
- - - - diffuse fibrosis (M9654/3) 201.7
- - - - reticular type (M9655/3) 201.7
- - - predominance (M9651/3) 201.4
- - lymphocytic-histiocytic predominance
  (M9651/3) 201.4
- - mixed cellularity (M9652/3) 201.6
- - nodular sclerosis (M9656/3) 201.5
- - - cellular phase (M9657/3) 201.5
- Hodgson's 441.6
- - ruptured 441.5
- Hoffa's 272.8
- Hoffa-Kastert 272.8
- Holla (see also Spherocytosis) 282.0
- hoof and mouth 078.4
- hookworm (see also Ancylostomiasis)
  126.9
- Horton's 446.5
- Huebner-Herter 579.0
- Huntington's 333.4
- Hurler's 277.5
- Hutchinson's
- - meaning
- - - angioma serpiginosum 709.1
- - - cheiropompholyx 705.8
- - - prurigo estivalis 692.7
- Hutchinson-Boeck 135
- Hutchinson-Gilford 259.8
- hyaline (diffuse) (generalized) 728.9
- - membrane (lung) 769
- hydatid (see also Echinococcus) 122.9
- Hyde's 698.3
- hyperkinetic - see also Hyperkinesia
- - heart 429.8
- hypertensive (see also Hypertension)
  401.9
- hypophysis 253.9
- Iceland 049.8 † 323.4*
- I-cell 272.7
- ill-defined 799.8
- inclusion 078.5
- - salivary gland 078.5
- infective NEC 136.9
- inguinal gland 289.9
- internal semilunar cartilage, cystic 717.5
- intervertebral disc 722.9
- - with myelopathy 722.7 † 336.3*
- intestine 569.9
- - functional 564.9
- - - congenital 751.3
- - - psychogenic 306.4
- - organic 569.9
- - protozoal NEC 007.9
- iris 364.9

Disease - *continued*
- iron
- − − metabolism 275.0
- − − storage 275.0
- − Iselin's 732.5
- − itai-itai 985.5
- − Jadassohn-Pellizari's 701.3
- − Jakob-Creutzfeldt 046.1 † 331.5*
- − − with dementia 290.1
- − Jaksch-Luzet 285.8
- − Janet's 300.8
- − Jansky-Bielschowsky 330.1
- − jaw NEC 526.9
- − − fibrocystic 526.2
- − Jensen's 363.0
- − Jeune's 756.4
- − jigger 134.1
- − joint NEC 719.9
- − − Charcot's 094.0 † 713.5*
- − − degenerative 715.9
- − − − multiple 715.0
- − − − spine 721.9
- − − hypertrophic (chronic) (degenerative) 715.9
- − − − spine 721.9
- − − sacroiliac 724.6
- − − spine NEC 724.9
- − − − sacroiliac 724.6
- − Jungling's 135
- − Kahler's (M9730/3) 203.0
- − Kaposi's 757.3
- − − lichen ruber moniliformis 697.8
- − − xeroderma pigmentosum 757.3
- − Kaschin-Beck 716.0
- − Katayama 120.2
- − kidney (functional) (pelvis) (see also Disease, renal) 593.9
- − − cystic (multiple), congenital 753.1
- − − fibrocystic (congenital) 753.1
- − − in gout 274.1 † 583.8*
- − − polycystic (congenital) 753.1
- − Kienbock's 732.3
- − Kimmelstiel(-Wilson) 250.3 † 581.8*
- − kissing 075
- − Klebs' (see also Nephritis) 583.9
- − Klippel's 723.8
- − Koebner's 757.3
- − Kohler's
- − − patellar 732.4
- − − tarsal navicular 732.5
- − Korsakoff's (nonalcoholic) 294.0
- − − alcoholic 291.1
- − Kostman's 288.0
- − Krabbe's 330.0
- − Kraepelin-Morel (see also Schizophrenia) 295.9
- − Kraft-Weber-Dimitri 759.6

Disease - *continued*
- − Kuf's 330.1
- − Kugelberg-Welander 335.1
- − Kummell's 721.7
- − kuru 046.0 † 323.0*
- − Kussmaul's 446.0
- − Kyasanur Forest 065.2
- − Kyrle's 701.1
- − labyrinth, ear 386.8
- − lacrimal system 375.9
- − Lafora's 333.2
- − Landry's 357.0
- − Lane's 569.8
- − Larsen-Johansson 732.4
- − larynx 478.7
- − Legg(-Calve)-Perthes 732.1
- − legionnaire's 482.8
- − Leigh's 330.8
- − Leiner's 695.8
- − lens (eye) 366.9
- − Letterer-Siwe's (M9722/3) 202.5
- − Lewandowsky's 017.0
- − Libman-Sacks 710.0 † 424.9*
- − Lichtheim's - see Degeneration, combined
- − ligament 728.9
- − Lignac's 270.0
- − Lindau's 759.6
- − Lindau-von Hippel 759.6
- − lip NEC 528.5
- − lipoid-storage NEC 272.7
- − Little's - see Palsy, cerebral
- − liver 573.9
- − − chronic 571.9
- − − − alcoholic 571.3
- − − cystic, congenital 751.6
- − − fibrocystic (congenital) 751.6
- − − glycogen storage 271.0
- − − organic 573.9
- − − polycystic (congenital) 751.6
- − Lobo's 116.2
- − Lobstein's 756.5
- − Lorain's 253.3
- − Ludwig's 528.3
- − luetic - see Syphilis
- − lumbosacral region 724.6
- − lung 518.8
- − − congenital 748.6
- − − cystic 518.8
- − − − congenital 748.4
- − − fibroid (chronic) (see also Fibrosis, lung) 515
- − − fluke 121.2
- − − − oriental 121.2
- − − in
- − − − amyloidosis 277.3 † 517.8*
- − − − polymyositis 710.4 † 517.8*

Disease - *continued*
- Nairobi sheep 066.1
- nasal 478.1
- navel (newborn) NEC 779.8
- nemaline body 359.0
- neoplastic, generalized (M8000/6) 199.0
- nerve - see Disorder, nerve
- nervous system (central) (peripheral) 349.9
- - autonomic, peripheral 337.9
- - congenital 742.9
- - inflammatory - see Encephalitis
- - parasympathetic 337.9
- - specified NEC 349.8
- - sympathetic 337.9
- - vegetative 337.9
- Nettleship's 757.3
- Neumann's 694.4
- neuromuscular system NEC 358.9
- Newcastle 077.8 † 372.0*
- Nicolas(-Durand)-Favre 099.1
- Niemann-Pick 272.7
- nipple 611.9
- - Paget's (M8540/3) 174.0
- nonarthropod-borne NEC 078.8
- - central nervous system NEC 049.9
- - enterovirus NEC 078.8
- nonautoimmune hemolytic 283.1
- nose 478.1
- nucleus pulposus - see Disease, intervertebral disc
- nutritional 269.9
- oast-house urine 270.2
- oesophagus 530.9
- Oguchi's 368.6
- Ohara's 021
- Ollier's 756.4
- Opitz's 289.5
- Oppenheim's 358.8
- Oppenheim-Urbach 250.7 † 709.8*
- optic nerve NEC 377.4
- orbit 376.9
- Ormond's 593.4
- Osgood's tibia 732.4
- Osgood-Schlatter 732.4
- Osler-Rendu 448.0
- Osler-Vaquez (M9950/1) 238.4
- osteofibrocystic 252.0
- Otto's 715.3
- outer ear 380.9
- ovary NEC 620.9
- - cystic 620.2
- - noninflammatory 620.9
- - - specified NEC 620.8
- - polycystic 256.4
- Owren's (see also Defect, coagulation 286.3

Disease - *continued*
- Paget's
- - with infiltrating duct carcinoma of the breast (M8541/3) - see Neoplasm, breast, malignant
- - bone 731.0
- - - osteosarcoma in (M9184/3) - see Neoplasm, bone, malignant
- - breast (M8540/3) 174.0
- - extramammary (M8542/3) - see also Neoplasm, skin, malignant
- - - anus 154.3
- - - - skin 173.5
- - malignant (M8540/3)
- - - breast 174.0
- - - specified site NEC (M8542/3) - see Neoplasm, skin, malignant
- - - unspecified site 174.0
- - mammary (M8540/3) 174.0
- - nipple (M8540/3) 174.0
- palate (soft) 528.9
- pancreas 577.9
- - cystic 577.2
- - - congenital 751.7
- - fibrocystic 277.0
- Panner's 732.3
- panvalvular - see Endocarditis, mitral
- parametrium 629.9
- parasitic NEC 136.9
- - cerebral NEC 123.9
- - intestinal NEC 129
- - mouth 112.0
- - skin NEC 134.9
- - specified type - see Infestation
- - tongue 112.0
- parathyroid (gland) 252.9
- Parkinson's 332.0
- parodontal 523.9
- Parrot's 090.0
- Parry's 242.0
- Parson's 242.0
- Pavy's 593.6
- Paxton's 111.2
- pearl-workers' 730.1
- Pelizaeus-Merzbacher 330.0
- Pellegrini-Stieda 726.6
- pelvis, pelvic
- - female NEC 629.9
- - - specified NEC 629.8
- - gonococcal (acute) 098.1
- - - chronic or duration of 2 months or over 098.3
- - inflammatory 614.9
- - - with
- - - - abortion - see categories 634-639, fourth digit .0
- - - - ectopic gestation 639.0

Disease - *continued*
- pelvis - *continued*
- - inflammatory - *continued*
- - - acute 614.3
- - - chronic 614.4
- - - complicating pregnancy 646.6
- - - - fetus or newborn 760.8
- - - puerperal, postpartum, childbirth 670
- - - specified NEC 614.8
- - organ, female NEC 629.9
- - peritoneum, female NEC 629.9
- penis 607.9
- - inflammatory 607.2
- peptic NEC 536.9
- periapical tissues NEC 522.9
- periodic (familial) (Reimann's) NEC 277.3
- periodontal NEC 523.9
- - specified NEC 523.8
- periosteum 733.9
- peripheral
- - arterial 443.9
- - autonomic nervous system 337.9
- - nerves - see Polyneuropathy
- - vascular NEC 443.9
- peritoneum 568.9
- - pelvic, female NEC 629.9
- Perthes' 732.1
- Petit's (see also Hernia, diaphragm) 553.3
- Peutz-Jeghers 759.6
- Peyronie's 607.8
- Pfeiffer's 075
- pharynx 478.2
- Phoca's 610.1
- Pick's
- - brain 331.1
- - - dementia in 290.1
- - liver 423.2
- Pierson's 732.1
- pigeon fanciers' 495.2
- pineal gland 259.8
- pink 985.0
- Pinkus's 697.1
- pinworm 127.4
- pituitary (gland) 253.9
- pituitary-snuff-takers' 495.8
- placenta
- - complicating pregnancy or childbirth 656.7
- - fetus or newborn 762.2
- pleura (cavity) (see also Pleurisy) 511.0
- Plummer's 242.3
- pneumatic
- - drill 994.9
- - hammer 994.9

Disease - *continued*
- policeman's 729.2
- Pollitzer's 705.8
- polycystic (congenital) 759.8
- - kidney or renal 753.1
- - liver or hepatic 751.6
- - lung or pulmonary 518.8
- - - congenital 748.4
- - ovary, ovaries 256.4
- - spleen 759.0
- Pompe's 271.0
- Poncet's 015.9
- Posadas-Wernicke 114
- Pott's 015.0 † 730.4*
- Poulet's 714.2
- pregnancy NEC (see also Pregnancy) 646.9
- Preiser's 733.0
- Pringle's 759.5
- prostate 602.9
- - specified type NEC 602.8
- protozoal NEC 136.8
- - intestine, intestinal NEC 007.9
- pseudo-Hurler's 272.7
- psychiatric (see also Psychosis) 298.9
- psychotic (see also Psychosis) 298.9
- Puente's 528.5
- puerperal NEC (see also Puerperal) 674.9
- pulmonary - see also Disease, lung
- - artery 417.9
- - heart 416.9
- - valve (see also Endocarditis, pulmonary) 424.3
- pulp (dental) NEC 522.9
- pulseless 446.7
- Putnam's - see Degeneration, combined
- Pyle's 756.8
- pyramidal tract NEC 333.9
- Quervain's 727.0
- Quincke's 995.1
- Quinquaud's 704.0
- rag-sorters' 022.1
- Raynaud's 443.0
- Recklinghausen's (M9540/1) 237.7
- - bones 252.0
- Reclus's 610.1
- - cystic 610.1
- rectum NEC 569.4
- Reichmann's 536.8
- Reiter's 099.3
- renal (functional) (pelvis) 593.9
- - with
- - - edema (see also Nephrosis) 581.9
- - - lesion of interstitial nephritis 583.8
- - - stated generalized cause - see Nephritis

Disease - *continued*
 − renal - *continued*
 − − acute - see Nephritis, acute
 − − chronic - see Nephritis, chronic
 − − complicating pregnancy or puerperium
 NEC 646.2
 − − − with hypertension - see Toxemia, of
 pregnancy
 − − − fetus or newborn 760.1
 − − cystic, congenital 753.1
 − − fibrocystic (congenital) 753.1
 − − hypertensive (see also Hypertension,
 kidney) 403.9
 − − polycystic (congenital) 753.1
 − − subacute 581.9
 − − tubular (see also Nephrosis, tubular)
 584.5
 − Rendu-Osler-Weber 448.0
 − renovascular (arteriosclerotic) (see also
 Hypertension, kidney) 403.9
 − respiratory (tract) 519.9
 − − acute or subacute NEC
 − − − due to fumes or vapours 506.3
 − − chronic 519.9
 − − − arising in the perinatal period 770.7
 − − − due to fumes or vapours 506.4
 − − due to
 − − − external agents 508.9
 − − − − specified NEC 508.8
 − − − fumes or vapours 506.9
 − − − − acute or subacute NEC 506.3
 − − − − chronic 506.4
 − − upper (acute) (infectious) NEC 465.9
 − − − multiple sites NEC 465.8
 − − − noninfectious NEC 478.9
 − − − streptococcal 034.0
 − retina, retinal NEC 362.9
 − − Batten's or Batten-Mayou 330.1 †
 362.7*
 − − vascular lesion 362.1
 − rheumatic 716.9
 − − heart - see Disease, heart, rheumatic
 − rheumatoid (heart) - see Arthritis,
 rheumatoid
 − rickettsial NEC 083.9
 − − specified type NEC 083.8
 − Riedel's 245.3
 − Riga-Fede 529.0
 − Riggs' 523.4
 − Ritter's 695.8
 − Roble's 125.3 † 360.1*
 − Roger's 745.4
 − Rokitansky's (see also Necrosis, liver)
 570
 − Romberg's 349.8
 − Rosenthal's 286.2
 − Rossbach's 536.8

Disease - *continued*
 − Rossbach's - *continued*
 − − psychogenic 306.4
 − Roth-Bernhardt 355.1
 − Rust's 015.0 † 720.8*
 − sacroiliac NEC 724.6
 − Saint Palogren's 723.1
 − salivary gland or duct NEC 527.9
 − − inclusion 078.5
 − − virus 078.5
 − Sander's 297.1
 − Sandhoff's 272.7
 − sandworm 126.9
 − Savill's 695.8
 − Schamberg's 709.0
 − Schaumann's 135
 − Schenck's 117.1
 − Scheuermann's 732.0
 − Schilder(-Flatau) 341.1
 − Schimmelbusch's 610.1
 − Schlatter's tibia 732.4
 − Schlatter-Osgood 732.4
 − Schmorl's 722.3
 − Scholz's 330.0
 − Schonlein(-Henoch) 287.0
 − Schuller-Christian 277.8
 − Schultz's 288.0
 − Schwalbe-Ziehen-Oppenheimer 333.6
 − sclera 379.1
 − scrofulous 017.2
 − scrotum 608.9
 − sebaceous glands NEC 706.9
 − semilunar cartilage, cystic 717.5
 − seminal vesicle 608.9
 − Senear-Usher 694.4
 − serum NEC 999.5
 − Sever's 732.5
 − Sezary's (M9701/3) 202.2
 − Shaver's 503
 − Sheehan's 253.2
 − shipyard 077.1 † 370.4*
 − sickle cell (Hb C) (Hb D) (Hb E) (Hb G)
 (Hb J) (Hb K) (Hb O) (Hb P) (high fetal
 gene) 282.6
 − − with other abnormal hemoglobin NEC
 282.6
 − − elliptocytosis 282.6
 − − spherocytosis 282.6
 − − thalassemia 282.4
 − silo-fillers' 506.9
 − simian B 054.3 † 323.4*
 − Simmond's 253.2
 − Simons' 272.6
 − Sinding-Larsen 732.4
 − sinus - see also Sinusitis
 − − brain 437.9
 − Sirkari's 085.0

Disease - *continued*
- sixth 057.8
- Sjogren's 710.2
- - with lung involvement 710.2 † 517.8*
- Skevas-Zerfus 989.5
- skin NEC 709.9
- - due to metabolic disorder 277.9
- Sneddon-Wilkinson 694.1
- specific NEC - see Syphilis
- Spielmeyer-Stock 330.1
- Spielmeyer-Vogt 330.1
- spinal (cord) NEC 336.9
- - congenital 742.9
- spine 733.9
- - joint (see also Disease, joint) 724.9
- - tuberculous 015.0 † 730.4*
- spinocerebellar 334.9
- - specified NEC 334.8
- spleen 289.5
- - amyloid 277.3
- - organic 289.5
- - polycystic 759.0
- - postinfectional 289.5
- sponge-divers' 989.5
- Stanton's 025
- Stargardt's 362.7
- Steinert's 359.2
- Stevens-Johnson 695.1
- Sticker's 057.0
- Still's 714.3
- Stokes' 242.0
- Stokes-Adams 426.9
- Stokvis(-Talma) 289.7
- stomach NEC 537.9
- - functional 536.9
- - - psychogenic 306.4
- stonemasons' 502
- storage
- - glycogen (see also Disease, glycogen storage) 271.0
- - mucopolysaccharide 277.5
- striatopallidal system NEC 333.9
- Strumpell-Marie 720.0
- Stuart-Prower 286.3
- Sturge(-Weber)(-Dimitri) 759.6
- Sudeck's 733.7
- supporting structures of teeth NEC 525.9
- suprarenal (gland) (capsule) 255.9
- Sutton and Gull's - see Hypertension, kidney
- Sutton's 709.0
- sweat glands NEC 705.9
- sweating 078.2
- Swift(-Feer) 985.0
- swimming-pool (bacillus) 031.1
- sympathetic nervous system 337.9
- synovium 727.9

Disease - *continued*
- syphilitic - see Syphilis
- systemic tissue mast cell (M9741/3) 202.6
- Taenzer's 757.4
- Takayasu's (pulseless) 446.7
- Talma's 728.8
- Tangier 272.5
- Taylor's 701.8
- Tay-Sachs 330.1
- tear duct 375.6
- tendon 727.9
- - inflammatory NEC 727.9
- testis 608.9
- Thomsen's 359.2
- Thomson's 757.3
- Thornwaldt's 478.2
- throat 478.2
- - septic 034.0
- thrombo-embolic (see also Embolism) 444.9
- thymus (gland) 254.9
- thyroid (gland) NEC 246.9
- - heart (see also Hyperthyroidism) 242.9 † 425.7*
- Tietze's 733.6
- Tommaselli's
- - correct substance properly administered 599.7
- - overdose or wrong substance given or taken 961.4
- tongue 529.9
- tonsils, tonsillar (and adenoids) 474.9
- tooth, teeth 525.9
- - hard tissues NEC 521.9
- - pulp NEC 522.9
- trachea 519.1
- tricuspid - see Endocarditis, tricuspid
- triglyceride-storage, type I, II, III 272.7
- trophoblastic (see also Hydatidiform mole) 630
- tsutsugamushi 081.2
- tube (fallopian), noninflammatory 620.9
- - specified NEC 620.8
- tuberculous NEC (see also Tuberculosis) 011.9
- tubo-ovarian
- - inflammatory (see also Salpingo-oophoritis) 614.2
- - noninflammatory 620.9
- - - specified NEC 620.8
- tubotympanic, chronic 382.1
- tympanum 385.9
- Uhl's 746.8
- umbilicus (newborn) NEC 779.8
- Underwood's 778.1
- Unverricht(-Lundborg) 333.2

Disease - *continued*
- Urbach-Oppenheim 250.7 † 709.8*
- Urbach-Wiethe 272.8
- ureter 593.9
- urethra 599.9
- - specified NEC 599.8
- urinary 599.9
- - bladder 596.9
- - - specified NEC 596.8
- - tract 599.9
- Usher-Senear 694.4
- uterus 625.9
- - infective (see also Endometritis) 615.9
- - inflammatory (see also Endometritis) 615.9
- - noninflammatory 621.9
- - - specified NEC 621.8
- uveal tract (anterior) 364.9
- - posterior 363.9
- vagabonds' 132.1
- vagina, vaginal
- - inflammatory 616.9
- - - specified NEC 616.8
- - noninflammatory 623.9
- - - specified NEC 623.8
- Valsuani's 648.2
- valve, valvular - see Endocarditis
- Van Bogaert-Nijssen(-Peiffer) 330.0
- Van Neck's 732.1
- Vaquez's (M9950/1) 238.4
- Vaquez-Osler (M9950/1) 238.4
- vas deferens 608.9
- vascular 459.9
- - arteriosclerotic - see Arteriosclerosis
- - hypertensive - see Hypertension
- - obliterative 447.1
- - - peripheral 443.9
- - occlusive 459.9
- - peripheral (occlusive) 443.9
- vasomotor 443.9
- vasospastic 443.9
- vein 459.9
- venereal 099.9
- - specified nature or type NEC 099.8
- Verneuil's 095
- Verse's 275.4 † 722.9*
- vertebra, vertebral NEC 733.9
- - disc - see Disease, intervertebral disc
- vibration NEC 994.9
- Vidal's 698.3
- Vincent's 101
- Virchow's 733.9
- virus (filtrable) NEC 078.8
- - arbovirus NEC 066.9
- - arthropod-borne NEC 066.9
- - nonarthropod-borne NEC 078.8
- - - central nervous system NEC 049.9

Disease - *continued*
- virus - *continued*
- - suspected damage to fetus affecting management of pregnancy 655.3
- vitreous 379.2
- vocal cords 478.5
- Vogt's (Cecile) 333.7
- Vogt-Spielmeyer 330.1
- von Bechterew's 720.0
- von Economo 049.8 † 323.4*
- von Gierke's 271.0
- von Graefe's 378.8
- von Hippel's 759.6
- von Hippel-Lindau 759.6
- von Jaksch's 285.8
- von Recklinghausen's (M9540/1) 237.7
- - bones 252.0
- von Recklinghausen-Appelbaum 275.0
- von WILLEBRAND(-→Jurgens') 286.4
- Vrolik's 756.5
- vulva
- - inflammatory 616.9
- - - specified NEC 616.8
- - noninflammatory 624.9
- - - specified NEC 624.8
- Waldenstrom's (osteochondrosis) 732.1
- Wardrop's (with lymphangitis) 681.9
- wasting NEC 799.4
- Waterhouse-Friderichsen 036.3 † 255.5*
- Weber-Christian 729.3
- Weil's 100.0
- - of lung 100.0
- Werdnig-Hoffmann 335.0
- Werlhof's (see also Purpura, thrombocytopenic) 287.3
- Wermer's 258.0
- Werner's 259.8
- Wernicke-Posadas 114
- Whipple's 040.2
- whipworm 127.3
- white blood cells NEC 288.9
- white-spot 701.0
- Whitmore's 025
- Wilson's 275.1
- winter vomiting 078.8
- Wolman's 272.7
- woolsorters' 022.1
- Ziehen-Oppenheim 333.6
- zoonotic, bacterial NEC 027.9
- - specified type NEC 027.8
Disfigurement (due to scar) 709.2
- problem NEC V49.8
- - head V48.6
- - limb V49.4
- - neck V48.7
- - trunk V48.7
Disgerminoma - see Dysgerminoma

Disinsertion, retina 361.0
Disintegration, complete, of the body 799.8
– traumatic 869.1
Dislocatable hip, congenital 754.3
Dislocation (articular) (closed) (simple) 839.8

Note – The following fourth-digit subdivisions are for use with categories 830–835, 837 and 838:
   .0 Simple
   .1 Compound
"Simple" includes closed, complete, partial, uncomplicated, and unspecified dislocation.
"Compound" includes dislocation specified as infected or open and dislocation with foreign body.

Dislocation - *continued*
– with fracture - see Fracture
– acromioclavicular (joint) 831.-
– anatomical site
– – specified (simple) NEC 839.6
– – – compound 839.7
– – unspecified or ill-defined (simple) 839.8
– – – compound 839.9
– ankle (scaphoid bone) 837.-
– arm (simple) 839.8
– – compound 839.9
– astragalus 837.-
– atlantoaxial (simple) 839.0
– – compound 839.1
– atlas (simple) 839.0
– – compound 839.1
– axis (simple) 839.0
– – compound 839.1
– back (simple) 839.8
– – compound 839.9
– breast bone (simple) 839.6
– – compound 839.7
– capsule, joint - code by site under Dislocation
– carpal (bone) 833.-
– carpometacarpal (joint) 833.-
– cartilage (joint) - code by site under Dislocation
– – knee - see Tear, meniscus
– cervical, cervicodorsal, or cervicothoracic (spine) (vertebrae) 839.0
– – compound 839.1
– chronic - see Dislocation, recurrent
– clavicle 831.-
– coccyx (simple) 839.4
– – compound 839.5

Dislocation - *continued*
– collar bone 831.-
– compound (open) NEC 839.9
– congenital NEC 755.8
– coracoid 831.-
– costal cartilage (simple) 839.6
– – compound 839.7
– costochondral (simple) 839.6
– – compound 839.7
– cricoarytenoid articulation (simple) 839.6
– – compound 839.7
– cricothyroid articulation (simple) 839.6
– – compound 839.7
– dorsal vertebrae (simple) 839.2
– – compound 839.3
– elbow 832.-
– – congenital 754.8
– – recurrent 718.3
– eye 360.8
– eyeball 360.8
– femur
– – distal end (simple) 836.5
– – – compound 836.6
– – proximal end 835.-
– fibula
– – distal end 837.-
– – proximal end (simple) 836.5
– – – compound 836.6
– finger(s) 834.-
– foot 838.-
– forearm (simple) 839.8
– – compound 839.9
– fracture - see Fracture
– glenoid 831.-
– habitual - see Dislocation, recurrent
– hand (simple) 839.8
– – compound 839.9
– hip 835.-
– – congenital 754.3
– – recurrent 718.3
– humerus
– – distal end 832.-
– – proximal end 831.-
– infracoracoid 831.-
– innominate (pubic junction) (sacral junction) 839.6
– – acetabulum 835.-
– – compound 839.7
– interphalangeal (joint)
– – finger or hand 834.-
– – foot or toe 838.-
– jaw (cartilage) (meniscus) 830.-
– knee (simple) 836.5
– – compound 836.6
– – congenital 754.4
– – habitual 718.3
– – old 718.2

Dislocation - *continued*
− knee - *continued*
− − recurrent 718.3
− lacrimal gland 375.1
− leg (simple) 839.8
− − compound 839.9
− lens (complete) (crystalline) (partial) 379.3
− − congenital 743.3
− − traumatic 921.3
− ligament - code by site under Dislocation
− lumbar (vertebrae) 839.2
− − compound 839.3
− lumbosacral (vertebrae) 839.2
− − compound 839.3
− − congenital 756.1
− mandible 830.-
− maxilla (inferior) 830.-
− meniscus (knee) - see Tear, meniscus
− − other sites - code by site under Dislocation
− metacarpal (bone)
− − distal end 834.-
− − proximal end 833.-
− metacarpophalangeal (joint) 834.-
− metatarsal (bone) 838.-
− metatarsophalangeal (joint) 838.-
− midcarpal (joint) 833.-
− midtarsal (joint) 838.-
− multiple locations (except fingers only or toes only) (simple) 839.8
− − compound 839.9
− navicular (bone) foot 837.-
− neck (simple) 839.0
− − compound 839.1
− nose (simple) 839.6
− − compound 839.7
− not recurrent, not current injury 718.2
− occiput from atlas (simple) 839.0
− − compound 839.1
− old - see Dislocation, recurrent
− paralytic (flaccid) (spastic) 718.2
− patella (simple) 836.3
− − compound 836.4
− − congenital 755.6
− pathological NEC 718.2
− − lumbosacral joint 724.6
− − sacroiliac 724.6
− − spine 724.8
− pelvis (simple) 839.6
− − acetabulum 835.-
− − compound 839.7
− phalanx
− − finger or hand 834.-
− − foot or toe 838.-
− prosthesis, internal - see Complications, mechanical

Dislocation - *continued*
− radiocarpal (joint) 833.-
− radioulnar (joint)
− − distal 833.-
− − proximal 832.-
− radius
− − distal end 833.-
− − proximal end 832.-
− recurrent 718.3
− − elbow 718.3
− − hip 718.3
− − joint NEC 718.3
− − knee 718.3
− − patella 718.3
− − sacroiliac 724.6
− − shoulder 718.3
− rib (cartilage) 839.6
− − compound 839.7
− − congenital 756.3
− sacrococcygeal (simple) 839.4
− − compound 839.5
− sacro-iliac (joint) (ligament) 839.4
− − compound 839.5
− − congenital 755.6
− − recurrent 724.6
− sacrum (simple) 839.4
− − compound 839.5
− scaphoid (bone)
− − ankle or foot 837.-
− − wrist 833.-
− scapula 831.-
− semilunar cartilage, knee - see Tear, meniscus
− septal cartilage (nose) 839.6
− − compound 839.7
− septum (nasal) (old) 470
− sesamoid bone - code by site under Dislocation
− shoulder (blade) (ligament) 831.-
− − chronic 718.3
− − recurrent 718.3
− skull (see also Injury, intracranial) 854.0
− spine (see also Dislocation, vertebrae) 839.4
− − congenital 756.1
− spontaneous 718.2
− sternoclavicular (joint) (simple) 839.6
− − compound 839.7
− sternum (simple) 839.6
− − compound 839.7
− subglenoid 831.-
− symphysis
− − jaw 830.-
− − mandibular 830.-
− − pubis (simple) 839.6
− − − compound 839.7
− tarsal (bone) (joint) 838.-

Dislocation - *continued*
- tarsometatarsal (joint) 838.-
- temporomandibular (joint) 830.-
- thigh
- - distal end (simple) 836.5
- - - compound 836.6
- - proximal end 835.-
- thoracic (vertebrae) 839.2
- - compound 839.3
- thumb 834.-
- thyroid cartilage (simple) 839.6
- - compound 839.7
- tibia
- - distal end 837.-
- - proximal end (simple) 836.5
- - - compound 836.6
- tibiofibular (joint)
- - distal 837.-
- - superior (simple) 836.5
- - - compound 836.6
- toe(s) 838.-
- trachea (simple) 839.6
- - compound 839.7
- ulna
- - distal end 833.-
- - proximal end 832.-
- vertebrae (articular process) (body) 839.4
- - cervical, cervicodorsal or cervicothoracic (simple) 839.0
- - - compound 839.1
- - compound NEC 839.5
- - congenital 756.1
- - specified region NEC (simple) 839.4
- - - compound 839.5
- wrist (scaphoid) (semilunar) (carpal bone) 833.-
- xiphoid cartilage (simple) 839.6
- - compound 839.7
Disorder - see also Disease
- accommodation 367.5
- adrenogenital 255.2
- affective (see also Psychosis, affective) 296.9
- aggressive, unsocialized 312.0
- allergic - see Allergy
- amino-acid
- - metabolism NEC (see also Disturbance, metabolism, amino-acid) 270.9
- - neonatal, transitory 775.8
- - renal transport NEC 270.0
- - transport NEC 270.9
- anaerobic glycolysis with anemia 282.3
- articulation - see Disorder, joint
- balance
- - acid-base 276.9

Disorder - *continued*
- balance - *continued*
- - acid-base - *continued*
- - - mixed 276.4
- - electrolyte 276.9
- - fluid 276.9
- behavior NEC - see Disturbance, conduct
- bilirubin excretion 277.4
- bipolar (alternating) 296.5
- - currently
- - - depressed 296.3
- - - manic 296.2
- - mixed 296.4
- bladder 596.9
- - functional NEC 596.5
- - specified NEC 596.8
- bone NEC 733.9
- brachial plexus 353.0
- breast 611.9
- - puerperal, postpartum 676.3
- - specified NEC 611.8
- Briquet's 300.8
- bursa 727.9
- - shoulder region 726.1
- carbohydrate metabolism, congenital 271.9
- cardiac, functional 427.9
- cardiovascular system 429.2
- - psychogenic 306.2
- cartilage NEC 733.9
- - articular 718.0
- cervical
- - region NEC 723.9
- - root (nerve) NEC 353.2
- character NEC 301.9
- coagulation (factor) (see also Defect, coagulation) 286.9
- - neonatal, transitory 776.3
- coccyx 724.7
- colon 569.9
- - functional 564.9
- - - congenital 751.3
- conduct (see also Disturbance, conduct) 312.9
- - adjustment reaction 309.3
- - compulsive 312.2
- - hyperkinetic 314.2
- convulsive (secondary) (see also Convulsions) 780.3
- cranial nerve - see Disorder, nerve, cranial
- degradation
- - branched chain amino-acid 270.3
- dentition 520.6
- depressive NEC 311
- developmental, specific NEC 315.9
- - associated with hyperkinesia 314.1

Disorder - *continued*
- developmental - *continued*
- - language 315.3
- - learning 315.2
- - - arithmetical 315.1
- - - reading 315.0
- - mixed 315.5
- - motor coordination 315.4
- - specified NEC 315.8
- - speech 315.3
- digestive 536.9
- - fetus or newborn 777.9
- - - specified NEC 777.8
- - psychogenic 306.4
- - system, psychogenic 306.4
- electrolyte NEC 276.9
- emotional (see also Disorder, mental, nonpsychotic) 300.9
- endocrine 259.9
- esophagus 530.9
- - psychogenic 306.4
- eustachian tube NEC 381.9
- factor, coagulation (see also Defect, coagulation) 286.9
- fascia 728.9
- gastric (functional) 536.9
- - motility 536.8
- - psychogenic 306.4
- - secretion 536.8
- gastrointestinal (functional) NEC 536.9
- - psychogenic 306.4
- gender-role 302.6
- genitourinary system
- - female 629.9
- - male 608.9
- - psychogenic 306.5
- heart action 427.9
- hematological, transient neonatal 776.9
- - specified NEC 776.8
- hematopoietic organs 289.9
- hemorrhagic NEC 287.9
- - due to circulating anticoagulants 286.5
- hemostasis (see also Defect, coagulation) 286.9
- immune mechanism (immunity) 279.9
- - specified NEC 279.8
- integument, fetus or newborn 778.9
- - specified NEC 778.8
- intestinal 569.9
- - functional NEC 564.9
- - - postoperative NEC 564.4
- - psychogenic 306.4
- joint NEC 719.9
- - psychogenic 306.0
- - temporomandibular 524.6
- kidney 593.9
- - functional 588.9

Disorder - *continued*
- kidney - *continued*
- - functional - *continued*
- - - specified NEC 588.8
- lactation 676.9
- ligament 728.9
- ligamentous attachments, peripheral - see also Enthesopathy
- - spine 720.1
- limb NEC 729.9
- - psychogenic 306.0
- lipid
- - metabolism, congenital 272.9
- - storage 272.7
- lipoprotein deficiency, familial 272.5
- low back 724.9
- - psychogenic 306.0
- lumbosacral
- - plexus 353.1
- - root (nerve) NEC 353.4
- manic 296.0
- meniscus NEC 718.0
- menopausal 627.9
- - specified NEC 627.8
- menstrual 626.9
- - psychogenic 306.5
- - specified NEC 626.8
- mental (nonpsychotic) 300.9
- - affecting management of pregnancy, childbirth or puerperium 648.4
- - due to or associated with drug consumption NEC 292.9
- - neurotic (see also Neurosis) 300.9
- - presenile, psychotic 290.1
- - previous, affecting management of pregnancy, childbirth or puerperium V23.8
- - psychoneurotic (see also Neurosis) 300.9
- - psychotic (see also Psychosis) 298.9
- - senile, psychotic NEC 290.2
- - specific, following organic brain damage 310.9
- - - cognitive or personality change NEC 310.1
- - - frontal lobe syndrome 310.0
- - - postconcussional syndrome 310.2
- - - specified NEC 310.8
- metabolism NEC 277.9
- - calcium 275.4
- - complicating abortion - see categories 634-639, fourth digit .4
- - congenital 277.9
- - copper 275.1
- - in labor and delivery 669.0
- - iron 275.0
- - magnesium 275.2

Disorder - *continued*
- personality 301.9
- - affective 301.1
- - agressive 301.3
- - amoral 301.7
- - anancastic 301.4
- - anankastic 301.4
- - antisocial 301.7
- - asocial 301.7
- - asthenic 301.6
- - compulsive 301.4
- - cyclothymic 301.1
- - dyssocial 301.7
- - emotional instability 301.5
- - explosive 301.3
- - following organic brain damage 310.1
- - histrionic 301.5
- - hyperthymic 301.1
- - hypothymic 301.1
- - hysterical 301.5
- - immature 301.8
- - inadequate 301.6
- - labile 301.5
- - moral deficiency 301.7
- - obsessional 301.4
- - obsessive(-compulsive) 301.4
- - paranoid 301.0
- - passive(-dependent) 301.6
- - passive-aggressive 301.8
- - pathological NEC 301.9
- - pseudosocial 301.7
- - psychopathic 301.9
- - schizoid 301.2
- - unstable 301.5
- pigmentation, choroid (congenital) 743.5
- pituitary, thalamic 253.9
- - anterior NEC 253.4
- - iatrogenic 253.7
- porphyrin metabolism 277.1
- postmenopausal 627.9
- - specified NEC 627.8
- psychic, with disease classified elsewhere 316
- psychogenic NEC (see also Condition) 300.9
- - anxiety 300.0
- - appetite 307.5
- - asthenic 300.5
- - cardiovascular (system) 306.2
- - compulsive 300.3
- - cutaneous 306.3
- - depressive 300.4
- - digestive (system) 306.4
- - dysmennorrheic 306.5
- - dyspneic 306.1
- - endocrine (system) 306.6
- - eye 306.7

Disorder - *continued*
- psychogenic NEC - *continued*
- - feeding 307.5
- - functional NEC 306.9
- - gastric 306.4
- - gastrointestinal (system) 306.4
- - genitourinary (system) 306.5
- - heart (function) (rhythm) 306.2
- - hyperventilatory 306.1
- - hypochondriacal 300.7
- - hysterical 300.1
- - intestinal 306.4
- - joint 306.0
- - learning 315.2
- - limb 306.0
- - lymphatic (system) 306.8
- - menstrual 306.5
- - micturition 306.5
- - monoplegic NEC 306.0
- - motor 307.9
- - muscle 306.0
- - musculoskeletal 306.0
- - neurocirculatory 306.2
- - obsessive 300.3
- - occupational 300.8
- - organ or part of body NEC 306.9
- - organs of special sense 306.7
- - paralytic NEC 306.0
- - phobic 300.2
- - physical NEC 306.9
- - pruritic 306.3
- - rectal 306.4
- - respiratory (system) 306.1
- - rheumatic 306.0
- - sexual (function) 302.7
- - skin (allergic) (pruritic) (eczematous) 306.3
- - sleep 307.4
- - specified part of body NEC 306.8
- - stomach 306.4
- psychomotor NEC 307.9
- - hysterical 300.1
- psychoneurotic (see also Neurosis) 300.9
- - mixed NEC 300.8
- psychophysiologic (see also Disorder, psychogenic) 306.9
- psychosexual identity 302.6
- psychosomatic NEC (see also Disorder, psychogenic) 306.9
- purine metabolism 277.2
- pyrimidine metabolism 277.2
- reflex 796.1
- renal function, impaired 588.9
- - specified NEC 588.8
- respiration, respiratory NEC 519.9
- - psychogenic 306.1
- sacrum 724.6

Disorder - *continued*
- seizure 780.3
- sense of smell 781.1
- - psychogenic 306.7
- sexual function, psychogenic 302.7
- skin NEC 709.9
- - fetus or newborn 778.9
- - - specified NEC 778.8
- - psychogenic (allergic) (eczematous)
  (pruritic) 306.3
- sleep 780.5
- - nonorganic origin 307.4
- speech NEC 784.5
- spine NEC 724.9
- - ligamentous or muscular
  attachments,peripheral 720.1
- steroid metabolism NEC 255.2
- stomach (functional) (see also Disorder,
  gastric) 536.9
- substitution 300.1
- synovium 727.9
- temperature regulation, fetus or newborn
  778.4
- tendon 727.9
- - shoulder region 726.1
- thoracic root (nerve) NEC 353.3
- thyrocalcitonin secretion 246.0
- thyroid (gland) NEC 246.9
- tooth NEC
- - development NEC 520.9
- - - specified NEC 520.8
- - eruption 520.6
- - - with abnormal position 524.3
- tubular, phosphate-losing 588.0
- unsocialized aggressive 312.0
- visual cortex 377.7
Displacement, displaced
- acquired traumatic of bone, cartilage,
  joint, tendon NEC (without fracture) -
  see Dislocation
- - with fracture - see Fracture
- adrenal gland (congenital) 759.1
- appendix retrocecal (congenital) 751.5
- auricle (congenital) 744.2
- bladder (acquired) 596.8
- - congenital 753.8
- brachial plexus (congenital) 742.8
- brain stem, caudal 742.4
- canuliculus (lacrimalis) 743.6
- cardia through oesophageal hiatus 750.6
- cerebellum, caudal 742.4
- cervix (see also Malposition, uterus)
  621.6
- colon (congenital) 751.4
- device, implant or graft - see
  Complications, mechanical
- epithelium

Displacement - *continued*
- epithelium - *continued*
- - columnar of cervix 622.1
- - cuboidal, beyond limits of external os
  752.8
- esophageal mucosa into cardia of
  stomach, congenital 750.4
- esophagus (acquired) 530.8
- - congenital 750.4
- eyeball (acquired) (old) 376.3
- - congenital 743.8
- - current 871.3
- fallopian tube (acquired) 620.4
- - congenital 752.1
- - opening (congenital) 752.1
- gallbladder (congenital) 751.6
- gastric mucosa 750.7
- - into
- - - duodenum 750.7
- - - esophagus 750.7
- - - Meckel's diverticulum 750.7
- globe (acquired) (old) (lateral) 376.3
- - current 871.3
- heart (congenital) 746.8
- - acquired 429.8
- hymen (upward) (congenital) 752.4
- intervertebral disc (with neuritis,
  radiculitis, sciatica, or other pain) 722.2
- - with myelopathy (any site) 722.7 †
  336.3*
- - cervical, cervicodorsal, cervicothoracic
  722.0
- - - due to major trauma - see
  Dislocation, cervical
- - due to major trauma - see Dislocation,
  vertebrae
- - lumbar, lumbosacral 722.1
- - - due to major trauma - see
  Dislocation, lumbar
- - thoracic, thoracolumbar 722.1
- - - due to major trauma - see
  Dislocation, thoracic
- kidney (acquired) 593.0
- - congenital 753.3
- lachrymal, lacrimal apparatus or duct
  (congenital) 743.6
- macula (congenital) 743.5
- Meckel's diverticulum (congenital) 751.0
- nail (congenital) 757.5
- - acquired 703.8
- oesophagus (acquired) 530.8
- - congenital 750.4
- opening of Wharton's duct in mouth
  750.2
- organ or site, congenital NEC - see
  Malposition, congenital
- ovary (acquired) 620.4

Displacement - *continued*
- ovary - *continued*
- - congenital 752.0
- - free in peritoneal cavity 752.0
- - into hernial sac 620.4
- oviduct (acquired) 620.4
- - congenital 752.1
- parotid gland (congenital) 750.2
- punctum lacrimale (congenital) 743.6
- sacro-iliac (joint) (congenital) 755.6
- - current injury - see Dislocation, sacro-iliac
- - old 724.6
- spleen, congenital 759.0
- stomach (congenital) 750.7
- sublingual duct (congenital) 750.2
- tongue (downward) 750.1
- tooth, teeth 524.3
- trachea (congenital) 748.3
- ureter or ureteric opening or orifice (congenital) 753.4
- uterine opening of oviducts or fallopian tubes 752.1
- uterus, uterine (see also Malposition, uterus) 621.6
- ventricular septum 746.8
- - with rudimentary ventricle 746.8
Disproportion 653.9
- affecting fetus or newborn 763.1
- caused by
- - conjoined twins 653.7
- - contraction pelvis (general) 653.1
- - - inlet 653.2
- - - outlet 653.3
- - fetal
- - - ascites 653.7
- - - hydrocephalus 653.6
- - - hydrops 653.7
- - - meningomyelocele 653.7
- - - sacral teratoma 653.7
- - - tumor 653.7
- - hydrocephalic fetus 653.6
- - pelvis, pelvic, abnormality (bony) NEC 653.0
- - unusually large fetus 653.5
- causing obstructed labor 660.1
- cephalopelvic, normally formed fetus 653.4
- fetal NEC 653.5
- fetopelvic, normally formed fetus 653.4
- fetus or newborn 763.1
- mixed maternal and fetal origin, normally formed fetus 653.4
- pelvis, pelvic (bony) NEC 653.1
- specified NEC 653.8
Disruptio uteri - see Rupture, uterus
Disruption

Disruption - *continued*
- family V61.0
- ligament(s) - see also Sprain
- - knee
- - - current injury - see Dislocation, knee
- - - old 717.8
- marital V61.1
- - involving
- - - divorce V61.0
- - - estrangement V61.0
- wound
- - episiotomy 674.2
- - operation 998.3
- - - cesarean 674.1
- - perineal (obstetric) 674.2
Dissatisfaction with
- employment V62.2
- school environment V62.3
Dissecting - see condition
Dissection
- aorta 441.0
- vascular 459.9
- wound - see Wound, open
Disseminated - see condition
Dissociation
- auriculoventricular or atrioventricular (any degree) 426.8
- interference 426.8
Dissociative reaction, state 300.1
Dissolution, vertebra 733.0
Distension
- abdomen 787.3
- bladder 596.8
- cecum 569.8
- colon 569.8
- gallbladder (see also Disease, gallbladder) 575.8
- intestine 569.8
- kidney 593.8
- liver 573.9
- seminal vesicle 608.8
- stomach 536.8
- - acute 536.1
- - psychogenic 306.4
- ureter 593.8
- uterus 621.8
Distichia, distichiasis (eyelid) 743.6
Distoma hepaticum infestation 121.3
Distomiasis 121.9
- bile passages 121.3
- - due to Clonorchis sinensis 121.1
- hemic 120.9
- hepatic 121.3
- - due to Clonorchis sinensis 121.1
- intestinal 121.4
- liver 121.3

Distortion - *continued*
- skull bone(s) - *continued*
- - with - *continued*
- - - encephalocele 742.0
- - - hydrocephalus 742.3
- - - - with spina bifida 741.0
- - - microcephalus 742.1
- spinal cord 742.5
- spine 756.1
- spleen 759.0
- sternum 756.3
- thorax (wall) 756.3
- thymus (gland) 759.2
- thyroid (gland) 759.2
- - cartilage 748.3
- tibia 755.6
- toe(s) 755.6
- tongue 750.1
- trachea (cartilage) 748.3
- ulna 755.5
- ureter 753.4
- - causing obstruction 753.2
- urethra 753.8
- - causing obstruction 753.6
- uterus 752.3
- vagina 752.4
- vein (peripheral) 747.6
- - great 747.4
- - portal 747.4
- - pulmonary 747.4
- vena cava (inferior) (superior) 747.4
- vertebra 756.1
- vulva 752.4
- wrist (bones) (joint) 755.5
Distress
- abdomen 789.0
- epigastric 789.0
- fetal (syndrome) 768.4
- - affecting management of pregnancy or childbirth 656.3
- - liveborn infant 768.4
- - - first noted
- - - - before onset of labor 768.2
- - - - during labor or delivery 768.3
- - stillborn infant (death before onset of labor) 768.0
- - - death during labor 768.1
- gastrointestinal (functional) 536.9
- - psychogenic 306.4
- intestinal (functional) NEC 564.9
- - psychogenic 306.4
- intrauterine - see Distress, fetal
- maternal 669.0
- respiratory 786.0
- - adult, syndrome 518.5
- - fetus or newborn 770.8
- - syndrome (idiopathic) (newborn) 769

Distress - *continued*
- stomach 536.9
- - psychogenic 306.4
Distribution vessel, atypical 747.6
- coronary artery 746.8
- spinal 747.6
Districhiasis 704.2
Disturbance - see also Disease
- absorption NEC 579.9
- - calcium 269.3
- - carbohydrate 579.8
- - fat 579.8
- - protein 579.8
- - vitamin (see also Deficiency, vitamin) 269.2
- acid-base equilibrium 276.9
- activity and attention, simple, with hyperkinesis 314.0
- assimilation, food 579.9
- auditory nerve, except deafness 388.5
- behavior - see Disturbance, conduct
- blood clotting (mechanism) (see also Defect, coagulation) 286.9
- cerebral nerve NEC 352.9
- circulatory 459.9
- conduct 312.9
- - adjustment reaction 309.3
- - compulsive 312.2
- - hyperkinetic 314.2
- - mixed with emotions 312.3
- - socialized 312.1
- - specified NEC 312.8
- - unsocialized 312.0
- coordination 781.3
- cranial nerve NEC 352.9
- deep sensibility - see Disturbance, sensation
- digestive 536.9
- - psychogenic 306.4
- electrolyte - see Imbalance, electrolyte
- emotions specific to childhood and adolescence 313.9
- - with
- - - anxiety and fearfulness 313.0
- - - misery and unhappiness 313.1
- - - sensitivity 313.2
- - - shyness 313.2
- - - social withdrawal 313.2
- - involving relationship problems 313.3
- - mixed 313.8
- - specified NEC 313.8
- endocrine (gland) 259.9
- - neonatal, transitory 775.9
- - - specified NEC 775.8
- equilibrium 780.4
- feeding 783.3
- - infant or elderly 783.3

Disturbance - *continued*
- feeding - *continued*
- - infant or elderly - *continued*
- - - newborn 779.3
- - - nonorganic origin 307.5
- - psychogenic, NEC 307.5
- fructose metabolism 271.2
- gait 781.2
- - hysterical 300.1
- gastric (functional) 536.9
- - motility 536.8
- - psychogenic 306.4
- - secretion 536.8
- gastrointestinal (functional) 536.9
- - psychogenic 306.4
- habit, child 307.9
- hearing, except deafness 388.4
- heart, functional (conditions in 426, 427, 428)
- - due to presence of (cardiac) prosthesis 429.4
- - postoperative (immediate) 997.1
- - - long term effect of cardiac surgery 429.4
- hormones 259.9
- innervation uterus, sympathetic, parasympathetic 621.8
- keratinization NEC
- - gingiva 523.1
- - lip 528.5
- - oral (mucosa) (soft tissue) 528.7
- - tongue 528.7
- learning, specific NEC 315.2
- memory (see also Amnesia) 780.9
- - mild, following organic brain damage 310.1
- mental (see also Disorder, mental) 300.9
- - associated with diseases classified elsewhere 316
- metabolism 277.9
- - amino-acid 270.9
- - - aromatic 270.2
- - - branched-chain 270.3
- - - straight-chain 270.7
- - - sulfur-bearing 270.4
- - ammonia 270.6
- - arginine 270.6
- - arginosuccinic acid 270.6
- - carbohydrate NEC 271.9
- - cholesterol 272.9
- - citrulline 270.6
- - complicating abortion - see categories 634-639, fourth digit .4
- - cystathionine 270.4
- - fat 272.9
- - general 277.9
- - glutamine 270.7

Disturbance - *continued*
- metabolism - *continued*
- - glycine 270.7
- - histidine 270.5
- - homocystine 270.4
- - in labor or delivery 669.0
- - iron 275.0
- - isoleucine 270.3
- - leucine 270.3
- - lipoid 272.9
- - lysine 270.7
- - methionine 270.4
- - neonatal, transitory 775.9
- - - specified NEC 775.8
- - ornithine 270.6
- - phosphate 275.3
- - phosphatides 275.3
- - serine 270.7
- - sodium NEC 276.9
- - threonine 270.7
- - tryptophan 270.2
- - tyrosine 270.2
- - urea cycle 270.6
- - valine 270.3
- motor 796.1
- nervous functional 799.2
- neuromuscular mechanism (eye) due to syphilis 094.8
- nutritional 269.9
- - nail 703.8
- ocular motion 378.8
- - psychogenic 306.7
- oculogyric 378.8
- - psychogenic 306.7
- oculomotor 378.8
- - psychogenic 306.7
- olfactory nerve 781.1
- optic nerve 377.4
- oral epithelium, including tongue 528.7
- personality (pattern) (trait) (see also Disorder, personality) 301.9
- - following organic brain damage 310.1
- polyglandular 258.9
- psychomotor 307.9
- pupillary 379.4
- reflex 796.1
- rhythm, heart 427.9
- salivary secretion 527.7
- sensation (cold) (heat) (localization) (tactile discrimination, localization) (texture) (vibratory) NEC 782.0
- - hysterical 300.1
- - skin 782.0
- - smell 781.1
- - taste 781.1
- sensory - see Disturbance, sensation

Disturbance - *continued*
- situational (transient) (see also Reaction, adjustment) 309.9
- - acute 308.3
- sleep 780.5
- - nonorganic origin 307.4
- sociopathic 301.7
- speech NEC 784.5
- - developmental 315.3
- - - associated with hyperkinesis 314.1
- stomach (functional) (see also Disturbance, gastric) 536.9
- sympathetic (nerve) 337.9
- temperature sense 782.0
- - hysterical 300.1
- tooth
- - eruption 520.6
- - formation 520.4
- - structure, hereditary NEC 520.5
- touch - see Disturbance, sensation
- vascular 459.9
- - arteriosclerotic - see Arteriosclerosis
- vasomotor 443.9
- vasospastic 443.9
- vision, visual NEC 368.9
Diuresis 788.4
Divers'
- palsy or paralysis 993.3
- squeeze 993.3
Diverticula, diverticulitis, diverticulosis, diverticulum (acute) (multiple) (perforated) (ruptured) 562.1
- appendix (noninflammatory) 543
- bladder (sphincter) 596.3
- - congenital 753.8
- bronchus (congenital) 748.3
- - acquired 494
- calyx, calyceal (kidney) 593.8
- cardia (stomach) 537.1
- cecum 562.1
- - congenital 751.5
- colon 562.1
- - congenital 751.5
- duodenum 562.0
- - congenital 751.5
- epiphrenic (esophagus) 530.6
- esophagus (congenital) 750.4
- - acquired 530.6
- - epiphrenic 530.6
- - pulsion 530.6
- - traction 530.6
- - Zenker's 530.6
- eustachian tube 381.8
- fallopian tube 620.8
- gastric 537.1
- heart (congenital) 746.8
- ileum 562.0

Diverticula - *continued*
- intestine (large) 562.1
- - congenital 751.5
- - small 562.0
- jejunum 562.0
- kidney (pelvis) (calyces) 593.8
- - with calculus 592.0
- Meckel's (displaced) (hypertrophic) 751.0
- oesophagus - see Diverticulum, esophagus
- organ or site, congenital NEC - see Distortion
- pericardium (congenital) (cyst) 746.8
- pharyngo-esophageal (pulsion) 530.6
- pharynx (congenital) 750.2
- pulsion (esophagus) 530.6
- rectosigmoid 562.1
- - congenital 751.5
- rectum 562.1
- seminal vesicle 608.0
- sigmoid 562.1
- - congenital 751.5
- stomach (acquired) 537.1
- - congenital 750.7
- trachea (congenital) 748.3
- - acquired 519.1
- traction (esophagus) 530.6
- ureter (acquired) 593.8
- - congenital 753.4
- ureterovesical orifice 593.8
- urethra (acquired) 599.2
- - congenital 753.8
- ventricle, left (congenital) 746.8
- vesical 596.3
- - congenital 753.8
- Zenker's (esophagus) 530.6
Division
- cervix uteri 622.8
- external os into two openings by frenum 752.4
- glans penis 752.8
- hymen 752.4
- labia minora (congenital) 752.4
- ligament (partial or complete) (current) - see also Sprain, strain
- - with open wound - see Wound, open
- muscle (partial or complete) (current) - see also Sprain, strain
- - with open wound - see Wound, open
- nerve - see Injury, nerve, by site
- spinal cord - see Injury, spinal, by region
- vein 459.9
Divorce V61.0
Dizziness 780.4
- hysterical 300.1
- psychogenic 306.9

Doehle-Heller aortitis 093.1 † 447.7*
Dog bite - see Wound, open
Dolichocephaly 754.0
Dolichocolon 751.5
Dolichostenomelia 759.8
Donohue's syndrome 259.8
Donor V59.9
– blood V59.0
– bone V59.2
– – marrow V59.3
– cornea V59.5
– kidney V59.4
– lymphocyte V59.8
– organ V59.9
– – specified NEC V59.8
– potential, examination of V70.8
– skin V59.1
– specified organ or tissue NEC V59.8
Donovanosis 099.2
Double
– albumin 273.8
– aortic arch 747.2
– auditory canal 744.2
– auricle (heart) 746.8
– bladder 753.8
– external os 752.4
– kidney with double pelvis (renal) 753.3
– meatus urinarius 753.8
– monster 759.4
– organ or site not listed here - see
  Accessory
– orifice
– – heart valve NEC 746.8
– – – pulmonary 746.0
– pelvis (renal) with double ureter 753.4
– tongue 750.1
– ureter (one or both sides) 753.4
– – with double pelvis (renal) 753.4
– urethra 753.8
– urinary meatus 753.8
– uterus 752.2
– – with doubling of cervix and vagina
  752.2
– – in pregnancy or childbirth 654.0
– – – fetus or newborn 763.8
– vagina 752.4
– – with doubling of cervix and uterus
  752.2
– vision 368.2
– vulva 752.4
Douglas' pouch, cul-de-sac - see condition
Down's disease or syndrome 758.0
Dracontiasis 125.7
Dracunculiasis 125.7
Dracunculosis 125.7
Drainage
– abscess (spontaneous) - see Abscess

Drainage - *continued*
– anomalous
– – pulmonary veins to hepatic veins or
  right atrium 747.4
– stump (amputation) (surgical) 997.6
– suprapubic, bladder 596.8
Dream state, hysterical 300.1
Drepanocytic anemia (see also Disease,
  sickle cell) 282.6
Dreschlera (infection) 118
– hawaiiensis 117.8
Dressler's syndrome (see also Insufficiency,
  coronary) 411
Drift, ulnar 736.0
Drinking (alcohol)
– excessive, to excess NEC 305.0
– – continual 303
– – habitual 303
Drop
– finger 736.2
– foot 736.7
– toe 735.8
– wrist 736.0
Dropped
– dead 798.1
– heart beats 426.6
Dropsy, dropsical 782.3
– abdomen 789.5
– brain - see Hydrocephalus
– cardiac, heart (see also Failure, heart,
  congestive) 428.0
– cardiorenal 404.9
– fetus or newborn 778.0
– – due to iso-immunisation 773.3
– gangrenous (see also Gangrene) 785.4
– lung 514
– malarial (see also Malaria) 084.9
– pericardium (see also Pericarditis) 423.9
Drowned, drowning 994.1
Drowsiness 780.0
Drug
– addiction (see also Dependence) 304.9
– adverse effect nec, correct substance
  properly administered 995.2
– dependence (see also Dependence) 304.9
– habit (see also Dependence) 304.9
– overdose - see Table of drugs and
  chemicals
– poisoning - see Table of drugs and
  chemicals
– wrong substance given or taken in error -
  see Table of drugs and chemicals
Drunkenness 305.0
– acute in alcoholism 303
– chronic 303
– pathologic 291.4
Drusen

Drusen - *continued*
- optic disc 377.2
- retina (degenerative) 362.5
Drusenfieber 075
Dry - see also condition
- socket (teeth) 526.5
Dryness
- larynx 478.7
- mouth 527.7
- nose 478.1
- throat 478.2
Duane's syndrome 378.7
Dubin-Johnson disease or syndrome 277.4
Dubois' disease 090.5
Duchenne's
- locomotor ataxia 094.0
- muscular dystrophy 359.1
- paralysis 335.2
- syndrome 335.2
Duchenne-Aran muscular atrophy 335.1
Duchenne-Griesinger disease 359.1
Ducrey's
- bacillus 099.0
- chancre 099.0
Duct, ductus - see condition
Duengero 061
Duhring's disease 694.0
Dukes(-Filatow) disease 057.8
Dullness, cardiac (increased) (decreased)
785.3
Dumbness (see also Aphasia) 784.3
Dumdum fever 085.0
Dumping syndrome (postgastrectomy)
564.2
Duodenitis (nonspecific) (peptic) 535.6
Duodenocholangitis (see also Cholecystitis)
575.8
Duodenum, duodenal - see condition
Duplay's disease, periarthritis or syndrome
726.2
Duplex - see also Accessory
- kidney 753.3
- placenta - see Placenta, abnormal
Duplication - see also Accessory
- anus 751.5
- appendix 751.5
- biliary duct (any) 751.6
- bladder 753.8
- cecum 751.5
- - and appendix 751.5
- cystic duct 751.6
- digestive organs 751.8
- esophagus 750.4
- frontonasal process 756.0
- gallbladder 751.6
- intestine (large) (small) 751.5
- kidney 753.3

Duplication - *continued*
- liver 751.6
- oesophagus 750.4
- pancreas 751.7
- penis 752.8
- respiratory organs NEC 748.9
- salivary duct 750.2
- spinal cord (incomplete) 742.5
- stomach 750.7
Dupuytren's
- contraction 728.6
- disease 728.6
- fracture 824.4
- - ankle 824.4
- - - open 824.5
- - fibula 824.4
- - - open 824.5
- - open 824.5
- - radius 813.4
- - - open 813.5
- muscle contracture 728.6
Durand-Nicolas-Favre disease 099.1
Duroziez's disease 746.5
Dust reticulation 504
Dutton's
- disease 086.9
- relapsing fever (West African) 087.1
Dwarfism 259.4
- achondroplastic 756.4
- congenital 259.4
- constitutional 259.4
- hypophyseal 253.3
- infantile 259.4
- Lorain(-Levi) type 253.3
- metatropic 756.4
- nephrotic-glycosuric (with
hypophosphatemic rickets) 270.0
- nutritional 263.2
- ovarian 758.6
- pancreatic 577.8
- pituitary 253.3
- psychosocial 259.4
- renal 588.0
Dyke-Young anemia (secondary)
(symptomatic) 283.9
Dysacousis 388.4
Dysadrenocortism 255.9
Dysarthria 784.5
Dysautonomia (see also Neuropathy,
peripheral, autonomic) 337.9
- familial 742.8
Dysbarism 993.3
Dysbasia 719.7
- angiosclerotica intermittens 443.9
- hysterical 300.1
- lordotica (progressiva) 333.6
- nonorganic origin 307.9

Dysbasia - *continued*
- psychogenic 307.9
Dyscalculia 315.1
Dyschezia (see also Constipation) 564.0
Dyschondroplasia (with hemangiomata)
  756.4
Dyschondrosteosis 756.5
Dyschromia 709.0
Dyscranio-pyo-phalangy 759.8
Dyscrasia
- blood 289.9
- - with antepartum hemorrhage 641.3
- - fetus or newborn NEC 776.9
- - puerperal, postpartum 666.3
- ovary 256.8
- pluriglandular 258.9
- polyglandular 258.9
Dysendocrinism 259.9
Dysentery, dysenteric (bilious) (catarrhal)
  (diarrhea) (epidemic) (gangrenous)
  (hemorrhagic) (infectious) (sporadic)
  (tropical) (ulcerative) 009.0
- abscess, liver (see also Abscess, amebic)
  006.3
- amebic (see also Amebiasis) 006.9
- - with abscess - see Abscess, amebic
- - acute 006.0
- - chronic 006.1
- arthritis 009.0 † 711.3*
- - bacillary 004.9 † 711.3*
- asylum 004.9
- bacillary 004.9
- - arthritis 004.9 † 711.3*
- - Boyd 004.2
- - Flexner 004.1
- - Schmitz(-Stutzer) 004.0
- - Shiga 004.0
- - Shigella 004.9
- - - group A 004.0
- - - group B 004.1
- - - group C 004.2
- - - group D 004.3
- - - specified type NEC 004.8
- - Sonne 004.3
- - specified type NEC 004.8
- bacterium 004.9
- balantidial 007.0
- Balantidium coli 007.0
- Boyd's 004.2
- Chilomastix 007.8
- Chinese 004.9
- choleriform 001.1
- coccidial 007.2
- Dientameba fragilis 007.8
- due to specified organism NEC - see
  Enteritis, infectious
- Embadomonas 007.8

Dysentery - *continued*
- Entameba, entamebic - see Dysentery,
  amebic
- Flexner's 004.1
- Flexner-Boyd 004.2
- Giardia lamblia 007.1
- giardial 007.1
- Hiss-Russell 004.1
- Lamblia 007.1
- leishmanial 085.0
- malarial (see also Malaria) 084.6
- metazoal 127.9
- Monilia 112.8
- protozoal NEC 007.9
- Russell's 004.8
- Salmonella 003.0
- schistosomal 120.1
- Schmitz(-Stutzer) 004.0
- Shiga 004.0
- Shigella NEC (see also Dysentery,
  bacillary) 004.9
- Sonne 004.3
- strongyloidiasis 127.2
- trichomonal 007.3
- tuberculous 014
- viral (see also Enteritis, viral) 008.8
Dysesthesia 782.0
- hysterical 300.1
Dysfibrinogenemia (congenital) 286.3
Dysfunction
- adrenal 255.9
- bladder 596.5
- bleeding, uterus 626.8
- cerebral 348.3
- colon 564.9
- - psychogenic 306.4
- colostomy or enterostomy 569.6
- cystic duct (see also Disease, gallbladder)
  575.8
- endocrine NEC 259.9
- endometrium 621.8
- enteric stoma 569.6
- gallbladder (see also Disease,
  gallbladder) 575.8
- gastrointestinal 536.9
- gland, glandular NEC 259.9
- heart 427.9
- hemoglobin 288.8
- hepatic 573.9
- hypophysis 253.9
- kidney (see also Disease, renal) 593.9
- labyrinthine 386.5
- liver 573.9
- - constitutional 277.4
- ovary 256.9
- - specified NEC 256.8
- papillary muscle 427.9

Dysfunction - *continued*
- pineal gland 259.8
- pituitary (gland) 253.9
- placental - see Placenta, insufficiency
- polyglandular 258.9
- pylorus 537.9
- rectum 564.9
- - psychogenic 306.4
- segmental 739.9
- senile 797
- somatic 739.9
- stomach 536.9
- - psychogenic 306.4
- suprarenal 255.9
- symbolic NEC 784.6
- temporomandibular (joint) (joint-pain-syndrome) 524.6
- testicular 257.9
- thyroid 246.9
- - complicating pregnancy, childbirth or puerperium 648.1
- uterus, complicating delivery 661.9
- - fetus or newborn 763.7
- - hypertonic 661.4
- - hypotonic 661.2
- - - primary 661.0
- - - secondary 661.1
Dysgenesis
- gonadal (due to chromosomal anomaly) 758.6
- - pure 752.7
- ovarian 758.6
- renal 753.0
- reticular 279.2
- seminiferous tubule 758.6
Dysgerminoma (M9060/3)
- specified site - see Neoplasm, malignant
- unspecified site
- - female 183.0
- - male 186.9
Dysgeusia 781.1
Dysgraphia 781.3
Dyshidrosis 705.8
Dysidrosis 705.8
Dysinsulinism 251.8
Dyskaryotic cervical smear 795.0
Dyskeratosis (see also Keratosis) 701.1
- cervix 622.1
- congenital 757.3
- follicularis 757.3
- uterus NEC 621.8
Dyskinesia 781.3
- biliary 575.8
- esophagus 530.5
- hysterical 300.1
- intestinal 564.8
- nonorganic origin 307.9

Dyskinesia - *continued*
- orofacial 333.8
- psychogenic 307.9
Dyslalia 784.5
- developmental 315.3
Dyslexia 784.6
- developmental 315.0
- secondary to organic lesion 784.6
Dysmaturity (see also Immaturity) 765.1
- lung 770.4
Dysmenorrhea (exfoliative) (membranous) (primary) 625.3
- essential 625.3
- psychogenic 306.5
Dysmetria 781.3
Dysnomia 784.3
Dysorexia 783.0
- hysterical 300.1
Dysostosis
- cleidocranial, cleidocranialis 755.5
- craniofacial 756.0
- mandibulofacial, incomplete 756.0
- multiplex 277.5
Dyspareunia (female) 625.0
- male 608.8
- psychogenic 302.7
Dyspepsia (allergic) (congenital) (functional) (gastrointestinal) (neurogenic) (occupational) (reflex) 536.8
- atonic 536.8
- - psychogenic 306.4
- diarrhea
- - psychogenic 306.4
- intestinal 564.8
- - psychogenic 306.4
- nervous 306.4
- neurotic 306.4
- psychogenic 306.4
Dysphagia 787.2
- functional 300.1
- hysterical 300.1
- nervous 300.1
- psychogenic 306.4
- sideropenic 280
Dysphagocytosis, congenital 288.1
Dysphasia 784.5
Dysphonia 784.4
- functional 300.1
- hysterical 300.1
- psychogenic 306.1
- spastica 478.7
Dyspituitarism 253.9
Dysplasia - see also Anomaly
- brain 742.9
- bronchopulmonary, fetus or newborn 770.7
- cervix (uteri) 622.1

Dysplasia - *continued*
- chondroectodermal 756.5
- chondromatose 756.4
- dentinal 520.5
- diaphysial, progressive 756.5
- ectodermal (anhidrotic) (Bason)
  (Clouston) (congenital) (Feinmesser)
  (hereditary) (hidrotic) (Marshall)
  (Robinson) 757.3
- epiphysealis 756.9
- - multiplex 756.5
- - punctata 756.5
- epiphysis 756.9
- - multiple 756.5
- epithelial, uterine cervix 622.1
- eye 743.1
- fibrous
- - bone NEC 733.2
- - diaphysial, progressive 756.5
- - jaw 526.8
- - monostotic 733.2
- - polyostotic 756.5
- hip, congenital 755.6
- joint 755.8
- leg 755.6
- lung 748.5
- mammary (gland) (benign) 610.9
- - cystic 610.1
- - specified NEC 610.8
- metaphyseal 756.9
- monostotic fibrous 733.2
- muscle 756.8
- nervous system (general) 742.9
- neuro-ectodermal 759.6
- oculodentodigital 759.8
- periosteum 733.9
- polyostotic fibrous 756.5
- retinal 743.5
- spinal cord 742.9
- thymic, with immunodeficiency 279.2
- vagina 623.0
Dyspnea (nocturnal) (paroxysmal) 786.0
- asthmatic (bronchial) 493.9
- - with bronchitis 493.9
- - - chronic 491.2
- - cardiac (see also Failure, ventricular,
  left) 428.1
- cardiac (see also Failure, ventricular, left)
  428.1
- functional 300.1
- hyperventilation 786.0
- hysterical 300.1
- newborn 770.8
- psychogenic 306.1
- uremic - see Uremia
Dyspraxia 781.3
- syndrome 315.4

Dysproteinemia 273.8
Dysrhythmia
- cardiac 427.9
- - postoperative 997.1
- - - long term effect of cardiac surgery
  429.4
- cerebral or cortical 348.3
Dyssocial behavior, without manifest
  psychiatric disorder V71.0
Dyssynergia
- biliary (see also Disease, biliary) 576.8
- cerebellaris myoclonica 334.2
Dysthyroidism 246.9
Dystocia 661.9
- affecting fetus or newborn 763.1
- cervical 661.0
- - fetus or newborn 763.7
- contraction ring 661.4
- - fetus or newborn 763.7
- fetal 660.9
- - fetus or newborn 763.1
- maternal 660.9
- - fetus or newborn 763.1
- positional 660.0
- - fetus or newborn 763.1
- shoulder (girdle) 660.4
- - fetus or newborn 763.1
- uterine NEC 661.4
- - fetus or newborn 763.7
Dystonia
- deformans progressive 333.6
- lenticularis 333.6
- musculorum deformans 333.6
- torsion (idiopathic) 333.6
- - fragments 333.8
- - symptomatic 333.7
Dystonic movements 781.0
Dystrophy, dystrophia 783.9
- adiposogenital 253.8
- Becker's type 359.1
- breviocollis 756.1
- cervical (sympathetic) NEC 337.9
- choroid (central aerolar) (generalized)
  (gyrate) (hereditary) (peripapillary)
  363.5
- cornea (endothelial) (epithelial)
  (granular) (hereditary) (lattice) (macular)
  371.5
- Duchenne's 359.1
- due to malnutrition 263.9
- Erb's 359.1
- familial
- - hyperplastic periosteal 756.5
- - osseous 756.5
- Fuch's 371.5
- Gower's muscular 359.1
- hair 704.2

Dystrophy - *continued*
- Landouzy-Dejerine 359.1
- Leyden-Moebius 359.1
- muscular 359.1
- − congenital (hereditary) (progressive) 359.1
- − − myotonic 359.2
- − distal 359.1
- − Duchenne type 359.1
- − Erb type 359.1
- − facioscapulohumeral 359.1
- − Gower's 359.1
- − hereditary (progressive) 359.1
- − Landouzy-Dejerine type 359.1
- − limb-girdle 359.1
- − myotonic 359.2
- − progressive (hereditary) 359.1
- − − Charcot-Marie(-Tooth) type 356.1
- − pseudohypertrophic (infantile) 359.1
- myocardium, myocardial (see also Degeneration, myocardial) 429.1
- myotonic 359.2
- myotonica 359.2
- nail 703.8
- − congenital 757.5
- nutritional 263.9
- ocular 359.1

Dystrophy - *continued*
- oculocerebrorenal 270.8
- oculopharyngeal 359.1
- ovarian 620.8
- papillary (and pigmentary) (see also Acanthosis) 701.1
- pituitary (gland) 253.8
- polyglandular 258.8
- retinal (albipunctate) (pigmentary) (vitelliforme) (hereditary) 362.7
- − in
- − − − cerebral lipidoses 330.1 † 362.7*
- − − − systemic lipidoses 272.7 † 362.7*
- Salzmann's nodular 371.4
- scapuloperoneal 359.1
- skin NEC 709.9
- sympathetic (reflex) (see also Neuropathy, peripheral, autonomic) 337.9
- tapetoretinal 362.7
- thoracic asphyxiating 756.8
- unguium 703.8
- − congenital 757.5
- vitreoretinal 362.7
- vulva 624.0
Dysuria 788.1
- psychogenic 306.5

E

Eale's disease 362.1
Ear - see also condition
– piercing V50.3
– tropical 111.8
– wax 380.4
Earache 388.7
Eberth's disease 002.0
Ebstein's
– anomaly (heart) 746.2
– disease, meaning diabetes 250.3 † 581.8*
Eccentro-osteochondrodysplasia 277.5

Ecchondroma (M9210/0) - see Neoplasm,
  bone, benign
Ecchondrosis (M9210/1) 238.0
Ecchordosis physaliphora 756.0
Ecchymosis (multiple) 459.8
– conjunctiva 372.7
– eye (traumatic) 921.0
– eyelids (traumatic) 921.0
– newborn 772.6
– spontaneous 782.7
– traumatic - see Contusion
Echinococciasis - see Echinococcus
Echinococcosis - see Echinococcus

Echinococcus (infection) 122.9
– granulosus 122.4
– – liver 122.0
– – lung 122.1
– – specified site NEC 122.3
– – thyroid 122.2
– liver NEC 122.8
– – multilocularis 122.5
– lung NEC 122.9
– – multilocularis 122.6
– multilocularis 122.7
– – liver 122.5
– – specified site NEC 122.6
– orbit 122.9 † 376.1*
– specified site NEC 122.9
– – granulosus 122.3
– – multilocularis 122.6
– thyroid NEC 122.9
– – granulosus 122.2
– – multilocularis 122.6
Echinorhynchiasis 127.7
Echinostomiasis 121.8
Echolalia 784.6
Eclampsia, eclamptic (coma) (convulsions)
  (delirium) 780.3

Eclampsia - *continued*
– female, child-bearing age NEC - see
  Eclampsia, pregnancy
– gravidarum - see Eclampsia, pregnancy
– male 780.3
– not associated with pregnancy or
  childbirth 780.3
– pregnancy, childbirth or puerperium
  642.6
– – with pre-existing hypertension 642.7
– – fetus or newborn 760.0
– uremic 586
Economic circumstance affecting care
  V60.9
Economo's disease 049.8 † 323.4*
Ectasia, ectasis
– aorta, (see also Aneurysm, aorta) 441.6
– – ruptured 441.5
– breast 610.4
– capillary 448.9
– cornea 371.7
– duct 610.4
– mammary duct 610.4
– papillary 448.9
– sclera 379.1
Ecthyma 686.8
– contagiosum 051.2
– gangrenosum 686.0
– infectiosum 051.2
Ectocardia 746.8
Ectodermal dysplasia, congenital 757.3
Ectodermosis erosiva pluriorificialis 695.1
Ectopic, ectopia (congenital) 759.8
– abdominal viscera 751.8
– – due to defect in anterior abdominal
    wall 756.8
– ACTH syndrome 255.0
– anus 751.5
– auricular beats 427.6
– beats 427.6
– bladder 753.5
– bone and cartilage in lung 748.6
– brain 742.4
– breast tissue 757.6
– cardiac 746.8
– cerebral 742.4
– cordis 746.8
– endometrium 617.9
– gastric mucosa 750.7
– gestation - see Pregnancy, ectopic

Ectopic - *continued*
- heart 746.8
- hormone secretion NEC 259.3
- kidney (crossed) (pelvis) 753.3
- lens 743.3
- lentis 743.3
- mole - see Pregnancy, ectopic
- organ or site NEC - see Malposition, congenital
- pancreas 751.7
- pregnancy - see Pregnancy, ectopic
- pupil 364.7
- renal 753.3
- testis 752.5
- ureter 753.4
- ventricular beats 427.6
- vesicae 753.5
Ectromelia 755.4
- lower limb 755.3
- upper limb 755.2
Ectropion 374.1
- anus 569.4
- cervix 622.0
- - with mention of cervicitis 616.0
- congenital 743.6
- eyelid (cicatricial) (paralytic) (senile) (spastic) 374.1
- - congenital 743.6
- iris 364.5
- lip (congenital) 750.2
- - acquired 528.5
- rectum 569.4
- urethra 599.8
- uvea 364.5
Eczema (acute) (allergic) (chronic) (erythematous) (fissum) (occupational) (rubrum) (squamous) 692.9
- atopic 691.8
- contact NEC 692.9
- dermatitis NEC 692.9
- due to specified cause - see Dermatitis, due to
- dyshydrotic 705.8
- - external ear 380.2
- flexural 691.8
- gouty 274.8
- herpeticum 054.0
- hypertrophicum 701.8
- hypostatic - see Varicose vein
- impetiginous 684
- infantile (due to any substance) (intertriginous) (seborrheic) 691.8
- intertriginous NEC 692.9
- - infantile 691.8
- intrinsic 691.8
- lichenified NEC 692.9
- marginatum 110.3

Eczema - *continued*
- nummular NEC 692.9
- pustular 686.8
- seborrheic 690
- - infantile 691.8
- solare 692.7
- stasis - see Varicose vein
- vaccination, vaccinatum 999.0
- varicose - see also Varicose vein
Eddowes' disease or syndrome 756.5
Edema, edematous 782.3
- with nephritis (see also Nephrosis) 581.9
- angioneurotic (allergic) (any site) (with urticaria) 995.1
- - hereditary 277.6
- angiospastic 443.9
- Berlin's (traumatic) 921.3
- brain 348.5
- - due to birth injury 767.8
- - fetus or newborn 767.8
- cardiac (see also Failure, heart, congestive) 428.0
- cardiovascular (see also Failure, heart, congestive) 428.0
- cerebral - see Edema, brain
- cerebrospinal vessel - see Edema, brain
- cervix (uteri) (acute) 622.8
- - puerperal, postpartum 674.8
- circumscribed, acute 995.1
- - hereditary 277.6
- complicating pregnancy 646.1
- - with hypertension - see Toxemia, of pregnancy
- conjunctiva 372.7
- connective tissue 782.3
- cornea 371.2
- due to lymphatic obstruction 457.1
- epiglottis - see Edema, glottis
- essential, acute 995.1
- - hereditary 277.6
- extremities, lower - see Edema, legs
- eyelid NEC 374.8
- familial, hereditary (legs) 757.0
- famine 262
- fetus or newborn 778.5
- gestational 646.1
- - with hypertension - see Toxemia, of pregnancy
- glottis, glottic, glottidis (obstructive) (passive) 478.6
- - allergic 995.1
- - - hereditary 277.6
- - due to external agent - see condition, respiratory, acute, due to
- heart (see also Failure, heart, congestive) 428.0
- heat 992.7

Edema - *continued*
- hereditary (legs) 757.0
- inanition 262
- infectious 782.3
- iris 364.4
- joint 719.0
- larynx - see Edema, glottis
- legs 782.3
- - due to venous obstruction 459.2
- - hereditary 757.0
- localized 782.3
- - due to venous obstruction 459.2
- - - lower extremity 459.2
- lower extremities - see Edema, legs
- lung 514
- - acute 518.4
- - - with heart condition or failure (see
      also Failure, ventricular, left) 428.1
- - - chemical (due to fumes or vapors)
      506.1
- - - due to
- - - - external agent(s) NEC 508.9
- - - - - specified NEC 508.8
- - - - fumes or vapors (chemical)
        (inhalation) 506.1
- - - - radiation 508.0
- - chemical (acute) 506.1
- - - chronic 506.4
- - chronic 514
- - - chemical (due to fumes or vapors)
      506.4
- - - due to
- - - - external agent(s) NEC 508.9
- - - - - specified NEC 508.8
- - - - fumes or vapors (chemical)
        (inhalation) 506.4
- - - - radiation 508.1
- - due to
- - - external agent NEC 508.9
- - - high altitude 993.2
- - - near drowning 994.1
- - terminal 514
- lymphatic 457.1
- - due to mastectomy 457.0
- macula 362.5
- malignant (see also Gas gangrene) 040.0
- Milroy's 757.0
- nasopharynx 478.2
- nutritional 262
- - with dyspigmentation, skin and hair
    260
- optic disc or nerve 377.0
- orbit 376.3
- - circulatory 459.8
- penis 607.8
- periodic 995.1
- - hereditary 277.6

Edema - *continued*
- pharynx 478.2
- pitting 782.3
- pulmonary - see Edema, lung
- Quincke's 995.1
- - hereditary 277.6
- renal (see also Nephrosis) 581.9
- retina 362.8
- salt 276.0
- scrotum 608.8
- seminal vesicle 608.8
- spermatic cord 608.8
- spinal cord 336.1
- starvation 262
- subglottic - see Edema, glottis
- supraglottic - see Edema, glottis
- testis 608.8
- toxic NEC 782.3
- traumatic NEC 782.3
- tunica vaginalis 608.8
- vas deferens 608.8
- vulva (acute) 624.8
Edentia (complete) (partial) (see also
  Absence, tooth) 520.0
- congenital (deficiency of tooth buds)
  520.0
- due to accident, extraction, or local
  periodontal disease 525.1
Edsall's disease 992.2
Educational handicap V62.3
Edward's syndrome 758.2
Effect, adverse NEC
- abnormal gravitational (G) forces or
  states 994.9
- altitude (high) - see Effect, adverse, high
  altitude
- anesthetic
- - in labor and delivery NEC 668.9
- - - fetus or newborn 763.5
- antitoxin - see Complications, vaccination
- atmospheric pressure 993.9
- - due to explosion 993.4
- - high 993.3
- - low - see Effect, adverse, high altitude
- - specified effect NEC 993.8
- biological, correct substance properly
  administered (see also Effect, adverse,
  drug) 995.2
- blood (derivatives) (serum) (transfusion)
  - see Complications, transfusion
- chemical substance NEC 989.9
- - specified - see Table of drugs and
    chemicals
- cobalt, radioactive 990
- cold (temperature) (weather) 991.9
- - chilblains 991.5
- - frostbite - see Frostbite

Effect - *continued*
- cold - *continued*
- - specified effect NEC 991.8
- drugs and medicaments NEC 995.2
- - correct substance properly
  administered 995.2
- - overdose or wrong substance given or
  taken 977.9
- - - specified drug - see Table of drugs
  and chemicals
- electric current (shock) 994.8
- - burn - see Burn
- electricity (shock) 994.8
- - burn - see Burn
- exertion (excessive) 994.5
- exposure 994.9
- - exhaustion 994.4
- external cause NEC 994.9
- fallout (radioactive) NEC 990
- fluoroscopy NEC 990
- foodstuffs
- - allergic reaction (see also Allergy,
  food) 693.1
- - noxious 988.9
- - - specified type NEC (see also
  Poisoning, by name of noxious
  foodstuff) 988.8
- gases, fumes, or vapors - see Table of
  drugs and chemicals
- glue (airplane) sniffing 304.6
- heat - see Heat
- high altitude NEC 993.2
- - anoxia 993.2
- - on
- - - ears 993.0
- - - sinuses 993.1
- - polycythemia 289.0
- hot weather - see Heat
- hunger 994.2
- immunization - see Complications,
  vaccination
- immunological agents - see
  Complications, vaccination
- implantation (removable) of isotope or
  radium NEC 990
- infrared (radiation) (rays) NEC 990
- - dermatitis or eczema 692.8
- infusion - see Complications, infusion
- ingestion or injection of isotope
  (therapeutic) NEC 990
- irradiation NEC 990
- isotope (radioactive) NEC 990
- lack of care of infants 995.5
- lightning 994.0
- - burn - see Burn
- lirugin - see Complications, vaccination

Effect - *continued*
- medicinal substance, correct, properly
  administered (see also Effect, adverse,
  drug) 995.2
- mesothorium NEC 990
- motion 994.6
- overheated places - see Heat
- polonium NEC 990
- psychosocial, of work environment V62.1
- radiation (diagnostic) (fallout) (infrared)
  (natural source) (therapeutic) (tracer)
  (ultraviolet) (X-ray) NEC 990
- - dermatitis or eczema - see Dermatitis,
  due to, radiation
- - fibrosis of lungs 508.1
- - pneumonitis 508.0
- - pulmonary manifestations
- - - acute 508.0
- - - chronic 508.1
- - suspected damage to fetus affecting
  management of pregnancy 655.6
- radioactive substance NEC 990
- - dermatitis or eczema 692.8
- radioactivity NEC 990
- radiotherapy NEC 990
- - dermatitis or eczema 692.8
- radium NEC 990
- roentgen rays NEC 990
- roentgenography NEC 990
- roentgenoscopy NEC 990
- serum (prophylactic) (therapeutic) NEC
  999.5
- specified NEC 995.8
- - external cause NEC 994.9
- teletherapy NEC 990
- thirst 994.3
- transfusion - see Complications,
  transfusion
- ultraviolet (radiation) (rays) NEC 990
- - burn - see also Burn
- - - from sun 692.7
- - dermatitis or eczema - see Dermatitis,
  due to, ultraviolet rays
- uranium NEC 990
- vaccine (any) - see Complications,
  vaccination
- weightlessness 994.9
- whole blood - see Complications,
  transfusion
- work environment V62.1
- X-rays NEC 990
- - dermatitis or eczema 692.8

Effects, late - see Late effect

Effort syndrome (aviators') (psychogenic)
306.2

Effusion

Effusion - *continued*
- amniotic fluid - see Rupture, membranes, premature
- brain (serous) 437.9
- bronchial (see also Bronchitis) 490
- cerebral 437.9
- cerebrospinal (see also Meningitis) 322.9
- - vessel 437.9
- chest - see Effusion, pleura
- intracranial 437.9
- joint 719.0
- meninges (see also Meningitis) 322.9
- pericardium, pericardial (see also, pericarditis) 423.9
- peritoneal (chronic) 568.8
- pleura, pleurisy, pleuritic, pleuropericardial 511.9
- - fetus or newborn 511.9
- - nontuberculous 511.9
- - - bacterial 511.1
- - pneumococcal 511.1
- - staphylococcal 511.1
- - streptococcal 511.1
- - tuberculous 012.0
- - - primary progressive 010.1
- pulmonary - see Effusion, pleura
- spinal (see also Meningitis) 322.9
- thorax, thoracic - see Effusion, pleura
Egg shell nails 703.8
- congenital 757.5
Egyptian splenomegaly 120.1
Ehlers-Danlos syndrome 756.8
Eichstedt's disease 111.0
Eisenmenger's defect, complex, or syndrome 745.4
Ejaculation semen, painful 608.8
- psychogenic 306.5
Ekbom syndrome 333.9
El Tor cholera 001.1
Elastic skin 757.3
- acquired 701.8
Elastofibroma (M8820/0) - see Neoplasm, connective tissue, benign
Elastoma 757.3
- juvenile 757.3
Elastomyofibrosis 425.3
Elastosis
- actinic, solar 692.7
- atrophicans 701.8
- perforans serpiginosa 701.1
- senilis 701.8
Elbow - see condition
Electric current, electricity, effects (concussion) (fatal) (nonfatal) (shock) 994.8
- burn - see Burn
Electrocution 994.8

Electrolyte imbalance 276.9
Elephantiasis (nonfilarial) 457.1
- arabum (see also Infestation, filarial) 125.9
- congenital (any site) 757.3
- due to
- - Brugia (malayi) 125.1
- - mastectomy operation 457.0
- - Wuchereria (bancrofti) 125.0
- - - malayi 125.1
- eyelid 374.8
- filarial (see also Infestation, filarial) 125.9
- filariensis (see also Infestation, filarial) 125.9
- glandular 457.1
- graecorum 030.9
- lymphangiectatic 457.1
- lymphatic vessel 457.1
- - due to mastectomy operation 457.0
- scrotum 457.1
- streptococcal 457.1
- surgical 997.9
- - postmastectomy 457.0
- telangiectodes 457.1
- vulva (nonfilarial) 624.8
Elevated - see Elevation
Elevation
- antibody titer 795.7
- basal metabolic rate 794.7
- blood pressure (see also Hypertension) 401.9
- - reading (incidental) (isolated) (nonspecific), no diagnosis of hypertension 796.2
- body temperature (of unknown origin) (see also Pyrexia) 780.6
- conjugate eye 378.8
- diaphragm, congenital 756.6
- immunoglobulin level 795.7
- lactic acid dehydrogenase (LDH) level 790.4
- scapula, congenital 755.5
- sedimentation rate 790.1
- transaminase level 790.4
- venous pressure 459.8
Elliptocytosis (congenital) (hereditary) 282.1
- Hb C (disease) 282.7
- hemoglobin disease 282.7
- sickle cell (disease) 282.6
Ellison-Zollinger syndrome 251.5
Ellis-van Creveld syndrome 756.5
Elongated - see Elongation
Elongation (congenital) - see also Distortion
- bone 756.9
- cervix (uteri) 752.4

Elongation - *continued*
− cervix - *continued*
− − acquired 622.6
− − hypertrophic 622.6
− colon 751.5
− common bile duct 751.6
− cystic duct 751.6
− frenulum, penis 752.8
− labia minora, acquired 624.8
− ligamentum patellae 756.8
− petiolus (epiglottidis) 748.3
− tooth, teeth 520.2
− uvula 750.2
− − acquired 528.9
Emaciation (due to malnutrition) 261
Embadomoniasis 007.8
Embedded tooth, teeth 520.6
− with abnormal position (same or adjacent
    tooth) 524.3
Embolic - see condition
Embolism (septic) 444.9
− with
− − abortion - see categories 634-639 -
    fourth digit .6
− − ectopic gestation 639.6
− air (any site) 958.0
− − with
− − − abortion - see categories 634-639,
    fourth digit .6
− − due to implanted device 996.7
− − following infusion, perfusion or
    transfusion 999.1
− − in pregnancy, childbirth or puerperium
    673.0
− − traumatic 958.0
− amniotic fluid (pulmonary) 673.1
− − with abortion - see categories 634-639,
    fourth digit .6
− aorta, aortic 444.1
− − abdominal 444.0
− − bifurcation 444.0
− − saddle 444.0
− − thoracic 444.1
− artery 444.9
− − auditory, internal 433.8
− − basilar (see also Occlusion, artery,
    basilar) 433.0
− − carotid (common) (internal) (see also
    Occlusion, artery, carotid) 433.1
− − cerebellar (anterior inferior) (posterior
    inferior) (superior) 433.8
− − cerebral (see also Embolism, brain)
    434.1
− − choroidal (anterior) 433.8
− − communicating posterior 433.8
− − coronary (see also Infarct,
    myocardium) 410

Embolism - *continued*
− artery - *continued*
− − extremity (lower) (upper) 444.2
− − hypophyseal 433.8
− − mesenteric (with gangrene) 557.0
− − ophthalmic 362.3
− − peripheral 444.2
− − pontine 433.8
− − precerebral NEC - see Occlusion,
    artery, precerebral NEC
− − pulmonary - see Embolism, pulmonary
− − renal 593.8
− − retinal 362.3
− − specified NEC 444.8
− − vertebral (see also Occlusion, artery,
    vertebral) 433.2
− birth, mother - see Embolism, obstetrical
− blood clot
− − with
− − − abortion - see categories 634-639,
    fourth digit .6
− − in pregnancy, childbirth or puerperium
    673.2
− brain 434.1
− − puerperal, postpartum, childbirth
    674.0
− capillary 448.9
− cardiac (see also Infarct, myocardium)
    410
− carotid (artery) (common) (internal) (see
    also Occlusion, artery, carotid) 433.1
− cavernous sinus (venous) - see Embolism,
    intracranial venous sinus
− cerebral (see also Embolism, brain) 434.1
− coronary (artery or vein) (systemic) (see
    also Infarct, myocardium) 410
− due to presence of any device, implant or
    graft (classifiable to 996.0-996.5) 996.7
− extremities 444.2
− eye 362.3
− fat (cerebral) (pulmonary) (systemic)
    958.1
− − complicating delivery 673.8
− femoral 444.2
− − vein 453.8
− following infusion, perfusion or
    transfusion
− − air 999.1
− − thrombus 999.2
− heart (fatty) (see also Infarct,
    myocardium) 410
− hepatic (vein) 453.0
− in pregnancy, childbirth or puerperium
    (pulmonary) - see Embolism, obstetrical
− intestine (artery) (vein) (with gangrene)
    557.0

Embolism - *continued*
- intracranial (see also Embolism, brain) 434.1
- − − venous sinus (any) 325
- − − − nonpyogenic 437.8
- kidney (artery) 593.8
- lateral sinus (venous) - see Embolism, intracranial venous sinus
- longitudinal sinus (venous) - see Embolism, intracranial venous sinus
- lower extremity 444.2
- lung (massive) - see Embolism, pulmonary
- meninges (see also Embolism, brain) 434.1
- mesenteric (artery) (vein) (with gangrene) 557.0
- multiple NEC 444.9
- obstetrical (pulmonary) 673.2
- − − air 673.0
- − − amniotic fluid (pulmonary) 673.1
- − − blood clot 673.2
- − − cardiac 674.8
- − − fat 673.8
- − − heart 674.8
- − − pyemic 673.3
- − − septic 673.3
- − − specified NEC 674.8
- ophthalmic 362.3
- paradoxical NEC 444.9
- penis 607.8
- peripheral arteries NEC 444.2
- pituitary 253.8
- portal (vein) 452
- postoperative 997.2
- precerebral artery (see also Occlusion, artery, precerebral NEC) 433.9
- puerperal - see Embolism, obstetrical
- pulmonary (artery) (vein) 415.1
- − − with
- − − − abortion - see categories 634-639 - fourth digit .6
- − − − ectopic gestation 639.6
- − − in pregnancy, childbirth or puerperium - see Embolism, obstetrical
- pyemic (multiple) 038.9
- − − with
- − − − abortion - see categories 634-639 - fourth digit .6
- − − − ectopic gestation 639.6
- − − pneumococcal 038.2
- − − − with pneumonia 481
- − − puerperal, postpartum, childbirth (any organism) 673.3
- − − specified organism NEC 038.8
- − − staphylococcal 038.1
- − − streptococcal 038.0

Embolism - *continued*
- renal (artery) 593.8
- − − vein 453.3
- retina, retinal 362.3
- septicemic - see Embolism, pyemic
- sinus - see Embolism, intracranial venous sinus
- soap, with abortion - see categories 634-639, fourth digit .6
- spinal cord 437.8
- − − pyogenic origin 324.1
- spleen, splenic (artery) 444.8
- thrombus (thromboembolism) following infusion, perfusion or transfusion 999.2
- vein 453.9
- − − cerebral (see also Embolism, brain) 434.1
- − − coronary (see also Infarct, myocardium) 410
- − − hepatic 453.0
- − − mesenteric (with gangrene) 557.0
- − − portal 452
- − − pulmonary - see Embolism, pulmonary
- − − renal 453.3
- − − specified NEC 453.8
- − − vena(e) cava(e) 453.2
- vessels of brain (see also Embolism, brain) 434.1
Embolus - see Embolism

Embryoma (M9080/1) - see also Neoplasm, uncertain behavior
- benign (M9080/0) - see Neoplasm, benign
- kidney (M8960/3) 189.0
- liver (M8970/3) 155.0
- malignant (M9080/3) - see also Neoplasm, malignant
- − − kidney (M8960/3) 189.0
- − − liver (M8970/3) 155.0
- − − testis (M9070/3) 186.9
- − − − undescended 186.0
- testis (M9070/3) 186.9
- − − undescended 186.0
Embryonic
- circulation 747.9
- heart 747.9
- vas deferens 752.8
Embryopathia NEC 759.9
Embryotomy 763.8
Embryotoxon 743.4

Emesis (see also Vomiting) 787.0
- gravidarum - see Hyperemesis, gravidarum
Emotionality, pathological 301.3
Emotogenic disease (see also Disorder, psychogenic) 306.9

Emphysema (atrophic) (bullous) (chronic)
(diffuse) (essential) (hypertrophic)
(interlobular) (lung) (obstructive)
(panacinar) (panlobar) (postural)
(pulmonary) (senile) (subpleural)
(unilobular) (vesicular) 492
– cellular tissue (traumatic) 958.7
– – surgical 998.8
– compensatory 518.2
– congenital 770.2
– conjunctiva 372.8
– connective tissue (traumatic) 958.7
– – surgical 998.8
– due to
– – fumes or vapors 506.4
– eye 376.8
– eyelid 374.8
– – surgical 998.8
– – traumatic 958.7
– fetus or newborn 770.2
– interstitial 518.1
– – congenital 770.2
– – fetus or newborn 770.2
– laminated tissue 958.7
– – surgical 998.8
– mediastinal 518.1
– – fetus or newborn 770.2
– orbit, orbital 376.8
– subcutaneous 958.7
– – due to trauma 958.7
– – surgical 998.8
– surgical 998.8
– thymus (gland) (congenital) 254.8
– traumatic 958.7
Empyema (chest) (diaphragmatic) (double)
(encapsulated) (general) (interlobar)
(lung) (mesial) (necessitatis) (perforating
chest wall) (pleura) (pneumococcal)
(residual) (sacculated) (streptococcal)
(supradiaphragmatic) 510.9
– with fistula 510.0
– accessory sinus (chronic) (see also
Sinusitis) 473.9
– acute 510.9
– – with fistula 510.0
– antrum (chronic) (see also Sinusitis,
maxillary) 473.0
– brain (any part) (see also Abscess, brain)
324.0
– ethmoidal (chronic) (sinus) (see also
Sinusitis, ethmoidal) 473.2
– extradural (see also Abscess, extradural)
324.9
– frontal (chronic) (sinus) (see also
Sinusitis, frontal) 473.1
– gallbladder (see also Cholecystitis, acute)
575.0

Empyema - *continued*
– mastoid (process) (acute) 383.0
– maxilla, maxillary 526.4
– – sinus (chronic) (see also Sinusitis,
maxillary) 473.0
– nasal sinus (chronic) (see also Sinusitis)
473.9
– sinus (see also Sinusitis) 473.9
– sphenoidal (sinus) (see also Sinusitis,
sphenoidal) 473.3
– subarachnoid (see also Abscess,
extradural) 324.9
– subdural (see also Abscess, extradural)
324.9
– tuberculous 012.0
– ureter (see also Ureteritis) 593.8
– ventricular (see also Abscess, brain)
324.0
Enameloma 520.2
Encephalitis (chronic) (hemorrhagic)
(idiopathic) (nonepidemic) (spurious)
(subacute) 323.9
– acute - see also Encephalitis, viral
– – disseminated (postinfectious) NEC
136.9 † 323.6*
– – – postimmunization or
postvaccination 323.5
– – inclusion body 049.8 † 323.4*
– – inclusional 049.8 † 323.4*
– – necrotizing 049.8 † 323.4*
– arboviral, arbovirus NEC 064 † 323.3*
– arthropod-borne NEC 064 † 323.3*
– Australian 062.4 † 323.3*
– California (virus) 062.5 † 323.3*
– Central European 063.2 † 323.3*
– Czechoslovakian 063.2 † 323.3*
– Dawson's (inclusion body) 046.2 † 323.1*
– due to
– – actinomycosis 039.8 † 323.4*
– – toxoplasmosis (acquired) 130 † 323.4*
– – – congenital (active) 771.2 † 323.4*
– endemic 049.8 † 323.4*
– epidemic 049.8 † 323.4*
– equine (acute) (infectious) (viral) 062.9 †
323.3*
– – Eastern 062.2 † 323.3*
– – Venezuelan 066.2 † 323.3*
– – Western 062.1 † 323.3*
– Far Eastern 063.0 † 323.3*
– following vaccination or other
immunization procedure 323.5
– herpes 054.3 † 323.4*
– Ilheus (virus) 062.8 † 323.3*
– infectious (acute) (virus) NEC 049.8 †
323.4*
– influenzal 487.8 † 323.4*
– – lethargic 049.8 † 323.4*

Encephalitis - *continued*
- Japanese (B type) 062.0 † 323.3*
- la Crosse 062.5 † 323.3*
- Langat 063.8 † 323.3*
- lead 984.- † 323.7*
- lethargic (acute) (infectious) (influenzal)
  049.8 † 323.4*
- louping ill 063.1 † 323.3*
- lupus 710.0
- lymphatica 049.0 † 321.6*
- Mengo 049.8 † 323.4*
- meningococcal 036.1 † 323.4*
- mumps 072.2 † 323.4*
- Murray Valley 062.4 † 323.3*
- myoclonic 049.8 † 323.4*
- Negishi virus 064 † 323.3*
- otitic NEC 382.4 † 323.4*
- parasitic NEC 123.9 † 323.4*
- periaxialis (concentrica) (diffuse) 341.1
- postchickenpox 052 † 323.6*
- postimmunization 323.5
- postinfectious NEC 136.9 † 323.6*
- postmeasles 055.0 † 323.6*
- postvaccinal 323.5
- postvaricella 052 † 323.6*
- postviral NEC 079.9 † 323.6*
- - postexanthematous 057.9 † 323.6*
- - - specified NEC 057.8 † 323.6*
- Powassan 063.8 † 323.3*
- Rio Bravo 049.8 † 323.4*
- rubella 056.0 † 323.4*
- Russian
- - autumnal 062.0 † 323.3*
- - spring-summer type (taiga) 063.0 †
  323.3*
- saturnine 984.- † 323.7*
- serous 048 † 323.4*
- St. Louis type 062.3 † 323.3*
- summer 062.0 † 323.3*
- suppurative 324.0
- syphilitic 094.8 † 323.4*
- - congenital 090.4 † 323.4*
- torula, torular 117.5 † 323.4*
- toxic NEC 989.9 † 323.7*
- toxoplasmic (acquired) 130 † 323.4*
- - congenital (active) 771.2 † 323.4*
- trichinosis 124 † 323.4*
- trypanosomiasis 086.- † 323.4*
- tuberculous 013.8 † 323.4*
- type
- - B 062.0 † 323.3*
- - C 062.3 † 323.3*
- Vienna type 049.8 † 323.4*
- viral, virus 049.9 † 323.4*
- - arthropod-borne NEC 064 † 323.3*
- - - vector unknown 064 † 323.3*
- - specified type NEC 049.8 † 323.4*

Encephalocele 742.0
Encephalomalacia (brain) (cerebellar)
  (cerebral) (see also Softening, brain) 434.9
Encephalomeningitis - see
  Meningo-encephalitis
Encephalomeningocele 742.0
Encephalomeningomyelitis - see
  Meningo-encephalitis
Encephalomeningopathy (see also
  Meningo-encephalitis) 349.9
Encephalomyelitis (chronic)
  (granulomatous) (hemorrhagic
  necrotizing, acute) (myalgic, benign) (see
  also Encephalitis) 323.9
- acute disseminated (postinfectious)
  136.9 † 323.6*
- - postimmunization 323.5
- due to or resulting from vaccination (any)
  323.5
- postchickenpox 052 † 323.6*
- postmeasles 055.0 † 323.6*
- postvaccinal 323.5
- rubella 056.0 † 323.4*
Encephalomyelocele 742.0
Encephalomyelomeningitis - see
  Meningo-encephalitis
Encephalomyeloneuropathy (see also
  Encephalomyelitis) 349.9
Encephalomyelopathy (see also
  Encephalomyelitis) 349.9
Encephalomyeloradiculoneuritis (acute)
  357.0
Encephalomyeloradiculopathy (see also
  Encephalomyelitis) 349.9
Encephalopathia hyperbilirubinemica,
  newborn 774.7
- due to isoimmunization (conditions in
  773.0-773.2) 773.4
Encephalopathy (acute) (toxic) 348.3
- anoxic - see Damage, brain, anoxic
- arteriosclerotic 437.0
- congenital 742.9
- demyelinating callosal 341.8
- due to
- - birth injury 767.8
- - hyperinsulinism - see Hyperinsulinism
- - influenza (virus) 487.8
- - lack of vitamin (see also Deficiency,
  vitamin) 269.2
- - serum (nontherapeutic) (therapeutic)
  999.5
- - syphilis 094.8 † 323.4*
- - trauma (postconcussional) 310.2
- - - current 850
- - - - with skull fracture - see Fracture,
  skull
- - vaccination 999.5

Encephalopathy - *continued*
- hepatic 572.2
- hyperbilirubinemic, newborn 774.7
- - due to isoimmunization (conditions in
    773.0-773.2) 773.4
- hypertensive 437.2
- hypoglycemic 251.2
- hypoxic - see Damage, brain, anoxic
- infantile cystic necrotizing (congenital)
    341.8
- lead 984.- † 323.7*
- leucopolio 330.0
- necrotizing, subacute 330.8
- pellagrous 265.2
- portosystemic 572.2
- postcontusional 310.2
- saturnine 984.- † 323.7*
- spongioform, subacute (viral) 046.1 †
    331.5*
- subcortical progressive (Schilder) 341.1
- traumatic (postconcussional) 310.2
- - current 850
- - - with skull fracture - see Fracture,
    skull
- vitamin B deficiency NEC 266.9
- Wernicke's 265.1
Encephalorrhagia (see also Hemorrhage,
  brain) 432.9
Enchondroma (M9220/0) - see Neoplasm,
  bone, benign
- multiple, congenital 756.4
Enchondromatosis (cartilaginous)
  (multiple) 756.4
Enchondroses multiple (cartilaginous)
  756.4
Encopresis (see also Incontinence, feces)
  787.6
- nonorganic origin 307.7
Encounter with health services for
  administrative purpose only V68.9
- specified reason NEC V68.8
Encystment - see Cyst
Endarteritis (bacterial, subacute) (infective)
  (septic) 447.6
- brain, cerebral or cerebrospinal 437.4
- deformans - see Arteriosclerosis
- embolic (see also Embolism) 444.9
- obliterans - see also Arteriosclerosis
- - pulmonary 417.8
- retina 362.1
- senile - see Arteriosclerosis
- syphilitic 093.8
- - brain or cerebral 094.8
- - congenital 090.5
- - spinal 094.8
- tuberculous 017.8
Endemic - see condition

Endocarditis (chronic) (indeterminate)
  (interstitial) (marantic) (nonbacterial
  thrombotic) (residual) (sclerotic) 424.9
  (sclerous) (senile) (valvular)
- with rheumatic fever (conditions in 390)
- - active - see Endocarditis, acute,
    rheumatic
- - inactive or quiescent (with chorea)
    397.9
- acute or subacute 421.9
- - rheumatic (aortic) (mitral)
    (pulmonary) (tricuspid) 391.1
- - - with chorea (acute) (rheumatic)
    (Sydenham's) 392.0
- aortic (heart) (nonrheumatic) (valve)
    424.1
- - with
- - - mitral disease 396
- - - - active or acute 391.1
- - - - - with chorea (acute)
      (rheumatic) (Sydenham's)
      392.0
- - - rheumatic fever (conditions in 390)
- - - - active - see Endocarditis, acute,
      rheumatic
- - - - inactive or quiescent (with
      chorea) 395.9
- - - - - with mitral disease 396
- - acute or subacute 421.9
- - arteriosclerotic 424.1
- - congenital 746.8
- - rheumatic 395.9
- - - with mitral disease 396
- - - - active or acute 391.1
- - - - - with chorea (acute)
      (rheumatic) (Sydenham's)
      392.0
- - - active or acute 391.1
- - - - with chorea (acute) (rheumatic)
      (Sydenham's) 392.0
- - specified cause NEC 424.1
- - syphilitic 093.2 † 424.1*
- arteriosclerotic 424.9
- atypical verrucous (Libman-Sacks)
    710.0 † 424.9*
- bacterial (acute) (any valve) (chronic)
    (subacute) 421.0
- candidal 112.8 † 421.1*
- congenital 425.3
- Coxsackie 074.2 † 421.1*
- due to prosthetic cardiac valve 996.6
- fetal 425.3
- gonococcal 098.8 † 421.1*
- infectious or infective (acute) (any valve)
    (chronic) (subacute) 421.0
- lenta (acute) (any valve) (chronic)
    (subacute) 421.0

Endocarditis - *continued*
- Libman-Sacks 710.0 † 424.9*
- Loeffler's 421.0
- malignant (acute) (any valve) (chronic) (subacute) 421.0
- meningococcal 036.4 † 421.1*

- mitral (chronic) (double) (fibroid) (heart) (inactive) (valve) (with chorea) 394.9
- - with
- - - aortic valve disease 396
- - - - active or acute 391.1
- - - - - with chorea (acute) (rheumatic) (Sydenham's) 392.0
- - - rheumatic fever (conditions in 390)
- - - - active - see Endocarditis, acute, rheumatic
- - - - inactive or quiescent (with chorea) 394.9
- - - - - with aortic valve disease 396
- - active or acute 391.1
- - - with chorea (acute) (rheumatic) (Sydenham's) 392.0
- - arteriosclerotic 424.0
- - congenital 746.8
- - nonrheumatic 424.0
- - - acute or subacute 421.9
- monilial 112.8 † 421.1*
- mycotic (acute) (any valve) (chronic) (subacute) 421.0
- pneumococcic (acute) (any valve) (chronic) (subacute) 421.0

- pulmonary (chronic) (heart) (valve) 424.3
- - with rheumatic fever (conditions in 390)
- - - active - see Endocarditis, acute, rheumatic
- - - inactive or quiescent (with chorea) 397.1
- - acute or subacute 421.9
- - - rheumatic 391.1
- - - - with chorea (acute) (rheumatic) (Sydenham's) 392.0
- - arteriosclerotic 424.3
- - congenital 746.0
- - rheumatic (chronic) (inactive) (with chorea) 397.1
- - - active or acute 391.1
- - - - with chorea (acute) (rheumatic) (Sydenham's) 392.0
- - syphilitic 093.2 † 424.3*
- purulent (acute) (any valve) (chronic) (subacute) 421.0
- rheumatic (chronic) (inactive) (with chorea) 397.9

Endocarditis - *continued*
- rheumatic - *continued*
- - active or acute (aortic) (mitral) (pulmonary) (tricuspid) 391.1
- - - with chorea (acute) (rheumatic) (Sydenham's) 392.0
- septic (acute) (any valve) (chronic) (subacute) 421.0
- streptococcal (acute) (any valve) (chronic) (subacute) 421.0
- subacute - see Endocarditis, acute
- suppurative (acute) (any valve) (chronic) (subacute) 421.0
- syphilitic NEC 093.2 † 424.9*
- toxic (see also Endocarditis, acute) 421.9
- tricuspid (chronic) (heart) (inactive) (rheumatic) (valve) (with chorea) 397.0
- - with rheumatic fever (conditions in 390)
- - - active - see Endocarditis, acute, rheumatic
- - - inactive or quiescent (with chorea) 397.0
- - active or acute 391.1
- - - with chorea (acute) (rheumatic) (Sydenham's) 392.0
- - arteriosclerotic 424.2
- - congenital 746.8
- - nonrheumatic 424.2
- - - acute or subacute 421.9
- - specified cause, except rheumatic 424.2
- tuberculous (see also Tuberculosis, endocarditis) 017.8 † 424.9*
- typhoid 002.0 † 421.1*
- ulcerative (acute) (any valve) (chronic) (subacute) 421.0
- vegetative (acute) (any valve) (chronic) (subacute) 421.0
- verrucous (acute) (any valve) (chronic) (subacute) NEC 710.0 † 424.9*
- - nonbacterial 710.0 † 424.9*
- - nonrheumatic 710.0 † 424.9*
Endocardium, endocardial - see also condition
- cushion defect 745.6
Endocervicitis (see also Cervicitis) 616.0
- due to
- - intrauterine (contraceptive) device 996.6
- hyperplastic 616.0
Endocrine - see condition
Endocrinopathy, pluriglandular 258.9
Endodontitis 522.0
Endomastoiditis 383.9
Endometrioma 617.9
Endometriosis 617.9

Endometriosis - *continued*
- fallopian tube 617.2
- in scar or skin 617.6
- intestine 617.5
- ovary 617.1
- pelvic peritoneum 617.3
- rectovaginal septum 617.4
- specified site NEC 617.8
- stromal (M8931/1) 236.0
- uterus 617.0
- vagina 617.4
Endometritis (nonspecific) (purulent) (septic) (suppurative) 615.9
- with
- - abortion - see categories 634-639, fourth digit .0
- - ectopic gestation 639.0
- acute 615.0
- blenorrhagic 098.1 † 615.9*
- - acute 098.1 † 615.0*
- - chronic or duration of 2 months or over 098.3 † 615.1*
- cervix, cervical (see also Cervicitis) 616.0
- - hyperplastic 616.0
- chronic 615.1
- complicating pregnancy 646.6
- - fetus or newborn 760.8
- gonorrheal 098.1 † 615.9*
- - acute 098.1 † 615.0*
- - chronic or duration of 2 months or over 098.3 † 615.1*
- hyperplastic 621.3
- - cervix 616.0
- polypoid - see Endometritis, hyperplastic
- puerperal, postpartum, childbirth 670
- senile (atrophic) 615.9
- subacute 615.0
- tuberculous 016.4
Endometrium - see condition
Endomyocarditis - see Endocarditis
Endomyofibrosis 425.0
Endomyometritis (see also Endometritis) 615.9
Endopericarditis - see Endocarditis
Endoperineuritis - see Disorder, nerve
Endophlebitis (see also Phlebitis) 451.9
Endophthalmia 360.0
- gonorrheal 098.4 † 360.0*
Endophthalmitis (acute) (infective) (metastatic) (purulent) (subacute) 360.0
- parasitic 360.1
- purulent 360.0
- sympathetic 360.1
Endosalpingioma (M9111/1) 236.2
Endosteitis - see Osteomyelitis
Endothelioma, bone (M9260/3) - see Neoplasm, bone, malignant

Endotheliosis 287.8
- hemorrhagic infectional 287.8
Endotrachelitis (see also Cervicitis) 616.0
Enema rash 692.8
Engelmann's disease 756.5
Engman's disease 690
Engorgement
- breast 611.7
- - newborn 778.7
- - puerperal, postpartum 676.2
- lung 514
- pulmonary 514
- stomach 536.8
- venous, retina 362.3
Enlargement, enlarged - see also Hypertrophy
- adenoids (and tonsils) 474.1
- alveolar ridge 525.8
- apertures of diaphragm (congenital) 756.6
- blind spot, visual field 368.4
- gingival 523.8
- heart, cardiac (see also Hypertrophy, cardiac) 429.3
- lacrimal gland, chronic 375.0
- liver (see also Hypertrophy, liver) 789.1
- lymph gland or node 785.6
- organ or site, congenital NEC - see Anomaly, specified type NEC
- parathyroid (gland) 252.0
- prostate, simple 600
- spleen - see Splenomegaly
- thymus (gland) (congenital) 254.0
- thyroid (gland) (see also Goiter) 240.9
- tongue 529.8
- tonsils (and adenoids) 474.1
- uterus 621.2
Enophthalmos 376.5
Entamebiasis - see Amebiasis
Entamebic - see Amebiasis
Entanglement
- umbilical cord(s) 663.3
- - with compression 663.2
- - affecting fetus or newborn 762.5
- - around neck (with compression) 663.1
- - of twins in monoamniotic sac 663.2
Enteralgia 789.0
Enteric - see condition
Enteritis (acute) (choleraic) (congestive) (diarrheal) (epidemic) (exudative) (follicular) (hemorrhagic) (infantile) (lienteric) (perforative) (presumed infectious) (pseudomembranous) (zymotic) (see also Note at category 009.3) 009.1Note at category 009.3) 009.3
- adaptive 564.1
- aertrycke infection 003.0

Enteropathy - *continued*
- gluten 579.0
- hemorrhagic, terminal 557.0
- protein-losing 579.8
Enteroperitonitis (see also Peritonitis)
  567.9
Enteroptosis 569.8
Enterorrhagia 578.9
Enterospasm 564.1
- psychogenic 306.4
Enterostenosis (see also Obstruction,
  intestine) 560.9
Enthesopathy 726.9
- ankle and tarsus 726.7
- elbow region 726.3
- hip 726.5
- knee 726.6
- peripheral NEC 726.8
- shoulder region 726.1
- - adhesive 726.0
- spinal 720.1
- wrist and carpus 726.4
Entrance, air into vein - see Embolism, air
Entrapment, nerve - see Neuropathy,
  entrapment
Entropion (cicatricial) (eyelid) (paralytic)
  (senile) (spastic) 374.0
- congenital 743.6
Enucleated eye
- traumatic, current 871.3
Enuresis 788.3
- habit disturbance 307.6
- nocturnal 788.3
- - psychogenic 307.6
- nonorganic origin 307.6
- psychogenic 307.6
Eosinophilia 288.3
- allergic 288.3
- hereditary 288.3
- pulmonary 518.3
- tropical 518.3
Ependymitis (acute) (cerebral) (chronic)
  (granular) (see also Meningitis) 322.9
Ependymoblastoma (M9392/3)
- specified site - see Neoplasm, malignant
- unspecified site 191.9
Ependymoma (epithelial) (malignant)
  (M9391/3)
- anaplastic type (M9392/3)
- - specified site - see Neoplasm,
    malignant
- - unspecified site 191.9
- benign (M9391/0)
- - specified site - see Neoplasm, benign
- - unspecified site 225.0
- myxopapillary (M9394/1) 237.5
- papillary (M9393/1) 237.5

Ependymoma - *continued*
- specified site - see Neoplasm, malignant
- unspecified site 191.9
Ependymopathy 349.2
Ephelides, ephelis 709.0
Epiblepharon (congenital) 743.6
Epicanthus, epicanthic fold (eyelid)
  (congenital) 743.6
Epicondylitis (elbow) 726.3
Epicystitis (see also Cystitis) 595.9
Epidemic - see condition
Epidermidalization, cervix 622.1
Epidermis, epidermal - see condition
Epidermodysplasia verruciformis 078.1
Epidermolysis
- bullosa 757.3
- necroticans combustiformis 695.1
- - due to drug
- - - correct substance properly
    administered 695.1
- - - overdose or wrong substance given
    or taken 977.9
- - - - specified drug - see Table of drugs
    and chemicals
Epidermophytid - see Dermatophytosis
Epidermophytosis (infected) - see
  Dermatophytosis
Epididymis - see condition
Epididymitis (acute) (nonvenereal)
  (recurrent) (residual) 604.9
- with abscess 604.0
- blennorrhagic 098.0
- - chronic or duration of 2 months or over
    098.2
- caseous 016.2 † 604.9*
- gonococcal 098.0
- - chronic or duration of 2 months or over
    098.2
- syphilitic 095
- tuberculous 016.2 † 604.9*
Epididymo-orchitis (see also Epididymitis)
  604.9
- with abscess 604.0
Epidural - see condition
Epigastritis (see also Gastritis) 535.5
Epigastrium, epigastric - see condition
Epigastrocele - see Hernia, ventral
Epiglottiditis (acute) 464.3
- chronic 476.1
Epiglottis - see condition
Epiglottitis (acute) 464.3
- chronic 476.1
Epignathus 759.4
Epilepsia
- partialis continua 345.7
- procursiva 345.8
Epilepsy, epileptic (idiopathic) 345.9

Epilepsy - *continued*
- abdominal 345.5
- absence 345.0
- akinetic 345.0
- automatism 345.4
- Bravais-jacksonian 345.5
- cerebral 345.9
- climacteric 345.9
- clonic 345.1
- clouded state 345.9
- coma 345.3
- communicating 345.4
- convulsions 345.9
- cortical (focal) (motor) 345.5
- cysticercosis 123.1
- deterioration 294.1
- due to syphilis 094.8
- equivalent 345.5
- fit 345.9
- focal (motor) 345.5
- generalized 345.9
- - convulsive 345.1
- - flexion 345.1
- - nonconvulsive 345.0
- grand mal 345.1
- jacksonian (motor) (sensory) 345.5
- Kojevnikov's 345.7
- Kojewnikoff's 345.7
- limbic system 345.4
- major 345.1
- minor 345.0
- mixed (type) 345.9
- motor partial 345.5
- musicogenic 345.1
- myoclonus, myoclonic 345.1
- - progressive (familial) 333.2
- parasitic NEC 123.9
- partial (focalized) 345.5
- - with
- - - impairment of consciousness 345.4
- - - memory and ideational disturbances 345.4
- - secondarily generalized 345.4
- peripheral 345.9
- petit mal 345.0
- progressive (familial) myoclonic 333.2
- psychomotor 345.4
- psychosensory 345.4
- reflex 345.1
- senile 345.9
- somatomotor 345.5
- somatosensory 345.5
- specified type NEC 345.8
- status (grand mal) 345.3
- - focal motor 345.7
- - petit mal 345.2
- - psychomotor 345.7

Epilepsy - *continued*
- status - *continued*
- - temporal lobe 345.7
- symptomatic 345.9
- temporal lobe 345.4
- tonic(-clonic) 345.1
- traumatic (injury unspecified) 907.0
- - injury specified - code to late effect of specified injury
- twilight 293.0
- uncinate (gyrus) 345.4
- Unverricht(-Lundborg) (familial myoclonic) 333.2
- visceral 345.5
- visual 345.5
Epiloia 759.5
Epimenorrhea 626.2
Epipharyngitis (see also Nasopharyngitis) 460
Epiphora 375.2
Epiphyseolysis, epiphysiolysis (see also Osteochondrosis) 732.9
Epiphysitis (see also Osteochondrosis) 732.9
- juvenile 732.6
- syphilitic (congenital) 090.0
- vertebral 732.0
Epiplocele (see also Hernia) 553.9
Epiploitis (see also Peritonitis) 567.9
Epiplosarcomphalocele - see Hernia, umbilicus
Episcleritis 379.0
- gouty 274.8 † 379.0*
- periodica fugax 379.0
- - angioneurotic - see Edema, angioneurotic
- suppurative 379.0
- syphilitic 095 † 379.0*
- tuberculous 017.3 † 379.0*
Episode
- brain (see also Disease, cerebrovascular, acute) 436
- cerebral (see also Disease, cerebrovascular, acute) 436
- depersonalization (in neurotic state) 300.6
- psychotic (see also Psychosis) 298.9
- - organic, transient 293.9
- schizophrenic (acute) NEC 295.4
Epispadias
- female 753.8
- male 752.6
Episplenitis 289.5
Epistaxis (multiple) 784.7
- vicarious menstruation 626.8
Epithelioma (malignant) (M8011/3) - see also Neoplasm, malignant

Epithelioma - *continued*
- adenoides cysticum (M8100/0) - see Neoplasm, skin, benign
- basal cell (M8090/3) - see Neoplasm, skin, malignant
- benign (M8011/0) - see Neoplasm, benign
- Bowen's (M8081/2) - see Neoplasm, skin, in situ
- calcifying (benign) (Malherbe) (M8110/0) - see Neoplasm, skin, benign
- external site - see Neoplasm, skin, malignant
- intraepidermal, Jadassohn (M8096/0) - see Neoplasm, skin, benign
- squamous cell (M8070/3) - see Neoplasm, malignant
Epithelium, epithelial - see condition
Epituberculosis (with atelectasis) (allergic) 010.8
Eponychia 757.5
Epstein's
- nephrosis or syndrome (see also Nephrosis) 581.9
- pearl 528.4
Epulis (gingiva) (giant cell) 523.8
Equinia 024
Equinovarus (congenital) 754.5
- acquired 736.7
Equivalent
- convulsive (abdominal) 345.5
- epileptic (psychic) 345.5
Erb(-Duchenne) paralysis (birth injury) (newborn) 767.6
Erb's
- disease 359.1
- palsy, paralysis (brachial) (birth) (newborn) 767.6
- - spinal (spastic) syphilitic 094.8
- pseudohypertrophic muscular dystrophy 359.1
Erb-Goldflam disease or syndrome 358.0
Erection, painful (persistent) 607.3
Ergosterol deficiency (vitamin D) 268.9
- with
- - osteomalacia 268.2
- - rickets (see also Rickets) 268.0
Ergotism 988.2
- from ergot used as drug (migraine therapy)
- - correct substance properly administered 349.8
- - overdose or wrong substance given or taken 975.0
Erichsen's disease 300.1
Erosio interdigitalis blastomycetica 112.3
Erosion

Erosion - *continued*
- artery 447.2
- bone 733.9
- bronchus 519.1
- cartilage (joint) 733.9
- cervix (uteri) (acquired) (chronic) (congenital) 622.0
- - with mention of cervicitis 616.0
- cornea (recurrent) (see also Keratitis) 371.4
- - traumatic 918.1
- dental (idiopathic) (occupational) 521.3
- duodenum, postpyloric - see Ulcer, duodenum
- esophagus 530.8
- gastric - see Ulcer, stomach
- intestine 569.8
- lymphatic vessel 457.8
- oesophagus 530.8
- pylorus, pyloric (ulcer) - see Ulcer, stomach
- spine, aneurysmal 094.8
- spleen 289.5
- stomach - see Ulcer, stomach
- teeth (idiopathic) (occupational) 521.3
- - due to
- - - medicine 521.3
- - - persistent vomiting 521.3
- urethra 599.8
- uterus 621.8
- vertebra 733.9
Erotomania 302.8
Error, refractive 367.9
Eructation 787.3
- nervous 306.4
- psychogenic 306.4
Eruption
- creeping 126.9
- drug - see Dermatitis, due to drug
- Hutchinson, summer 692.7
- Kaposi varicelliform 054.0
- napkin (psoriasiform) 691.0
- polymorphous
- - light (sun) 692.7
- - - other 692.8
- ringed 695.8
- skin (see also Dermatitis) 782.1
- - creeping (meaning hookworm) 126.9
- - due to
- - - prophylactic inoculation or vaccination against disease - see Dermatitis, due to vaccine
- - - smallpox vaccination NEC - see Dermatitis, due to vaccine
- - erysipeloid 027.1
- - feigned 698.4
- - Kaposi's varicelliform 054.0

Eruption - *continued*
- skin - *continued*
- - lichenoid, axilla 698.3
- - toxic NEC 695.0
- tooth, teeth
- - accelerated 520.6
- - delayed 520.6
- - disturbance of 520.6
- - in abnormal sequence 520.6
- - incomplete 520.6
- - late 520.6
- - partial 520.6
- - premature 520.6
- vesicular 709.8
Erysipelas (gangrenous) (infantile) (newborn) (phlegmonous) (suppurative) 035
- external ear 035 † 380.1*
- puerperal, postpartum, childbirth 670
Erysipelatoid (Rosenbach's) 027.1
Erysipeloid (Rosenbach's) 027.1
Erythema, erythematous (infectional) 695.9
- ab igne - code by site under Burn 949.1
- annulare (centrifugum) (rheumaticum) 695.0
- arthriticum epidemicum 026.1
- brucellum (see also Brucellosis) 023.9
- due to
- - chemical (contact) NEC 692.4
- - - internal 693.8
- - drug (internal use) 693.0
- - - contact 692.3
- elevatum diutinum 695.8
- endemic 265.2
- epidemic, arthritic 026.1
- figuratum perstans 695.0
- gluteal 691.0
- heat - code by site under Burn 949.1
- ichthyosiforme congenitum 757.1
- induratum (primary) (scrofulosorum) 017.1
- - nontuberculous 695.2
- infectiosum 057.0
- inflammation NEC 695.9
- intertrigo 695.8
- iris 695.1
- lupus (local) (see also Lupus) 695.4
- marginatum 695.0
- medicamentosum - see Dermatitis, due to drug
- migrans 529.1
- multiforme 695.1
- - bullosum 695.1
- - conjunctiva 695.1
- - exudativum (hebra) 695.1
- - pemphigoides 694.5
- napkin 691.0

Erythema - *continued*
- neonatorum 778.8
- nodosum 695.2
- - tuberculous 017.1
- palmar 695.0
- pernio 991.5
- rash, newborn 778.8
- scarlatiniform (recurrent) (exfoliative) 695.0
- solare 692.7
- streptogenes 696.5
- toxic, toxicum NEC 695.0
- - newborn 778.8
- tuberculous (primary) 017.0
Erythematosus - see condition
Erythematous - see condition
Erythermalgia (primary) 443.8
Erythralgia 443.8
Erythrasma 039.0
Erythredema 985.0
- polyneuritica 985.0
- polyneuropathy 985.0
Erythremia (acute) (M9841/3) 207.0
- chronic (M9842/3) 207.1
- secondary 289.0
Erythroblastopenia 284.8
Erythroblastosis (fetalis) (newborn) 773.2
- due to
- - ABO
- - - antibodies 773.1
- - - incompatibility, maternal/fetal 773.1
- - - isoimmunization 773.1
- - Rh
- - - antibodies 773.0
- - - incompatibility, maternal/fetal 773.0
- - - isoimmunization 773.0
Erythrocyanosis (crurum) 443.8
Erythrocythemia - see Erythremia
Erythrocytosis (megalosplenic)
- familial 289.6
- oval, hereditary (see also Elliptocytosis) 282.1
Erythroderma (see also Erythema) 695.9
- desquamativum 695.8
- exfoliative 695.8
- ichthyosiform, congenital 757.1
- neonatorum 778.8
- psoriaticum 696.1
- secondary 695.9
Erythrogenesis imperfecta 284.0
Erythroleukemia (M9840/3) 207.0
Erythromelalgia 443.8
Erythrophagocytosis 289.9
Erythrophobia 300.2
Erythroplakia

Erythroplakia - *continued*
– oral mucosa 528.7
Erythroplasia (Queyrat) (M8080/2)
– specified site - see Neoplasm, skin, in situ
– unspecified site 233.5
Eso-enteritis - see Enteritis
Esophagectasis 530.8
Esophagismus 530.5
Esophagitis (acute) (alkaline) (chemical)
  (chronic) (infectional) (necrotic) (peptic)
  (postoperative) (reflux) 530.1
– tuberculous 017.8 † 530.1*
Esophagomalacia 530.8
Esophagostomiasis 127.7
Esophagotracheal - see condition
Esophagus - see condition
Esophoria 378.4
– convergence, excess 378.8
– divergence, insufficiency 378.8
Esotropia (alternating) (monocular) 378.0
– intermittent 378.2
Espundia 085.5
Essential - see condition
Esthesioneuroblastoma (M9522/3) 160.0
Esthesioneurocytoma (M9521/3) 160.0
Esthesioneuroepithelioma (M9523/3)
  160.0
Esthiomene 099.1
Estivo-autumnal
– fever 084.0
– malaria 084.0
Estrangement V61.0
Estriasis 134.0
Ethanolaminuria 270.8
Ethanolism (see also Alcoholism) 303
Etherism 304.6
Ethmoid, ethmoidal - see condition
Ethmoiditis (chronic) (purulent)
  (nonpurulent) (see also Sinusitis,
  ethmoidal) 473.2
– influenzal 487.1
– Woakes 471.1
Ethylism (see also Alcoholism) 303
Eulenburg's disease 359.2
Eunuchism 257.2
Eunuchoidism 257.2
– hypogonatropic 257.2
European blastomycosis 117.5
Eustachian - see condition
Euthyroidism 244.9
Evaluation for suspected condition (see also
  Observation) V71.9
– specified condition NEC V71.8
Eventration
– colon into chest - see Hernia, diaphragm
– diaphragm (congenital) 756.6
Eversion

Eversion - *continued*
– bladder 596.8
– cervix (uteri) 622.0
– – with mention of cervicitis 616.0
– foot NEC 736.7
– – congenital 755.6
– punctum lacrimale (postinfectional)
  (senile) 375.5
– ureter (meatus) 593.8
– urethra (meatus) 599.8
– uterus 618.1
Evisceration
– birth injury 767.8
– bowel (congenital) - see Hernia,
  abdomen
– congenital (see also Hernia, abdomen)
  553.2
– operative wound 998.3
– traumatic NEC 869.1
– – eye 871.3
Evulsion - see Avulsion
Ewing's
– angioendothelioma (M9260/3) - see
  Neoplasm, bone, malignant
– sarcoma (M9260/3) - see Neoplasm,
  bone, malignant
– tumor (M9260/3) - see Neoplasm, bone,
  malignant
Exaggerated lumbosacral angle (with
  impinging spine) 756.1
Examination (general) (routine) (of) (for)
  V70.0
– allergy V72.7
– cervical papanicolaou smear V76.2
– dental V72.2
– ear V72.1
– eye V72.0
– following
– – accident (motor vehicle) V71.4
– – inflicted injury (victim or culprit) NEC
  V71.6
– – rape or seduction, alleged (victim or
  culprit) V71.5
– – treatment (for) V67.9
– – – combined V67.6
– – – fracture V67.4
– – – mental disorder V67.3
– – – specified condition NEC V67.5
– follow-up (routine) (following) V67.9
– – chemotherapy V67.2
– – postpartum V24.2
– – psychotherapy V67.3
– – radiotherapy V67.1
– – surgery V67.0
– gynecological V72.3
– – for contraceptive maintenance V25.4
– health - see Examination, medical

Excess - *continued*
- secretion - *continued*
- − sweat 780.8
- short
- − organ or site, congenital NEC - see Anomaly, specified type NEC
- − umbilical cord
- − − affecting fetus or newborn 762.6
- − − in pregnancy or childbirth 663.4
- skin, eyelid 743.6
- − acquired 374.3
- sodium 276.0
- sputum 786.4
- sweating 780.8
- thirst 783.5
- − due to deprivation of water 994.3
- vitamin
- − A (dietary) 278.2
- − − administered as drug (chronic) (prolonged excessive intake) 278.2
- − − − reaction to sudden overdose 963.5
- − D (dietary) 278.4
- − − administered as drug (chronic) (prolonged excessive intake) 278.4
- − − − reaction to sudden overdose 963.5
Excitability, abnormal, under minor stress 309.2
Excitation
- catatonic 295.2
- psychogenic 298.1
- reactive (from emotional stress, psychological trauma) 298.1
Excitement
- manic 296.0
- mental
- − reactive (from emotional stress, psychological trauma) 298.1
- state
- − reactive (from emotional stress, psychological trauma) 298.1
Excoriation (traumatic) (see also Injury, superficial) 919.-
- neurotic 698.4
Excyclophoria 378.4
Excyclotropia 378.3
Exencephalus 742.0
Exercise
- breathing V57.0
- remedial NEC V57.1
- therapeutic NEC V57.1
Exfoliation, teeth due to systemic causes 525.0
Exfoliative - see condition
Exhaustion, exhaustive (physical NEC) 780.7

Exhaustion - *continued*
- battle (see also Reaction, stress, acute) 308.9
- cardiac (see also Failure, heart) 428.9
- delirium (see also Reaction, stress, acute) 308.9
- due to
- − cold 991.8
- − excessive exertion 994.5
- − exposure 994.4
- fetus or newborn 779.8
- heart (see also Failure, heart) 428.9
- heat - see Heat, exhaustion
- manic 296.0
- maternal, complicating delivery 669.8
- − affecting fetus or newborn 763.8
- mental 300.5
- myocardium, myocardial (see also Failure, heart) 428.9
- nervous 300.5
- old age 797
- postinfectional NEC 780.7
- psychogenic 300.5
- psychosis (see also Reaction, stress, acute) 308.9
- senile 797
- − dementia 290.0
Exhibitionism 302.4
Exomphalos 756.7
- meaning hernia - see Hernia, umbilicus
Exophoria 378.4
- convergence, insufficiency 378.8
- divergence, excess 378.8
Exophthalmos 376.3
- congenital 743.6
- hyperthyroidism 242.0
- intermittent NEC 376.3
- malignant 242.0
- pulsating 376.3
- − endocrine NEC 259.9 † 376.2*
- − thyrotoxic 242.- † 376.2*
- thyroid 242.0
Exostosis 726.9
- cartilaginous (M9210/0) - see Neoplasm, bone, benign
- congenital 756.4
- external ear canal 380.8
- gonococcal 098.8
- jaw (bone) 526.8
- multiple (cancellous) (hereditary) 756.4
- orbit 376.4
- osteocartilaginous (M9210/0) - see Neoplasm, bone, benign
- syphilitic 095 † 730.8*
Exotropia (alternating) (monocular) 378.1
- intermittent 378.2
Explanation of

F

F U O (see also Pyrexia) 780.6
Faber's syndrome 280
Fabry's disease 272.7
Face, facial - see condition
Facet of cornea 371.4
Faciocephalalgia, autonomic (see also
  Neuropathy, peripheral, autonomic) 337.9
Factor, psychic, associated with diseases
  classified elsewhere 316
Failure, failed
– attempted abortion (legal) 638.-
– cardiac (see also Failure, heart) 428.9
– cardiorenal (chronic) 428.9
– – hypertensive 404.9
– cardiorespiratory (see also Failure, heart)
  799.1
– – specified during or due to a procedure
  997.1
– – – long-term effect of cardiac surgery
  429.4
– cardiovascular (chronic) (see also Failure,
  heart) 428.9
– cerebrovascular 437.8
– cervical dilatation in labor 661.0
– – fetus or newborn 763.7
– circulation, circulatory (peripheral) 785.5
– – fetus or newborn 779.8
– compensation - see Disease, heart
– congestive (see also Failure, heart,
  congestive) 428.0
– coronary (see also Insufficiency,
  coronary) 411
– descent of head (at term) 652.5
– – fetus or newborn 763.1
– – in labor 660.1
– engagement of head NEC 652.5
– – in labor 660.1
– fetal head to enter pelvic brim 652.5
– – in labor 660.1
– – – fetus or newborn 763.1
– forceps NEC 660.7
– – fetus or newborn 763.1
– heart (acute) (sudden) 428.9
– – with
– – – acute pulmonary edema - see
  Failure, ventricular, left
– – – decompensation (see also Failure,
  heart, congestive) 428.0
– – – dilatation - see Disease, heart
– – arteriosclerotic 440.9

Failure - *continued*
– heart - *continued*
– – complicating
– – – abortion - see categories 630-639,
  fourth digit .8
– – – delivery (cesarean) (instrumental)
  669.4
– – – ectopic or molar pregnancy 639.8
– – – obstetric anesthesia or sedation
  668.1
– – – surgery 997.1
– – congestive 428.0
– – – with
– – – – rheumatic fever (conditions in
  390)
– – – – – active 391.8
– – – – – inactive or quiescent (with
  chorea) 398.9
– – – fetus or newborn 779.8
– – – hypertensive (see also
  Hypertension, heart) 402.9
– – – rheumatic (chronic) (inactive) (with
  chorea) 398.9
– – – – active or acute 391.8
– – – – – with chorea 392.0
– – degenerative (see also Degeneration,
  myocardial) 429.1
– – due to presence of (cardiac) prosthesis
  429.4
– – fetus or newborn 779.8
– – high output - see Disease, heart
– – hypertensive (see also Hypertension,
  heart) 402.9
– – left (ventricular) (see also Failure,
  ventricular, left) 428.1
– – organic - see Disease, heart
– – postoperative (immediate) 997.1
– – – long term effect of cardiac surgery
  429.4
– – rheumatic (chronic) (inactive) 398.9
– – right (ventricular) (secondary to left
  heart failure, conditions in 428.1) (see
  also Failure, heart, congestive) 428.0
– – senile 797
– – specified during or due to a procedure
  997.1
– – – long term effect of cardiac surgery
  429.4
– – thyrotoxic (see also Thyrotoxicosis)
  242.9 † 425.7*

Falling, any organ or part - see Prolapse
Fallopian
- insufflation V26.2
- tube - see condition
Fallot's tetrad or tetralogy 745.2
Fallout, radioactive (adverse effect) NEC
  990
False - see also condition
- joint 733.8
- labor (pains) 644.0
- opening, urinary 752.8
- passage, urethra (prostatic) 599.4
- positive
- - serological test for syphilis 795.6
- - Wasserman reaction 795.6
- pregnancy 300.1
Family, familial - see also condition
- disruption V61.0
- planning advice V25.0
- problem V61.9
- - specified NEC V61.8
Famine 994.2
- edema 262
Fanconi(-de Toni)(-Debre) syndrome
  270.0
Fanconi's anemia 284.0
Farcin 024
Farcy 024
Farmers'
- lung 495.0
- skin 692.7
Farsightedness 367.0
Fascia - see condition
Fasciculation 781.0
Fasciculitis optica 377.3
Fasciitis 729.4
- nodular 728.7
- perirenal 593.4
- plantar 728.7
- traumatic (old) 728.7
- - current - code by site under Sprain,
    strain
Fascioliasis 121.3
Fasciolopsiasis 121.4
Fasciolopsis, small intestine 121.4
Fat
- excessive 278.0
- - in heart (see also Degeneration,
    myocardial) 429.1
- general 278.0
- in stool 792.1
- localized (pad) 278.1
- - heart (see also Degeneration,
    myocardial) 429.1
- - knee 729.3
- - retropatellar 729.3
- pad 278.1

Fatal syncope 798.1
Fatigue 780.7
- combat (see also Reaction, stress, acute)
  308.9
- during pregnancy 646.8
- heat (transient) 992.6
- muscle 729.8
- myocardium (see also Failure, heart)
  428.9
- nervous 300.5
- neurosis 300.5
- operational 300.8
- posture 729.8
- psychogenic (general) 300.5
- senile 797
- syndrome 300.5
- voice 784.4
Fatness 278.0
Fatty - see also condition
- apron 278.1
- degeneration - see Degeneration, fatty
- heart (enlarged) (see also Degeneration,
  myocardial) 429.1
- liver 571.8
- - alcoholic 571.0
- necrosis - see Degeneration, fatty
Fauces - see condition
Faucitis 478.2
Faulty - see also condition
- position of teeth 524.3
Favism 282.2
- anemia 282.2
Favus 110.9
- beard 110.0
- capitis 110.0
- corporis 110.5
- eyelid 110.8
- foot 110.4
- hand 110.2
- scalp 110.0
- specified site NEC 110.8
Fear
- complex 300.2
- reaction 300.2
Feared complaint unfounded V65.5
Febricula (continued) (simple) (see also
  Pyrexia) 780.6
Febrile (see also Pyrexia) 780.6
Febris (see also Fever) 780.6
- aestiva - see Fever, hay
- flava (see also Fever, yellow) 060.9
- melitensis 023.0
- pestis (see also Plague) 020.9
- puerperalis 670
- recurrens (see also Fever, relapsing)
  087.9
- - pediculo vestimenti, causa 087.0

Febris - *continued*
- rubra 034.1
- typhoidea 002.0
- typhosa 002.0
Fecal - see condition
Fecalith (impaction) 560.3
- appendix 543
- congenital 777.1
Feeble rapid pulse due to shock following
   injury 958.4
Feeble-minded 317
Feeding
- faulty 783.3
- improper 783.3
- problem (elderly) 783.3
- - infant 783.3
- - nonorganic 307.5
Feer's disease 985.0
Feet - see condition
Feigned illness V65.2
Feil-Klippel syndrome 756.1
Feinmesser's (hidrotic) ectodermal
   dysplasia 757.3
Felix's disease 732.1
Felon (with lymphangitis) 681.0
Felty's syndrome 714.1
Feminization, testicular 257.8
Femur, femoral - see condition
Fenestration, fenestrated - see also
   Imperfect, closure
- aorta-pulmonary 745.0
- aorticopulmonary 745.0
- cusps, heart valve NEC 746.8
- - pulmonary 746.0
- hymen 752.4
- pulmonic cusps 746.0
Fermentation (gastric) (gastrointestinal)
   (stomach) 536.8
- intestine 564.8
Fetalis uterus 752.3
Fetid
- breath 784.9
- sweat 705.8
Fetishism 302.8
Fetus, fetal - see also condition
- type lung tissue 770.4
Fever 780.6
- with chills 780.6
- - in malarial regions 084.6
- abortus NEC 023.9
- Aden 061
- African tick-borne 087.1
- American
- - mountain tick 066.1
- - spotted 082.0
- and ague (see also Malaria) 084.6
- aphthous 078.4

Fever - *continued*
- arbovirus hemorrhagic 065.9
- Assam 085.0
- Australian A or Q 083.0
- Bangkok hemorrhagic 065.4
- bilious, hemoglobinuric 084.8
- blackwater 084.8
- blister 054.9
- boutonneuse 082.1
- brain 323.9
- breakbone 061
- Bullis 082.8
- Bunyamwera 066.3
- Burdwan 085.0
- Bwamba 066.3
- Cameroon (see also Malaria) 084.6
- Canton 081.9
- cat scratch 078.3
- cerebral 323.9
- cerebrospinal (meningococcal) (see also
   Meningitis) 036.0 † 320.5*
- Chagres 084.0
- Chandipura 066.8
- Changuinola 066.0
- Charcot's (biliary) (hepatic)
   (intermittent) (see also
   Choledocholithiasis) 574.5
- Chikungunya (viral) 066.3
- - hemorrhagic 065.4
- childbed 670
- Chitral 066.0
- Colombo 002.9
- Colorado tick (virus) 066.1
- congestive
- - malarial (see also Malaria) 084.6
- - remittent (see also Malaria) 084.6
- Congo virus 065.0
- continued malarial 084.0
- Corsican (see also Malaria) 084.6
- Crimean hemorrhagic 065.0
- Cyprus (see also Brucellosis) 023.9
- dandy 061
- deer fly 021
- dehydration, newborn 778.4
- dengue (virus) 061
- - hemorrhagic 065.4
- desert 114
- due to heat 992.0
- Dumdum 085.0
- enteric 002.0
- ephemeral (of unknown origin) (see also
   Pyrexia) 780.6
- erysipelatous (see also Erysipelas) 035
- estivo-autumnal (malarial) 084.0
- famine - see also Fever, relapsing
- - meaning typhus - see Typhus
- Far Eastern hemorrhagic 065.0

Fever - *continued*
- Fort Bragg 100.8
- gastroenteric 002.0
- gastromalarial (see also Malaria) 084.6
- Gibraltar (see also Brucellosis) 023.9
- glandular 075
- Guama (viral) 066.3
- Haverhill 026.1
- hay (allergic) 477.9
- - with asthma (bronchial) 493.0
- - due to
- - - allergen other than pollen 477.8
- - - pollen, any plant or tree 477.0
- heat (effects) 992.0
- hematuric, bilious 084.8
- hemoglobinuric (malarial) 084.8
- - bilious 084.8
- hemorrhagic (arthropod-borne) NEC 065.9
- - with renal syndrome 078.6 † 581.8*
- - arenaviral 078.7
- - Argentinian 078.7
- - Bangkok 065.4
- - Bolivian 078.7
- - Central Asian 065.0
- - Chikungunya 065.4
- - Crimean 065.0
- - dengue (virus) 065.4
- - epidemic 078.6 † 581.8*
- - - of Far East 065.0
- - Far Eastern 065.0
- - Junin virus 078.7
- - Korean 078.6 † 581.8*
- - Machupo virus 078.7
- - mite-borne 065.8
- - mosquito-borne 065.4
- - Omsk 065.1
- - Philippine 065.4
- - Russian (Yaroslav) 078.6 † 581.8*
- - Singapore 065.4
- - Southeast Asia 065.4
- - Thailand 065.4
- - tick-borne NEC 065.3
- hepatic (see also Cholecystitis) 575.8
- - intermittent (see also Choledocholithiasis) 574.5
- herpetic (see also Herpes) 054.9
- Hyalomma tick 065.0
- inanition 780.6
- infective NEC 136.9
- intermittent (bilious) (see also Malaria) 084.6
- - hepatic (see also Choledocholithiasis) 574.5
- - of unknown origin (see also Pyrexia) 780.6
- - pernicious 084.0

Fever - *continued*
- iodide
- - correct substance properly administered 780.6
- - overdose or wrong substance given or taken 975.5
- Japanese river 081.2
- jungle yellow 060.0
- Katayama 120.2
- Kedani 081.2
- Kenya 082.1
- Lassa 078.8
- Lone Star 082.8
- lung - see Pneumonia
- malaria, malarial (see also Malaria) 084.6
- Malta (see also Brucellosis) 023.9
- Marseilles 082.1
- marsh (see also Malaria) 084.6
- Mayaro (viral) 066.3
- Mediterranean (see also Brucellosis) 023.9
- - familial 277.3
- - tick 082.1
- meningeal - see Meningitis
- metal fumes 985.8
- Meuse 083.1
- Mexican - see Typhus, Mexican
- mianeh 087.1
- miasmatic (see also Malaria) 084.6
- miliary 078.2
- milk, female 672
- mill 504
- Monday 504
- mosquito-borne NEC 066.3
- - hemorrhagic 065.4
- mountain
- - meaning
- - - Rocky Mountain spotted 082.0
- - - undulant fever (see also Brucellosis) 023.9
- - tick (American) 066.1
- Mucambo (viral) 066.3
- mud 100.8
- nine-mile 083.0
- non-exanthematous tick 066.1
- North Asian tick-borne typhus 082.2
- O'nyong-nyong (viral) 066.3
- Omsk hemorrhagic 065.1
- Oropouche (viral) 066.3
- Oroya 088.0
- paludal (see also Malaria) 084.6
- Panama 084.0
- pappataci 066.0
- paratyphoid 002.9
- - A 002.1
- - B 002.2
- - C 002.3

Fever - *continued*
- sun 061
- swamp 100.8
- sweating 078.2
- Tahyna 062.5 † 323.3*
- tertian - see Malaria, tertian
- Thailand hemorrhagic 065.4
- thermic 992.0
- three-day 066.0
- – with Coxsackie exanthem 074.8
- tick
- – American mountain 066.1
- – Colorado 066.1
- – Kemerovo 066.1
- – Quaranfil 066.1
- tick-bite NEC 066.1
- tick-borne NEC 066.1
- – hemorrhagic NEC 065.3
- trench 083.1
- tsutsugamushi 081.2
- typhogastric 002.0
- typhoid (abortive) (ambulant) (any site) (hemorrhagic) (infection) (intermittent) (malignant) (rheumatic) 002.0
- typhomalarial (see also Malaria) 084.6
- typhus - see Typhus
- undulant (see also Brucellosis) 023.9
- unknown origin (see also Pyrexia) 780.6
- uremic - see Uremia
- uveoparotid 135
- valley 114
- Venezuelan equine 066.2
- Volhynian 083.1
- Wesselsbron (viral) 066.3
- West
- – African 084.8
- – Nile (viral) 066.3
- Whitmore's 025
- Wolhynian 083.1
- worm 128.9
- yellow 060.9
- – jungle 060.0
- – sylvatic 060.0
- – urban 060.1
- Zika (viral) 066.3

Fibrillation
- atrial or auricular (established) 427.3
- cardiac 427.4
- coronary (see also Infarct, myocardium) 410
- heart 427.4
- muscular 728.9
- ventricular 427.4

Fibrin
- ball or bodies, pleural (sac) 511.0
- chamber, anterior (eye) (gelatinous exudate) 364.0

Fibrinogenolysis - see Fibrinolysis
Fibrinogenopenia (see also Defect, coagulation) 286.9
- acquired 286.6
- congenital 286.3
Fibrinolysis (hemorrhagic) (acquired) 286.6
- with
- – abortion - see categories 634-639, fourth digit .1
- – ectopic gestation 639.1
- antepartum or intrapartum 641.3
- – fetus or newborn 762.1
- newborn, transient 776.2
- postpartum 666.3
Fibrinopenia (hereditary) (see also Defect, coagulation) 286.3
- acquired 286.7
Fibrinopurulent - see condition
Fibrinous - see condition
Fibroadenoma (M9010/0)
- cellular intracanalicular (M9020/0) 217
- giant (intracanalicular) (M9020/0) 217
- intracanalicular (M9011/0)
- – cellular (M9020/0) 217
- – giant (M9020/0) 217
- – specified site - see Neoplasm, benign
- – unspecified site 217
- juvenile (M9030/0) 217
- pericanalicular (M9012/0)
- – specified site - see Neoplasm, benign
- – unspecified site 217
- phyllodes (M9020/0) 217
- prostate 600
- specified site - see Neoplasm, benign
- unspecified site 217
Fibroadenosis, breast (chronic) (cystic) (diffuse) (periodic) (segmental) 610.2
Fibroangioma (M9160/0) - see also Neoplasm, benign
- juvenile (M9160/0)
- – specified site - see Neoplasm, benign
- – unspecified site 210.7
Fibrochondrosarcoma (M9220/3) - see Neoplasm, cartilage, malignant
Fibrocystic
- disease 277.0
- – bone NEC 733.2
- – breast 610.1
- – jaw 526.2
- – kidney (congenital) 753.1
- – liver 751.6
- – lung 518.8
- – – congenital 748.4
- – pancreas 277.0
- kidney (congenital) 753.1
Fibroelastosis (cordis) (endocardial) (endomyocardial) 425.3

Fibroid (tumor) (M8890/0) - see also
 Neoplasm, connective tissue, benign
- disease, lung (chronic) (see also Fibrosis,
 lung) 515
- heart (disease) (see also Myocarditis)
 429.0
- in pregnancy or childbirth 654.1
- - causing obstructed labor 660.2
- - fetus or newborn 763.8
- induration, lung (chronic) (see also
 Fibrosis, lung) 515
- liver - see Cirrhosis, liver
- lung (see also Fibrosis, lung) 515
- pneumonia (chronic) (see also Fibrosis,
 lung) 515
- uterus 218
Fibrolipoma (M8851/0) 214
Fibroliposarcoma (M8850/3) - see
 Neoplasm, connective tissue, malignant
Fibroma (M8810/0) - see also Neoplasm,
 connective tissue, benign
- ameloblastic (M9330/0) 213.1
- - upper jaw (bone) 213.0
- bone (nonossifying) 733.9
- - ossifying (M9262/0) - see Neoplasm,
 bone, benign
- cementifying (M9274/0) - see Neoplasm,
 bone, benign
- chondromyxoid (M9241/0) - see
 Neoplasm, bone, benign
- desmoplastic (M8823/1) - see Neoplasm,
 connective tissue, uncertain behavior
- fascial (M8813/0) - see Neoplasm,
 connective tissue, benign
- invasive (M8821/1) - see Neoplasm,
 connective tissue, uncertain behavior
- molle (M8851/0) 214
- myxoid (M8811/0) - see Neoplasm,
 connective tissue, benign
- nasopharynx, nasopharyngeal (juvenile)
 (M9160/0) 210.7
- nonosteogenic (nonossifying) - see
 Dysplasia, fibrous
- odontogenic (M9321/0) 213.1
- - upper jaw (bone) 213.0
- ossifying (M9262/0) - see Neoplasm,
 bone, benign
- periosteal (M8812/0) - see Neoplasm,
 bone, benign
- prostate 600
- soft (M8851/0) 214
Fibromatosis
- abdominal (M8822/1) - see Neoplasm,
 connective tissue, uncertain behavior
- aggressive (M8821/1) - see Neoplasm,
 connective tissue, uncertain behavior
- gingival 523.8

Fibromatosis - *continued*
- subcutaneous pseudosarcomatous
 (proliferative) 728.7
Fibromyoma (M8890/0) - see also
 Neoplasm, connective tissue, benign
- uterus (corpus) 218
- - in pregnancy or childbirth 654.1
- - - causing obstructed labor 660.2
- - - fetus or newborn 763.8
Fibromyositis 729.1
- scapulohumeral 726.2
Fibromyxolipoma (M8852/0) 214
Fibromyxoma (M8811/0) - see Neoplasm,
 connective tissue, benign
Fibromyxosarcoma (M8811/3) - see
 Neoplasm, connective tissue, malignant
Fibroodontoma, ameloblastic (M9290/0)
 213.1
- upper jaw (bone) 213.0
Fibroosteoma (M9262/0) - see Neoplasm,
 bone, benign
Fibroplasia, retrolental 362.2
Fibropurulent - see condition
Fibrosarcoma (M8810/3) - see also
 Neoplasm, connective tissue, malignant
- ameloblastic (M9330/3) 170.1
- - upper jaw (bone) 170.0
- congenital (M8814/3) - see Neoplasm,
 connective tissue, malignant
- fascial (M8813/3) - see Neoplasm,
 connective tissue, malignant
- infantile (M8814/3) - see Neoplasm,
 connective tissue, malignant
- odontogenic (M9330/3) 170.1
- - upper jaw (bone) 170.0
- periosteal (M8812/3) - see Neoplasm,
 bone, malignant
Fibrosclerosis
- breast 610.3
- penis (corpora cavernosa) 607.8
Fibrosis, fibrotic
- adrenal (gland) 255.8
- amnion 658.8
- anal papillae 569.4
- anus 569.4
- appendix, appendiceal, noninflammatory
 543
- arteriocapillary - see Arteriosclerosis
- bladder 596.8
- - panmural 595.1
- bone, diffuse 756.5
- breast 610.3
- capillary - see also Arteriosclerosis
- - lung (chronic) (see also Fibrosis, lung)
 515
- cardiac (see also Myocarditis) 429.0
- cervix 622.8

Fibrosis - *continued*
- chorion 658.8
- corpus cavernosum 607.8
- cystic (of pancreas) 277.0
- due to (presence of) any device, implant or graft 996.7
- ejaculatory duct 608.8
- endocardium (see also Endocarditis) 424.9
- endomyocardial 425.0
- epididymis 608.8
- eye muscle 378.6
- heart (see also Myocarditis) 429.0
- hepatolienal - see Cirrhosis, liver
- hepatosplenic - see Cirrhosis, liver
- intrascrotal 608.8
- kidney (see also Sclerosis, renal) 587

- liver - see Cirrhosis, liver
- lung (atrophic) (capillary) (chronic) (confluent) (massive) (perialveolar) (peribronchial) 515
- - with
- - - anthracosilicosis 500
- - - anthracosis 500
- - - asbestosis 501
- - - bagassosis 495.1
- - - bauxite 503
- - - berylliosis 503
- - - byssinosis 504
- - - calcicosis 502
- - - chalicosis 502
- - - dust reticulation 504
- - - farmers' lung 495.0
- - - gannister disease 502
- - - graphite 503
- - - pneumoconiosis NEC 505
- - - pneumosiderosis 503
- - - siderosis 503
- - - silicosis 502
- - diffuse (idiopathic) (interstitial) 516.3
- - due to fumes or vapors (chemical) (inhalation) 506.4
- - following radiation 508.1
- - postinflammatory 515
- - silicotic 502
- - tuberculous 011.4
- lymphatic gland 289.3
- median bar 600

- mediastinum (idiopathic) 519.3
- meninges 349.2
- myocardium, myocardial (see also Myocarditis) 429.0
- oviduct 620.8
- pancreas 577.8
- penis 607.8
- periappendiceal 543

Fibrosis - *continued*
- perineum, in pregnancy or childbirth 654.8
- - causing obstructed labor 660.2
- - - fetus or newborn 763.1
- placenta - see Placenta, abnormal
- pleura 511.0
- prostate (chronic) 600
- pulmonary (see also Fibrosis, lung) 515
- rectal sphincter 569.4
- retroperitoneal, idiopathic 593.4
- scrotum 608.8
- seminal vesicle 608.8
- senile 797
- skin NEC 709.2
- spermatic cord 608.8
- spleen 289.5
- - bilharzial 120.- † 289.5*
- subepidermal nodular (M8832/0) -see neoplasm, skin, benign 216.9
- submucous NEC 709.2
- - oral 528.8
- - tongue 528.8
- testis 608.8
- - chronic, due to syphilis 095
- thymus (gland) 254.8
- tunica vaginalis 608.8
- uterus (non neoplastic) 621.8
- - bilharzial 120.- † 621.8*
- vagina 623.8
- valve, heart (see also Endocarditis) 424.9
- vas deferens 608.8
- vein 459.8
- - lower extremities 459.8
Fibrositis (periarticular) (rheumatoid) 729.0
- humeroscapular region 726.2
- nodular, chronic
- - Jaccoud 714.4
- - rheumatoid 714.4
- scapulohumeral 726.2
Fibrothorax 511.0
Fibrotic - see Fibrosis
Fibrous - see condition
Fibroxanthoma (M8831/0) - see also Neoplasm, connective tissue, benign
- atypical (M8831/1) - see Neoplasm, connective tissue, uncertain behavior
- malignant (M8831/3) - see Neoplasm, connective tissue, malignant
Fibroxanthosarcoma (M8831/3) - see Neoplasm, connective tissue, malignant
Fiedler's
- disease 100.0
- myocarditis (acute) 422.9
Fifth disease 057.0
Filaria, filarial - see Infestation, filarial
Filariasis (see also Infestation, filarial) 125.9

Filariasis - *continued*
- bancroftian 125.0
- due to
- - bancrofti 125.0
- - Brugia (Wuchereria) (malayi) 125.1
- - malayi 125.1
- - Wuchereria (bancrofti) 125.0
- - - malayi 125.1
- Malayan 125.1
- Ozzardi 125.5
- specified type NEC 125.6
Filatov's disease 075
File-cutters' disease 984.-
- specified type of lead - see Table of drugs and chemicals
Fimbrial cyst 752.3
Fimbriated hymen 752.4
Financial problem affecting care V60.2
Finger - see condition
Fire, Saint Anthony's (see also Erysipelas) 035
Fish hook stomach 537.8
Fish-meal workers' lung 495.8
Fissure, fissured
- anus, anal 565.0
- - congenital 751.5
- buccal cavity 528.9
- ear, lobule (congenital) 744.2
- epiglottis (congenital) 748.3
- larynx 478.7
- - congenital 748.3
- lip 528.5
- - congenital 749.1
- - - with cleft palate 749.2
- nipple 611.2
- - puerperal, postpartum 676.1
- palate (congenital) 749.0
- - with cleft lip 749.2
- postanal 565.0
- rectum 565.0
- skin 709.8
- spine (congenital) 741.9
- - with hydrocephalus 741.0
- tongue (acquired) 529.5
- - congenital 750.1
Fistula 686.9
- abdomen (wall) 569.8
- - bladder 596.2
- - intestine 569.8
- - ureter 593.8
- - uterus 619.2
- abdominorectal 569.8
- abdominosigmoidal 569.8
- abdominothoracic 510.0
- abdominouterine 619.2
- - congenital 752.3
- abdominovesical 596.2

Fistula - *continued*
- accessory sinuses (see also Sinusitis) 473.9
- actinomycotic - see Actinomycosis
- alveolar
- - antrum (see also Sinusitis, maxillary) 473.0
- - process 522.7
- anorectal 565.1
- antrobuccal (see also Sinusitis, maxillary) 473.0
- antrum (see also Sinusitis, maxillary) 473.0
- anus, anal (recurrent) (infectional) 565.1
- - congenital 751.5
- - tuberculous 014
- aorta-duodenal 447.2
- appendix, appendicular 543
- arteriovenous (acquired)
- - brain 437.3
- - - congenital 747.8
- - - ruptured (see also Hemorrhage, subarachnoid) 430
- - congenital 747.6
- - - brain 747.8
- - - coronary 746.8
- - - pulmonary 747.3
- - - specified site NEC 747.8
- - coronary 414.1
- - - congenital 746.8
- - pulmonary 417.0
- - - congenital 747.3
- - surgically created (for dialysis) V45.1
- - - complication NEC 996.7
- - - - infection 996.6
- - - - mechanical 996.1
- - traumatic - see Injury, blood vessel
- artery 447.2
- aural 383.8
- - congenital 744.4
- auricle 380.3
- - congenital 744.4
- Bartholin's gland 619.9
- bile duct (see also Fistula, biliary) 576.4
- biliary (duct) (tract) 576.4
- bladder (sphincter) 596.2
- - into seminal vesicle 596.2
- bone 733.9
- brain 348.8
- - arteriovenous 437.8
- - - congenital 747.8
- branchial (cleft) 744.4
- branchiogenous 744.4
- breast 611.0
- - puerperal, postpartum 675.1
- bronchial 510.0

Fistula - *continued*
- bronchocutaneous, bronchomediastinal, bronchopleural, bronchopleuromediastinal (infective) 510.0
- − tuberculous 011.3
- broncho-esophageal (see also Fistula, esophagobronchial) 530.8
- buccal cavity (infective) 528.3
- canal ear 380.8
- carotid-cavernous (see also Hemorrhage, brain, traumatic) 853.0
- cecosigmoidal 569.8
- cecum 569.8
- cerebrospinal (fluid) 349.8
- cervical, lateral 744.4
- cervicoaural 744.4
- cervicosigmoidal 619.1
- cervicovesical 619.0
- cervix 619.9
- chest (wall) 510.0
- cholecystocolic (see also Fistula, gallbladder) 575.5
- cholecystocolonic (see also Fistula, gallbladder) 575.5
- cholecystoduodenal (see also Fistula, gallbladder) 575.5
- cholecysto-enteric (see also Fistula, gallbladder) 575.5
- cholecystogastric (see also Fistula, gallbladder) 575.5
- cholecystointestinal (see also Fistula, gallbladder) 575.5
- choledochoduodenal (see also Fistula, gallbladder) 576.4
- cholocolic (see also Fistula, gallbladder) 575.5
- coccyx 685.1
- − with abscess 685.0
- colon 569.8
- colostomy 569.6
- common duct (see also Fistula, gallbladder) 576.4
- congenital, site not listed - see Anomaly, specified type NEC
- coronary, arteriovenous 414.1
- − congenital 746.8
- costal region 510.0
- cul-de-sac, Douglas' 619.9
- cutaneous 686.9
- cystic duct (see also Fistula, gallbladder) 575.5
- − congenital 751.6
- dental 522.7
- diaphragm 510.0
- − bronchovisceral 510.0
- − pleuroperitoneal 510.0

Fistula - *continued*
- diaphragm - *continued*
- − pulmonoperitoneal 510.0
- duodenum 537.4
- ear (external) 380.8
- enterocolic 569.8
- entero-uterine 619.1
- − congenital 752.3
- enterovaginal 619.1
- − congenital 752.4
- epididymis 608.8
- − tuberculous 016.2 † 608.8*
- esophagobronchial 530.8
- − congenital 750.3
- esophagocutaneous 530.8
- esophagopleural-cutaneous 530.8
- esophagotracheal 530.8
- − congenital 750.3
- esophagus 530.8
- − congenital 750.4
- ethmoid (see also Sinusitis, ethmoidal) 473.2
- eyeball (cornea) (sclera) 360.3
- eyelid 373.1
- fallopian tube (external) 619.2
- fecal 569.8
- − congenital 751.5
- from periapical lesion 522.7
- frontal sinus (see also Sinusitis, frontal) 473.1
- gallbladder 575.5
- − with calculus, cholelithiasis, stones (see also Cholelithiasis) 574.2
- gastric 537.4
- gastrocolic 537.4
- − congenital 750.7
- − tuberculous 014
- gastroenterocolic 537.4
- gastrojejunal 537.4
- gastrojejunocolic 537.4
- genital tract-skin (female) 619.2
- hepatopleural 510.0
- hepatopulmonary 510.0
- ileorectal 569.8
- ileosigmoidal 569.8
- ileovesical 596.1
- ileum 569.8
- in ano 565.1
- − tuberculous 014
- inner ear (labyrinth) 386.4
- intestine 569.8
- intestinocolonic (abdominal) 569.8
- intestinoureteral 593.8
- intestinouterine 619.1
- intestinovaginal 619.1
- intestinovesical 596.1
- involving female genital tract 619.9

Fistula - *continued*
- involving female genital tract - *continued*
- - digestive-genital 619.1
- - genital tract-skin 619.2
- - specified site NEC 619.8
- - urinary-genital 619.0
- ischiorectal (fossa) 566
- jejunum 569.8
- joint 719.8
- - tuberculous - see Tuberculosis, joint
- kidney 593.8
- labium (majus) (minus) 619.9
- labyrinth 386.4
- lacrimal (gland) (sac) 375.6
- lacrimonasal duct 375.6
- laryngotracheal 748.3
- larynx 478.7
- lip 528.5
- - congenital 750.2
- lumbar, tuberculous 015.0 † 730.4*
- lung 510.0
- lymphatic 457.8
- mamillary 611.0
- mammary (gland) 611.0
- - puerperal, postpartum 675.1
- mastoid (process) (region) 383.1
- maxillary (see also Sinusitis, maxillary) 473.0
- mediastinal 510.0
- mediastinobronchial 510.0
- mediastinocutaneous 510.0
- middle ear 385.8
- mouth 528.3
- nasal 478.1
- - sinus (see also Sinusitis) 473.9
- nasopharynx 478.2
- nipple - see Fistula, breast
- nose 478.1
- oesophagobronchial 530.8
- - congenital 750.3
- oesophagocutaneous 530.8
- oesophagopleural-cutaneous 530.8
- oesophagotracheal 530.8
- - congenital 750.3
- oesophagus 530.8
- - congenital 750.4
- oral (cutaneous) 528.3
- - maxillary (see also Sinusitis, maxillary) 473.0
- - nasal (with cleft palate) 749.0
- orbit, orbital 376.0
- oro-antral (see also Sinusitis, maxillary) 473.0
- oviduct (external) 619.2
- pancreatic 577.8
- pancreaticoduodenal 577.8
- parotid (gland) 527.4

Fistula - *continued*
- parotid - *continued*
- - region 528.3
- pelvo-abdomino-intestinal 569.8
- penis 607.8
- perianal 565.1
- pericardium (pleura) (sac) - see Pericarditis
- pericecal 569.8
- perineorectal 569.8
- perineosigmoidal 569.8
- perineum, perineal (with urethral involvement) NEC 599.1
- - tuberculous 017.8
- - ureter 593.8
- perirectal 565.1
- - tuberculous 014
- peritoneum (see also Peritonitis) 567.2
- periurethral 599.1
- pharyngo-esophageal 478.2
- pharynx 478.2
- - branchial cleft (congenital) 744.4
- pilonidal (infected) (rectum) 685.1
- - with abscess 685.0
- pleura, pleural, pleurocutaneous, pleuroperitoneal 510.0
- - stomach 510.0
- - tuberculous 012.0
- postauricular 383.8
- postoperative
- - persistant 998.6
- preauricular (congenital) 744.4
- prostate 602.8
- pulmonary 510.0
- - arteriovenous 417.0
- - - congenital 747.3
- - tuberculous (see also Tuberculosis, pulmonary) 011.9
- pulmonoperitoneal 510.0
- rectolabial 619.1
- rectosigmoid 569.8
- - intercommunicating 569.8
- rectoureteral 593.8
- rectourethral 599.1
- - congenital 753.8
- rectouterine 619.1
- - congenital 752.3
- rectovaginal 619.1
- - congenital 752.4
- - old, postpartal 619.1
- - tuberculous 014
- rectovesical 596.1
- - congenital 753.8
- rectovesicovaginal 619.1
- rectovulval 619.1
- - congenital 752.4
- rectum (to skin) 565.1

Fistula - *continued*
- rectum - *continued*
- - tuberculous 014
- renal 593.8
- retroauricular 383.8
- salivary duct or gland 527.4
- - congenital 750.2
- scrotum (urinary) 608.8
- - tuberculous 016.3
- semicircular canals 386.4
- sigmoid 569.8
- - vesicoabdominal 596.1
- skin 686.9
- - ureter 593.8
- - vagina 619.2
- splenocolic 289.5
- stercoral 569.8
- stomach 537.4
- sublingual gland 527.4
- - congenital 750.2
- submaxillary
- - gland 527.4
- - - congenital 750.2
- - region 528.3
- thoracic 510.0
- - duct 457.8
- thoracicoabdominal 510.0
- thoracicogastric 510.0
- thoracicointestinal 510.0
- thorax 510.0
- thyroglossal duct 759.2
- thyroid 246.8
- trachea (congenital) (external) (internal) 748.3
- tracheo-esophageal 530.8
- - congenital 750.3
- - following tracheostomy 519.0
- traumatic
- - arteriovenous - see also Injury, blood vessel
- - - brain - see Injury, intracranial
- tuberculous - code by site under Tuberculosis
- typhoid 002.0
- umbilical 759.8
- umbilico-urinary 753.8
- urachus 753.7
- ureter (persistent) 593.8
- ureteroabdominal 593.8
- ureterorectal 593.8
- ureterosigmoido-abdominal 593.8
- ureterovaginal 619.0
- ureterovesical 596.2
- urethra 599.1
- - congenital 753.8
- - tuberculous 016.1
- urethroperineal 599.1

Fistula - *continued*
- urethroperineovesical 596.2
- urethrorectal 599.1
- - congenital 753.8
- urethroscrotal 608.8
- urethrovaginal 619.0
- urethrovesical 596.2
- urinary (persistent) (recurrent) 599.1
- - tract 599.1
- uteroabdominal 619.2
- - congenital 752.3
- uteroenteric 619.1
- uterointestinal 619.1
- - congenital 752.3
- uterorectal 619.1
- - congenital 752.3
- utero-ureteric 619.0
- uterovaginal 619.8
- uterovesical 619.0
- - congenital 752.3
- uterus 619.9
- vagina (wall) 619.9
- - postpartal, old 619.9
- vaginocutaneous (postpartal) 619.2
- vaginoperineal 619.2
- vesical NEC 596.2
- vesico-abdominal 596.2
- vesicocervicovaginal 619.0
- vesicocolic 596.1
- vesico-enteric 596.1
- vesico-intestinal 596.1
- vesicometrorectal 619.1
- vesicoperineal 596.2
- vesicorectal 596.1
- - congenital 753.8
- vesicosigmoidal 596.1
- vesicosigmoidovaginal 619.1
- vesico-ureteral 596.2
- vesico-ureterovaginal 619.0
- vesico-urethral 596.2
- vesico-urethrorectal 596.1
- vesico-uterine 619.0
- - congenital 752.3
- vesicovaginal 619.0
- vulvorectal 619.1
- - congenital 752.4
Fit 780.3
- apoplectic (see also Disease, cerebrovascular, acute) 436
- epileptic (see also Epilepsy) 345.9
- fainting 780.2
- hysterical 300.1
- newborn 779.0
Fitting (of)
- artificial
- - arm (complete) (partial) V52.0
- - breast V52.4

Fitting - *continued*
- artificial - *continued*
- - eye V52.2
- - leg (complete) (partial) V52.1
- colostomy belt V53.5
- contact lenses V53.1
- dentures V52.3
- device NEC V53.9
- - abdominal V53.5
- - nervous system V53.0
- - orthodontic V53.4
- - orthotic V53.1
- - prosthetic V52.9
- - - breast V52.4
- - - dental V52.3
- - - specified NEC V52.8
- - special senses V53.0
- - substitution
- - - auditory V53.0
- - - visual V53.0
- - urinary V53.6
- glasses (reading) V53.1
- hearing aid V53.2
- ileostomy device V53.5
- intestinal appliance NEC V53.5
- orthopedic (device) V53.7
- - brace V53.7
- - cast V53.7
- - corset V53.7
- - shoes V53.7
- pacemaker (cardiac) V53.3
- prosthesis V52.9
- - breast V52.4
- - specified NEC V52.8
- spectacles V53.1
- wheelchair V53.8
Fitzhugh-Curtis syndrome 098.8
Fixation
- joint - see Ankylosis
- larynx 478.7
- pupil 364.7
- stapes 385.2
- - deafness (see also Deafness, conductive) 389.0
- uterus (acquired) - see Malposition, uterus
- vocal cord 478.5
Flaccid - see also condition
- foot 736.7
- forearm 736.0
- palate, congenital 750.2
Flail
- chest 807.4
- - newborn 767.3
- joint (paralytic) 718.8
Flajani's disease 242.0
Flat

Flat - *continued*
- chamber (eye) 360.3
- chest, congenital 754.8
- foot (acquired) (fixed type) (painful) (postural) 734
- - congenital 754.6
- - rachitic 268.1
- organ or site, congenital NEC - see Anomaly, specified type NEC
- pelvis 738.6
- - with disproportion 653.2
- - - causing obstructed labor 660.1
- - - fetus or newborn 763.1
- - congenital 755.6
Flatau-Schilder disease 341.1
Flattening
- head, femur 736.3
- hip 736.3
- lip (congenital) 744.8
- nose (congenital) 754.0
Flatulence 787.3
Flatus 787.3
- vaginalis 629.8
Flax-dressers' disease 504
Flea bite - see Injury, superficial
Fleischer's ring 275.1
Fleischer-Kayser ring 275.1
Fleischner's disease 732.3
Fleshy mole 631
Flexibilitas cerea - see Catalepsy
Flexion
- cervix (see also Malposition, uterus) 621.6
- contracture, joint (see also Contraction, joint) 718.4
- deformity, joint (see also Contraction, joint) 718.4
- - hip, congenital 754.3
- uterus (see also Malposition, uterus) 621.6
- - lateral - see Lateroversion, uterus
Flexner's
- bacillus 004.1
- diarrhea (ulcerative) 004.1
- dysentery 004.1
Flexner-Boyd dysentery 004.2
Flexure - see condition
Floater, vitreous 379.2
Floating
- cartilage (joint) 718.0
- - knee 717.6
- gallbladder (congenital) 751.6
- kidney (see also Lesion, kidney) 593.0
- - congenital 753.3
- rib 756.3
- spleen 289.5
Flooding 626.2

Floor - see condition
Flu - see also Influenza
- gastric NEC 008.8
Fluctuating blood pressure 796.4
Fluid
- abdomen 789.5
- chest (see also Pleurisy, with effusion)
  511.9
- heart (see also Failure, heart, congestive)
  428.0
- joint 719.0
- loss (acute) 276.5
- lung - see also Edema, lung
- - encysted 511.8
- peritoneal cavity 789.5
- pleural cavity (see also Pleurisy, with
  effusion) 511.9
Flukes NEC (see also Infestation, flukes)
  121.9
- blood NEC (see also Infestation,
  schistosoma) 120.9
- liver 121.3
Fluor (vaginalis) 623.5
- trichomonal or due to Trichomonas
  (vaginalis) 131.0
Fluorosis (dental) (chronic) 520.3
Flushing 782.6
Flutter
- atrial or auricular 427.3
- heart 427.4
- ventricular 427.4
Fochier's abscess - code by site under
  Abscess
Focus, Assmann's 011.0
Folds, anomalous - see also Anomaly,
  specified type NEC
- epicanthic 743.6
- heart 746.8
Folie a deux 297.3
Follicle
- cervix (nabothian) (ruptured) 616.0
- nabothian 616.0
Folliclis (primary) 017.0
Follicular - see condition
Folliculitis 704.8
- abscedens et suffodiens 704.8
- decalvans 704.0
- gonorrheal (acute) 098.0
- - chronic or duration of 2 months or over
  098.2
- keloid, keloidalis 706.1
- pustular 704.8
- ulerythematosa reticulata 701.8
Folling's disease 270.1
Food
- asphyxia (from aspiration or inhalation)
  (see also Asphyxia, food) 933.1

Food - *continued*
- choked on (see also Asphyxia, food)
  933.1
- deprivation 994.2
- - specified kind of food NEC 269.8
- lack of 994.2
- strangulation or suffocation (see also
  Asphyxia, food) 933.1
Foot - see condition
Foramen ovale (nonclosure) (patent)
  (persistent) 745.5
Forbe's glycogen storage disease 271.0
Forbes-Albright syndrome 253.1
Forced birth or delivery NEC 669.8
- affecting fetus or newborn, NEC 763.8
Forceps delivery NEC 669.5
- fetus or newborn 763.2
Fordyce's disease (mouth) 750.2
Fordyce-Fox disease 705.8
Forearm - see condition
Foreign body
- accidently left during a procedure 998.4
- anterior chamber (eye) - see Foreign
  body, intraocular
- ciliary body (eye) - see Foreign body,
  intraocular
- entering through orifice
- - accessory sinus 932
- - air passage (upper) 933.0
- - - lower 934.8
- - alimentary canal 938
- - alveolar process 935.0
- - antrum (Highmore) 932
- - anus 937
- - appendix 936
- - asphyxia due to (see also Asphyxia,
  food) 933.1
- - auditory canal 931
- - auricle 931
- - bladder 939.0
- - bronchioles 934.8
- - bronchus (main) 934.1
- - buccal cavity 935.0
- - canthus (inner) 930.1
- - cecum 936
- - cervix (canal) uterine 939.1
- - coil, ileocecal 936
- - colon 936
- - conjunctiva 930.1
- - conjunctival sac 930.1
- - cornea 930.0
- - digestive organ or tract NEC 938
- - duodenum 936
- - ear (external) 931
- - esophagus 935.1
- - eye (external) NEC 930.9
- - - combined sites 930.8

Foreign body - *continued*
- retained - *continued*
- - vitreous - *continued*
- - - magnetic 360.5
- retina - see Foreign body, intraocular
- superficial, without major open wound (see also Injury, superficial) 919.-
- swallowed NEC 938
- vitreous (humor) - see Foreign body, intraocular
Formation
- hyalin in cornea 371.4
- sequestrum in bone (due to infection) 730.1
- valve
- - colon, congenital 751.5
- - ureter (congenital) 753.2
Fort Bragg fever 100.8
Fossa - see also condition
- pyriform - see condition
Fothergill's
- disease, meaning scarlatina anginosa 034.1
- neuralgia (see also Neuralgia, trigeminal) 350.1
Foul breath 784.9
Found dead (cause unknown) 798.9
Foundling V20.0
Fournier's disease 608.8
Fourth
- cranial nerve - see condition
- disease 057.8
- molar 520.1
Foville's syndrome 344.8
Fox's
- disease 705.8
- impetigo 684
Fox-Fordyce disease 705.8
Fracture (abduction) (adduction) (avulsion) (compression) (crush) (dislocation) (oblique) (separation) 829.-

---

Note − For fracture of any of the following sites with fracture of other bones − *see* Fracture, multiple.

The following fourth-digit subdivisions are for use with those categories in 805–829 for which a more detailed fourth-digit subdivision is not provided and indicated below:
    .0 Closed
    .1 Open
"Closed" includes the following descriptions of fractures, with or without delayed healing, unless they are specified as open or compound:
    comminuted
    depressed

elevated
fissured
greenstick
impacted
linear
march
simple
slipped epiphysis
spiral
unspecified.
"Open" includes the following descriptions of fractures, with or without delayed healing:
    compound
    infected
    missile
    puncture
    with foreign body.

Fracture - *continued*
- with
- - internal injuries in the same region (classifiable to 860-869) - code by site under Injury, internal 869.-
- - - pelvic region - see Fracture, pelvis

- acetabulum (with visceral injury) 808.0
- - open 808.1
- acromion (process) 811.-

- alveolus 802.8
- - open 802.9
- ankle (closed) 824.8
- - bimalleolar 824.4
- - - open 824.5
- - bone (closed) 825.2
- - - open 825.3
- - open 824.9
- - talus 825.2
- - - open 825.3
- - trimalleolar 824.6
- - - open 824.7
- antrum 801.-
- arm 818.-
- - and leg(s) (any bones) 828.-
- - both (any bones) (with ribs) (with sternum) 819.-
- - lower 813.0
- - - open 813.1
- - upper - see Fracture, humerus

- astragalus (closed) 825.2
- - open 825.3
- axis - see Fracture, vertebra, cervical
- back - see Fracture, vertebra
- Barton's 813.4
- - open 813.5
- basal (skull) 801.-

Fracture - *continued*
- Bennett's (see also Fracture, metacarpus) 815.-
- bimalleolar (closed) 824.4
- - open 824.5
- bone NEC 829.-
- - birth injury, NEC 767.3
- - pathological (cause unknown) 733.1
- boot top - see Fracture, fibula
- breast bone - see Fracture, sternum
- bucket handle (semilunar cartilage) - see Tear, meniscus
- calcaneus (closed) 825.0
- - open 825.1
- capitellum (humerus) 812.4
- - open 812.5
- carpal bone(s) 814.-
- cartilage, knee (semilunar) - see Tear, meniscus
- cervical - see Fracture, vertebra, cervical
- chauffeur's 813.4
- - open 813.5
- clavicle (acromial end) (interligamentous) (shaft) 810.-
- - birth injury 767.2
- clay-shovellers' - see Fracture, vertebra, cervical
- coccyx - see Fracture, vertebra, coccyx
- collar bone 810.-
- Colles' (reversed) 813.4
- - open 813.5
- comminuted - code as Fracture, by site, closed 829.-
- congenital 756.9
- costochondral junction - see Fracture, rib
- costosternal junction - see Fracture, rib
- cranium - see Fracture, skull
- cricoid cartilage 807.5
- - open 807.6
- cuboid (ankle) (closed) 825.2
- - open 825.3
- cuneiform
- - foot (closed) 825.2
- - - open 825.3
- - wrist 814.-
- due to
- - birth injury - see Birth injury, fracture
- - gunshot - code as Fracture, open
- Dupuytren's (ankle) (fibula) 824.4
- - open 824.5
- - radius 813.4
- - - open 813.5
- elbow (supracondylar) 812.4
- - open 812.5
- ethmoid (bone) (sinus) 801.-
- face bone(s) (closed) NEC 802.8
- - with

Fracture - *continued*
- face bone(s) - *continued*
- - with - *continued*
- - - other bone(s) 804.-
- - - skull bone(s) 803.-
- - - - involving other bone(s) 804.-
- - open 802.9
- femur, femoral (closed) 821.0
- - cervicotrochanteric 820.0
- - - open 820.1
- - condyles, epicondyles 821.2
- - - open 821.3
- - distal end 821.2
- - - open 821.3
- - epiphysis
- - - capital 820.0
- - - - open 820.1
- - - head 820.0
- - - - open 820.1
- - - lower 821.2
- - - - open 821.3
- - - trochanteric 820.0
- - - - open 820.1
- - - upper 820.0
- - - - open 820.1
- - head 820.0
- - - open 820.1
- - lower end or extremity 821.2
- - - open 821.3
- - neck 820.8
- - - base 820.0
- - - - open 820.1
- - - extracapsular 820.2
- - - - open 820.3
- - - intertrochanteric (section) 820.2
- - - - open 820.3
- - - intracapsular 820.0
- - - - open 820.1
- - - intratrochanteric 820.2
- - - - open 820.3
- - - midcervical 820.0
- - - - open 820.1
- - - open 820.9
- - - transcervical 820.0
- - - - open 820.1
- - - transtrochanteric 820.2
- - - - open 820.3
- - open 821.1
- - peritrochanteric 820.2
- - - open 820.3
- - shaft (lower third) (middle third) (upper third) 821.0
- - - open 821.1
- - subcapital 820.0
- - - open 820.1
- - subtrochanteric (region) (section) 820.2

Fracture - *continued*
− femur - *continued*
− − subtrochanteric - *continued*
− − − open 820.3
− − transepiphyseal 820.0
− − − open 820.1
− − T-shaped, into knee joint 821.2
− − − open 821.3
− fibula (styloid) (with tibia) (closed) 823.0
− − distal end 824.8
− − − open 824.9
− − epiphysis
− − − lower 824.8
− − − − open 824.9
− − − upper 823.0
− − − − open 823.1
− − head - see Fracture, fibula, upper end
− − involving ankle 824.2
− − − open 824.3
− − lower end or extremity 824.8
− − − open 824.9
− − malleolus 824.2
− − − open 824.3
− − open NEC 823.1
− − proximal end 823.0
− − − open 823.1
− − shaft 823.2
− − − open 823.3
− − upper end or extremity 823.0
− − − open 823.1
− finger(s), of one hand 816.-
− − with
− − − metacarpal bone(s), of same hand 817.-
− − − thumb of same hand 816.-
− foot, except toe(s) alone (closed) 825.2
− − open 825.3
− forearm (closed) NEC 813.0
− − open 813.1
− fossa, anterior, middle, or posterior 801.-
− frontal (bone) 800.-
− − sinus 801.-
− glenoid (cavity) (scapula) 811.-
− greenstick - code as Fracture, closed 829.-
− hand, one 815.-
− − carpals 814.-
− − metacarpals 815.-
− − multiple, bones of one hand 817.-
− − phalanges 816.-
− healing or old with complications - code by nature of the complication
− heel bone (closed) 825.0
− − open 825.1
− hip (see also Fracture, femur, neck) 820.8
− − open 820.9
− humerus (closed) 812.2

Fracture - *continued*
− humerus - *continued*
− − anatomical neck - see Fracture, humerus, upper end
− − articular process - see Fracture, humerus, lower end
− − distal end - see Fracture, humerus, lower end
− − epiphysis
− − − lower - see Fracture, humerus, lower end
− − − upper - see Fracture, humerus, upper end
− − external condyle - see Fracture, humerus, lower end
− − great tuberosity - see Fracture, humerus, upper end
− − internal epicondyle - see Fracture, humerus, lower end
− − lesser tuberosity - see Fracture, humerus, upper end
− − lower end (articular process) or extremity 812.4
− − − open 812.5
− − open NEC 812.3
− − proximal end - see Fracture, humerus, upper end
− − shaft 812.2
− − − open 812.3
− − surgical neck - see Fracture, humerus, upper end
− − T-shaped - see Fracture, humerus, lower end
− − tuberosity - see Fracture, humerus, upper end
− − upper end or extremity 812.0
− − − open 812.1
− hyoid bone 807.5
− − open 807.6
− hyperextension 813.4
− − open 813.5
− ilium (with visceral injury) 808.4
− − open 808.5
− impaction, impacted - code as Fracture, closed 829.-
− incus 801.-
− innominate bone (with visceral injury) 808.4
− − open 808.5
− instep, of one foot (closed) 825.2
− − with toe(s) of same foot 827.-
− − open 825.3
− internal
− − ear 801.-
− − semilunar cartilage, knee (current) - see Tear, meniscus
− ischium (with visceral injury) 808.4

Note – Multiple fractures of sites classifiable to the same three- or four-digit category are coded to that category, except for sites classifiable to 810–818 or 820–827 in different limbs.

Multiple fractures of sites classifiable to different fourth-digit subdivisions within the same three-digit category should be dealt with according to the coding rules.

Multiple fractures of sites classifiable to different three-digit categories (identifiable from the listing under "Fracture"), and of sites classifiable to 810–818 or 820–827 in different limbs should be coded according to the following list, which should be referred to in the following priority order: skull or face bones, pelvis or vertebral column, legs, arms.

Fracture - *continued*
- multiple - *continued*
- - pelvis with other bone(s) except skull or face bone(s) (site(s) classifiable to 808 with site(s) classifiable to 805, 806, 807 or 810-829) 809.-
- - skull, specified or unspecified bone(s), or face bone(s) with any other bone(s) (site(s) classifiable to 800-803 with site(s) classifiable to 805-829) 804.-
- - vertebral column with other bone(s) except skull or face bone(s) (site(s) classifiable to 805 or 806 with site(s) classifiable to 807, 808 or 810-829) 809.-
- nasal (bone(s)) (closed) 802.0
- - open 802.1
- - sinus 801.-
- navicular
- - tarsal (closed) 825.2
- - - open 825.3
- - wrist 814.-
- neck - see Fracture, vertebra, cervical
- neural arch - see Fracture, vertebra
- nose, nasal (bone) (septum) (closed) 802.0
- - open 802.1
- occiput 801.-
- odontoid process - see Fracture, vertebra, cervical
- olecranon (ulna) 813.0
- - open 813.1
- orbit, orbital (bone) (region) (closed) 802.8
- - floor (blow-out) (closed) 802.6
- - - open 802.7
- - open 802.9
- - roof (closed) 801.-
- - specified part NEC 802.8
- - - open 802.9
- os
- - calcis (closed) 825.0
- - - open 825.1
- - magnum 814.-
- - pubis (with visceral injury) 808.2
- - - open 808.3
- osseous
- - auditory meatus 801.-
- - labyrinth 801.-
- ossicles, auditory 801.-
- palate (closed) 802.8
- - open 802.9
- parietal bone 800.-
- patella 822.-
- pathological (cause unknown) 733.1
- pedicle (of vertebral arch) - see Fracture, vertebra

Fracture - *continued*
- pelvis, pelvic (bone(s)) (multiple) (with visceral injury) 808.8
- - open 808.9
- - rim 808.4
- - - open 808.5
- phalanx, phalanges, of one
- - foot 826.-
- - - with bone(s) of same lower limb 827.-
- - hand 816.-
- - - with metacarpal bone(s) of same hand 817.-
- pisiform 814.-
- pond 800.-
- Pott's 824.4
- - open 824.5
- prosthetic device, internal - see Complications, mechanical
- pubis (with visceral injury) 808.2
- - open 808.3
- radius (with ulna) (closed) 813.0
- - distal end - see Fracture, radius, lower end
- - epiphysis
- - - lower - see Fracture, radius, lower end
- - - upper - see Fracture, radius, upper end
- - head - see Fracture, radius, upper end
- - lower end or extremity 813.4
- - - open 813.5
- - neck - see Fracture, radius, upper end
- - open NEC 813.1
- - proximal end - see Fracture, radius, upper end
- - shaft 813.2
- - - open 813.3
- - upper end 813.0
- - - open 813.1
- ramus
- - inferior or superior (with visceral injury) 808.8
- - - open 808.9
- - mandible 802.2
- - - open 802.3
- rib(s) (closed) 807.0
- - with flail chest (open) 807.4
- - open 807.1
- root, tooth 873.6
- - complicated 873.7
- sacrum - see Fracture, vertebra, sacrum
- scaphoid
- - ankle (closed) 825.2
- - - open 825.3
- - wrist 814.-

Fracture - *continued*
- scapula (acromial or acromion process) (body) (glenoid (cavity)) (neck) 811.-
- semilunar
- - bone, wrist 814.-
- - cartilage (knee) (interior) - see Tear, meniscus
- sesamoid bone
- - ankle 825.2
- - other - code by site under Fracture
- - wrist 814
- shoulder 812.0
- - blade 811.-
- - open 812.1
- sinus (ethmoid) (frontal) (maxillary) (nasal) (sphenoidal) 801.-
- skull (multiple NEC) 803.-

Note – The following fourth-digit subdivisions are for use with categories 800–801 and 803–804:
   .0 *Closed without mention of intracranial injury*
   .1 *Closed with intracranial injury*
   .2 *Open without mention of intracranial injury*
   .3 *Open with intracranial injury*
"Intracranial injury" includes any condition classifiable to 850–854.

Fracture - *continued*
- skull - *continued*
- - with
- - - face bone(s) 803.-
- - - - involving other bone(s) 804.-
- - base 801.-
- - birth injury 767.3
- - face bones - see Fracture, face bones
- - vault 800.-
- Smith's 813.4
- - open 813.5
- sphenoid 801.-
- spine - see Fracture, vertebra
- spinous process - see Fracture, vertebra
- spontaneous (cause unknown) 733.1
- stapes 801.-
- stave (see also Fracture, metacarpal) 815.-
- sternum (closed) 807.2
- - with flail chest (open) 807.4
- - open 807.3
- supracondylar, elbow 812.4
- - open 812.5
- symphysis pubis (with visceral injury) 808.2
- - open 808.3

Fracture - *continued*
- talus (ankle bone) (closed) 825.2
- - open 825.3
- tarsus, tarsal bone(s) (with metatarsus) of one foot (closed) NEC 825.2
- - open 825.3
- temporal bone (styloid) 801.-
- tendon - see Sprain, strain
- thigh - see Fracture, femur, shaft
- thumb (and finger(s)) of one hand 816.-
- - with metacarpal bone(s) of same hand 817.-
- thyroid cartilage 807.5
- - open 807.6
- tibia (with fibula) (closed) 823.0
- - condyles - see Fracture, tibia, upper end
- - distal end 824.8
- - - open 824.9
- - epiphysis
- - - lower 824.8
- - - - open 824.9
- - - upper - see Fracture, tibia, upper end
- - head (involving knee joint) - see Fracture, tibia, upper end
- - intercondyloid eminence - see Fracture, tibia, upper end
- - involving ankle 824.0
- - - open 824.1
- - lower end or extremity (anterior lip) (posterior lip) 824.8
- - - open 824.9
- - malleolus 824.0
- - - open 824.1
- - open NEC 823.1
- - proximal end - see Fracture, tibia, upper end
- - shaft 823.2
- - - open 823.3
- - spine - see Fracture, tibia, upper end
- - tuberosity - see Fracture, tibia, upper end
- - upper end or extremity 823.0
- - - open 823.1
- toe(s), of one foot 826.-
- - with bone(s) of same lower limb 827.-
- tooth (root) 873.6
- - complicated 873.7
- trachea 807.5
- - open 807.6
- transverse process - see Fracture, vertebra
- trapezium 814.-
- trapezoid bone 814.-
- trimalleolar (closed) 824.6
- - open 824.7

Fracture - *continued*
- trochanter (closed) (greater) (lesser) 820.2
- − open 820.3
- trunk (closed) 809.0
- − open 809.1
- tuberosity (external) - code by site under Fracture
- ulna (with radius) (closed) 813.0
- − coronoid process - see Fracture, ulna, upper end
- − distal end - see Fracture, ulna, lower end
- − epiphysis
- − − lower - see Fracture, ulna, lower end
- − − upper - see Fracture, ulna, upper end
- − head - see Fracture, ulna, lower end
- − lower end 813.4
- − − open 813.5
- − olecranon process - see Fracture, ulna, upper end
- − open NEC 813.1
- − proximal end - see Fracture, ulna, upper end
- − shaft 813.2
- − − open 813.3
- − styloid process - see Fracture, ulna, lower end
- − transverse - code by site under Fracture, ulna
- − upper end 813.0
- − − open 813.1
- unciform 814.-
- vertebra, vertebral (back) (body) (column) (neural arch) (pedicle) (spinous process) (transverse process) (closed) 805.8
- − with
- − − hematomyelia - code by region under Fracture, vertebra, with spinal cord lesion
- − − injury to
- − − − cauda equina 806.6
- − − − − open 806.7
- − − − nerve - code by region under Fracture, vertebra, with spinal cord lesion
- − − paralysis - code by region under Fracture, vertebra, with spinal cord lesion
- − − paraplegia - code by region under Fracture, vertebra, with spinal cord lesion
- − − quadriplegia - code by region under Fracture, vertebra, with spinal cord lesion

Fracture - *continued*
- vertebra - *continued*
- − with - *continued*
- − − spinal concussion - code by region under Fracture, vertebra, with spinal cord lesion
- − − spinal cord lesion NEC 806.8
- − − − open 806.9
- − − specified region - code as Fracture, vertebra, by region, with spinal cord lesion
- − atlanto-axial - see Fracture, vertebra, cervical
- − cervical (hangman) (teardrop) 805.0
- − − with spinal cord lesion 806.0
- − − − open 806.1
- − − open 805.1
- − coccyx 805.6
- − − with spinal cord lesion 806.6
- − − − open 806.7
- − − open 805.7
- − dorsal 805.2
- − − with spinal cord lesion 806.2
- − − − open 806.3
- − − open 805.3
- − fetus or newborn 767.4
- − lumbar 805.4
- − − with spinal cord lesion 806.4
- − − − open 806.5
- − − open 805.5
- − open NEC 805.9
- − sacrum 805.6
- − − with spinal cord lesion 806.6
- − − − open 806.7
- − − open 805.7
- − thoracic 805.2
- − − with spinal cord lesion 806.2
- − − − open 806.3
- − − open 805.3
- vertex 800.-
- vomer (bone) 802.0
- − open 802.1
- wrist 814.-
- xiphoid (process) - see Fracture, sternum
- zygoma (closed) 802.4
- − open 802.5
Fragilitas
- crinium 704.2
- ossium 756.5
- − with blue sclerotics 756.5
- unguium 703.8
- − congenital 757.5
Fragility
- bone 756.5
- − with deafness and blue sclera 756.5
- capillary (hereditary) 287.8
- hair 704.2

Furuncle - see also Carbuncle
- eyelid 373.1
- lacrimal
- - gland 375.0
- - passages (duct) (sac) 375.3
- orbit, orbital 376.0
Furunculosis (see also Carbuncle) 680.9
- external auditory meatus 680.0 † 380.1*
Fusarium (infection) 118
Fusion, fused (congenital)
- anal (and urogenital canal) 751.5
- aorta and pulmonary artery 745.0
- astragaloscaphoid 755.6
- atria 745.5
- atrium and ventricle 745.6
- auditory canal 744.0
- auricles, heart 745.5
- binocular with defective stereopsis 368.3
- bone 756.9
- cervical spine - see Fusion, spine
- choanal 748.0
- cusps, heart valve NEC 746.8
- - mitral 746.8
- - tricuspid 746.8
- ear ossicles 744.0
- fingers 755.1
- hymen 752.4
- joint (acquired) - see also Ankylosis
- - congenital 755.8
- kidneys (incomplete) 753.3
- labium (majus) (minus) 752.4
- larynx and trachea 748.3
- limb 755.8
- - lower 755.6
- - upper 755.5
- lobes, lung 748.5

Fusion - *continued*
- lumbosacral (acquired) 724.6
- - congenital 756.1
- - surgical V45.4
- nares 748.0
- nose, nasal 748.0
- nostril(s) 748.0
- organ or site not listed - see Anomaly, specified type NEC
- ossicles 756.9
- - auditory 744.0
- pulmonary valve segment 746.0
- pulmonic cusps 746.0
- ribs 756.3
- sacro-iliac (joint) (acquired) 724.6
- - congenital 755.6
- - surgical V45.4
- spine (acquired) 724.9
- - arthrodesis status V45.4
- - congenital 756.1
- - postoperative status V45.4
- sublingual duct with submaxillary duct at opening in mouth 750.2
- testis 752.8
- toes 755.1
- tooth, teeth 520.2
- trachea and esophagus 750.3
- twins 759.4
- vagina 752.4
- valve cusps - see Fusion, cusps
- ventricles, heart 745.4
- vertebra (arch) - see Fusion, spine
- vulva 752.4
Fusospirillosis (mouth) (tongue) (tonsil) 101

G

Gafsa boil 085.1
Gain
- weight (abnormal) (excessive) (see also Weight, gain) 783.1
Gaisbock's disease 289.0
Gait
- abnormality 781.2
- - hysterical 300.1
- ataxic 781.2
- - hysterical 300.1
- disturbance 781.2
- - hysterical 300.1
- paralytic 781.2
- spastic 781.2
- staggering 781.2
- - hysterical 300.1
Galactocele (breast) (infected) 611.5
- puerperal, postpartum 676.8
Galactophoritis 611.0
- puerperal, postpartum 675.2
Galactorrhea 676.6
- not associated with childbirth 611.6
Galactosemia 271.1
Galactosuria 271.1
Galacturia 791.1
- bilharziasis 120.0
Galen's vein - see condition
Gall duct - see condition
Gallbladder - see also condition
- acute (see also Disease, gallbladder) 575.9
Gallop rhythm 427.8
Gallstone (cholemic) (colic) (impacted) (see also Cholelithiasis) 574.2
- causing intestinal obstruction (see also Impaction, intestine) 560.3
Gammopathy, monoclonal (benign) 273.1
- associated with lymphoplasmacytic dyscrasia 273.1
Gamna's disease 289.5
Gandy-Nanta disease 289.5
Gang activity, without manifest psychiatric disorder V71.0
Gangliocytoma (M9490/0) - see Neoplasm, connective tissue, benign
Ganglioglioma (M9505/1) - see Neoplasm, uncertain behavior
Ganglion (compound) (diffused) (joint) (tendon (sheath)) 727.4
- of yaws (early) (late) 102.6

Ganglion - *continued*
- tuberculous 015.9
Ganglioneuroblastoma (M9490/3) - see Neoplasm, connective tissue, malignant
Ganglioneuroma (M9490/0) - see also Neoplasm, connective tissue, benign
- malignant (M9490/3) - see Neoplasm, connective tissue, malignant
Ganglioneuromatosis (M9491/0) - see Neoplasm, connective tissue, benign
Ganglionitis
- fifth nerve (see also Neuralgia, trigeminal) 350.1
- gasserian 350.1
- geniculate (see also Neuralgia, trigeminal) 351.1
- - herpetic 053.1 † 351.1*
- - newborn 767.5
- herpes zoster 053.1 † 351.1*
- herpetic geniculate 053.1 † 351.1*
Gangliosidosis 330.1
Gangosa 102.5
Gangrene, gangrenous (cutaneous) (dry) (infected) (local) (moist) (septic) (skin) (spreading cutaneous) (stasis) (ulcer) (ulcerative) 785.4
- with diabetes (mellitus) 250.6 † 785.4*
- abdomen (wall) 785.4
- alveolar 526.5
- anus 569.4
- appendices epiploicae - see Gangrene, mesentery
- appendix 540.9
- - with perforation, peritonitis, or rupture 540.0
- arteriosclerotic (general) (senile) 440.2 † 785.4*
- auricle 785.4
- Bacillus welchii (see also Gangrene, gas) 040.0
- bile duct (see also Cholecystitis) 576.8
- bladder 595.8
- bowel, cecum, or colon - see Gangrene, intestine
- Clostridium perfringens or welchii (see also Gangrene, gas) 040.0
- connective tissue 785.4
- cornea (see also Keratitis) 371.4
- corpora cavernosa 607.2
- - noninfective 607.8

Gangrene - *continued*
- cutaneous, spreading 785.4
- decubital - see Ulcer, decubitus
- diabetic (any site) 250.6 † 785.4*
- dropsical 785.4
- emphysematous (see also Gangrene, gas) 040.0
- epidemic 988.2
- epididymis (infectional) (see also Epididymitis) 604.9
- extremity (lower) (upper) 785.4
- gallbladder or duct (see also Cholecystitis, acute) 575.0
- gas (bacillus) 040.0
- - with
- - - abortion - see categories 634-639, fourth digit .0
- - - ectopic gestation 639.0
- - puerperal, postpartum, childbirth 670
- hernia - see Hernia, by site, gangrenous
- intestine, intestinal (hemorrhagic) (massive) 557.0
- - with
- - - mesenteric embolism 557.0
- - - obstruction (see also Obstruction, intestine) 560.9
- liver 573.8
- lung 513.0
- Meleney's 686.0
- mesentery 557.0
- - with
- - - embolism 557.0
- - - intestinal obstruction (see also Obstruction, intestine) 560.9
- mouth 528.1
- omphalocele 551.1
- ovary (see also Salpingo-oophoritis) 614.2
- pancreas 577.0
- penis 607.2
- - noninfective 607.8
- perineum 785.4
- pharynx 462
- presenile 443.1
- pulmonary 513.0
- pulp 522.1
- Raynaud's 443.0 † 785.4*
- rectum 569.4
- retropharyngeal 478.2
- rupture - see Hernia, by site, gangrenous
- scrotum 608.4
- - noninfective 608.8
- senile 440.2 † 785.4*
- spermatic cord 608.4
- - noninfective 608.8
- spine 785.4
- spirochetal NEC 104.8

Gangrene - *continued*
- spreading cutaneous 785.4
- stomach 537.8
- symmetrical 443.0 † 785.4*
- testis (infectional) (see also Orchitis) 604.9
- - noninfective 608.8
- throat 462
- thyroid (gland) 246.8
- tuberculous NEC (see also Tuberculosis) 011.9
- tunica vaginalis 608.4
- - noninfective 608.8
- umbilicus 785.4
- uterus (see also Endometritis) 615.9
- vas deferens 608.4
- - noninfective 608.8
- vulva (see also Vulvitis) 616.1
Gannister disease 502
Ganser's syndrome, hysterical 300.1

Gardner-Diamond syndrome 287.2
Gargoylism 277.5
Garre's
- disease 730.1
- osteitis (sclerosing) 730.1
- osteomyelitis 730.1
Garrod's pad, knuckle 728.7
Gartner's duct
- cyst 752.1
- persistent 752.8
Gas
- asphyxia, asphyxiation, inhalation, poisoning, suffocation NEC 987.9
- - specified gas - see Table of drugs and chemicals
- bacillus gangrene or infection - see Gas gangrene
- gangrene 040.0
- - with
- - - abortion - see categories 634-639, fourth digit .0
- - - ectopic gestation 639.0
- - puerperal, postpartum, childbirth 670
- on stomach 787.3
- pains 787.3
Gastralgia 536.8
- psychogenic 307.8
Gastrectasis 536.1
- psychogenic 306.4

Gastric - see condition
Gastrinoma (M8153/1)
- malignant (M8153/3)
- - pancreas 157.4
- - specified site NEC - see Neoplasm, malignant
- - unspecified site 157.4

Gastrinoma - *continued*
- specified site - see Neoplasm, uncertain behavior
- unspecified site 235.5
Gastritis (simple) 535.5
- acute 535.0
- alcoholic 535.3
- allergic 535.4
- atrophic 535.1
- chronic (atrophic) 535.1
- due to diet deficiency 269.9 † 535.4*
- giant hypertrophic 535.2
- hypertrophic (mucosa) 535.2
- nervous 306.4
- spastic 536.8
- superficial 535.4
- tuberculous 017.8
Gastrocarcinoma (M8010/3) 151.9
Gastrocolic - see condition
Gastrocolitis - see Enteritis
Gastrodisciasis 121.8
Gastroduodenitis (see also Gastritis) 535.5
- infectional 535.0
- virus, viral 008.8
- - specified type 008.6
Gastrodynia 536.8
Gastroenteritis (acute) (catarrhal) (congestive) (epidemic) (hemorrhagic) (presumed infectious) (zymotic) (see also Enteritis and note at category 009.3) 009.1
- allergic 558
- chronic 558
- dietetic 558
- due to food poisoning (see also Poisoning, food) 005.9
- infectious (see also Enteritis, infectious) 009.0
- noninfectious 558
- salmonella 003.0
- septic (see also Enteritis, infectious) 009.0
- toxic 558
- viral NEC (see also Enteritis, infectious) 008.8
- - specified type 008.6
Gastro-enterocolitis - see Enteritis
Gastro-enteroptosis 569.8
Gastrohepatitis (see also Gastritis) 535.5
Gastro-intestinal - see condition
Gastrojejunal - see condition
Gastrojejunitis 535.5
Gastrojejunocolic - see condition
Gastroliths 537.8
Gastromalacia 537.8
Gastroptosis 537.5
Gastrorrhagia (see also Hematemesis) 578.0

Gastrorrhea 536.8
- psychogenic 306.4
Gastroschisis (congenital) 756.7
- acquired 569.8
Gastrospasm (neurogenic) (reflex) 536.8
- neurotic 306.4
- psychogenic 306.4
Gastrostaxis (see also Hematemesis) 578.0
Gastrostenosis 537.8
Gastrosuccorrhea (continuous) (intermittent) 536.8
- neurotic 306.4
- psychogenic 306.4
Gaucher's
- disease (adult) (infantile) 272.7
- splenomegaly 272.7
Gee(-Herter)(-Thaysen) disease 579.0
Gelineau's syndrome 347
Gemination, tooth, teeth 520.2
Gemistocytoma (M9411/3)
- specified site - see Neoplasm, malignant
- unspecified site 191.9
General, generalized - see condition
Genital - see condition
Genitoanorectal syndrome 099.1
Genitourinary system - see condition
Genu
- congenital 755.6
- extrorsum, introrsum (acquired) 736.6
- - congenital 755.6
- - late effects of rickets 268.1
- - rachitic (old) 268.1
- recurvatum (acquired) 736.5
- - congenital 754.4
- - late effects of rickets 268.1
- valgum, varum (acquired) 736.4
- - congenital 755.6
- - late effects of rickets 268.1
Geographic tongue 529.1
Geotrichosis 117.9
- intestine 117.9
- lung 117.9
- mouth 117.9
Gephyrophobia 300.2
Gerbode's defect 745.4
Gerhardt's syndrome 478.3
Gerlier's disease 078.8
German measles 056.9
Germinoblastoma (diffuse) (M9614/3) 202.8
- follicular (M9692/3) 202.0
Germinoma (M9064/3) - see Neoplasm, malignant
Gerontoxon 371.4
Gestation (period) - see also Pregnancy
- ectopic - see Pregnancy, ectopic
Ghon tubercle primary infection 010.0

Ghost
− teeth 520.4
− vessels 370.6
Ghoul hand 102.3
Giant
− cell
− − epulis 523.8
− − peripheral granuloma 523.8
− colon (congenital) 751.3
− esophagus (congenital) 750.4
− kidney 753.3
− oesophagus (congenital) 750.4
− urticaria 995.1
− − hereditary 277.6
Giardiasis 007.1
Gibert's disease 696.3
Giddiness 780.4
− hysterical 300.1
− psychogenic 306.9
Gierke's disease 271.0
Gigantism (hypophyseal) 253.0
Gilbert's cholemia or disease 277.4
Gilchrist's disease 116.0
Gilford-Hutchinson disease 259.8
Gilles de la Tourette's disease 307.2
Gingivitis 523.1
− acute 523.0
− − necrotizing 101
− chronic 523.1
− desquamative 523.1
− expulsiva 523.4
− hyperplastic 523.1
− marginal, simple 523.1
− pellagrous 265.2
− ulcerative 523.1
− − acute necrotizing 101
− Vincent's 101
Gingivoglossitis 529.0
Gingivopericementitis 523.4
Gingivosis 523.1
Gingivostomatitis 523.1
− herpetic 054.2
Giovannini's disease 117.9
Gland, glandular - see condition
Glanders 024
Glanzmann's disease or thrombasthenia 287.1
Glass-blowers' disease 527.1
Glaucoma 365.9
− absolute 360.4
− acute 365.2
− − narrow angle 365.2
− − secondary 365.6
− angle-closure (acute) (chronic) (intermittent) 365.2
− borderline 365.0
− capsulare 365.5

Glaucoma - *continued*
− chronic 365.1
− − noncongestive 365.1
− − open angle 365.1
− − simple 365.1
− closed angle 365.2
− congenital 743.2
− corticosteroid-induced 365.3
− hypersecretion 365.8
− in
− − aniridia 743.4 † 365.4*
− − axenfeld's anomaly 743.4 † 365.4*
− − concussion of globe 365.6
− − congenital syndromes NEC 759.8 † 365.4*
− − disorder of lens NEC 365.5
− − hypermature cataract 365.5
− − iridocyclitis 365.6
− − ocular disorders NEC 365.6
− − postdislocation of lens 365.5
− − pseudoexfoliation of capsule 365.5
− − retinal vein occlusion 365.6
− − Rieger's anomaly 743.4 † 365.4*
− − rubeosis of iris 365.6
− − tumor of globe 365.6
− infantile 743.2
− low tension 365.1
− malignant 365.2
− narrow angle 365.2
− newborn 743.2
− noncongestive (chronic) 365.1
− nonobstructive 365.1
− obstructive 365.6
− − due to lens changes 365.5
− open angle 365.1
− phacolytic 365.5
− pigmentary 365.1
− postinfectious 365.6
− secondary NEC 365.6
− simple (chronic) 365.1
− simplex 365.1
− suspect 365.0
− syphilitic 095 † 365.6*
− traumatic 365.6
− − newborn 767.8
− tuberculous 017.3 † 365.6*
Glaucomatous flecks (subscapular) 366.3
Gleet 098.2
Glenard's disease 569.8
Glioblastoma (multiforme) (M9440/3)
− with sarcomatous component (M9442/3)
− − specified site - see Neoplasm, malignant
− − unspecified site 191.9
− giant cell (M9441/3)
− − specified site - see Neoplasm, malignant

Glioblastoma - *continued*
– giant cell - *continued*
– – unspecified site 191.9
– specified site - see Neoplasm, malignant
– unspecified site 191.9
Glioma (malignant) (M9380/3)
– astrocytic (M9400/3)
– – specified site - see Neoplasm,
    malignant
– – unspecified site 191.9
– mixed (M9382/3)
– – specified site - see Neoplasm,
    malignant
– – unspecified site 191.9
– nose 748.1
– specified site NEC - see Neoplasm,
    malignant
– subependymal (M9383/1) 237.5
– unspecified site 191.9
Gliomatosis cerebri (M9381/3) 191.0
Glioneuroma (M9505/1) - see Neoplasm,
    uncertain behavior
Gliosarcoma (M9380/3)
– specified site - see Neoplasm, malignant
– unspecified site 191.9
Gliosis (cerebral) 349.8
– spinal 336.0
Glisson's cirrhosis - see Cirrhosis, portal
Globinuria 791.2
Globus 306.4
– hystericus 300.1
Glomangioma (M8712/0) 228.0
Glomangiosarcoma (M8710/3) - see
    Neoplasm, connective tissue, malignant
Glomerular nephritis (see also Nephritis)
    583.9
Glomerulitis (see also Nephritis) 583.9
Glomerulonephritis (see also Nephritis)
    583.9
Glomerulosclerosis (see also Sclerosis,
    renal) 587
– intercapillary 250.3 † 581.8*
Glossalgia 529.6
Glossitis 529.0
– areata exfoliativa 529.1
– atrophic 529.4
– benign migratory 529.1
– gangrenous 529.0
– Hunter's 529.4
– median rhomboid 529.2
– Moeller's 529.4
– pellagrous 265.2
Glossodynia 529.6
– exfoliativa 529.4
Glossophytia 529.3
Glossoplegia 529.8
Glossopyrosis 529.6

Glossy skin 701.9
Glottis - see condition
Glottitis - see Glossitis
Glucagonoma (M8152/0)
– malignant (M8152/3)
– – pancreas 157.4
– – specified site NEC - see Neoplasm,
    malignant
– – unspecified site 157.4
– pancreas 211.7
– specified site NEC - see Neoplasm,
    benign
– unspecified site 211.7
Glucoglycinuria 270.7
Glue
– ear 381.2
– sniffing (airplane glue) 304.6
Glycinemia 270.7
Glycinuria (renal) 270.0
Glycogen
– infiltration (see also Disease, glycogen
    storage) 271.0
– storage disease (see also Disease,
    glycogen storage) 271.0
Glycogenosis (diffuse) (generalized) (with
    hepatic cirrhosis) (see also Disease,
    glycogen storage) 271.0
– cardiac 271.0 † 425.7*
Glycopenia 251.2
Glycosuria 791.5
– renal 271.4
Gnathostoma spinigerum (infection)
    (infestation) 128.1
– wandering swellings from 128.1
Gnathostomiasis 128.1

Goiter (adolescent) (colloid) (diffuse)
    (dipping) (due to iodine deficiency)
    (endemic) (heart) (hyperplastic) (internal)
    (intrathoracic) (juvenile) (mixed type)
    (parenchymatous) (plunging) (sporadic)
    (subclavicular) (substernal) 240.9 Note at
    category 009.3) 009.3
– with
– – hyperthyroidism (recurrent) (see also
    Goiter, toxic) 242.0
– – – adenomatous 242.3
– – – nodular 242.3
– – thyrotoxicosis (see also Goiter, toxic)
    242.0
– – – adenomatous 242.3
– – – nodular 242.3
– adenomatous (see also Goiter, nodular)
    241.9
– cancerous (M8000/3) 193
– congenital 246.1
– cystic (see also Goiter, nodular) 241.9

Goiter - *continued*
- due to enzyme defect in synthesis of thyroid hormone 246.1
- dyshormonogenic 246.1
- exophthalmic 242.0
- fibrous 245.3
- lingual 759.2
- lymphadenoid 245.2
- malignant (M8000/3) 193
- multinodular (nontoxic) 241.1
- - toxic or with hyperthyroidism 242.2
- nodular (nontoxic) 241.9
- - with
- - - hyperthyroidism 242.3
- - - thyrotoxicosis 242.3
- - endemic 241.9
- - exophthalmic 242.0
- - sporadic 241.9
- - toxic 242.3
- nontoxic 241.9
- - multinodular 241.1
- - uninodular 241.0
- pulsating 242.0
- simple 240.0
- toxic 242.0
- - adenomatous 242.3
- - multinodular 242.2
- - nodular 242.3
- - uninodular 242.1
- uninodular (nontoxic) 241.0
- - toxic or with hyperthyroidism 242.1

Goldberg-Maxwell syndrome 257.8
Goldblatt
- hypertension 440.1
- kidney 440.1
Goldenhaar's syndrome 756.0
Goldflam-Erb disease or syndrome 358.0
Goldscheider's disease 757.3
Goldstein's disease 448.0
Golfers' elbow 726.3
Gonadoblastoma (M9073/1)
- specified site - see Neoplasm, uncertain behavior
- unspecified site
- - female 236.2
- - male 236.4
Gonecystitis (see also Vesiculitis) 608.0

Gongylonemiasis 125.6
- mouth 125.6
Goniosynechiae 364.7
Gonococcemia 098.8
Gonococcus, gonococcal (disease) (infection) (see also Condition) 098.0
- anus 098.7
- bursa 098.5 † 727.3*
- chronic NEC 098.2

Gonococcus - *continued*
- complicating pregnancy, childbirth or puerperium 647.1
- - fetus or newborn 760.2
- conjunctiva, conjunctivitis (neonatorum) 098.4 † 372.0*
- endocardium 098.8 † 421.1*
- eye (newborn) 098.4 † 372.0*
- fallopian tubes (chronic) 098.3 † 614.-*
- - acute 098.1 † 614.0*
- genito-urinary (organ) (system) (tract) (acute) (see also Gonorrhea) 098.0
- - lower 098.0
- - - chronic 098.2
- - upper 098.1
- - - chronic 098.3
- heart 098.8 † 421.1*
- joint 098.5 † 711.4*
- lymphatic (gland) (node) 098.8
- meninges 098.8 † 320.7*
- pelvis (acute) 098.1
- - chronic or duration of 2 months or over 098.3
- pharynx 098.6
- pyosalpinx (chronic) 098.3 † 614.-*
- - acute 098.1 † 614.0*
- rectum 098.7
- skin 098.8
- specified site NEC 098.8
- tendon sheath 098.5 † 727.0*
- urethra (acute) 098.0
- - chronic or duration of 2 months or over 098.2
- vulva (acute) 098.0
- - chronic or duration of 2 months or over 098.2
Gonocytoma (M9073/1)
- specified site - see Neoplasm, uncertain behavior
- unspecified site
- - female 236.2
- - male 236.4
Gonorrhea 098.0
- acute 098.0
- Bartholin's gland (acute) 098.0
- - chronic or duration of 2 months or over 098.2
- bladder (acute) 098.1 † 595.4*
- - chronic or duration of 2 months or over 098.3 † 595.4*
- cervix (acute) 098.1 † 616.0*
- - chronic or duration of 2 months or over 098.3 † 616.0*
- chronic 098.2
- complicating pregnancy, childbirth or puerperium 647.1
- - fetus or newborn 760.2

Gonorrhea - *continued*
- conjunctiva, conjunctivitis (neonatorum) 098.4 † 372.0*
- Cowper's gland (acute) 098.0
- - chronic or duration of 2 months or over 098.2
- duration two months or over 098.2
- fallopian tube (chronic) 098.3 † 614.-*
- - acute 098.1 † 614.0*
- genitourinary system (organ) (system) (tract) (acute) 098.0
- - chronic 098.2
- - duration two months or over 098.2
- kidney (acute) 098.1 † 583.8*
- - chronic or duration of 2 months or over 098.3 † 583.8*
- ovary (acute) 098.1 † 614.0*
- - chronic or duration of 2 months or over 098.3 † 614.-*
- pelvis (acute) 098.1
- - chronic or duration of 2 months or over 098.3
- penis (acute) 098.0
- - chronic or duration of 2 months or over 098.2
- prostate (acute) 098.1 † 601.4*
- - chronic or duration of 2 months or over 098.3 † 601.4*
- seminal vesicle (acute) 098.1 † 608.0*
- - chronic or duration of 2 months or over 098.3 † 608.0*
- specified site not listed - see Gonococcus
- spermatic cord (acute) 098.1
- - chronic or duration of 2 months or over 098.3
- urethra (acute) 098.0
- - chronic or duration of 2 months or over 098.2
- vagina (acute) 098.0
- - chronic or duration of 2 months or over 098.2
- vas deferens (acute) 098.1
- - chronic or duration of 2 months or over 098.3
- vulva (acute) 098.0
- - chronic or duration of 2 months or over 098.2
Goodpasture's syndrome 446.2
Gopalan's syndrome 266.2
Gorlin-Chaudry-Moss syndrome 759.8
Gougerot-Carteaud disease or syndrome 701.8
Goundou 102.6
Gout, gouty 274.9
- lead 984.-
- - specified type of lead - see Table of drugs and chemicals

Gout - *continued*
- saturnine 984.-
- - specified type of lead - see Table of drugs and chemicals
- syphilitic 095
- tophi NEC 274.0 † 712.0*
- - ear 274.8 † 380.8*
- - heart 274.8 † 425.7*
Gower's muscular dystrophy 359.1
Gradenigo's syndrome 382.0
Grain
- handlers' disease or lung 495.8
- mite 133.8
Grand mal (idiopathic) 345.1
Granite workers' lung 502
Granular - see also condition
- kidney (contracting) (see also Sclerosis, renal) 587
- liver - see Cirrhosis, liver
Granulation tissue - see also Granuloma
- abnormal or excessive 701.5
Granulocytopenia, granulocytopenic (primary) 288.0
- malignant 288.0
Granuloma 686.1
- abdomen 568.8
- annulare 695.8
- apical 522.6
- aural 380.2
- beryllium (skin) 709.4
- bone 730.1
- - eosinophilic 277.8
- - from residual foreign body 730.9
- canaliculus lacrimalis 375.8
- cerebral 348.8
- coccidioidal (primary) (progressive) 114
- - lung 114
- - meninges 114
- colon 569.8
- conjunctiva 372.6
- dental 522.6
- ear, middle (see also Otitis, media) 385.8
- eosinophilic 277.8
- - bone 277.8
- - lung 277.8
- - oral mucosa 528.9
- eyelid 373.8
- facial
- - lethal midline 446.3
- - malignant 446.3
- foot NEC 686.1
- foreign body (in soft tissue) NEC 728.8
- - in operation wound 998.4
- - skin 709.4
- gangraenescens 446.3
- giant cell (central) (reparative) (jaw) 526.3

Granuloma - *continued*
- giant cell - *continued*
- - gingiva 523.8
- - peripheral (gingiva) 523.8
- gland (lymph) 289.3
- Hodgkin's (M9661/3) 201.1
- ileum 569.8
- infectious NEC 136.9
- inguinale (Donovan) 099.2
- - venereal 099.2
- intestine 569.8
- iridocyclitis 364.1
- jaw (bone) 526.3
- - reparative giant cell 526.3
- kidney (see also Infection, kidney) 590.9
- lacrimal sac (nonspecific) 375.8
- larynx 478.7
- lethal midline 446.3
- lipid 999.9
- liver 572.8
- lung (infectious) (see also Fibrosis, lung) 515
- - coccidioidal 114
- - eosinophilic 277.8
- Majocchi's 110.6
- malignant of face 446.3
- mandible 526.3
- midline 446.3
- monilial 112.3
- operation wound 998.5
- - foreign body 998.4
- - stitch 998.4
- - talc 998.7
- oral mucosa, pyogenic 528.9
- orbit, orbital 376.1
- paracoccidioidal 116.1
- penis 099.2
- periapical 522.6
- peritoneum 568.8
- - due to ova of helminths NEC (see also Helminthiasis) 128.9
- postmastoidectomy cavity 383.3
- prostate 601.8
- pudendi (ulcerating) 099.2
- pudendorum (ulcerative) 099.2
- pulp, internal (tooth) 521.4
- pyogenic, pyogenicum (skin) 686.1
- - of maxillary alveolar ridge 522.6
- - oral mucosa 528.9
- rectum 569.4
- reticulohistiocytic 277.8
- rubrum nasi 705.8
- schistosoma 120.9
- septic (skin) 686.1
- silica (skin) 709.4
- sinus (accessory) (infectional) (nasal) (see also Sinusitis) 473.9

Granuloma - *continued*
- skin (pyogenicum) 686.1
- - from foreign body or material 709.4
- spine
- - syphilitic (epidural) 094.8
- - tuberculous 015.0 † 730.4*
- stich (postoperative) 998.4
- suppurative (skin) 686.1
- swimming pool 031.1
- talc 728.8
- - in operation wound 998.7
- telangiectaticum (skin) 686.1
- trichophyticum 110.6
- tropicum 102.4
- umbilicus 686.1
- - newborn 771.4
- urethra 599.8
- vagina 099.2
- venereum 099.2
- vocal cords 478.5
Granulomatosis NEC 686.1
- infantiseptica 771.2
- miliary 027.0
- necrotizing, respiratory 446.4
- progressive septic 288.1
- Wegener's 446.4
Granulomatous tissue - see Granuloma
Granulosis rubra nasi 705.8
Graphite fibrosis (of lung) 503
Graphospasm 300.8
- organic 333.8
Grating scapula 733.9
Gravel (urinary) (see also Calculus) 592.9
Graves' disease 242.0
Gravis - see condition
Grawitz tumor (M8312/3) 189.0
Grayness, hair (premature) 704.3
- congenital 757.4
Green sickness 280
Greenfield's disease 330.0
Greenstick fracture - code as Fracture, closed
Griesinger's disease (see also Ancylostomiasis) 126.9
Grinders'
- asthma 502
- lung 502
- phthisis 011.4
Grinding, teeth 306.8
Grip
- Dabney's 074.1
- devil's 074.1
Grippe, grippal - see also Influenza
- Balkan 083.0
- summer 074.8
Grippy cold 487.1
Groin - see condition

Growing pains, children 781.9
Growth (fungoid) (neoplastic) (new)
  (M8000/1) - see also Neoplasm,
  unspecified nature
- adenoid (vegetative) 474.2
- benign (M8000/0) - see Neoplasm,
  benign
- malignant (M8000/3) - see Neoplasm,
  malignant
- rapid, childhood V21.0
- secondary (M8000/6) - see Secondary
  neoplasm
Gruber's hernia - see Hernia, abdominal
Gruby's disease 110.0
Gubler-Millard paralysis 344.8
Guerin-Stern syndrome 754.8
Guillain-Barre disease or syndrome 357.0
Guinea worms (infection) (infestation)
  125.7
Gull and Sutton's disease - see
  Hypertension, kidney
Gull's disease 244.8
Gum - see condition
Gumboil 522.7
Gumma (syphilitic) 095
- artery 093.8
- - cerebral or spinal 094.8
- bone 095
- - of yaws (late) 102.6
- brain 094.8
- cauda equina 094.8
- central nervous system 094.9
- ciliary body 095 † 364.1*
- congenital 090.5
- - testicle 090.5
- eyelid 095 † 373.5*
- heart 093.8
- intracranial 094.8
- iris 095 † 364.1*
- kidney 095
- larynx 095
- leptomeninges 094.2 † 320.7*

Gumma - *continued*
- liver 095
- meninges 094.2 † 320.7*
- myocardium 093.8
- nasopharynx 095
- neurosyphilitic 094.9
- nose 095
- orbit 095 † 376.1*
- palate (soft) 095
- penis 095
- pericardium 093.8
- pharynx 095
- pituitary 095
- scrofulous 017.0
- skin 095
- specified site NEC 095
- spinal cord 094.8
- tongue 095
- tonsil 095
- trachea 095
- tuberculous 017.0
- ulcerative due to yaws 102.4
- ureter 095
- yaws 102.4
- - bone 102.6
Gunn's syndrome 742.8
Gunshot wound - see also Wound, open
- fracture - code as Fracture, open
- internal organs (abdomen, chest or
  pelvis) - see Injury, internal, by site, with
  open wound
- intracranial 851.1
Gynandrism 752.7
Gynandroblastoma (M8632/1)
- specified site - see Neoplasm, uncertain
  behavior
- unspecified site
- - female 236.2
- - male 236.4
Gynecomastia 611.1
Gynephobia 300.2
Gyrate scalp 757.3

H

H disease 270.0
Habit, habituation
− chorea 307.2
− disturbance, child 307.9
− drug - see Dependence, drug
− laxative 305.9
− spasm 307.2
− tic 307.2
Haff disease 985.1
Hageman factor defect, deficiency or
disease (see also Defect, coagulation)
286.3
Haglund's disease or osteochondrosis 732.5
Hailey-Hailey disease 757.3
Hair - see also condition
− plucking 307.9
Hairball in stomach 935.2
Hairy black tongue 529.3
Half vertebra 756.1
Halitosis 784.9
Hallerman-Streiff syndrome 756.0
Hallervorden-Spatz disease 333.0
Hallopeau's
− acrodermatitis 696.1
− disease 701.0
Hallucination (auditory) (gustatory)
(olfactory) (tactile) 780.1
− visual 368.1
Hallucinosis 298.9
− alcoholic (acute) 291.3
− induced by drug 292.1
Hallus - see Hallux
Hallux 735.9
− malleus (acquired) 735.3
− rigidus (acquired) 735.2
− − congenital 755.6
− − late effects of rickets 268.1
− valgus (acquired) 735.0
− − congenital 755.6
− varus (acquired) 735.1
− − congenital 755.6
Hamartoblastoma 759.6
Hamartoma 759.6
− epithelial (gingival), odontogenic, central
or peripheral (M9321/0) 213.1
− − upper jaw (bone) 213.0
Hamman-Rich syndrome 516.3
Hammer toe (acquired) 735.4
− congenital 755.6
− late effects of rickets 268.1

Hand - see condition
Hand-Schuller-Christian disease or
syndrome 277.8
Hanging (asphyxia) (strangulation)
(suffocation) 994.7
Hangnail (with lymphangitis) 681.0
Hangover (alcohol) 305.0
Hanot's cirrhosis or disease - see Cirrhosis,
biliary
Hanot-Chauffard(-Troisier) syndrome
275.0
Hansen's disease 030.9
− benign (form) 030.1
− malignant (form) 030.0
Harada's syndrome 363.2
Hardening
− artery - see Arteriosclerosis
− brain 348.8
− liver 571.8
Harelip (complete) (incomplete) 749.1
− with cleft palate 749.2
Harlequin (fetus) (color change syndrome)
757.1
Harley's disease 283.2
Harris's lines 733.9
Hart's disease 270.0
Hartnup's disease 270.0
Harvester lung 495.0
Hashimoto's disease or struma 245.2
Hass's disease or osteochondrosis 732.3
Hassal-Henle bodies or warts (cornea)
371.4
Haut mal 345.1
Haverhill fever 026.1
Hawkins's keloid 701.4
Hayem-Widal syndrome 283.9
Haygarth's nodosities 715.0
Hazard-Crile tumor (M8350/3) 193
Hb (abnormal)
− disease - see Disease, hemoglobin
− trait - see Trait
Head - see condition
Headache 784.0
− allergic 346.2
− cluster 346.2
− emotional 307.8
− histamine 346.2
− lumbar puncture 349.0
− migraine 346.9
− nonorganic origin 307.8

Headache - *continued*
- postspinal 349.0
- psychogenic 307.8
- sick 346.1
- spinal fluid loss 349.0
- tension 307.8
- vascular 784.0
- - migraine type 346.9
- vasomotor 346.9
Health
- advice V65.4
- checkup V70.0
- education V65.4
- instruction V65.4
- services provided because (of)
- - boarding school residence V60.6
- - holiday relief for person providing
  home care V60.5
- - inadequate
- - - housing V60.1
- - - resources V60.2
- - lack of housing V60.0
- - no care available in home V60.4
- - person living alone V60.3
- - poverty V60.2
- - residence in institution V60.6
- - specified cause NEC V60.8
Healthy
- infant
- - accompanying sick mother V65.0
- - receiving care V20.1
- person accompanying sick person V65.0
Heart - see condition
Heartburn 787.1
- psychogenic 306.4
Heat (effects) 992.9
- apoplexy 992.0
- burn - see also Burn
- - from sun 692.7
- collapse 992.1
- cramps 992.2
- dermatitis or eczema 692.8
- edema 992.7
- erythema - code by site under Burn 949.1
- excessive 992.9
- - specified effect NEC 992.8
- exhaustion 992.5
- - anhydrotic 992.3
- - due to
- - - salt (and water) depletion 992.4
- - - water depletion 992.3
- - - - with salt depletion 992.4
- fatigue (transient) 992.6
- fever 992.0
- hyperpyrexia 992.0
- prickly 705.1
- prostration - see Heat, exhaustion

Heat - *continued*
- pyrexia 992.0
- rash 705.1
- specified effect NEC 992.8
- stroke 992.0
- sunburn 692.7
- syncope 992.1
Heavy-for-dates (fetus or infant) 766.1
- exceptionally 766.0
- 4500g or more 766.0
Hebephrenia, hebephrenic (acute) 295.1
- dementia (praecox) 295.1
- schizophrenia 295.1
Heberden's
- disease 715.0
- nodes 715.0
Hebra, nose 040.1
Hebra's
- disease
- - meaning
- - - dermatitis exfoliativa 695.8
- - - erythema multiforme exudativum
  695.1
- - - pityriasis rubra 695.8
- - pityriasis 695.8
- prurigo 698.2
Heel - see condition
Heerfordt's disease 135
Hegglin's anomaly or syndrome 288.2
Heidenhain's disease 290.1
- with dementia 290.1
Heilmeyer-Schoner disease (M9842/3)
  207.1
Heine-Medin disease 045.9 † 323.2*
Heinz-body anemia, congenital 282.7
Heller's disease or syndrome 299.1
Helminthiasis (see also Infestation) 128.9
- Ancylostoma (see also Ancylostoma)
  126.9
- intestinal NEC 127.9
- - mixed types (intestinal) (types
  classifiable to more than one of the
  titles 120.0-127.7) 127.8
- - specified type NEC 127.7
- mixed types (intestinal) (types classifiable
  to more than one of the titles
  120.0-127.7) 127.8
- necator (americanus) 126.1
- specified type NEC 128.8
Heloma 700
Hemangioblastoma (M9161/1) - see also
  Neoplasm, connective tissue, uncertain
  behavior
- malignant (M9161/3) - see Neoplasm,
  connective tissue, malignant
Hemangioblastomatosis cerebelloretinal
  759.6

Hemangioendothelioma (M9130/1) - see
also Neoplasm, uncertain behavior
− benign (M9130/0) 228.0
− bone (diffuse) (M9130/3) - see
Neoplasm, bone, malignant
− malignant (M9130/3) - see Neoplasm,
connective tissue, malignant
− nervous system (M9130/0) 228.0
Hemangiofibroma (M9160/0) - see
Neoplasm, benign
Hemangiolipoma (M8861/0) 214
Hemangioma (M9120/0) 228.0
− arteriovenous (M9123/0) 228.0
− capillary (M9131/0) 228.0
− cavernous (M9121/0) 228.0
− infantile (M9131/0) 228.0
− intramuscular (M9132/0) 228.0
− juvenile (M9131/0) 228.0
− malignant (M9120/3) - see Neoplasm,
connective tissue, malignant
− plexiform (M9131/0) 228.0
− racemose (M9123/0) 228.0
− sclerosing (M8832/0) - see Neoplasm,
skin, benign
− simplex (M9131/0) 228.0
− venous (M9122/0) 228.0
− verrucous keratotic (M9142/0) 228.0
Hemangiomatosis (systemic) 757.3
− involving single site - see Hemangioma
Hemangiopericytoma (M9150/1) - see also
Neoplasm, connective tissue, uncertain
behavior
− benign (M9150/0) - see Neoplasm,
connective tissue, benign
− malignant (M9150/3) - see Neoplasm,
connective tissue, malignant
Hemangiosarcoma (M9120/3) - see
Neoplasm, connective tissue, malignant
Hemarthrosis (nontraumatic) 719.1
− traumatic - see Sprain, by site
Hematemesis 578.0
− with ulcer - code by site under Ulcer, with
hemorrhage 533.9
− newborn 772.4
− − due to swallowed maternal blood 777.3
Hematidrosis 705.8
Hematinuria (see also Hemoglobinuria)
791.2
− malarial 084.8
− paroxysmal 283.2
Hematite miners' lung 503
Hematocele 608.8
− cord, male 608.8
− female NEC 629.0
− ischiorectal 569.8
− male NEC 608.8
− ovary 629.0

Hematocele - continued
− pelvis, pelvic
− − female 629.0
− − − with ectopic pregnancy, NEC 633.9
− − male 608.8
− periuterine 629.0
− retrouterine 629.0
− scrotum 608.8
− spermatic cord (diffuse) 608.8
− testis 608.8
− tunica vaginalis 608.8
− uterine ligament 629.0
Hematocephalus 742.4
Hematochyluria (see also Infestation,
filarial) 125.9
Hematocolpos 626.8
Hematocornea 371.1
Hematogenous - see condition
Hematoma (traumatic) (skin surface intact)
- see also Contusion
− with
− − crush injury - see Crush
− − fracture - see Fracture
− − injury of internal organs - see Injury,
internal, by site
− − nerve injury - see Injury, nerve
− − open wound - see Wound, open
− aorta, dissecting 441.0
− arterial (complicating trauma) 904.9
− − specified site - see Injury, blood vessel
− auricle 380.3
− birth injury 767.8
− brain 853.0
− − with
− − − cerebral laceration or contusion (see
also Laceration, cerebral) 851.0
− − − open intracranial wound 853.1
− − − skull fracture - see Fracture, skull
− − fetus or newborn NEC 767.0
− − nontraumatic (see also Hemorrhage,
brain) 431
− − − epidural or extradural 432.0
− − − newborn NEC 772.8
− − − subarachnoid, arachnoid or
meningeal (see also Hemorrhage,
subarachnoid) 430
− − − subdural (see also Hemorrhage,
subdural) 432.1
− − subarachnoid, arachnoid or meningeal
- see Hematoma, subarachnoid
− − subdural, epidural or extradural - see
Hematoma, subdural
− breast (nontraumatic) 611.8
− broad ligament (nontraumatic) 620.7
− − traumatic - see Injury, internal, broad
ligament
− calcified NEC 959.9

Hematoma - *continued*
- vulva - *continued*
- - fetus or newborn 767.8
Hematometra 621.4
Hematomyelia 336.1
- with fracture, vertebra (conditions in 805-) (see also Fracture, vertebra, by region, with spinal cord lesion) 806.8
- fetus or newborn 767.4
Hematomyelitis 323.9
Hematoperitoneum - see Hemoperitoneum
Hematopneumothorax (see also Hemothorax) 511.8
Hematoporphyria (congenital) 277.1
- acquired 277.1
Hematoporphyrinuria (congenital) 277.1
- acquired 277.1
Hematorachis, hematorrhachis 336.1
- fetus or newborn 767.4
Hematosalpinx 620.8
- infectional (see also Salpingo-oophoritis) 614.2
Hematospermia 608.8
Hematothorax (see also Hemothorax) 511.8
Hematuria (essential) (idiopathic) 599.7
- endemic 120.0
- intermittent 599.7
- malarial 084.8
- paroxysmal 599.7
- sulphonamide, sulfonamide
- - correct substance properly administered 599.7
- - overdose or wrong substance given or taken 961.0
- tropical 120.0
- tuberculous 016.9
Hemballism(us) 333.5
Hemeralopia (night blindness) 368.6
- meaning day blindness 368.1
- vitamin A deficiency 264.5 † 368.6*
Hemianalgesia (see also Disturbance, sensation) 782.0
Hemianencephaly 740.0
Hemianesthesia (see also Disturbance, sensation) 782.0
Hemianopia, hemianopsia (binasal) (bitemporal) (nasal) (peripheral) (heteronymous) (homonymous) 368.4
- syphilitic 095 † 368.4*
Hemiathetosis 781.0
Hemiatrophy 799.8
- cerebellar 334.8
- face 349.8
- - progressive 349.8
- fascia 728.9
- leg 728.2
- tongue 529.8

Hemicardia 746.8
Hemicephalus, hemicephaly 740.0
Hemichorea 333.5
Hemicrania 346.9
- congenital malformation 740.0
Hemidystrophy - see Hemiatrophy
Hemiectromelia 755.4
Hemihypalgesia (see also Disturbance, sensation) 782.0
Hemihypertrophy (congenital) 759.8
- cranial 756.0
Hemihypesthesia (see also Disturbance, sensation) 782.0
Hemimelia 755.4
- lower limb 755.3
- upper limb 755.2
Hemiparalysis (see also Hemiplegia) 342.9
Hemiparesis (see also Hemiplegia) 342.9
Hemiparesthesia (see also Disturbance, sensation) 782.0
Hemiplegia 342.9
- acute (see also Disease, cerebrovascular, acute) 436
- alternans facialis 344.8
- apoplectic (see also Disease, cerebrovascular, acute) 436
- arteriosclerotic 437.0
- ascending (spinal) NEC 344.8
- attack (see also Disease, cerebrovascular, acute) 436
- brain, cerebral (current episode) 437.8
- cerebral (current episode) 437.8
- congenital (cerebral) (spastic) (spinal) 343.1
- cortical (current episode) 437.8
- embolic (current episode) (see also Embolism, brain) 434.1
- flaccid 342.0
- hypertensive (current episode) 437.8
- hysterical 300.1
- infantile (postnatal) 343.4
- middle alternating NEC 344.8
- newborn NEC 767.0
- seizure (current episode) (see also Disease, cerebrovascular, acute) 436
- spastic 342.1
- - congenital or infantile 343.1
- thrombotic (current episode) (see also Thrombosis, brain) 434.0
Hemisection, spinal cord - code by region under Fracture, vertebra, with spinal cord lesion
Hemispasm 781.0
- facial 781.0
Hemisporosis 117.9
Hemitremor 781.0
Hemivertebra 756.1

Hemochromatosis 275.0
– with refractory anemia 285.0
– diabetic 275.0
– hereditary 275.0
– liver 275.0
– myocardium 275.0
– primary idiopathic 275.0
– secondary 275.0
Hemodialysis V56.0
Hemoglobin - see also condition
– abnormal (disease) - see Disease,
  hemoglobin
– AS genotype 282.5
– fetal, hereditary persistence 282.7
– low NEC 285.9
– S (Hb S), heterozygous 282.5
Hemoglobinemia 283.2
– due to blood transfusion 999.8
– paroxysmal 283.2
Hemoglobinopathy (mixed) NEC 282.7
– with thalassemia 282.4
– sickle-cell 282.6
– – with thalassemia 282.4
Hemoglobinuria 791.2
– with anemia, hemolytic, acquired
  (chronic) NEC 283.2
– cold (agglutinin) (paroxysmal) (with
  Raynaud's syndrome) 283.2
– due to
– – exertion 283.2
– – hemolysis 283.2
– intermittent 283.2
– malarial 084.8
– march 283.2
– nocturnal (paroxysmal) 283.2
– paroxysmal (cold) (nocturnal) 283.2

Hemolymphangioma (M9175/0) 228.1
Hemolysis
– fetal - see Jaundice, fetus or newborn
– intravascular
– – with
– – – abortion - see categories 634-639,
      fourth digit .1
– – – ectopic gestation 639.1
– – – hemorrhage of pregnancy 641.3
– – – – fetus or newborn 762.1
– – postpartum 666.3
– neonatal - see Jaundice, fetus or newborn
Hemolytic - see condition

Hemopericardium (with effusion) 423.0
– newborn 772.8
– traumatic (see also Hemothorax,
  traumatic) 860.2
– – with open wound into thorax 860.3
Hemoperitoneum 568.8
– infectional (see also Peritonitis) 567.2

Hemoperitoneum - *continued*
– traumatic - see Injury, internal,
  peritoneum
Hemophilia (familial) (hereditary) 286.0
– A 286.0
– B 286.1
– C 286.2
– calcipriva (see also Fibrinolysis) 286.7
– classical 286.0
– nonfamilial (see also Fibrinolysis) 286.7
– vascular 286.4
Hemophilus influenzae NEC (see also
  Condition) 041.5
Hemophthalmos 360.4
Hemopneumothorax (see also Hemothorax)
  511.8
– traumatic 860.4
– – with open wound into thorax 860.5
Hemoptysis 786.3
– newborn 770.3
– tuberculous - code by type under
  tuberculosis, pulmonary 011.9
Hemorrhage, hemorrhagic 459.0
– abdomen 459.0
– accidental, antepartum 641.2
– – fetus or newborn 762.1
– adenoid 474.8
– adrenal (capsule) (gland) 255.4
– – medulla 255.4
– – newborn 772.5
– after labor - see Hemorrhage, postpartum
– alveolar
– – lung, newborn 770.3
– – process 525.8
– alveolus 525.8
– amputation stump (surgical) 998.1
– – secondary, delayed 997.6
– anemia (chronic) 280
– – acute 285.1
– antepartum - see Hemorrhage, pregnancy
– anus (sphincter) 569.3
– apoplexy (stroke) (see also Hemorrhage,
  brain) 432.9
– arachnoid - see Hemorrhage,
  subarachnoid
– artery 459.0
– – brain (see also Hemorrhage, brain)
  431
– – middle meningeal - see Hemorrhage,
  subarachnoid
– basilar (ganglion) (see also Hemorrhage,
  brain) 431
– bladder 596.8
– bowel 578.9
– – newborn 772.4
– brain (miliary) (nontraumatic) 431
– – due to

Hemorrhage - *continued*
- brain - *continued*
- - due to - *continued*
- - - birth injury 767.0
- - - rupture of aneurysm (congenital)
    (see also Hemorrhage,
    subarachnoid) 430
- - - - mycotic 431
- - - syphilis 094.8
- - epidural or extradural - see
    Hemorrhage, extradural
- - fetus NEC 767.0
- - newborn (traumatic) NEC 767.0
- - - anoxic NEC 772.8
- - puerperal, postpartum, childbirth
    674.0
- - subarachnoid, arachnoid or meningeal
    - see Hemorrhage, subarachnoid
- - subdural - see Hemorrhage, subdural
- - traumatic NEC 853.0
- - - with
- - - - cerebral laceration or contusion
    (see also Laceration, cerebral)
    851.0
- - - - open intracranial wound 853.1
- - - - skull fracture - see Fracture, skull
- - - - subarachnoid, subdural or
    extradural - see Hemorrhage,
    subarachnoid, traumatic
- breast 611.7
- bronchial tube - see Hemorrhage, lung
- bronchopulmonary - see Hemorrhage,
    lung
- bronchus - see Hemorrhage, lung
- bulbar (see also Hemorrhage, brain) 431
- capillary 448.9
- - primary 287.8
- cardiovascular (see also Carditis) 429.8
- cecum 578.9
- cephalic (see also Hemorrhage, brain)
    431
- cerebellar (see also Hemorrhage, brain)
    431
- cerebellum (see also Hemorrhage, brain)
    431
- cerebral (see also Hemorrhage, brain)
    431
- - fetus or newborn (anoxic) (traumatic)
    767.0
- cerebromeningeal (see also Hemorrhage,
    brain) 431
- cerebrospinal (see also Hemorrhage,
    brain) 431
- cerebrum (see also Hemorrhage, brain)
    431
- cervix (uteri) (stump) NEC 622.8
- cesarean section wound 674.3

Hemorrhage - *continued*
- chamber anterior (eye) 364.4
- childbirth - see Hemorrhage,
    complicating delivery
- choroid (expulsive) 363.6
- ciliary body 364.4
- cochlea 386.8
- colon - see Hemorrhage, intestine
- complicating
- - delivery 641.9
- - - associated with
- - - - afibrinogenemia 641.3
- - - - - fetus or newborn 763.8
- - - - coagulation defect 641.3
- - - - - fetus or newborn 763.8
- - - - hyperfibrinolysis 641.3
- - - - - fetus or newborn 763.8
- - - - hypofibrinogenemia 641.3
- - - - - fetus or newborn 763.8
- - - due to
- - - - low-lying placenta 641.1
- - - - - fetus or newborn 762.0
- - - - placenta previa 641.1
- - - - - fetus or newborn 762.0
- - - - premature separation of placenta
    641.2
- - - - - fetus or newborn 762.1
- - - - retained
- - - - - placenta 666.0
- - - - - secundines 666.2
- - - - trauma 641.8
- - - - - fetus or newborn 763.8
- - - - uterine leiomyoma 641.8
- - - - - fetus or newborn 763.8
- - - fetus or newborn NEC 762.1
- - surgical procedure 998.1
- concealed NEC 459.0
- congenital 772.9
- conjunctiva 372.7
- - newborn 772.8
- cord, newborn 772.0
- - stump 772.3
- corpus luteum (ruptured) 620.1
- cortical (see also Hemorrhage, brain) 431
- cranial (see also Hemorrhage, brain)
    432.9
- cutaneous 287.2
- - newborn 772.6
- delayed
- - with
- - - abortion - see categories 634-639,
    fourth digit .1
- - - ectopic gestation 639.1
- - postpartum 666.2
- diathesis (familial) 287.9
- - newborn 776.0
- disease 287.9

Hemorrhage - *continued*
- disease - *continued*
- - newborn 776.0
- - specified type NEC 287.8
- due to (presence of) any device, implant or graft classifiable to 996.0-996.5 996.7
- duodenum, duodenal 537.8
- - ulcer - see Ulcer, duodenum, with hemorrhage
- dura mater - see Hemorrhage, subdural
- endotracheal - see Hemorrhage, lung
- epidural - see Hemorrhage, extradural
- episiotomy 674.3
- esophagus 530.8
- - varix 456.0
- excessive
- - with
- - - abortion - see categories 634-639, fourth digit .1
- - - ectopic gestation 639.1
- extradural (traumatic) 852.0
- - with
- - - cerebral laceration or contusion (see also Laceration, cerebral) 851.0
- - - open intracranial wound 852.1
- - - skull fracture - see Fracture, skull
- - birth injury 767.0
- - fetus or newborn (anoxic) (traumatic) 767.0
- - nontraumatic 432.0
- eye 379.8
- - fundus 362.8
- fallopian tube 620.8
- fetal-maternal 772.0
- - affecting management of pregnancy or puerperium 656.0
- fetus, fetal 772.0
- - from
- - - cut end of co-twin's cord 772.0
- - - placenta 772.0
- - - ruptured cord 772.0
- - - vasa praevia 772.0
- - into
- - - co-twin 772.0
- - - mother's circulation 772.0
- - - - affecting management of pregnancy or puerperium 656.0
- fibrinogenolysis (see also Fibrinolysis) 286.6
- fibrinolytic (acquired) (see also Fibrinolysis) 286.6
- fontanel 767.1
- from tracheostomy stoma 519.0
- fundus, eye 362.8
- funis
- - affecting fetus or newborn 772.0
- - complicating delivery 663.8

Hemorrhage - *continued*
- gastric (see also Hemorrhage, stomach) 578.9
- gastro-enteric 578.9
- - newborn 772.4
- gastrointestinal (tract) 578.9
- - newborn 772.4
- genitourinary (tract) NEC 599.8
- gingiva 523.8
- globe (eye) 360.4
- gravidarum - see Hemorrhage, pregnancy
- gum 523.8
- heart (see also Carditis) 429.8
- hypopharyngeal (throat) 459.0
- intermenstrual 626.8
- - irregular 626.6
- - regular 626.5
- internal (organs) NEC 459.0
- - capsule (see also Hemorrhage, brain) 431
- - ear 386.8
- - newborn 772.8
- intestine 578.9
- - congenital 772.4
- - newborn 772.4
- into
- - bladder wall 596.7
- - bursa 727.8
- - corpus luysii (see also Hemorrhage, brain) 431
- intra-abdominal 459.0
- intra-alveolar (lung), newborn 770.3
- intracerebral (see also Hemorrhage, brain) 431
- intracranial NEC (see also Hemorrhage, brain) 432.9
- intramedullary NEC 336.1
- intra-ocular 360.4
- intrapartum - see Hemorrhage, complicating delivery
- intrapelvic
- - female 629.8
- - male 459.0
- intraperitoneal 459.0
- intrapontine (see also Hemorrhage, brain) 431
- intra-uterine 621.4
- - complicating delivery - see Hemorrhage, complicating delivery
- - in pregnancy or childbirth - see Hemorrhage, pregnancy
- - postpartum - see Hemorrhage, postpartum
- intraventricular (see also Hemorrhage, brain) 431
- - fetus or newborn (anoxic) (traumatic) 772.1

Hemorrhage - *continued*
- intravesical 596.7
- iris (postinfectional) (postinflammatory) (toxic) 364.4
- joint (nontraumatic) 719.1
- kidney 593.8
- knee (joint) 719.1
- labyrinth 386.8
- lenticular striate artery (see also Hemorrhage, brain) 431
- ligature, vessel 998.1
- liver 573.8
- lung 786.3
- - newborn 770.3
- - tuberculous - code by type under Tuberculosis, pulmonary 011.9
- massive epicranial subaponeurotic, birth injury 767.1
- maternal, affecting fetus or newborn 762.1
- mediastinum - see Hemorrhage, lung
- medulla (see also Hemorrhage, brain) 431
- membrane (brain) (see also Hemorrhage, subarachnoid) 430
- - spinal cord - see Hemorrhage, spinal cord
- meninges, meningeal (brain) (middle) (see also Hemorrhage, subarachnoid) 430
- - spinal cord - see Hemorrhage, spinal cord
- mesentery 568.8
- metritis 626.8
- midbrain (see also Hemorrhage, brain) 431
- mole 631
- mouth 528.9
- mucous membrane NEC 459.0
- - newborn 772.8
- muscle 728.8
- nail (subungual) 703.8
- nasal turbinate 784.7
- - newborn 772.8
- nasopharynx 478.2
- navel 772.3
- newborn NEC 772.9
- nipple 611.7
- nose 784.7
- - newborn 772.8
- obstetrical surgical wound 674.3
- oesophagus 530.8
- - varix 456.0
- omentum 568.8
- - newborn 772.4
- optic nerve (sheath) 377.4
- orbit, orbital 376.3
- ovary 620.1

Hemorrhage - *continued*
- oviduct 620.8
- pancreas 577.8
- parathyroid (gland) (spontaneous) 252.8
- parturition - see Hemorrhage, complicating delivery
- penis 607.8
- pericardium, pericarditis 423.0
- perineal repair (obstetrical) 674.3
- peritoneum, peritoneal 459.0
- peritonsillar tissue 474.8
- - due to infection 475
- petechial 287.2
- pituitary (gland) 253.8
- placenta NEC 641.9
- - fetus or newborn 762.1
- - from surgical or instrumental damage 641.8
- - - fetus or newborn 762.1
- - previa 641.1
- - - fetus or newborn 762.0
- pleura - see Hemorrhage, lung
- polio-encephalitis superior 265.1
- polymyositis - see Polymyositis
- pons (see also Hemorrhage, brain) 431
- pontine (see also Hemorrhage, brain) 431
- postmenopausal 627.1
- postnasal 784.7
- postoperative 998.1
- postpartum (following delivery of placenta) 666.1
- - delayed or secondary 666.2
- - retained placenta 666.0
- - third stage 666.0
- pregnancy (antepartum) (intrapartum) (concealed) 641.9
- - accidental 641.2
- - - fetus or newborn 762.1
- - before 22 completed weeks' gestation 640.9
- - - fetus or newborn 762.1
- - due to
- - - afibrinogenemia, or other coagulation defect (conditions in category 286.-) 641.3
- - - - fetus or newborn 762.1
- - - coagulation defect 641.3
- - - - fetus or newborn 762.1
- - - hyperfibrinolysis 641.3
- - - - fetus or newborn 762.1
- - - hypofibrinogenemia 641.3
- - - - fetus or newborn 762.1
- - - leiomyoma, uterus 641.8
- - - - fetus or newborn 762.1
- - - marginal sinus (rupture) 641.2
- - - - fetus or newborn 762.1
- - - placenta previa 641.1

Hemorrhage - *continued*
- pregnancy - *continued*
- − due to - *continued*
- − − placenta previa - *continued*
- − − − fetus or newborn 762.0
- − − premature separation placenta
    (normally implanted) 641.2
- − − − fetus or newborn 762.1
- − − − threatened abortion 640.0
- − − − − fetus or newborn 762.1
- − − − trauma 641.8
- − − − − fetus or newborn 762.1
- − − early 640.9
- − − − fetus or newborn 762.1
- − − fetus or newborn NEC 762.1
- − − previous, affecting management of
    pregnancy, childbirth V23.4
- − − unavoidable - see Hemorrhage,
    pregnancy due to placenta previa
- prepartum - see Hemorrhage, pregnancy
- preretinal 362.8
- prostate 602.1
- puerperal (see also Hemorrhage,
    postpartum) 666.1
- pulmonary - see also Hemorrhage, lung
- − newborn (massive) 770.3
- purpura (primary) (see also Purpura,
    thrombocytopenic) 287.3
- rectum (sphincter) 569.3
- recurring, following initial hemorrhage at
    time of injury 958.2
- renal 593.8
- respiratory tract - see Hemorrhage, lung
- retina, retinal (vessels) 362.8
- − diabetic 250.4 † 362.0*
- retroperitoneal 459.0
- retroplacental (see also Placenta,
    separation) 641.2
- scalp 459.0
- − birth injury 767.1
- scrotum 608.8
- secondary (nontraumatic) 459.0
- − following initial hemorrhage at time of
    injury 958.2
- seminal vesicle 608.8
- skin 782.7
- − newborn 772.6
- spermatic cord 608.8
- spinal (cord) 336.1
- − fetus or newborn 767.4
- spleen 289.5
- stomach 578.9
- − newborn 772.4
- − ulcer - see Ulcer, stomach, with
    hemorrhage
- subarachnoid (nontraumatic) 430

Hemorrhage - *continued*
- subarachnoid - *continued*
- − fetus or newborn (anoxic) (traumatic)
    772.2
- − puerperal, postpartum, childbirth,
    pregnancy 674.0
- − traumatic 852.0
- − − with
- − − − cerebral laceration or contusion
        (see also Laceration, brain) 851.0
- − − − open intracranial wound 852.1
- − − − skull fracture - see Fracture, skull
- subconjunctiva 372.7
- subcortical (see also Hemorrhage, brain)
    431
- subcutaneous 782.7
- subdiaphragmatic 459.0
- subdural (nontraumatic) 432.1
- − birth injury 767.0
- − fetus or newborn (anoxic) (traumatic)
    767.0
- − spinal 336.1
- − traumatic 852.0
- − − with
- − − − cerebral laceration or contusion
        (see also Laceration, cerebral)
        851.0
- − − − open intracranial wound 852.1
- − − − skull fracture - see Fracture skull
- subhyaloid 362.8
- subperiosteal 733.9
- subretinal 362.8
- subtentorial (see also Hemorrhage,
    subdural) 432.1
- subungual 703.8
- suprarenal (capsule) (gland) 255.4
- − fetus or newborn 772.5
- tentorium (traumatic) NEC 853.0
- − with skull fracture - see Fracture, skull
- − fetus or newborn 767.0
- − nontraumatic - see Hemorrhage,
    subdural
- testis 608.8
- third stage 666.0
- thorax - see Hemorrhage, lung
- throat 784.8
- thymus (gland) 254.8
- thyroid (gland) 246.3
- − cyst 246.3
- tongue 529.8
- tonsil 474.8
- trachea - see Hemorrhage, lung
- traumatic - see also Nature of injury
- − brain - see Hemorrhage, brain,
    traumatic

Hemorrhage - *continued*
- traumatic - *continued*
- - recurring or secondary (following initial hemorrhage at time of injury) 958.2
- tuberculous NEC - code by type under Tuberculosis, pulmonary 011.9
- tunica vaginalis 608.8
- ulcer - code by site under Ulcer, with hemorrhage 533.9
- umbilical
- - after birth 772.3
- - cord
- - - after birth, newborn 772.3
- - - complicating delivery 663.8
- - - - affecting fetus or newborn 772.0
- - stump 772.3
- unavoidable (antepartum) (due to placenta previa) 641.1
- - fetus or newborn 762.0
- urethra (idiopathic) 599.8
- uterus uterine (abnormal) 626.9
- - climacteric 627.0
- - complicating delivery - see Hemorrhage, complicating delivery
- - functional or dysfunctional 626.8
- - in pregnancy - see Hemorrhage, pregnancy
- - intermenstrual 626.8
- - - irregular 626.6
- - - regular 626.5
- - postmenopausal 627.1
- - postpartum - see Hemorrhage, postpartum
- - prepubertal 626.8
- - pubertal 626.3
- vagina 623.8
- vas deferens 608.8
- vasa previa 663.5
- - affecting fetus or newborn 772.0
- ventricular (see also Hemorrhage, brain) 431
- vesical 596.8
- viscera 459.0
- - newborn 772.8
- vitreous (humor) (intra-ocular) 379.2
- vulva 624.8
Hemorrhoids 455.6
- bleeding, prolapsed, strangulated or ulcerated NEC 455.8
- complicating pregnancy and puerperium 671.8
- external 455.3
- - bleeding, prolapsed, strangulated or ulcerated 455.5
- - thrombosed 455.4
- internal 455.0

Hemorrhoids - *continued*
- internal - *continued*
- - bleeding, prolapsed, strangulated or ulcerated 455.2
- - thrombosed 455.1
- thrombosed NEC 455.7
Hemosalpinx 620.8
Hemosiderosis 275.0
- dietary 275.0
- pulmonary, idiopathic 275.0 † 516.1*
- transfusion 999.8
Hemothorax 511.8
- newborn 772.8
- nontuberculous 511.8
- - bacterial 511.1
- pneumococcal 511.1
- staphylococcal 511.1
- streptococcal 511.1
- traumatic 860.2
- - with
- - - open wound into thorax 860.3
- - - pneumothorax 860.4
- - - - with open wound into thorax 860.5
- tuberculous 012.0
Henoch(-Schonlein)
- disease or syndrome 287.0
- purpura 287.0
Henpue, henpuye 102.6
Hepar lobatum 095 † 573.2*
Hepatalgia 573.8
Hepatitis 573.3
- acute 570
- - alcoholic 571.1
- - infective 070.1 † 573.1*
- - - with hepatic coma 070.0 † 573.1*
- alcoholic 571.1
- amebic (see also Abscess, liver, amebic) 006.3
- anicteric, acute - see Hepatitis, viral
- antigen-associated (HAA) 070.3 † 573.1*
- - with hepatic coma 070.2 † 573.1*
- Australia-antigen (positive) 070.3 † 573.1*
- - with hepatic coma 070.2 † 573.1*
- catarrhal (acute) 070.1 † 573.1*
- - with hepatic coma 070.0 † 573.1*
- - newborn 070.1 † 573.1*
- - - with hepatic coma 070.0 † 573.1*
- cholangiolitic 573.8
- cholestatic 573.8
- chronic (active) (aggressive) (persistent) 571.4
- cytomegalic inclusion virus 078.5 † 573.1*
- diffuse 573.3
- due to
- - toxoplasmosis (acquired) 130 † 573.2*

Hepatitis - *continued*
- due to - *continued*
- - toxoplasmosis - *continued*
- - - congenital (active) 771.2 † 573.2*
- epidemic 070.1 † 573.1*
- - with hepatic coma 070.0 † 573.1*
- fetus or newborn 774.4
- fibrous (chronic) (see also Cirrhosis, liver) 571.4
- - acute 570
- from injection, inoculation or transfusion (blood) (plasma) (serum) (other substance) 070.3 † 573.1*
- - with hepatic coma 070.2 † 573.1*
- fulminant - see Hepatitis, viral
- hemorrhagic 573.8
- homologous serum 070.3 † 573.1*
- - with hepatic coma 070.2 † 573.1*
- hypertrophic (chronic) (see also Cirrhosis, liver) 571.4
- - acute 570
- in
- - infectious mononucleosis 075 † 573.1*
- - mumps 072.7 † 573.1*
- - toxoplasmosis 130 † 573.1*
- - yellow fever 060.- † 573.1*
- infectious, infective (acute) (chronic) (subacute) 070.1 † 573.1*
- - with hepatic coma 070.0 † 573.1*
- inoculation 070.3 † 573.1*
- - with hepatic coma 070.2 † 573.1*
- interstitial (chronic) 571.4
- - acute 570
- malarial 084.9 † 573.2*
- malignant (see also Necrosis, liver) 570
- neonatal (toxic) 774.4
- parenchymatous (acute) (see also Necrosis, liver) 570
- post-immunization 070.3 † 573.1*
- - with hepatic coma 070.2 † 573.1*
- post-transfusion 070.3 † 573.1*
- - with hepatic coma 070.2 † 573.1*
- recurrent 571.4
- serum 070.3 † 573.1*
- - with hepatic coma 070.2 † 573.1*
- subacute (see also Necrosis, liver) 570
- suppurative (diffuse) 572.0
- syphilitic (late) 095 † 573.2*
- - congenital (early) 090.0 † 573.2*
- - - late 090.5 † 573.2*
- - secondary 091.6 † 573.2*
- toxic 573.3
- - fetus or newborn 774.4
- tuberculous 017.8 † 573.2*
- viral, virus 070.9 † 573.1*
- - with hepatic coma 070.6 † 573.1*
- - Coxsackie 074.8 † 573.1*

Hepatitis - *continued*
- viral - *continued*
- - cytomegalic inclusion 078.5 † 573.1*
- - specified typype NEC 070.5 † 573.1*
- - - with hepatic coma 070.4 † 573.1*
- - type
- - - A 070.1 † 573.1*
- - - - with hepatic coma 070.0 † 573.1*
- - - B 070.3 † 573.1*
- - - - with hepatic coma 070.2 † 573.1*
Hepatization lung (acute) - see also Pneumonia, lobar
- chronic (see also Fibrosis, lung) 515
Hepatoblastoma (M8970/3) 155.0
Hepatocarcinoma (M8170/3) 155.0
Hepatocholangiocarcinoma (M8180/3) 155.0
Hepatocholangioma, benign (M8180/0) 211.5
Hepatocholangitis 573.8
Hepatocystitis (see also Cholecystitis) 575.1
Hepatolenticular degeneration 275.1
Hepatoma (malignant) (M8170/3) 155.0
- benign (M8170/0) 211.5
- congenital (M8970/3) 155.0
- embryonal (M8970/3) 155.0
Hepatomegalia glycogenica diffusa 271.0
Hepatomegaly (see also Hypertrophy, liver) 789.1
- congenital 751.6
- - syphilitic 090.0
Hepatoptosis 573.8
Hepatosis (toxic) 573.8
Hepatosplenomegaly 571.8
- hyperlipemic (Buerger-Grutz type) 272.3
Hereditary - see condition
Heredodegeneration, macular 362.7
Heredopathia atactica polyneuritiformis 356.3
Heredosyphilis (see also Syphilis, congenital) 090.9
Hermaphroditism (true) 752.7
- with specified chromosomal anomaly - see Anomaly, chromosomes, sex
Hernia, hernial (acquired) (recurrent) 553.9
- with obstruction (see also Hernia by site, with obstruction) 552.9
- - gangrenous (see also Hernia, by site, gangrenous) 551.9
- abdomen (wall) 553.2
- - with obstruction 552.2
- - gangrenous (with obstruction) 551.2
- abdominal, specified site NEC 553.8
- - with obstruction 552.8
- - gangrenous (with obstruction) 551.8
- appendix - see Hernia, abdominal
- bilateral (inguinal) - see Hernia, inguinal

Hernia - *continued*
- bladder (sphincter)
- – congenital (female) (male) 753.8
- – female 618.0
- – male 596.8
- brain, congenital 742.0
- cartilage, vertebra - see Displacement, intervertebral disc
- cerebral
- – congenital 742.0
- – endaural 742.0
- ciliary body 871.1
- colon - see Hernia, intestine
- Cooper's - see Hernia, abdominal
- crural - see Hernia, femoral
- diaphragm, diaphragmatic 553.3
- – with obstruction 552.3
- – congenital 756.6
- – gangrenous (with obstruction) 551.3
- – traumatic 862.0
- – – with open wound into cavity 862.1
- direct (inguinal) - see Hernia, inguinal
- diverticulum, intestine - see Hernia, intestine
- double (inguinal) - see Hernia, inguinal
- en glissade - see Hernia, inguinal
- epigastric - see Hernia, ventral
- esophageal hiatus - see also Hernia, hiatal
- – congenital 750.6
- external (inguinal) - see Hernia, inguinal
- fallopian tube 620.4
- fascia 728.8
- fat 729.3
- femoral 553.0
- – with obstruction 552.0
- – gangrenous (with obstruction) 551.0
- foramen magnum 348.4
- – congenital 742.0
- funicular (umbilical) - see also Hernia, umbilicus
- – spermatic (cord) - see Hernia, inguinal
- gangrenous (with obstruction) (see also Hernia, by site, gangrenous) 551.9
- gastrointestinal tract - see Hernia, intestine
- Gruber's - see Hernia, abdominal
- Hesselbach's - see Hernia, abdominal
- hiatal (esophageal) 553.3
- – with obstruction 552.3
- – congenital 750.6
- – gangrenous (with obstruction) 551.3
- incarcerated (see also Hernia, by site, with obstruction) 552.9
- – gangrenous (with obstruction) (see also Hernia, by site, gangrenous) 551.9
- incisional - see also Hernia, ventral
- – lumbar - see Hernia, abdominal

Hernia - *continued*
- indirect (inguinal) - see Hernia, inguinal
- inguinal (direct) (double) (external) (funicular) (indirect) (infantile) (internal) (interstitial) (oblique) (scrotal) (sliding) 550.9
- – with obstruction 550.1
- – gangrenous (with obstruction) 550.0
- internal - see also Hernia, abdominal
- – inguinal - see Hernia, inguinal
- interstitial - see also Hernia, intestine
- – inguinal - see Hernia, inguinal
- intervertebral cartilage or disc - see Displacement, intervertebral disc
- intestine, intestinal 553.9
- – with obstruction 552.9
- – gangrenous (with obstruction) 551.9
- intra-abdominal - see Hernia, intestine
- intraparietal - see Hernia, intestine
- iris 871.1
- irreducible (see also Hernia, by site, with obstruction) 552.9
- – gangrenous (with obstruction) (see also Hernia, by site, gangrenous) 551.9
- ischiatic - see Hernia, abdominal
- ischiorectal - see Hernia, abdominal
- lens 871.1
- linea (alba) (semilunaris) - see Hernia, ventral
- Littre's - see Hernia, intestine
- lumbar - see Hernia, abdominal
- lung (subcutaneous) 518.8
- mediastinum 519.3
- mesenteric (internal) - see Hernia, abdominal
- mesocolon - see Hernia, abdominal
- muscle (sheath) 728.8
- nucleus pulposus - see Displacement, intervertebral disc
- oblique (inguinal) - see Hernia, inguinal
- obstructive (see also Hernia, by site, with obstruction) 552.9
- – gangrenous (with obstruction) (see also Hernia, by site, gangrenous) 551.9
- obturator - see Hernia, abdominal
- oesophageal hiatus - see also Hernia, hiatal
- – congenital 750.6
- omental - see Hernia, abdominal
- ovary 620.4
- oviduct 620.4
- paraduodenal - see Hernia, abdominal
- paraesophageal - see also Hernia, hiatal
- – congenital 750.6
- paraumbilical - see Hernia, umbilicus
- parietal - see Hernia, intestine
- perineal - see Hernia, abdominal

Hernia - *continued*
- peritoneal - see Hernia, abdominal
- postoperative - see Hernia, ventral
- pregnant uterus 654.4
- prevesical 596.8
- properitoneal - see Hernia, abdominal
- pudendal - see Hernia, abdominal
- rectovaginal 618.6
- retroperitoneal - see Hernia, abdominal
- Richter's - see Hernia, intestine
- Rieux's, Riex's - see Hernia, abdominal
- sac condition (adhesion) (dropsy)
  (inflammation) (laceration)
  (suppuration) - code by site under Hernia
- sciatic - see Hernia, abdominal
- scrotum, scrotal - see Hernia, inguinal
- sliding (inguinal) - see also Hernia,
  inguinal
- - hiatus - see Hernia, hiatal
- spigelian - see Hernia, abdominal
- spinal 741.9
- - with hydrocephalus 741.0
- strangulated (see also Hernia, by site,
  with obstruction) 552.9
- - gangrenous (with obstruction) (see also
  Hernia, by site, gangrenous) 551.9
- supra-umbilicus - see Hernia, abdominal
- tendon 727.9
- testis (nontraumatic) 095
- Treitz's (fossa) - see Hernia, abdominal
- tunica vaginalis 752.8
- umbilicus, umbilical 553.1
- - with obstruction 552.1
- - gangrenous (with obstruction) 551.1
- ureter 593.8
- - with obstruction 593.4
- uterus 621.8
- - pregnant 654.4
- vaginal (posterior) 618.6
- Velpeau's - see Hernia, femoral
- ventral 553.2
- - with obstruction 552.2
- - gangrenous (with obstruction) 551.2
- vesical
- - congenital (female) (male) 753.8
- - female 618.0
- - male 596.8
- vitreous (into wound) 871.1
- - into anterior chamber 379.2
Herniation - see also Hernia
- brain (stem) 348.4
- cerebral 348.4
- mediastinum 519.3
- nucleus pulposus - see Displacement,
  intervertebral disc
Herpangina 074.0
Herpes, herpetic 054.9

Herpes - *continued*
- blepharitis (zoster) 053.2 † 373.5*
- - simplex 054.4 † 373.5*
- circinatus 110.5
- - bullosus 694.5
- circine 110.5
- conjunctivitis - see Herpetic
  keratoconjunctivitis
- cornea - see Herpetic keratitis
- encephalitis 054.3 † 323.4*
- eye (zoster) 053.2 † 373.5*
- - simplex 054.4 † 370.1*
- eyelid (zoster) 053.2 † 373.5*
- - simplex 054.4 † 373.5*
- febrilis 054.9
- fever 054.9
- geniculate ganglionitis 053.1 † 351.1*
- genital, genitalis 054.1
- gestationis 646.8
- gingivostomatitis 054.2
- iridocyclitis (simplex) 054.4 † 364.0*
- - zoster 053.2 † 364.0*
- iris (any site) 695.1
- iritis (simplex) 054.4 † 364.0*
- keratitis (simplex) 054.4 † 370.4*
- - dendritic 054.4 † 370.1*
- - disciform 054.4 † 370.5*
- - interstitial 054.4 † 370.5*
- - zoster 053.2 † 370.4*
- - - interstitial 053.2 † 370.5*
- keratoconjunctivitis (simplex) 054.4 †
  370.4*
- - zoster 053.2 † 370.4*
- labialis 054.9
- - meningococcal 036.8
- lip 054.9
- meningitis (simplex) 054.7 † 321.4*
- - zoster 053.0 † 321.3*
- ophthalmicus (zoster) 053.2 † 373.5*
- - simplex 054.4 † 373.5*
- penis 054.1
- pharyngitis 054.7
- scrotum 054.1
- septicemia 054.5
- simplex 054.9
- - complicated 054.8
- - - specified NEC 054.7
- - congenital 771.2
- - external ear 054.7 † 380.1*
- - keratitis 054.4 † 370.4*
- - - interstitial 054.4 † 370.5*
- - specified complication NEC 054.7
- - visceral 054.7
- stomatitis 054.2
- tonsurans 110.0
- - maculosus (of Hebra) 696.3
- visceral 054.7

Herpes - *continued*
- vulva 054.1
- whitlow 054.6
- zoster (see also Condition) 053.9
- - auricularis 053.7 † 380.1*
- - complicated 053.8
- - - specified NEC 053.7
- - eye(lid) 053.2 † 373.5*
- - geniculate 053.1 † 351.1*
- - keratitis 053.2 † 370.4*
- - - interstitial 053.2 † 370.5*
- - neuritis 053.1
- - ophthalmicus 053.2 † 373.5*
- - oticus 053.7 † 380.1*
- - specified complication NEC 053.7
- zosteriform, intermediate type 053.9
Herrick's anemia (see also Disease, sickle cell) 282.6
Hers's disease 271.0
Herter-Gee syndrome 579.0
Herxheimer's reaction 995.0
Hesselbach's hernia - see Hernia, abdominal

Heterochromia (congenital) 743.4
- cataract 366.3
- cyclitis 364.2
- hair 704.3
- iritis 364.2
- retained metallic foreign body 360.6
- - magnetic 360.5
- uveitis 364.2
Heterophoria 378.4
Heterophyes, small intestine 121.6
Heterophyiasis 121.6
Heteropsia 368.8
Heterotopia, heterotopic - see also Malposition, congenital
- cerebralis 742.4
- spinalis 742.5
Heterotropia 378.3
- intermittent 378.2
- vertical 378.3
Heubner's disease 094.8
Hexadactylism 755.0
Heyd's syndrome 572.4
Hibernoma (M8880/0) 214
Hiccough 786.8
- epidemic 078.8
- psychogenic 306.1
Hiccup (see also Hiccough) 786.8
Hidradenitis (suppurative) (axillaris) 705.8

Hidradenoma (nodular) (M8400/0) - see also Neoplasm, skin, benign
- clear cell (M8402/0) - see Neoplasm, skin, benign
- papillary (M8405/0) - see Neoplasm, skin, benign

Hidrocystoma (M8404/0) - see Neoplasm, skin, benign
High
- altitude effects 993.2
- - anoxia 993.2
- - on
- - - ears 993.0
- - - sinuses 993.1
- - polycythemia 289.0
- arch
- - foot 755.6
- - palate 750.2
- arterial tension (see also Hypertension) 401.9
- basal metabolic rate 794.7
- blood pressure (see also Hypertension) 401.9
- - reading (incidental) (isolated) (nonspecific), without diagnosis of hypertension 796.2
- diaphragm (congenital) 756.6
- head at term 652.5
- palate 750.2
- temperature (of unknown origin) (see also Pyrexia) 780.6
- thoracic rib 756.3
Hildenbrand's disease 081.9
Hill diarrhea 579.1
Hilliard's lupus 017.0
Hilum - see condition
Hip - see condition
Hippel's disease 759.6
Hippus 379.4
Hirschsprung's disease or megacolon 751.3
Hirsuties (see also Hypertrichosis) 704.1
Hirsutism (see also Hypertrichosis) 704.1
Hirudiniasis (external) (internal) 134.2
Hiss-Russell dysentery 004.1
Histidinemia 270.5
Histidinuria 270.5
Histiocytoma (M8832/0) - see also Neoplasm, skin, benign
- fibrous (M8830/0) - see also Neoplasm, skin, benign
- - atypical (M8830/1) - see Neoplasm, connective tissue, uncertain behavior
- - malignant (M8830/3) - see Neoplasm, connective tissue, malignant
Histiocytosis 277.8
- acute differentiated progressive (M9722/3) 202.5
- cholesterol 277.8
- lipid, lipoid (essential) 272.7
- malignant (M9720/3) 202.3
- X 277.8
- - acute (progressive) (M9722/3) 202.5
- - chronic 277.8

Histoplasmosis 115.9
- with pneumonia 115.9 † 484.7*
- African 115.1
- American 115.0
- Darling's 115.0
- large form 115.1
- lung 115.0
- small form 115.0
History (personal) of
- allergy to
- - analgesic agent NEC V14.6
- - anesthetic NEC V14.4
- - antibiotic agent NEC V14.1
- - anti-infective agent NEC V14.3
- - medicinal agents V14.9
- - - specified NEC V14.8
- - narcotic agent NEC V14.5
- - penicillin V14.0
- - serum V14.7
- - specified nonmedicinal agents V15.0
- - sulfonamides V14.2
- - vaccine V14.7
- arthritis V13.4
- congenital malformation V13.6
- contraception V15.7
- disease or disorder (of) V13.9
- - blood V12.3
- - blood-forming organs V12.3
- - circulatory system V12.5
- - digestive system V12.7
- - endocrine V12.2
- - genital system V13.2
- - hematological V12.3
- - immunity V12.2
- - infectious V12.0
- - mental V11
- - metabolic V12.2
- - musculoskeletal NEC V13.5
- - nervous system V12.4
- - obstetric V13.2
- - parasitic V12.0
- - respiratory system NEC V12.6
- - sense organs V12.4
- - skin V13.3
- - specified site or type NEC V13.8
- - subcutaneous tissue V13.3
- - trophoblastic V13.1
- - urinary system V13.0
- family of
- - allergy V19.6
- - anemia V18.2
- - arthritis V17.7
- - asthma V17.5
- - blindness V19.0
- - condition
- - - psychiatric V17.0
- - - skin V19.4

History - continued
- family of - continued
- - congenital anomalies V19.5
- - consanguinity V19.7
- - deafness V19.2
- - diabetes mellitus V18.0
- - disease or disorder (of)
- - - allergic V19.6
- - - blood NEC V18.3
- - - cardiovascular NEC V17.4
- - - digestive V18.5
- - - ear NEC V19.3
- - - endocrine V18.1
- - - eye NEC V19.1
- - - genitourinary NEC V18.7
- - - infectious V18.8
- - - ischemic heart V17.3
- - - kidney V18.6
- - - metabolic V18.1
- - - musculoskeletal NEC V17.8
- - - neurological NEC V17.2
- - epilepsy V17.2
- - hearing loss V19.2
- - Huntington's chorea V17.2
- - leukemia V16.6
- - malignant neoplasm (of) NEC V16.9
- - - breast (female) V16.3
- - - - male V16.8
- - - bronchus V16.1
- - - gastrointestinal tract V16.0
- - - genital organs V16.4
- - - hemopoietic NEC V16.7
- - - intrathoracic organs NEC V16.2
- - - lung V16.1
- - - lymphatic NEC V16.7
- - - respiratory organs NEC V16.2
- - - specified site NEC V16.8
- - - trachea V16.1
- - - urinary organs V16.5
- - mental retardation V18.4
- - psychiatric disorder V17.0
- - skin conditions V19.4
- - specified NEC V19.8
- - stroke (cerebrovascular) V17.1
- - visual loss V19.0
- injury NEC V15.5
- irradiation V15.3
- leukemia V10.6
- malignant neoplasm (of) V10.9
- - breast V10.3
- - bronchus V10.1
- - gastrointestinal tract V10.0
- - genital organs V10.4
- - hematopoietic NEC V10.7
- - intrathoracic organs NEC V10.2
- - lung V10.1
- - lymphatic NEC V10.7

History - *continued*
- malignant neoplasm - *continued*
- - respiratory organs NEC V10.2
- - skin V10.8
- - specified site NEC V10.8
- - trachea V10.1
- - urinary organs V10.5
- nutritional deficiency V12.1
- perinatal problems V13.7
- poisoning V15.6
- psychiatric disorder V11
- psychological trauma V15.4
- radiation therapy V15.3
- respiratory condition, chronic, NEC V17.6
- surgery (major) to
- - great vessels V15.1
- - heart V15.1
- - major organs NEC V15.2
His-Werner disease 083.1
Hives (bold) (see also Urticaria) 708.9
Hoarseness 784.4
Hobnail liver - see Cirrhosis, portal
Hobo V60.0
Hodgkin's
- disease (M9650/3) 201.9
- - lymphocytic
- - - depletion (M9653/3) 201.7
- - - - diffuse fibrosis (M9654/3) 201.7
- - - - reticular type (M9655/3) 201.7
- - - predominance (M9651/3) 201.4
- - lymphocytic-histiocytic predominance (M9651/3) 201.4
- - mixed cellularity (M9652/3) 201.6
- - nodular sclerosis (M9656/3) 201.5
- - - cellular phase (M9657/3) 201.5
- granuloma (M9661/3) 201.1
- lymphogranulomatosis (M9650/3) 201.9
- lymphoma (M9650/3) 201.9
- paragranuloma (M9660/3) 201.0
- sarcoma (M9662/3) 201.2

Hodgson's disease 441.6
- ruptured 441.5
Hoffa's disease 272.8
Hoffa-Kastert disease 272.8
Hoffman's syndrome 244.9 † 359.5*
- macula 362.5
- retina (macula) 362.5
- - round (without detachment) 361.3
Hoffman-Bouveret syndrome 427.2
Holla disease (see also Spherocytosis) 282.0

Hollow foot (congenital) 754.7
- acquired 736.7
Homesickness 309.8
Homocystinemia 270.4
Homocystinuria 270.4

Homologous serum jaundice (prophylactic) (therapeutic) 070.3 † 573.1*
- with hepatic coma 070.2 † 573.1*
Homosexuality 302.0
Honeycomb lung 518.8
- congenital 748.4
Hong Kong ear 117.3
Hooded
- clitoris 752.4
- penis 752.8
Hookworm (anemia) (disease) (infection) (infestation) - see Ancylostomiasis
Hordeolum (eyelid) (external) (internal) (recurrent) 373.1
Horn
- cutaneous 702
- - cheek 702
- - eyelid 702
- nail 703.8
- - congenital 757.5
- papillary 700
Horner's syndrome 337.9
- traumatic 954.0
Horseshoe kidney (congenital) 753.3
Horton's
- disease 446.5
- headache or neuralgia 346.2
Hospitalism in children NEC 309.8
Hourglass (contracture) - see also Contraction, hourglass
- stomach, congenital 750.7
- stricture - see Stricture, hourglass
Household, housing circumstance affecting care V60.9
- specified NEC V60.8
Housemaid's knee 727.2
Hudson-Stahli line (cornea) 371.1
Huebner-Herter disease 579.0
Human bite (open wound) - see also Wound, open
- intact skin surface - see Contusion
Humpback (acquired) 737.9
- congenital 756.1
Hunchback (acquired) 737.9
- congenital 756.1
Hunger 994.2
- air, psychogenic 306.1
Hunner's ulcer (see also Cystitis) 595.1
Hunt's
- neuralgia 053.1 † 351.1*
- syndrome (herpetic geniculate ganglionitis) 053.1 † 351.1*
- - dyssynergia cerebellaris myoclonica 334.2
Hunter's glossitis 529.4
Hunter-Hurler syndrome 277.5
Huntington's

Huntington's - *continued*
- chorea 333.4
- disease 333.4

Hurler's
- disease 277.5
- syndrome (in bones) 277.5

Hurthle cell
- adenocarcinoma (M8290/3) 193
- adenoma (M8290/0) 226
- carcinoma (M8290/3) 193
- tumor (M8290/0) 226

Hutchinson's
- disease meaning
- — angioma serpiginosum 709.1
- — cheiropompholyx 705.8
- — prurigo estivalis 692.7
- — summer eruption or summer prurigo 692.7
- melanotic freckle (M8742/2) - see Neoplasm, skin, in situ
- — malignant melanoma in (M8742/3) - see Melanoma
- teeth or incisors (congenital syphilis) 090.5

Hutchinson-Boeck disease or syndrome 135
Hutchinson-Gilford disease or syndrome 259.8
Hyalin plaque, sclera, senile 379.1

Hyaline
- degeneration (diffuse) (generalized) 728.8
- — localized - see Degeneration, by site
- membrane (disease) (lung) (pulmonary) 769

Hyalinosis cutis et mucosae 272.8
Hyalitis (asteroid) 379.2
- syphilitic 095 † 379.2*

Hydatid
- cyst or tumor - see Echinococcus
- mole - see Hydatidiform mole
- morgagni 752.8

Hydatidiform mole (benign) (complicating pregnancy) (delivered) (undelivered) 630
- invasive (M9100/1) 236.1
- malignant (M9100/1) 236.1
- previous, affecting management of pregnancy V23.1

Hydatidosis - see Echinococcus
Hyde's disease 698.3
Hydradenitis 705.8
Hydradenoma (M8400/0) - see Hidradenoma
Hydramnios 657
- fetus or newborn 761.3
Hydrancephaly 742.3
- with spina bifida 741.0
Hydranencephaly 742.3

Hydranencephaly - *continued*
- with spina bifida 741.0
Hydrargyrism NEC 985.0
Hydrarthrosis 719.0
- gonococcal 098.5 † 711.4*
- intermittent 719.3
- of yaws (early) (late) 102.6
- syphilitic 095
- — congenital 090.5
Hydremia 285.9
Hydrencephalocele (congenital) 742.0
Hydrencephalomeningocele (congenital) 742.0
Hydroa 694.0
- aestivale 692.7
- herpetiformis 694.0
- vacciniforme 692.7
Hydro-adenitis 705.8
Hydrocalycosis (see also Hydronephrosis) 591
Hydrocele (calcified) (chylous) (idiopathic) (infantile) (inguinal canal) (recurrent) (senile) (spermatic cord) (testis) (tunica vaginalis) 603.9
- canal of Nuck 629.1
- congenital 778.6
- encysted 603.0
- female NEC 629.8
- infected 603.1
- round ligament 629.8
- specified type NEC 603.8
- spinalis 741.9
- — with hydrocephalus 741.0
- vulva 624.8
Hydrocephalus (acquired) (external) (internal) (malignant) (noncommunicating) (obstructive) (recurrent) 331.4
- aqueduct Sylvius stricture (see also Hydrocephalus, congenital) 742.3
- causing disproportion 653.6
- — with obstructed labor 660.1
- — affecting fetus or newborn 763.1
- chronic (see also Hydrocephalus, congenital) 742.3
- communicating 331.3
- congenital (external) (internal) 742.3
- — with spina bifida 741.0
- due to toxoplasmosis (congenital) 771.2
- fetus (suspected), affecting management of pregnancy 655.0
- foramen Magendie block (acquired) 331.3
- — congenital (see also Hydrocephalus, congenital) 742.3
- newborn 742.3
- — with spina bifida 741.0

Hydrocephalus - *continued*
- syphilitic congenital 090.4
Hydrocolpos (congenital) 623.8
Hydrocystoma (M8404/0) - see Neoplasm, skin, benign
Hydro-encephalocele (congenital) 742.0
Hydro-encephalomeningocele (congenital) 742.0
Hydrohematopneumothorax (see also Hemothorax) 511.8
Hydromeningitis - see Meningitis
Hydromeningocele (spinal) 741.9
- with hydrocephalus 741.0
- cranial 742.0
Hydrometra 621.8
Hydrometrocolpos 623.8
Hydromicrocephaly 742.1
Hydromphalos (since birth) 757.3
Hydromyelia 742.5
Hydromyelocele 741.9
- with hydrocephalus 741.0
Hydronephrosis 591
- atrophic 591
- congenital 753.2
- early 591
- functionless (infected) 591
- infected 591
- intermittent 591
- primary 591
- secondary 591
- tuberculous 016.0
Hydropericarditis (see also Pericarditis) 423.9
Hydropericardium (see also Pericarditis) 423.9
Hydroperitoneum 789.5
Hydrophobia 071
Hydrophthalmos 743.2
Hydropneumohemothorax (see also Hemothorax) 511.8
Hydropneumopericarditis (see also Pericarditis) 423.9
Hydropneumopericardium (see also Pericarditis) 423.9
Hydropneumothorax 511.8
- nontuberculous 511.8
- - bacterial 511.1
- pneumococcal 511.1
- staphylococcal 511.1
- streptococcal 511.1
- traumatic 860.0
- - with open wound into thorax 860.1
- tuberculous 012.0
Hydrops 782.3
- abdominis 789.5
- amnii (complicating pregnancy) (see also Hydramnios) 657

Hydrops - *continued*
- articulorum intermittens 719.3
- cardiac (see also Failure, heart, congestive) 428.0
- endolymphatic 386.0
- fetal(is) or newborn (idiopathic) 778.0
- - due to iso-immunisation 773.3
- gallbladder (see also Disease, gallbladder) 575.3
- joint (see also Hydrarthrosis) 719.0
- labyrinth 386.0
- meningeal NEC 331.4
- nutritional 262
- pericardium - see Pericarditis
- pleura (see also Hydrothorax) 511.8
- renal (see also Nephrosis) 581.9
- spermatic cord (see also Hydrocele) 603.9
Hydropyonephrosis (see also Pyelitis) 590.8
- chronic 590.0
Hydrorhachis 742.5
Hydrorrhea (nasal) 478.1
- pregnancy - see Rupture, membranes, premature
Hydrosadenitis 705.8
Hydrosalpinx (fallopian tube) (follicularis) 614.1
Hydrothorax (double) (pleura) 511.8
- chylous (nonfilarial) 457.8
- - filarial (see also Infestation, filarial) 125.9
- nontuberculous 511.8
- - bacterial 511.1
- pneumococcal 511.1
- staphylococcal 511.1
- streptococcal 511.1
- traumatic 862.2
- - with open wound into thorax 862.3
- tuberculous 012.0
Hydroureter 593.5
- congenital 753.2
Hydroureteronephrosis (see also Hydronephrosis) 591
Hydrourethra 599.8
Hydroxykynureninuria 270.2
Hydroxyprolinemia 270.8
Hygroma (congenital) (cystic) (M9173/0) 228.1
- praepatellare, prepatellar 727.3
Hymen - see condition
Hymenolepiasis (diminuta) (infection) (infestation) (nana) 123.6
Hymenolepis (diminuta) (infection) (infestation) (nana) 123.6
Hypalgesia (see also Disturbance, sensation) 782.0
Hyperacidity (gastric) 536.8

Hyperacidity - *continued*
- psychogenic 306.4
Hyperactive, hyperactivity
- basal cell
- - uterine cervix 622.1
- cervix epithelial (basal) 622.1
- child 314.0
- gastrointestinal 536.8
- - psychogenic 306.4
- nasal mucous membrane 478.1
- stomach 536.8
- thyroid (gland) (see also
  Hyperthyroidism) 242.9
Hyperacusis 388.4
Hyperadrenalism 255.6
Hyperadrenocorticism 255.3
- congenital 255.2
- iatrogenic
- - correct substance properly
  administered 255.3
- - overdose or wrong substance given or
  taken 962.0
Hyperaffectivity 301.1
Hyperaldosteronism (primary) 255.1
Hyperalgesia (see also Disturbance,
  sensation) 782.0
Hyperalimentation 783.6
- carotin 278.3
- specified NEC 278.8
- vitamin
- - A 278.2
- - D 278.4
Hyperaminoaciduria
- arginine 270.6
- cystine 270.0
- lysine 270.7
- ornithine 270.6
Hyperammonemia (congenital) 270.6
Hyperazotemia 791.9
Hyperbetalipoproteinemia (familial) 272.0
- with prebetalipoproteinemia 272.2
Hyperbilirubinemia
- congenital 277.4
- constitutional 277.4
- neonatal (transient) (see also Jaundice,
  fetus or newborn 774.6
- - of prematurity 774.2
Hypercalcemia 275.4
Hypercalcinuria 275.4
Hypercapnia 786.0
Hypercarotinemia 278.3
Hypercementosis 521.5
Hyperchloremia 276.9
Hyperchlorhydria 536.8
- neurotic 306.4
- psychogenic 306.4
Hypercholesterinemia 272.0

Hypercholesterinemia - *continued*
- with hyperglyceridemia, endogenous
  272.2
- essential 272.0
- familial (essential) 272.0
- hereditary 272.0
- primary 272.0
- pure 272.0
Hypercholesterolemia - see
  Hypercholesterinemia
Hypercholesterolosis 272.0
Hyperchylia gastrica 536.8
- psychogenic 306.4
Hyperchylomicronemia 272.3
- familial 272.3
- - with hyperbetalipoproteinemia 272.3
Hypercorticosteronism
- correct substance properly administered
  255.3
- overdose or wrong substance given or
  taken 962.0
Hypercortisonism
- correct substance properly administered
  255.3
- overdose or wrong substance given or
  taken 962.0
Hyperelectrolythemia 276.9
Hyperemesis 536.2
- gravidarum (mild) 643.0
- - with
- - - carbohydrate depletion 643.1
- - - dehydration 643.1
- - - electrolyte imbalance 643.1
- - - metabolic disturbance 643.1
- - fetus or newborn 761.8
- - severe (with metabolic disturbance)
  643.1
- psychogenic 306.4
Hyperemia (acute) 780.9
- anal mucosa 569.4
- bladder 596.7
- cerebral 437.8
- conjunctiva 372.7
- ear internal, acute 386.3
- enteric 564.8
- eye 372.7
- eyelid (active) (passive) 374.8
- intestine 564.8
- iris 364.4
- kidney 593.8
- labyrinth 386.3
- liver (active) (passive) 573.8
- lung 514
- passive 780.9
- pulmonary 514
- renal 593.8
- retina 362.8

Hyperemia - *continued*
- stomach 537.8
Hyperesthesia (body surface) (see also Disturbance, sensation) 782.0
- larynx (reflex) 478.7
- - hysterical 300.1
- pharynx (reflex) 478.2
- - hysterical 300.1
Hyperestrogenism 256.0
Hyperextension, joint 718.8
Hyperfibrinolysis - see Fibrinolysis
Hyperfructosemia 271.2
Hyperfunction
- adrenal (cortex) 255.3
- - medulla 255.6
- - virilism 255.2
- ovarian 256.1
- pancreas 577.8
- parathyroid (gland) 252.0
- pituitary (gland) (anterior) 253.1
- testicular 257.0
Hypergammaglobulinemia 289.8
- polyclonal 273.0
- Waldenstrom's 273.0
Hyperglobulinemia 273.8
Hyperglycemia 790.6
- postpancreatectomy 251.3
Hyperglyceridemia 272.1
- endogenous 272.1
- essential 272.1
- familial 272.1
- hereditary 272.1
- mixed 272.3
- pure 272.1
Hyperglycinemia 270.7
Hypergonadism
- ovarian 256.1
- testicular (primary) 257.0
- - infantile 257.0
Hyperheparinemia (see also Circulating anticoagulants) 286.5
Hyperhidrosis, hyperidrosis 780.8
- psychogenic 306.3
Hyperhistidinemia 270.5
Hyperinsulinism NEC 251.1
- ectopic 251.1
- functional 251.1
- iatrogenic 251.0
- therapeutic misadventure (from administration of insulin) 962.3
Hyperkalemia 276.7
Hyperkeratosis (see also Keratosis) 701.1
- cervix 622.1
- congenital 757.3
- due to yaws (early) (late) (palmar or plantar) 102.3
- excentrica 757.3

Hyperkeratosis - *continued*
- figurata centrifuga atrophica 757.3
- follicularis 757.3
- - in cutem penetrans 701.1
- palmoplantaris climacterica 701.1
- pinta 103.1
- senile (with pruritus) 702
- universalis congenita 757.1
- vocal cord 478.5
- vulva 624.0
Hyperkinesia, hyperkinetic (disease) (reaction) (syndrome) 314.9
- with
- - conduct disorder 314.2
- - developmental delay 314.1
- - disturbance of activity and attention (simple) 314.0
- - specified manifestation NEC 314.8
- heart 429.8
- of childhood or adolescence NEC 314.9
Hyperlipemia - see Hyperlipidemia
Hyperlipidemia 272.4
- combined 272.4
- group
- - A 272.0
- - B 272.1
- - C 272.2
- - D 272.3
- mixed 272.2
- specified NEC 272.4
Hyperlipidosis 272.7
- hereditary 272.7
Hyperlipoproteinemia 272.4
- familial 272.4
- Fredrickson type
- - I 272.3
- - IIA 272.0
- - IIB 272.2
- - III 272.2
- - IV 272.1
- - V 272.3
- low-density-lipoid-type (LDL) 272.0
- very-low-density-lipoid-type (VLDL) 272.1
Hyperlysinemia 270.7
Hypermagnesemia 275.2
- neonatal 775.5
Hypermaturity (fetus or newborn) 766.2
Hypermenorrhea 626.2
Hypermethioninemia 270.4
Hypermetropia (congenital) 367.0
Hypermobility, hypermotility
- cecum 564.1
- coccyx 724.7
- colon 564.1
- - psychogenic 306.4
- gastrointestinal 536.8

Hyperplasia - *continued*
- pancreatic islet cells - *continued*
- - beta 251.1
- parathyroid (gland) 252.0
- persistent (primary) of vitreous 743.5
- pharynx (lymphoid) 478.2
- prostate (adenofibromatous) (nodular) 600
- renal artery 447.3
- reticulo-endothelial (cell) 289.9
- salivary gland (any) 527.1
- Schimmelbusch's 610.1
- suprarenal (capsule) (gland) 255.8
- thymus (gland) (persistent) 254.0
- thyroid (gland) (see also Goiter) 240.9
- tonsil (and adenoids) (lymphoid tissue) 474.1
- uterus, uterine 621.2
- - endometrium 621.3
- vulva 624.3
Hyperpnea (see also Hyperventilation) 786.0
Hyperpotassemia 276.7
Hyperprebetalipoproteinemia, familial 272.1
Hyperprolinemia 270.8
Hyperproteinemia 273.8
Hyperpyrexia 780.6
- heat (effects) 992.0
- malarial (see also Malaria) 084.6
- malignant, due to anesthetic 995.8
- rheumatic - see Fever, rheumatic
- unknown origin (see also Pyrexia) 780.6
Hyper-reflexia 796.1
Hypersalivation (see also Ptyalism) 527.7
Hypersecretion
- ACTH 255.3
- calcitonin 246.0
- corticoadrenal 255.3
- cortisol 255.0
- estrogen 256.0
- gastric 536.8
- - psychogenic 306.4
- gastrin 251.5
- glucagon 251.4
- hormone
- - ACTH 255.3
- - anterior pituitary 253.1
- - growth NEC 253.0
- - ovarian androgen 256.1
- - testicular 257.0
- - thyroid stimulating 242.8
- insulin - see Hyperinsulinism
- lacrimal glands 375.2
- medulloadrenal 255.6
- milk 676.6
- ovarian androgens 256.1

Hypersecretion - *continued*
- salivary gland (any) 527.7
- thyrocalcitonin 246.0
- upper respiratory 478.9
Hypersegmentation, hereditary 288.2
Hypersensitive, hypersensitiveness, hypersensitivity - see also Allergy
- carotid sinus 337.0
- colon 564.1
- - psychogenic 306.4
- drug (see also Allergy, drug) 995.2
- esophagus 530.8
- insect bites - see Injury, superficial
- labyrinth 386.5
- pain (see also Disturbance, sensation) 782.0
- pneumonitis NEC 495.9
- reaction 995.3
- - upper respiratory tract NEC 478.8
- stomach (allergic) (nonallergic) 536.8
- - psychogenic 306.4
Hypersomnia 780.5
- nonorganic origin 307.4
Hypersplenia 289.4
Hypersplenism 289.4
Hypersuprarenalism 255.3
Hypersusceptibility - see Allergy
Hypertelorism 756.0
Hypertension, hypertensive (arterial) (arteriolar) (degeneration) (disease) (essential) (fluctuating) (idiopathic) (intermittent) (labile) (orthostatic) (paroxysmal) (primary) (systemic) (vascular) 401.9

Note - The following fourth-digit subdivisions are for use with categories 401–405:
   .0 Specified as malignant
   .1 Specified as benign
   .9 Not specified as malignant or benign.

Hypertension - *continued*
- with
- - heart involvement (conditions in 428.-, 429.0-.3, .8, .9 due to hypertension) (see also Hypertension, heart) 402.-
- - renal sclerosis or failure (conditions in 585, 586, 587) (see also Hypertension, kidney) 403.-
- cardiorenal (disease) 404.-
- cardiovascular
- - disease (arteriosclerotic) (sclerotic) 402.-
- - renal (disease) (sclerosis) 404.-
- complicating pregnancy, childbirth or the puerperium 642.9

Hypertrophy - *continued*
- cardiac - *continued*
- - congenital NEC 746.8
- - fatty (see also Degeneration, myocardial) 429.1
- - hypertensive (see also Hypertension, heart) 402.9
- - rheumatic (with chorea) 398.9
- - - active or acute 391.8
- - - - with chorea 392.0
- - valve (see also Endocarditis) 424.9
- - - congenital NEC 746.8
- cartilage 733.9
- cecum 569.8
- cervix (uteri) 622.6
- - congenital 752.4
- - elongation 622.6
- clitoris (cirrhotic) 624.2
- - congenital 752.4
- colon 569.8
- - congenital 751.3
- conjunctiva, lymphoid 372.7
- corpora cavernosa 607.8
- duodenum 537.8
- endometrium (uterus) 621.3
- - cervix 622.6
- epididymis 608.8
- esophageal hiatus (congenital) 756.8
- - with hernia - see Hernia, diaphragm
- eyelid 374.3
- falx, skull 733.9
- fat pad
- - infrapatellar 729.3
- - knee 729.3
- - popliteal 729.3
- - prepatellar 729.3
- - retropatellar 729.3
- foot (congenital) 755.6
- frenum (tongue) 529.8
- - lip 528.5
- gallbladder or cystic duct (see also Disease, gallbladder) 575.8
- gastric mucosa 535.2
- gland, glandular (general) NEC 785.6
- gum (mucous membrane) 523.8
- heart (idiopathic) - see also Hypertrophy, cardiac
- - valve - see also Endocarditis
- - - congenital NEC 746.8
- hemifacial 754.0
- hepatic - see Hypertrophy, liver
- hiatus (esophageal) 756.8
- - with hernia - see Hernia, diaphragm
- hilus gland 785.6
- hymen, congenital 752.4
- ileum 569.8
- infrapatellar fat pad 729.3

Hypertrophy - *continued*
- intestine 569.8
- jejunum 569.8
- kidney (compensatory) 593.1
- - congenital 753.3
- labium (majus) (minus) 624.3
- ligament 728.9
- lingual tonsil (infectional) 474.1
- lip 528.5
- - congenital 744.8
- liver 789.1
- - acute 573.8
- - cirrhotic - see Cirrhosis, liver
- - congenital 751.6
- - fatty - see Fatty, liver
- lymph, lymphatic gland 785.6
- - tuberculous - see Tuberculosis, lymph gland
- mammary gland - see Hypertrophy, breast
- Meckel's diverticulum (congenital) 751.0
- median bar 600
- mediastinum 519.3
- meibomian gland 373.2
- meniscus, knee, congenital 755.6
- metatarsal head 733.9
- metatarsus 733.9
- mucous membrane
- - alveolar process 523.8
- - nose 478.1
- - of turbinate 478.0
- muscle 728.9
- muscular coat, artery 447.8
- myocardium (see also Hypertrophy, cardiac) 429.3
- - idiopathic 425.4
- myometrium 621.2
- nail 703.8
- - congenital 757.5
- nasal 478.1
- - alae 478.1
- - bone 738.0
- - cartilage 478.1
- - mucous membrane (septum) 478.1
- - sinus (see also Sinusitis) 473.9
- - turbinate 478.0
- nasopharynx, lymphoid (infectional) (tissue) (wall) 478.2
- neck uterus 622.6
- nipple 611.1
- normal aperture diaphragm (congenital) 756.6
- nose 478.1
- oesophageal hiatus 756.8
- organ or site, congenital NEC - see Anomaly, specified type NEC
- ovary 620.8

Hypertrophy - *continued*
- palate (hard) 526.8
- -- soft 528.9
- pancreas (congenital) 751.7
- papillae anal 569.4
- parathyroid (gland) 252.0
- parotid gland 527.1
- penis 607.8
- phallus 607.8
- pharyngeal tonsil 474.1
- pharynx 478.2
- -- lymphoid (infectional) (tissue) (wall)
    478.2
- pituitary (fossa) (gland) 253.8
- popliteal fat pad 729.3
- prepuce (congenital) 605
- -- female 624.2

- prostate (adenofibromatous)
    (asymptomatic) (benign) (early)
    (recurrent) 600
- -- congenital 752.8
- pseudomuscular 359.1

- pylorus (muscle) (sphincter) 537.0
- -- congenital 750.5
- -- infantile 750.5
- rectal sphincter 569.4
- rectum 569.4
- rhinitis (turbinate) 472.0
- salivary duct or gland 527.1
- -- congenital 750.2
- scaphoid (tarsal) 733.9
- scar 701.4
- scrotum 608.8
- sella turcica 253.8
- seminal vesicle 608.8
- sigmoid 569.8
- spermatic cord 608.8

- spleen - see Splenomegaly
- spondylitis 721.9
- stomach 537.8
- sublingual gland 527.1
- -- congenital 750.2
- submaxillary gland 527.1
- suprarenal (gland) 255.8
- tendon 727.9
- testis 608.8
- -- congenital 752.8

- thymic, thymus (gland) (congenital)
    254.0
- thyroid (gland) (see also Goiter) 240.9
- toe (congenital) 755.6
- -- acquired 735.8
- tongue 529.8
- -- congenital 750.1
- -- papillae (foliate) 529.3

Hypertrophy - *continued*
- tonsils (and adenoids) (faucial)
    (infectional) (lingual) (lymphoid)
    (pharyngeal) 474.1
- tunica vaginalis 608.8
- ureter 593.8
- urethra 599.8
- uterus 621.2
- -- neck 622.6
- uvula 528.9
- vagina 623.8
- vas deferens 608.8
- vein 459.8
- ventricle, ventricular (heart) - see also
    Hypertrophy, cardiac
- -- congenital 746.8
- -- in tetralogy of Fallot 745.2
- verumontanum 599.8
- vocal cord 478.5
- vulva 624.3
- -- stasis (nonfilarial) 624.3
Hypertropia 378.3
Hypertyrosinemia 270.2
Hyperuricemia 790.6
Hypervalinemia 270.3
Hyperventilation (tetany) 786.0
- hysterical 300.1
- psychogenic 306.1
- syndrome 306.1
Hyperviscidosis 277.0
Hypervitaminosis (dietary) NEC 278.8
- A 278.2
- -- reaction to sudden overdose 963.5
- D 278.4
- -- reaction to sudden overdose 963.5
- from excessive administration or use of
    vitamin preparations (chronic) 278.8
- -- reaction to sudden overdose 963.5
- K
- -- correct substance properly
    administered 278.8
- -- overdose or wrong substance given or
    taken 964.3
Hypervolemia 276.6
Hypesthesia (see also Disturbance,
    sensation) 782.0
- cornea 371.8
Hyphema 364.4
- traumatic 921.3
Hypoacidity gastric 536.8
- psychogenic 306.4
Hypoadrenalism, hypoadrenia 255.4
- tuberculous 017.6 † 255.4*
Hypoadrenocorticism 255.4
- pituitary 253.4
Hypoalbuminemia 273.8
Hypoalphalipoproteinemia 272.5

Hypobarism 993.2
Hypobaropathy 993.2
Hypobetalipoproteinemia (familial) 272.5
Hypocalcemia 275.4
– cow's milk 775.4
– dietary 269.3
– neonatal 775.4
– phosphate-loading (newborn) 775.4
Hypochloremia 276.9
Hypochlorhydria 536.8
– neurotic 306.4
– psychogenic 306.4
Hypocholesteremia 272.5
Hypochondria (reaction) 300.7
Hypochondriac 300.7
Hypochondriasis 300.7
Hypochromasia blood cells 280
Hypodontia (see also Anodontia) 520.0
Hypoeosinophilia 288.8
Hypoesthesia (see also Disturbance,
    sensation) 782.0
Hypofibrinogenemia (see also Defect,
    coagulation) 286.9
– acquired 286.6
– congenital 286.3
Hypofunction
– adrenal cortical 255.4
– cerebral 331.9
– corticoadrenal NEC 255.4
– intestinal 564.8
– labyrinth 386.5
– ovary 256.3
– pituitary (gland) (anterior) 253.2
– testicular 257.2
– – iatrogenic 257.1
– – postablative 257.1
– – postirradiation 257.1
– – postsurgical 257.1
Hypogammaglobulinemia 279.0
Hypogenitalism (male) (female)
    (congenital) 752.8
Hypoglycemia (spontaneous) 251.2
– coma 251.0
– due to insulin 251.0
– – therapeutic misadventure 962.3
– following gastrointestinal surgery 579.3
– in infant of diabetic mother 775.0
– infantile 251.2
– leucine-induced 270.3
– neonatal 775.6
– reactive 251.2
Hypogonadism
– female 256.3
– male 257.2
– ovarian (primary) 256.3
– pituitary 253.4
– testicular (primary) 257.2

Hypohidrosis 705.0
Hypoidrosis 705.0
Hypoinsulinemia, postsurgical 251.3
Hypokalemia 276.8
Hypoleukocytosis 288.8
Hypolipoproteinemia 272.5
Hypomagnesemia 275.2
– neonatal 775.4
Hypomania, hypomanic reaction 296.0
Hypomenorrhea 626.1
Hypometabolism 783.9
Hypomotility
– gastrointestinal (tract) 536.8
– – psychogenic 306.4
– intestine 564.8
– – psychogenic 306.4
– stomach 536.8
– – psychogenic 306.4
Hyponasality 784.4
Hyponatremia 276.1
Hypo-ovarianism 256.3
Hypo-ovarism 256.3
Hypoparathyroidism 252.1
– neonatal 775.4
Hypopharyngitis 462
Hypophoria 378.4
Hypophosphatasia 275.3
Hypophosphatemia (acquired)
    (nonfamilial) 275.3
– congenital 275.3
– familial 275.3
– renal 275.3
Hypophyseal, hypophysis - see also
    condition
– dwarfism 253.3
– gigantism 253.0
Hypopiesis - see Hypotension
Hypopinealism 259.8
Hypopituitarism (juvenile) 253.2
– induced by
– – hormone therapy 253.7
– – hypophysectomy 253.7
– – radiotherapy 253.7
– postpartum 253.2
Hypoplasia, hypoplasis 759.8
– adrenal (gland) 759.1
– alimentary tract 751.8
– – lower 751.2
– – upper 750.8
– anus, anal (canal) 751.2
– aorta, aortic 747.2
– – arch (tubular) 747.1
– – ascending, in hypoplastic left heart
        syndrome 746.7
– – orifice or valve 746.8
– – – in hypoplastic left heart syndrome
        746.7

Hypoplasia - *continued*
- appendix 751.2
- areola 757.6
- arm 755.2
- artery (peripheral) 747.6
- - brain 747.8
- - coronary 746.8
- - pulmonary 747.3
- - retinal 743.5
- - umbilical 747.5
- auditory canal 744.2
- - causing impairment of hearing 744.0
- biliary duct or passage 751.6
- bone NEC 756.9
- - face 756.0
- - mandible 524.0
- - marrow 284.9
- - maxilla 524.0
- - skull (see also Hypoplasia, skull) 756.0
- brain 742.1
- - gyri 742.2
- - part of 742.2
- breast (areola) 757.6
- bronchus 748.3
- cardiac 746.8
- - valve 746.8
- - - pulmonary 746.0
- carpus 755.2
- cartilaginous 756.9
- cecum 751.2
- cementum 520.4
- cephalic 742.1
- cerebellum 742.2
- cervix (uteri) 752.4
- clavicle 755.5
- coccyx 756.1
- colon 751.2
- corpus callosum 742.2
- cricoid cartilage 748.3
- digestive organ(s) or tract NEC 751.8
- - lower 751.2
- - upper 750.8
- ear (auricle) (lobe) 744.2
- - middle 744.0
- enamel of teeth (neonatal) (postnatal) (prenatal) 520.4
- endocrine (gland) NEC 759.2
- endometrium 621.8
- epididymis 752.8
- epiglottis 748.3
- erythroid, congenital 284.0
- esophagus 750.3
- eustachian tube 744.2
- eye 743.1
- - lid 743.6
- face 744.8
- - bone(s) 756.0

Hypoplasia - *continued*
- fallopian tube 752.1
- femur 755.3
- fibula 755.3
- finger 755.2
- focal dermal 757.3
- foot 755.3
- gallbladder 751.6
- genitalia, genital organ(s)
- - female 752.8
- - - external 752.4
- - - internal NEC 752.8
- - in adiposogenital dystrophy 253.8
- - male 752.8
- glottis 748.3
- hair 757.4
- hand 755.2
- heart 746.8
- - valve NEC 746.8
- - - pulmonary 746.0
- humerus 755.2
- intestine (small) 751.1
- - large 751.2
- iris 743.4
- jaw 524.0
- kidney(s) 753.0
- labium (majus) (minus) 752.4
- labyrinth, membranous 744.0
- larynx 748.3
- leg 755.3
- limb 755.4
- - lower 755.3
- - upper 755.2
- liver 751.6
- lung (lobe) 748.5
- mammary (areola) 757.6
- mandible, mandibular 524.0
- - unilateral condylar 526.8
- maxillary 524.0
- medullary 284.9
- megakaryocytic 287.3
- metacarpus 755.2
- metatarsus 755.3
- muscle 756.8
- - eye 743.6
- nail(s) 757.5
- nervous system NEC 742.8
- neural 742.8
- nose, nasal 748.1
- ophthalmic 743.1
- organ
- - of Corti 744.0
- - or site not listed - see Anomaly, specified type NEC
- osseous meatus (ear) 744.2
- ovary 752.0
- oviduct 752.1

Hypoplasia - *continued*
- pancreas 751.7
- parathyroid (gland) 759.2
- parotid gland 750.2
- patella 755.6
- pelvis, pelvic girdle 755.6
- penis 752.8
- peripheral vascular system 747.6
- pituitary (gland) 759.2
- pulmonary 748.5
- - arteriovenous 747.3
- - artery 747.3
- - valve 746.0
- radioulnar 755.2
- radius 755.2
- rectum 751.2
- respiratory system NEC 748.9
- rib 756.3
- sacrum 756.1
- scapula 755.5
- shoulder girdle 755.5
- skin 757.3
- skull (bone) 756.0
- - with
- - - anencephalus 740.0
- - - encephalocele 742.0
- - - hydrocephalus 742.3
- - - - with spina bifida 741.0
- - - microcephalus 742.1
- spinal (cord) (ventral horn cell) 742.5
- - vessel 747.6
- spine 756.1
- spleen 759.0
- sternum 756.3
- tarsus 755.3
- testis 752.8
- thymus (gland) 759.2
- thyroid (gland) 243
- - cartilage 748.3
- tibio-fibular 755.3
- toe 755.3
- tongue 750.1
- trachea (cartilage) (rings) 748.3
- Turner's 520.4
- ulna 755.2
- umbilical artery 747.5
- ureter 753.2
- uterus 752.3
- vagina 752.4
- vascular NEC 747.6
- - brain 747.8
- vein(s) (peripheral) 747.6
- - brain 747.8
- - great 747.4
- - portal 747.4
- - pulmonary 747.4
- vena cava (inferior) (superior) 747.4

Hypoplasia - *continued*
- vertebra 756.1
- vulva 752.4
- zonule (ciliary) 743.3
Hypopotassemia 276.8
Hypoproconvertinemia, congenital (see also Defect, coagulation) 286.3
Hypoproteinemia 273.8
Hypoproteinosis 260
Hypoprothrombinemia (congenital) (idiopathic) (see also Defect, coagulation) 286.3
- acquired 286.7
- newborn 776.3
Hypopyon (eye) (anterior chamber) 364.4
- iritis 364.0
- ulcer (cornea) 370.0
Hypopyrexia 780.9
Hyporeflex 796.1
Hyposecretion
- acth 253.4
- ovary 256.3
- salivary gland (any) 527.7
Hyposegmentation, hereditary 288.2
Hyposiderinemia 280
Hyposmolality 276.1
Hyposomnia 780.5
- nonorganic origin 307.4
Hypospadias (male) 752.6
- female 753.8
Hypospermatogenesis 606
Hyposphagma 372.7
Hypostasis pulmonary 514
Hypostatic - see condition
Hyposthenuria 593.8
Hyposuprarenalism 255.4
Hypotension (arterial) (constitutional) 458.9
- chronic 458.1
- maternal, syndrome (following labor and delivery) 669.2
- orthostatic (chronic) 458.0
- permanent idiopathic 458.1
- postural 458.0
Hypothermia (accidental) 991.6
- anesthetic 995.8
- neonatal NEC 778.3
- not associated with low environmental temperature 780.9
Hypothymergasia 296.1
Hypothyroidism (acquired) 244.9
- congenital 243
- due to
- - iodine (administration) (ingestion) 244.2
- - irradiation therapy 244.1
- - P-aminosalicylic acid (PAS) 244.3

Hypothyroidism - *continued*
- due to - *continued*
- - phenylbutazone 244.3
- - resorcinol 244.3
- - surgery 244.0
- iodine 244.2
- postsurgical 244.0
- specified cause NEC 244.8
Hypotonia, hypotonicity, hypotony
- bladder 596.4
- congenital 779.8
- - benign 358.8
- eye 360.3
- muscle 728.9
- uterus, uterine (contractions) - see
  Inertia, uterus
Hypotrichosis 704.0
- congenital 757.4
- lid, congenital 757.4
- postinfectional NEC 704.0
Hypotropia 378.3
Hypoventilation 786.0

Hypovitaminosis (see also Deficiency,
  vitamin) 269.2
Hypovolemia 276.5
- surgical shock 998.0
- traumatic (shock) 958.4
Hypoxia - see also Anoxia
- cerebral, during or resulting from a
  procedure NEC 997.0
- fetal - see Distress, fetal
- intra-uterine - see Distress, fetal
- myocardial (see also Insufficiency,
  coronary) 411
- newborn - see Asphyxia, newborn
Hypsarhythmia 345.6
Hysteralgia, pregnant uterus 646.8
Hysteria, hysterical (conversion)
  (dissociative state) 300.1
- anxiety 300.2
- psychosis, acute 298.1
Hystero-epilepsy 300.1
Hysterotomy, affecting fetus or newborn
  763.8

I

I.Q.
- under 20 318.2
- 20-34 318.1
- 35-49 318.0
- 50-70 317
I.R.D.S. 769
Ichthyosis (congenita) 757.1
- acquired 701.1
- fetalis gravior 757.1
- follicularis 757.1
- hystrix 757.3
- palmaris and plantaris 757.3
- simplex 757.1
- vera 757.1
Ichthyotoxism 988.0
- bacterial (see also Poisoning, food) 005.9
Icteroanemia, hemolytic (acquired) 283.9
- congenital (see also Sperocytosis) 282.0
Icterus (see also Jaundice) 782.4
- conjunctiva 782.4
- epidemic - see Icterus, infectious
- febrilis - see Icterus, infectious
- fetus or newborn - see Jaundice, fetus or newborn
- gravis (see also Necrosis, liver) 570
- - fetus or newborn NEC 773.2
- hematogenous (acquired) 283.9
- hemolytic (acquired) 283.9
- - congenital (see also Spherocytosis) 282.0
- hemorrhagic (acute) 100.0
- - leptospiral 100.0
- - spirochetal 100.0
- infectious 070.1 † 573.1*
- - with hepatic coma 070.0 † 573.1*
- - leptospiral 100.0
- - spirochetal 100.0
- intermittens juvenilis 277.4
- malignant (see also Necrosis, liver) 570
- neonatorum (see also Jaundice, fetus or newborn) 774.6
- pernicious (see also Necrosis, liver) 570
- spirochetal 100.0
Ictus solaris, solis 992.0
Id reaction (due to bacteria) 692.8
Idioglossia 307.0
Idiopathic - see condition
Idiosyncracy (see also Allergy) 995.3
- drug, medicament and biological - see Allergy, drug

Idiot, idiocy (congenital) 318.2
- amaurotic (Bielschowsky(-Jansky)) (family) (infantile (late)) (juvenile (late)) (Vogt-Spielmeyer) 330.1
Ileitis - see also Enteritis
- regional (ulcerative) 555.0
- terminal (ulcerative) 555.0
Ileocolitis - see Enteritis
Ileotyphus 002.0
Ileum - see condition
Ileus (adynamic) (bowel) (colon) (inhibitory) (intestine) (neurogenic) (paralytic) 560.1
- arteriomesenteric duodenal 537.2
- due to gallstone (in intestine) 560.3
- duodenal, chronic 537.2
- mechanical 560.9
- meconium 277.0 † 777.0*
- transitory of newborn 777.4
Iliac - see condition
Illegitimacy V61.6
Illness - see also Disease
- manic-depressive (see also Psychosis, manic-depressive) 296.6
Imbalance 781.2
- autonomic 337.9
- electrolyte 276.9
- - with hyperemesis gravidarum 643.1
- - complicating abortion - see categories 634-639, fourth digit .4
- - neonatal, transitory NEC 775.5
- endocrine 259.9
- eye muscle NEC 378.9
- hormone 259.9
- hysterical 300.1
- labyrinth 386.5
- posture 729.9
- sympathetic 337.9
Imbecile, imbecility 318.0
- moral 301.7
- old age 290.9
- senile 290.9
- specified I.Q. - see I.Q.
- unspecified I.Q. 318.0
Imbibition, cholesterol (gallbladder) 575.6
Imerslund(-Grasbeck) syndrome 281.1
Iminoacidopathy 270.8
Immature - see also Immaturity
- personality 301.8
Immaturity 765.1

Immaturity - *continued*
- extreme 765.0
- fetus or infant light-for-dates - see Light-for-dates
- lung, fetus or newborn 770.4
- organ or site NEC - see Hypoplasia
- pulmonary, fetus or newborn 770.4
- reaction 301.8
- sexual (female) (male) 259.0
Immersion 994.1
- foot 991.4
- hand 991.4
Immobile, immobility
- intestine 564.8
- joint - see Ankylosis
- syndrome (paraplegic) 728.3
Immunization
- ABO
- - affecting management of pregnancy 656.2
- - - fetus or newborn 773.1
- complication - see Complications, vaccination
- Rh factor
- - affecting management of pregnancy 656.1
- - - fetus or newborn 773.0
- - from transfusion 999.7
Immunotherapy, prophylactic V07.2
Impaction, impacted
- bowel, colon, rectum (fecal) 560.3
- calculus - see Calculus
- cerumen (ear) (external) 380.4
- cuspid 520.6
- - with abnormal position (same or adjacent tooth) 524.3
- dental 520.6
- - with abnormal position (same or adjacent tooth) 524.3
- fecal, feces 560.3
- fracture - code as Fracture, closed
- gallbladder (see also Cholelithiasis) 574.2
- gallstone(s) (see also Cholelithiasis) 574.2
- - in intestine (any part) 560.3
- intestine (calculus) (fecal) (gallstone) 560.3
- molar 520.6
- - with abnormal position (same or adjacent tooth) 524.3
- shoulder 660.4
- - affecting fetus or newborn 763.1
- tooth, teeth 520.6
- - with abnormal position (same or adjacent tooth) 524.3
- turbinate 733.9
Impaired, impairment (function)

Impaired - *continued*
- auditory discrimination 388.4
- hearing - see Deafness
- heart - see Disease, heart
- kidney (see also Disease, renal) 593.9
- - disorder resulting from 588.9
- - - specified NEC 588.8
- liver 573.8
- mastication 524.9
- mobility, ear ossicles 385.2
- myocardium, myocardial (see also Insufficiency, myocardial) 428.0
- rectal sphincter 787.9
- renal (see also Disease, renal) 593.9
- - disorder resulting from 588.9
- - - specified NEC 588.8
- vision NEC 369.9
Impaludism - see Malaria
Impediment, speech NEC 784.5
- psychogenic 307.9
- secondary to organic lesion 784.5
Imperception auditory (acquired) (congenital) (see also Deafness) 389.9
Imperfect
- aeration, lung (newborn) NEC 770.5
- closure (congenital)
- - alimentary tract NEC 751.8
- - - lower 751.5
- - - upper 750.8
- - atrioventricular ostium 745.6
- - branchial cleft or sinus 744.4
- - choroid 743.5
- - cricoid cartilage 748.3
- - cusps, heart valve NEC 746.8
- - - pulmonary 746.0
- - ductus
- - - arteriosus 747.0
- - - botalli 747.0
- - ear drum 744.2
- - - causing impairment of hearing 744.0
- - epiglottis 748.3
- - esophagus with communication to bronchus or trachea 750.3
- - eustachian valve 746.8
- - eyelid 743.6
- - foramen
- - - botalli 745.5
- - - ovale 745.5
- - genitalia, genital organ(s) or system
- - - female 752.8
- - - - external 752.4
- - - - internal NEC 752.8
- - - male 752.8
- - glottis 748.3
- - iris 743.4
- - kidney 753.3
- - larynx 748.3

Imperfect - *continued*
- closure - *continued*
- - lens 743.3
- - lip 749.1
- - - with cleft palate 749.2
- - nasal septum or sinus 748.1
- - nose 748.1
- - omphalomesenteric duct 751.0
- - optic nerve entry 743.5
- - organ or site not listed - see Anomaly, specified type NEC
- - ostium
- - - interatrial 745.5
- - - interauricular 745.5
- - - interventricular 745.4
- - palate 749.0
- - - with cleft lip 749.2
- - preauricular sinus 744.4
- - retina 743.5
- - roof of orbit 742.0
- - sclera 743.5
- - septum
- - - aortic 745.0
- - - aorticopulmonary 745.0
- - - atrial 745.5
- - - between aorta and pulmonary artery 745.0
- - - heart 745.9
- - - interatrial 745.5
- - - interauricular 745.5
- - - interventricular 745.4
- - - - in tetralogy of Fallot 745.2
- - - nasal 748.1
- - - ventricular 745.4
- - - - in tetralogy of Fallot 745.2
- - skull 756.0
- - - with
- - - - anencephalus 740.0
- - - - encephalocele 742.0
- - - - hydrocephalus 742.3
- - - - - with spina bifida 741.0
- - - - microcephalus 742.1
- - spine (with meningocele) 741.9
- - - with hydrocephalus 741.0
- - thyroid cartilage 748.3
- - trachea 748.3
- - tympanic membrane 744.2
- - - causing impairment of hearing 744.0
- - uterus (with communication to bladder, intestine or rectum) 752.3
- - uvula 749.0
- - - with cleft lip 749.2
- - vitelline duct 751.0
- erection 607.8
- fusion - see Imperfect closure
- intestinal canal 751.5
- poise 729.9

Imperfect - *continued*
- rotation - see Malrotation
- septum, ventricular 745.4
Imperfectly descended testis 752.5
Imperforate (congenital) - see also Atresia
- anus 751.2
- cervix (uteri) 752.4
- esophagus 750.3
- hymen 752.4
- jejunum 751.1
- oesophagus 750.3
- pharynx 750.2
- rectum 751.2
- urethra 753.6
- vagina 752.4
Impervious (congenital) - see also Atresia
- anus 751.2
- bile duct 751.6
- esophagus 750.3
- intestine (small) 751.1
- - large 751.5
- oesophagus 750.3
- rectum 751.2
- ureter 753.2
- urethra 753.6
Impetiginization of other dermatoses 684
Impetigo (any organism) (any site) (bullous) (circinate) (contagiosa) (neonatorum) (simplex) 684
- Bockhart's 704.8
- external ear 684 † 380.1*
- eyelid 684 † 373.5*
- Fox's 684
- furfuracea 696.5
- herpetiformis 694.3
- - non-obstetrical 694.3
- ulcerative 686.8
- vulgaris 684
Impingement, soft tissue between teeth 524.2
Implant, endometrial 617.9
Implantation
- anomalous - see also Anomaly, specified type NEC
- - ureter 753.4
- cyst
- - external area or site (skin) NEC 709.8
- - iris 364.6
- - vagina 623.8
- - vulva 624.8
- dermoid (cyst)
- - external area or site (skin) NEC 709.8
- - iris 364.6
- - vagina 623.8
- - vulva 624.8
- placenta, low or marginal - see Placenta previa

Impotence (sexual) (psychogenic) 302.7
− organic origin NEC 607.8
Impression, basilar 756.0
Imprisonment, anxiety concerning V62.5
Improper care (child) (newborn) 995.5
Improperly tied umbilical cord 772.3
Impulses, obsessional 300.3
Impulsive neurosis 300.3
Inaction, kidney (see also Disease, renal)
    593.9
Inactive - see condition
Inadequate, inadequacy
− biologic, constitutional, functional, or
    social 301.6
− cardiac and renal 404.9
− development
− − child 783.4
− − fetus 764.9
− − − affecting management of pregnancy
        656.5
− − genitalia
− − − after puberty NEC 259.0
− − − congenital - see Hypoplasia,
        genitalia
− − lungs 748.5
− − organ or site not listed - see Hypoplasia
− dietary 269.8
− household care, due to
− − family member
− − − handicapped or ill V60.4
− − − on vacation V60.5
− − − temporarily away from home V60.4
− − technical defects in home V60.1
− − temporary absence from home of
        person rendering care V60.4
− housing (heating) (space) V60.1
− material resources V60.2
− mental (see also Retardation, mental)
    319
− nervous system 799.2
− personality 301.6
− pulmonary
− − function 786.0
− − − newborn 770.8
− − ventilation, newborn 770.8
− respiration 786.0
− − newborn 770.8
Inanition 263.9
− with edema 262
− due to
− − deprivation of food 994.2
− − malnutrition 263.9
− fever 780.6
Inattention after or at birth 995.5
Incarceration, incarcerated
− colon (by hernia) - see also Hernia, by
    site, with obstruction

Incarceration - continued
− colon - continued
− − gangrenous - see Hernia, by site,
        gangrenous
− hernia - see also Hernia, by site, with
    obstruction
− − gangrenous - see Hernia, by site,
        gangrenous
− iris, in wound 871.1
− lens, in wound 871.1
− omentum (by hernia) - see also Hernia,
    by site, with obstruction
− − gangrenous - see Hernia, by site,
        gangrenous
− rupture (meaning hernia) (see also
    Hernia, by site, with obstruction) 552.9
− − gangrenous (see also Hernia, by site,
        gangrenous) 551.9
− uterus 621.8
− − gravid 654.3
− − − causing obstructed labor 660.2
− − − − fetus or newborn 763.1
Incident, cerebrovascular (see also Disease,
    cerebrovascular, acute) 436
Incineration (entire body) (from fire,
    conflagration, electricity or lightning)
    946.-
Incised wound
− external - see Wound, open
− internal organs (abdomen, chest or
    pelvis) - see Injury, internal, by site, with
    open wound
Incision, incisional
− hernia - see Hernia, ventral
− surgical, complication - see
    Complications, surgical procedure
− traumatic
− − external - see Wound, open
− − internal organs (abdomen, chest or
        pelvis) - see Injury, internal, by site,
        with open wound
Inclusion, gallbladder in liver (congenital)
    751.6
Incompatibility
− ABO
− − affecting management of pregnancy
        656.2
− − fetus 773.1
− − infusion or transfusion reaction 999.6
− − newborn 773.1
− blood (group) (Duffy) (K(ell)) (Kidd)
    (Lewis) (M) (S) NEC
− − affecting management of pregnancy
        656.2
− − fetus 773.2
− − infusion or transfusion reaction 999.6
− − newborn 773.2

Incompatibility - *continued*
- Rh (blood group) (factor)
- - affecting management of pregnancy 656.1
- - fetus 773.0
- - infusion or transfusion reaction 999.7
- - newborn 773.0
- rhesus - see Incompatibility, Rh
Incompetency, incompetent
- annular
- - aortic (valve) (see also Insufficiency, aortic) 424.1
- - mitral (valve) 424.0
- - pulmonary valve (heart) (see also Endocarditis, pulmonary) 424.3
- aortic (valve) (see also Insufficiency, aortic) 424.1
- - syphilitic 093.2 † 424.1*
- cardiac (orifice) 530.0
- - valve - see Endocarditis
- cervix, cervical (os) 622.5
- - in pregnancy 654.5
- - - fetus or newborn 761.0
- heart valve, congenital 746.8
- mitral (valve) - see Insufficiency, mitral
- pelvic fundus 618.8
- pulmonary valve (heart) (see also Endocarditis, pulmonary) 424.3
- tricuspid (annular) (valve) (see also Endocarditis, tricuspid) 397.0
- valvular - see Endocarditis

Incomplete - see also condition
- expansion lungs (newborn) NEC 770.5
- rotation - see Malrotation
Incontinence 788.3
- anal sphincter 787.6
- feces 787.6
- - due to hysteria 300.1
- - non-organic origin 307.7
- hysterical 300.1
- stress (female) 625.6
- - male 788.3
- urethral sphincter 788.3
- urine 788.3
- - male 788.3
- - neurogenic 788.3
- - nonorganic origin 307.6
- - stress (female) 625.6
- - - male 788.3

Incontinentia pigmenti 757.3
Incoordinate
- uterus (action) (contractions) 661.4
- - fetus or newborn 763.7
Incoordination, muscular 781.3
Increase, increased
- abnormal, in development 783.9

Increase - *continued*
- anticoagulants (antithrombin) (anti-VIIIA) (anti-IXA) (anti-XA) (anti-XIA) 286.5
- cold sense (see also Disturbance, sensation) 782.0
- estrogen 256.0
- function
- - adrenal (cortex) 255.3
- - - medulla 255.6
- - pituitary (gland) (anterior) (lobe) 253.1
- heat sense (see also Disturbance, sensation) 782.0
- intracranial pressure 348.2
- permeability
- - capillaries 448.9
- sphericity, lens 743.3
- splenic activity 289.4
- venous pressure 459.8
Incrustation, cornea, lead or zinc 930.0
Incyclophoria 378.4
Incyclotropia 378.3
Indeterminate sex 752.7
India rubber skin 757.3
Indigestion (bilious) (functional) 536.8
- acid 536.8
- due to decomposed food NEC 005.9
- fat 579.8
- nervous 306.4
- psychogenic 306.4
Indirect - see condition
Induced birth
- fetus or newborn 763.8
Induratio penis plastica 607.8
Induration, indurated
- brain 348.8
- breast (fibrous) 611.7
- - puerperal, postpartum 676.3
- broad ligament 620.8
- corpora cavernosa (penis) (plastic) 607.8
- liver (chronic) 573.8
- - acute 573.8
- lung (chronic) (fibroid) (see also Fibrosis, lung) 515
- - essential brown 275.0 † 516.1*
- penile 607.8
- phlebitic - see Phlebitis
- skin 782.8
Inebriety 305.0
Inefficiency, kidney (see also Disease, renal) 593.9
Inequality, leg (length) (acquired) 736.8
- congenital 755.3
Inertia
- bladder 596.4
- - neurogenic 344.6

Inertia - *continued*
- stomach 536.8
- - psychogenic 306.4
- uterus, uterine 661.2
- - fetus or newborn 763.7
- - primary 661.0
- - secondary 661.1
- vesical 596.4
- - neurogenic 344.6
Infancy, infantile - see also condition
- genitalia, genitals 259.0
- - in pregnancy or childbirth NEC 654.4
- - - causing obstructed labor 660.2
- - - - fetus or newborn 763.1
- - - fetus or newborn 763.8
- heart 746.9
- kidney 753.3
- lack of care 995.5
- os, uterus (see also Infantile genitalia) 259.0
- pelvis 738.6
- - with disproportion 653.1
- - - causing obstructed labor 660.1
- - - fetus or newborn 763.1
- penis 259.0
- testis 257.2
- uterus (see also Infantile genitalia) 259.0
- vulva 752.4
Infant - see also Infancy
- of diabetic mother (syndrome of) 775.0
Infantilism 259.9
- Brissaud's 244.9
- celiac 579.0
- intestinal 579.0
- pancreatic 577.8
- pituitary 253.3
- renal 588.0
Infants, healthy liveborn V39.-

Note – The following fourth-digit subdivisions are for use with categories V30–V39:
  .0 Born in hospital
  .1 Born before admission to hospital
  .2 Born outside hospital and not hospitalized.

Infants - *continued*
- multiple NEC V37.-
- - mates all live born V34.-
- - mates all stillborn V35.-
- - mates live and stillborn V36.-
- singleton V30.-
- twin NEC V33.-
- - mate live born V31.-
- - mate stillborn V32.-
Infarct, infarction

Infarct - *continued*
- adrenal (capsule) (gland) 255.4
- anterior NEC (see also Infarct, myocardium) 410
- appendices epiploicae 557.0
- bowel 557.0
- brain 434.9
- - embolic (see also Embolism, brain) 434.1
- - puerperal, postpartum, childbirth 674.0
- breast 611.8
- cardiac (see also Infarct, myocardium) 410
- cerebellar (see also Infarct, brain) 434.9
- - embolic (see also Embolism, brain) 434.1
- cerebral (see also Infarct, brain) 434.9
- - embolic (see also Embolism, brain) 434.1
- colon 557.0
- coronary artery (see also Infarct, myocardium) 410
- embolic (see also Embolism) 444.9
- fallopian tube 620.8
- heart (see also Infarct, myocardium) 410
- hepatic 573.4
- hypophysis (anterior lobe) 253.8
- intestine (acute) (agnogenic) (hemorrhagic) (nonocclusive) 557.0
- kidney 593.8
- liver 573.4
- lung (embolic) (thrombotic) 415.1
- - with
- - - abortion - see categories 634-639, fourth digit .6
- - - ectopic gestation 639.6
- - in pregnancy, childbirth or puerperium - see Embolism, obstetrical
- lymph node 457.8
- mesentery, mesenteric (embolic) (thrombotic) 557.0
- myocardium, myocardial (acute or with a stated duration of 8 weeks or less) 410
- - chronic or with a stated duration of over 8 weeks 414.8
- - healed or old, currently presenting no symptoms 412
- - past (diagnosed on ECG or other special investigation, but currently presenting no symptoms) 412
- - syphilitic 093.8
- omentum 557.0
- ovary 620.8
- papillary muscle - see Infarct, myocardium
- pituitary (gland) 253.8

Infarct - *continued*
- placenta (complicating pregnancy) 656.7
- – fetus or newborn 762.2
- posterior NEC (see also Infarct, myocardium) 410
- prostate 602.8
- pulmonary (artery) (vein) (hemorrhagic) 415.1
- – with
- – – abortion - see categories 634-639, fourth digit .6
- – – ectopic gestation 639.6
- – in pregnancy, childbirth or puerperium - see Embolism, obstetrical
- renal (see also Lesion, kidney) 593.8
- – embolic or thrombotic 593.8
- retina, retinal (artery) 362.8
- spinal (cord) (acute) (embolic) (nonembolic) 336.1
- spleen 289.5
- – embolic or thrombotic 444.8
- subchorionic - see Infarct, placenta
- subendocardial (see also Infarct, myocardium) 410
- suprarenal (capsule) (gland) 255.4
- thrombotic (see also Thrombosis) 453.9
- – artery, arterial - see Embolism
- thyroid (gland) 246.3
- ventricle (heart) (see also Infarct, myocardium) 410

Infecting - see condition

Infection, infected (opportunistic) 136.9
- with lymphangitis - see Lymphangitis
- abortion - see categories 634-639, fourth digit .0
- abscess (skin) - code by site under Abscess
- absidia 117.7
- Acanthocheilonema (perstans) 125.4
- – streptocerca 125.6
- accessory sinus (chronic) (see also Sinusitis) 473.9
- achorion - see Dermatophytosis
- Acremonium falciforme 117.4
- acromioclavicular 711.9
- Actinobacillus
- – lignieresii 027.8
- – mallei 024
- – muris 026.1
- Actinomadura - see Actinomycosis
- Actinomyces (israelii) - see also Actinomycosis
- – muris-ratti 026.1
- Actinomycetales (Actinomyces) (Actinomadura) (Nocardia) (Streptomyces) - see Actinomycosis

Infection - *continued*
- actinomycotic NEC (see also Actinomycosis) 039.9
- adenoid (and tonsil) (chronic) 474.0
- adenovirus NEC
- – in diseases classified elsewhere - see category 079-
- – unspecified nature or site 079.0
- Aerobacter aerogenes NEC 041.8
- aerogenes capsulatus (see also Gas gangrene) 040.0
- Ajellomyces dermatitidis 116.0
- alimentary canal NEC (see also Enteritis, infectious) 009.0
- Allescheria boydii 117.6
- Alternaria 118
- alveolus, alveolar (process) 522.4
- ameba, amebic (histolytica) 006.9
- – acute 006.0
- – chronic 006.1
- – free-living 136.2
- – hartmanni 007.8
- – specified
- – – site NEC 006.8
- – – type NEC 007.8
- amniotic fluid or cavity 658.4
- – fetus or newborn 762.7
- anal canal 569.4
- Angiostrongylus cantonensis 128.8
- Anisakiasis 127.1
- Anisakis larva 127.1
- anthrax (see also Anthrax) 022.9
- antrum (chronic) (see also Sinusitis, maxillary) 473.0
- anus (papillae) (sphincter) 569.4
- arbovirus (arbor virus) 066.9
- – specified type NEC 066.8
- argentophil-rod 027.0
- Ascaris lumbricoides 127.0
- Ascomycetes 117.4
- Aspergillus (flavus) (fumigatus) (terreus) 117.3
- atypical
- – acid-fast (bacilli) - see Mycobacterium, atypical
- – mycobacteria - see Mycobacterium, atypical
- auditory meatus (circumscribed) (diffuse) (external) 380.1
- auricle (ear) 380.1
- axillary gland 683
- Bacillus NEC 041.8
- – abortus 023.1
- – anthracis (see also Anthrax) 022.9
- – coli - see Infection, escherichia coli
- – coliform NEC 041.8
- – Ducrey's (any location) 099.0

Infection - *continued*
- congenital NEC - *continued*
- - clostridial 771.8
- - cytomegalovirus 771.1
- - Escherichia coli 771.8
- - hepatitis, viral 771.2
- - herpes simplex 771.2
- - listeriosis 771.2
- - malaria 771.2
- - poliomyelitis 771.2
- - rubella 771.0
- - Salmonella 771.8
- - streptococcal 771.8
- - toxoplasmosis 771.2
- - tuberculosis 771.2
- - urinary (tract) 771.8
- - vaccinia 771.2
- corpus luteum (see also Salpingo-oophoritis) 614.2
- Corynebacterium diphtheriae - see Diphtheria
- Coxsackie (see also Coxsackie) 079.2
- - in diseases classified elsewhere - see category 079-
- - meninges 047.0 † 321.1*
- - myocardium 074.2 † 422.0*
- - pericardium 074.2 † 420.0*
- - pharynx 074.0
- - specified disease NEC 074.8
- - unspecified nature or site 079.2
- Cryptococcus neoformans 117.5

- Cunninghamella 117.7
- cyst - see Cyst
- Cysticercus cellulosae 123.1
- cytomegalovirus
- - congenital 771.1
- dental 522.4
- Deuteromycetes 117.4
- Dipetalonema (perstans) 125.4
- - streptocerca 125.6
- diphtherial - see Diphtheria

- Diphyllobothrium (adult) (latum) (pacificum) 123.4
- - larval 123.5
- Diplogonoporus (grandis) 123.8
- Dipylidium (caninum) 123.8
- Dirofilaria 125.6
- Dracunculus medinensis 125.7
- Dreschlera 118
- - hawaiiense 117.8
- Ducrey's bacillus (any location) 099.0
- due to or resulting from
- - device, implant or graft (any) 996.6
- - injection, inoculation, infusion, transfusion, or vaccination (prophylactic) (therapeutic) 999.3

Infection - *continued*
- due to or resulting from - *continued*
- - injury NEC - code by site under Wound, open, complicated
- duodenum 535.6
- ear (middle) - see also Otitis media
- - external 380.1
- - inner 386.3
- Eaton's agent NEC 041.8
- Eberthella typhosa 002.0
- Echinococcus (see also Echinococcus) 122.9
- ECHO virus
- - in diseases classified elsewhere - see category 079-
- - unspecified nature or site 079.1
- endocardium - see Endocarditis, bacterial
- endocervix (see also Cervicitis) 616.0
- Entameba - see Infection ameba
- enteric (see also Enteritis, infectious) 009.0
- Enterobius vermicularis 127.4
- Entomophthora 117.7
- Epidermophyton - see Dermatophytosis
- episiotomy 674.3
- erysipeloid 027.1
- Erysipelothrix (insidiosa) (rhusiopathiae) 027.1
- Escherichia coli NEC 041.4
- - congenital 771.8
- - generalized 038.4
- - intestinal 008.0
- ethmoidal (chronic) (sinus) (see also Sinusitis, ethmoidal) 473.2
- eustachian tube (ear) 381.5
- external auditory canal (meatus) NEC 380.1
- eye NEC 360.0
- eyelid NEC 373.9
- fallopian tube (see also Salpingo-oophoritis) 614.2
- Fasciola
- - gigantica 121.3
- - hepatica 121.3
- Fasciolopsis (buski) 121.4
- fetus (intraamniotic) - see Infection, congenital
- filarial - see Infestation, filarial
- finger (skin) 686.9
- - abscess (with lymphangitis) 681.0
- - cellulitis (with lymphangitis) 681.0
- - distal closed space (with lymphangitis) 681.0
- fish tapeworm 123.4
- - larval 123.5
- flagellate, intestinal 007.9
- fluke - see Infestation, fluke

Infection - *continued*
- focal
-   - from tonsils 474.0
-   - teeth 522.4
- Fonsecaea
-   - compactum 117.2
-   - pedrosoi 117.2
- food (see also Poisoning, food) 005.9
- foot (skin) 686.9
-   - fungus 110.4
- Francisella tularensis 021
- frontal sinus (chronic) (see also Sinusitis, frontal) 473.1
- fungus NEC 117.9
-   - beard 110.0
-   - body 110.5
-   - dematiacious NEC 117.8
-   - foot 110.4
-   - groin 110.3
-   - hand 110.2
-   - nail 110.1
-   - pathogenic to compromised host only 118
-   - perianal (area) 110.3
-   - scalp 110.0
-   - skin 111.9
-    - foot 110.4
-    - hand 110.2
-   - toenails 110.1
-   - trachea 117.9
- Fusarium 118
- gallbladder (see also Cholecystitis, acute) 575.0
- gas bacillus (see also Gas gangrene) 040.0
- gastric 535.5
- gastroenteric (see also Enteritis, infectious) 009.0
- gastrointestinal (see also Enteritis, infectious) 009.0
- generalized NEC (see also Septicemia) 038.9
- genital organ or tract NEC
-   - with
-    - abortion - see categories 634-639, fourth digit .0
-    - ectopic gestation 639.0
-   - complicating pregnancy 646.6
-    - fetus or newborn 760.8
-   - male 608.4
-   - puerperal, postpartum, childbirth 670
-    - minor or localized 646.6
- Ghon tubercle, primary 010.0
- Giardia lamblia 007.1
- gingival 523.1
- Glenosporopsis amazonica 116.2
- Gnathostoma (spinigerum) 128.1
- Gongylonema 125.6

Infection - *continued*
- gonococcal NEC (see also Gonococcus) 098.0
- gram-negative bacilli NEC 041.8
- guinea worm 125.7
- gum 523.1
- heart (see also Carditis) 429.8
- helminths NEC 128.9
-   - intestinal 127.9
-    - mixed (types classifiable to more than one of the titles 120.0-127.7) 127.8
-    - specified type NEC 127.7
-   - specified type NEC 128.8
- Hemophilus influenzae NEC 041.5
- herpes (simplex) (see also Herpes) 054.9
-   - congenital 771.2
- Heterophyes heterophyes 121.6
- Histoplasma 115.9
-   - capsulatum 115.0
-   - duboisii 115.1
- hookworm (see also Ancylostomiasis) 126.9
- Hymenolepis 123.6
- hypopharynx 478.2
- inguinal glands 683
-   - due to soft chancre 099.0
- intestine, intestinal (see also Enteritis, infectious) 009.0
- intrauterine NEC 646.6
-   - specified infection NEC in fetus or newborn 771.8
- Isospora belli or hominis 007.2
- jaw (bone) (lower) (upper) 526.4
- joint - see Arthritis, infectious or infective
- kidney (cortex) (hematogenous) 590.9
-   - with
-    - abortion - see categories 634-639, fourth digit .8
-    - calculus 592.0
-    - ectopic gestation 639.8
-   - complicating pregnancy or puerperium 646.6
-    - fetus or newborn 760.1
-   - pelvis and ureter 590.3
- Klebsiella pneumoniae NEC 041.3
- knee (skin) NEC 686.9
-   - joint 711.9
- Koch's (see also Tuberculosis, pulmonary) 011.9
- labia (majora) (minora) (see also Vulvitis) 616.1
- lacrimal
-   - gland 375.0
-   - passages (duct) (sac) 375.3
- larynx NEC 478.7
- leg (skin) NEC 686.9

Infection - *continued*
- Leishmania (see also Leishmaniasis) 085.9
- - braziliensis 085.5
- - donovani 085.0
- - ethiopica 085.3
- - furunculosa 085.1
- - infantum 085.0
- - mexicana 085.4
- - tropica (minor) 085.1
- - - major 085.2
- Leptosphaeria senegalensis 117.4
- Leptospira (see also Leptospirosis) 100.9
- - australis 100.8
- - bataviae 100.8
- - pyrogenes 100.8
- - specified type NEC 100.8
- leptospirochetal NEC (see also Leptospirosis) 100.9
- Leptothrix - see Actinomycosis
- Listeria monocytogenes 027.2
- - congenital 771.2
- Loa loa 125.2
- - eyelid 125.2 † 373.6*
- Loboa loboi 116.2
- local, skin (staphylococcal) (streptococcal) NEC 686.9
- - abscess - code by site under Abscess
- - cellulitis - code by site under Cellulitis
- - ulcer (see also Ulcer, skin) 707.9
- Loefflerella
- - mallei 024
- - whitmori 025
- lung 518.8
- - atypical Mycobacterium 031.0
- - - tuberculous (see also Tuberculosis, pulmonary) 011.9
- - basilar 518.8
- - chronic 518.8
- - fungus NEC 117.9
- - spirochetal 104.8
- - virus - see Pneumonia, virus
- lymph gland (axillary) (cervical) (inguinal) 683
- - mesenteric 289.2
- lymphoid tissue, base of tongue or posterior pharynx, NEC 474.0
- Madurella
- - grisea 117.4
- - mycetomii 117.4
- major
- - following
- - - abortion - see categories 634-639, fourth digit .0
- - - ectopic gestation 639.0
- - puerperal, postpartum, childbirth 670
- malarial - see Malaria

Infection - *continued*
- Malassezia furfur 111.0
- Malleomyces
- - mallei 024
- - pseudomallei 025
- mammary gland 611.0
- - puerperal, postpartum 675.1
- Mansonella (ozzardi) 125.5
- mastoid (suppurative) - see Mastoiditis
- maxilla, maxillary 526.4
- - sinus (chronic) (see also Sinusitis, maxillary) 473.0
- mediastinum 519.2
- medina 125.7
- meibomian
- - cyst 373.1
- - gland 373.1
- meninges (see also Meningitis) 320.9
- meningococcal (see also Condition) 036.9
- - brain 036.1 † 323.4*
- - cerebrospinal 036.0 † 320.5*
- - endocardium 036.4 † 421.1*
- - generalized 036.2
- - meninges 036.0 † 320.5*
- - pericardium 036.4 † 420.0*
- - specified site NEC 036.8
- mesenteric lymph nodes or glands NEC 289.2
- Metagonimus 121.5
- metatarsophalangeal 711.9
- Microsporum, microsporic - see Dermatophytosis
- Mima polymorpha NEC 041.8
- mixed flora NEC 041.8
- Monilia (see also Candidiasis) 112.9
- - neonatal 771.7
- Monosporium apiospermum 117.6
- mouth NEC 528.9
- - parasitic 112.0
- mucor 117.7
- muscle NEC 728.8
- mycelium NEC 117.9
- mycetoma
- - actinomycotic NEC (see also Actinomycosis) 039.9
- - mycotic NEC 117.4
- Mycobacterium - see Mycobacterium
- mycoplasma NEC 041.8
- mycotic NEC 117.9
- - pathogenic to compromised host only 118
- - skin NEC 111.9
- - systemic 117.9
- myocardium NEC 422.9
- nail (chronic) (with lymphangitis) 681.9
- - finger 681.0
- - ingrowing 703.0

Infection - *continued*
- Rhinosporidium (seeberi) 117.0
- rhinovirus
- – in diseases classified elsewhere - see category 079-
- – unspecified nature or site 079.3
- Rhizopus 117.7
- rubella (see also Rubella) 056.9
- – congenital 771.0
- Saccharomyces (see also Candidiasis) 112.9
- Saksenaea 117.7
- salivary duct or gland (any) 527.2
- Salmonella (aertrycke) (callinarum) (choleraesuis) (enteritidis) (suipestifer) (typhimurium) 003.9
- – with
- – – gastroenteritis 003.0
- – – septicemia 003.1
- – – specified manifestation NEC 003.8
- – congenital 771.8
- – due to food (poisoning) (any serotype) (see also Poisoning, food, due to salmonella) 003.9
- – hirschfeldii 002.3
- – localized NEC 003.2
- – paratyphi 002.9
- – – A 002.1
- – – B 002.2
- – – C 002.3
- – schottmuelleri 002.2
- – typhi 002.0
- – typhosa 002.0
- saprophytic 136.8
- Schistosoma - see Infestation, Schistosoma
- Schmorl's bacillus 040.3
- scratch or other superficial injury - see Injury superficial
- scrotum (acute) NEC 608.4
- seminal vesicle (see also Vesiculitis) 608.0
- septic
- – generalized - see Septicemia
- – localized, skin (see also Abscess) 682.9
- septicemic - see Septicemia
- sheep liver fluke 121.3
- Shigella 004.9
- – boydii 004.2
- – dysenteriae 004.0
- – flexneri 004.1
- – group
- – – A 004.0
- – – B 004.1
- – – C 004.2
- – – D 004.3
- – schmitzii 004.0

Infection - *continued*
- Shigella - *continued*
- – shigae 004.0
- – sonnei 004.3
- – specified type NEC 004.8
- sinus (see also Sinusitis) 473.9
- – pilonidal 685.1
- – – with abscess 685.0
- – skin NEC 686.9
- Skene's duct or gland (see also Urethritis) 597.8
- skin (local) (staphylococcal) (streptococcal) NEC 686.9
- – abscess - code by site under Abscess
- – cellulitis - code by site under Cellulitis
- – due to fungus 111.9
- – – specified type NEC 111.8
- – mycotic 111.9
- – – specified type NEC 111.8
- – ulcer (see also Ulcer, skin) 707.9
- slow virus 046.9
- – specified condition 046.8
- Sparganum (mansoni) (proliferum) 123.5
- specific (see also Syphilis) 097.9
- – to perinatal period NEC 771.8
- spermatic cord NEC 608.4
- sphenoidal (sinus) (see also Sinusitis, sphenoidal) 473.3
- Spherophorus necrophorus 040.3
- spinal cord NEC (see also Encephalitis) 323.9
- – abscess 324.1
- – meninges - see Meningitis
- – streptococcal 320.2
- Spirillum
- – minus or minor 026.0
- – obermeieri 087.0
- spirochetal NEC 104.9
- – lung 104.8
- – specified nature or site NEC 104.8
- spleen 289.5
- Sporothrix schenckii 117.1
- Sporotrichum (schenckii) 117.1
- Sporozoa 136.8
- staphylococcal NEC 041.1
- – generalized (purulent) 038.1
- steatoma 706.2
- Stellantchasmus falcatus 121.6
- streptococcal NEC 041.0
- – congenital 771.8
- – generalized (purulent) 038.0
- Streptomyces - see Actinomycosis
- streptotrichosis - see Actinomycosis
- Strongyloides (stercoralis) 127.2
- stump (amputation) (surgical) 997.6
- subcutaneous tissue, local NEC 686.9
- submaxillary region 528.9

Infection - *continued*
- systemic - see Septicemia
- Taenia - see Infestation, Taenia
- Taeniarhyuchus saginatus 123.2
- tapeworm - see Infestation, tapeworm
- tendon (sheath) 727.8
- Ternidens diminutus 127.7
- testis (see also Orchitis) 604.9
- thigh (skin) 686.9
- threadworm 127.4
- throat 478.2
- - pneumococcal 462
- - staphylococcal 462
- - streptococcal 034.0
- - viral NEC (see also Pharyngitis) 462
- thyroglossal duct 529.8
- toe (skin) 686.9
- - abscess (with lymphangitis) 681.1
- - cellulitis (with lymphangitis) 681.1
- tongue NEC 529.0
- - parasitic 112.0
- tonsil (and adenoid) (faucial) (lingual) (pharyngeal) 474.0
- - acute or subacute 463
- tooth, teeth 522.4
- - periapical 522.4
- - peridental 523.3
- - socket 526.5
- Torula histolytica 117.5
- Toxocara (canis) (cati) (felis) 128.0
- Toxoplasma gondii 130
- trachea, chronic 491.8
- - fungus 117.9
- trematode NEC 121.9

- Treponema pallidum (see also Syphilis) 097.9
- Trichinella (spiralis) 124
- Trichomonas 131.9
- - cervix 131.0 † 616.0*
- - intestine 007.3
- - prostate 131.0 † 601.4*
- - specified sites NEC 131.8
- - urethra 131.0 † 597.8*
- - urogenitalis 131.0
- - vagina 131.0 † 616.1*
- - vulva 131.0 † 616.1*
- Trichophyton, trichophytic - see Dermatophytosis
- Trichosporon (beigelii) cutaneum 111.2

- Trichostrongylus 127.6
- Trichuris (trichiura) 127.3
- Trombicula (irritans) 133.8
- Trypanosoma (see also Trypanosomiasis) 086.9
- - cruzi 086.2
- tubal (see also Salpingo-oophoritis) 614.2

Infection - *continued*
- tuberculous NEC (see also Tuberculosis) 011.9
- tubo-ovarian (see also Salpingo-oophoritis) 614.2
- tunica vaginalis 608.4
- tympanic membrane 384.8
- typhoid (abortive) (ambulant) (bacillus) 002.0
- umbilicus 686.9
- - newborn NEC 771.4
- ureter 593.8
- urethra 597.8
- urinary (tract) NEC 599.0
- - with
- - - abortion - see categories 634-639, fourth digit .8
- - - ectopic gestation 639.8
- - complicating pregnancy, childbirth or puerperium 646.6
- - - asymptomatic 646.5
- - - fetus or newborn 760.1
- - newborn 771.8
- - tuberculous 016.1
- uterus, uterine (see also Endometritis) 615.9
- utriculus masculinus NEC 597.8
- vaccination 999.3
- vagina (granulation tissue) (wall) (see also Vaginitis) 616.1
- varicose veins - see Varicose vein
- vas deferens NEC 608.4
- verumontanum 597.8
- vesical (see also Cystitis) 595.9
- Vincent's (gums) (mouth) (tonsil) 101
- virus NEC 079.9
- - adenovirus
- - - in diseases classified elsewhere - see category 079-
- - - unspecified nature or site 079.0
- - central nervous system NEC 049.9
- - - enterovirus NEC 048
- - - - meningitis 047.9 † 321.7*
- - - - - specified type NEC 047.8 † 321.7*
- - - slow virus 046.9
- - - - specified condition NEC 046.8
- - chest 519.9
- - Coxsackie - see Infection, Coxsackie
- - ECHO
- - - in diseases classified elsewhere - see category 079-
- - - unspecified nature or site 079.1
- - in diseases classified elsewhere - see category 079-
- - intestine (see also Enteritis, viral) 008.8

Infection - *continued*
- virus NEC - *continued*
- - lung - see Pneumonia, virus
- - rhinovirus
- - - in diseases classified elsewhere - see category 079-
- - - unspecified nature or site 079.3
- - slow 046.9
- - - specified condition NEC 046.8
- - specified type NEC
- - - in diseases classified elsewhere - see category 079-
- - - unspecified nature or site 079.8
- - unspecified nature or site 079.9
- vulva (see also Vulvitis) 616.1
- whipworm 127.3
- Whitmore's bacillus 025
- wound (local) (post-traumatic) NEC 958.3
- - with
- - - dislocation - code as Dislocation, compound
- - - fracture - code as Fracture, open
- - - open wound - code as Wound, open, complicated
- - surgical 998.5
- Wuchereria 125.0
- - bancrofti 125.0
- - malayi 125.1
- yeast (see also Candidiasis) 112.9
- Yersinia pestis (see also Plague) 020.9
- Zeis' gland 373.1
- Zopfia senegalensis 117.4

Infective, infectious - see condition

Infertility
- female 628.9
- - associated with
- - - adhesions, peritubal 614.6 † 628.2*
- - - anomaly
- - - - cervical mucus 628.4
- - - - congenital
- - - - - cervix 628.4
- - - - - fallopian tube 628.2
- - - - - uterus 628.3
- - - - - vagina 628.4
- - - anovulation 628.0
- - - endometritis, tuberculous 016.4 † 628.3*
- - - Stein-Leventhal syndrome 256.4 † 628.0*
- - nonimplantation 628.3
- - origin
- - - cervical 628.4
- - - pituitary-hypothalamic 253.- † 628.1*
- - - specified NEC 628.8

Infertility - *continued*
- female - *continued*
- - origin - *continued*
- - - tubal (block) (occlusion) (stenosis) 628.2
- - - - adhesions 614.6 † 628.2*
- - - uterine 628.3
- - - vaginal 628.4
- - previous, requiring supervision of pregnancy V23.0
- male 606
Infestation 134.9
- Acanthocheilonema (perstans) 125.4
- - streptocerca 125.6
- Agamofilaria streptocerca 125.6
- Ancylostoma 126.9
- - americanus 126.1
- - braziliense 126.2
- - caninum 126.8
- - ceylanicum 126.3
- - duodenale 126.0
- Angiostrongylus cantonensis 128.8
- anisakiasis 127.1
- Anisakis larva 127.1
- arthropod NEC 134.1
- Ascaris lumbricoides 127.0
- Bacillus fusiformis 101
- Balantidium coli 007.0
- beef tapeworm 123.2
- Bothriocephalus (latus) 123.4
- - larval 123.5
- broad tapeworm 123.4
- - larval 123.5
- Brugia malayi 125.1
- candiru 136.8
- Capillaria
- - hepatica 128.8
- - philippinensis 127.5
- cat liver flukes 121.0
- cestodes NEC 123.9
- - specified type NEC 123.8
- chigger 133.8
- chigoe 134.1
- Chilomastix 007.8
- Clonorchis (sinensis) (liver) 121.1
- coccidia 007.2
- Cysticercus cellulosae 123.1
- Demodex folliculorum 133.8
- Dermatobia (hominis) 134.0
- Dibothriocephalus (latus) 123.4
- - larval 123.5
- Dicrocoelium dendriticum 121.8
- Diphyllobothrium (adult) (latum) (intestinal) (pacificum) 123.4
- - larval 123.5
- Diplogonoporus (grandis) 123.8
- Dipylidium (caninum) 123.8

Infestation - *continued*
- Phthirus (pubis) (any site) 132.2
- – with any infestation classifiable to
   132.0 and 132.1 132.3
- pinworm 127.4
- pork tapeworm (adult) 123.0
- protozoal NEC 136.8
- rat tapeworm 123.6
- roundworm (large) NEC 127.0
- sand flea 134.1
- saprophytic NEC 136.8
- Sarcoptes scabiei 133.0
- scabies 133.0
- Schistosoma 120.9
- – bovis 120.8
- – cercariae 120.3
- – hematobium 120.0
- – intercalatum 120.8
- – japonicum 120.2
- – mansoni 120.1
- – mattheii 120.8
- – specified
- – – site - see Schistosomiasis
- – – type NEC 120.8
- – spindale 120.8
- screw worms 134.0
- skin NEC 134.9
- Sparganum (mansoni) (proliferum) 123.5
- – larval 123.5
- specified type NEC 134.8
- Spirometra larvae 123.5
- Sporozoa NEC 136.8
- Stellantchasmus falcatus 121.6
- Strongyloides stercoralis 127.2
- Strongylus (gibsoni) 127.7
- Taenia 123.3
- – diminuta 123.6
- – echinococcus (see also Echinococcus)
   122.9
- – mediocanellata 123.2
- – nana 123.6
- – saginata 123.2
- – solium (intestinal form) 123.0
- – – larval form 123.1
- Taeniarhynchus saginatus 123.2
- tapeworm 123.9
- – beef 123.2
- – broad 123.4
- – – larval 123.5
- – dog 123.8
- – dwarf 123.6
- – fish 123.4
- – – larval 123.5
- – pork 123.0
- – rat 123.6
- Ternidens diminutus 127.7
- Tetranychus molestissimus 133.8

Infestation - *continued*
- threadworm 127.4
- tongue 112.0
- Toxocara (canis) (cati) (felis) 128.0
- trematode(s) NEC 121.9
- Trichina spiralis 124
- Trichinella spiralis 124
- Trichocephalus 127.3
- Trichomonas 131.9
- – cervix 131.0 † 616.0*
- – intestine 007.3
- – prostate 131.0 † 601.4*
- – specified site NEC 131.8
- – urethra 131.0 † 597.8*
- – urogenital 131.0
- – vagina 131.0 † 616.1*
- – vulva 131.0 † 616.1*
- Trichophyton - see Dermatophytosis
- Trichostrongylus (instabilis) 127.6
- Trichuris (trichiura) 127.3
- Trombicula (irritans) 133.8
- Trypanosoma - see Trypanosomiasis
- Tunga penetrans 134.1
- Uncinaria americana 126.1
- whipworm 127.3
- worms NEC 128.9
- Wuchereria 125.0
- – bancrofti 125.0
- – malayi 125.1

Infiltrate, infiltration
- with an iron compound 275.0
- amyloid (any site) (generalized) 277.3
- calcareous NEC 275.4
- – localized - see Degeneration by site
- calcium salt 275.4
- corneal 371.2
- eyelid 373.9
- glycogen, glycogenic (see also Disease,
   glycogen storage) 271.0
- heart, cardiac
- – fatty (see also Degeneration,
   myocardial) 429.1
- – glycogenic 271.0 † 425.7*
- inflammatory in vitreous 379.2
- kidney (see also Disease, renal) 593.9

- leukemic (M9800/3) - see Leukemia
- liver 573.8
- – fatty - see Fatty, liver
- – glycogen (see also Disease, glycogen
   storage) 271.0
- lung (eosinophilic) 518.3
- lymphatic (see also Leukemia, lymphatic)
   204.9
- – gland, pigmentary 289.3
- muscle, fatty 728.9
- myocardium, myocardial

Infiltrate - *continued*
- myocardium - *continued*
- - fatty (see also Degeneration,
    myocardial) 429.1
- - glycogenic 271.0 † 425.7*
- Ranke's primary 010.0
- thymus (gland) (fatty) 254.8
- vitreous humor 379.2
Infirmity 799.8
- senile 797
Inflammation, inflamed, inflammatory (with
  exudation)
- abducens (nerve) 378.8
- accessory sinus (chronic) (see also
  Sinusitis) 473.9
- adrenal (gland) 255.8
- alimentary canal - see Enteritis
- alveoli NEC 526.5
- - scorbutic 267
- - teeth 526.5
- anal canal 569.4
- antrum (chronic) (see also Sinusitis,
  maxillary) 473.0
- anus 569.4
- appendix (see also Appendicitis) 541
- arachnoid - see Meningitis
- areola 611.0
- - puerperal, postpartum 675.0
- areolar tissue NEC 686.9
- artery - see Arteritis
- auditory meatus (external) 380.1
- Bartholin's gland 616.8
- bile duct or passage (see also
  Cholecystitis) 576.1
- bladder (see also Cystitis) 595.9
- bone - see Osteomyelitis
- bowel - see Enteritis
- brain (see also Encephalitis) 323.9
- - membrane - see Meningitis
- breast 611.0
- - puerperal, postpartum 675.2
- broad ligament (see also Disease, pelvis,
  inflammatory) 614.4
- bronchi - see Bronchitis
- bursa - see Bursitis
- cecum (see also Appendicitis) 541
- cerebral (see also Encephalitis) 323.9
- - membrane - see Meningitis
- cerebrospinal - see also Meningitis
- - meningococcal 036.0 † 320.5*
- - tuberculous 013.8 † 323.4*
- cervix (uteri) (see also Cervicitis) 616.0
- chest 519.9
- choroid NEC 363.2
- colon - see Enteritis
- connective tissue (diffuse) NEC 728.9
- cornea (see also Keratitis) 370.9

Inflammation - *continued*
- corpora cavernosa 607.2
- cranial nerve - see Disorder, nerve,
  cranial
- diarrhea - see Diarrhea
- due to (presence of) any device, implant
  or graft classifiable to 996.0-996.5 996.6
- duodenum 535.6
- dura mater - see Meningitis
- ear (middle) - see also Otitis media
- - external 380.1
- - inner 386.3
- esophagus 530.1
- ethmoidal (chronic) (see also Sinusitis,
  ethmoidal) 473.2
- eustachian tube (catarrhal) 381.5
- extrarectal 569.4
- eyelid 373.9
- fallopian tube (see also
  Salpingo-oophoritis) 614.2
- fascia 728.9
- frontal (chronic) (sinus) (see also
  Sinusitis, frontal) 473.1
- gall duct (see also Cholecystitis) 575.1
- gallbladder (see also Cholecystitis, acute)
  575.0
- gastrointestinal - see Enteritis
- genital organ (internal) (diffuse) NEC
  614.9
- - male 608.4
- gland (lymph) (see also Lymphadenitis)
  289.3
- glottis (see also Laryngitis) 464.0
- heart (see also Carditis) 429.8
- hepatic duct (see also Cholecystitis) 576.8
- hernial sac - see Hernia, by site
- ileum (see also Enteritis) 009.1
- - terminal or regional 555.0
- intestine - see Enteritis
- jaw (acute) (bone) (chronic) (lower)
  (suppurative) (upper) 526.4
- jejunum - see Enteritis
- joint NEC 716.9
- - sacroiliac 720.2
- kidney (see also Nephritis) 583.9
- knee (joint) 716.6
- - tuberculous 015.2
- labium (majus) (minus) (see also
  Vulvitis) 616.1
- lacrimal
- - gland 375.0
- - passages (duct) (sac) 375.3
- larynx (see also Laryngitis) 464.0
- - diphtheritic 032.3
- leg NEC 686.9
- lip 528.5
- liver (capsule) (see also Hepatitis) 573.3

Inflammation - *continued*
- liver - *continued*
- − chronic 571.4
- lung (acute) (see also Pneumonia) 486
- − chronic 518.8
- lymph gland or node (see also Lymphadenitis) 289.3
- lymphatic vessel (see also Lymphangitis) 457.2
- maxilla, maxillary 526.4
- − sinus (chronic) (see also Sinusitis, maxillary) 473.0
- membranes of brain or spinal cord - see Meningitis
- meninges - see Meningitis
- mouth 528.0
- muscle 728.9
- myocardium (see also Myocarditis) 429.0
- nasal sinus (chronic) (see also Sinusitis) 473.9
- nasopharynx - see Nasopharyngitis
- navel 686.9
- − newborn NEC 771.4
- nerve NEC 729.2
- nipple 611.0
- − puerperal, postpartum 675.0
- nose 478.1
- − suppurative 472.0
- oculomotor (nerve) 378.8
- oesophagus 530.1
- optic nerve 377.3
- orbit (chronic) 376.1
- − acute 376.0
- ovary (see also Salpingo-oophoritis) 614.2
- oviduct (see also Salpingo-oophoritis) 614.2
- pancreas - see Pancreatitis
- parotid region 686.9
- pelvis, female (see also Disease, pelvis, inflammatory) 614.9
- penis 607.2
- perianal 569.4
- pericardium (see also Pericarditis) 423.9
- perineum (female) (male) 686.9
- perirectal 569.4
- peritoneum (see also Peritonitis) 567.9
- periuterine (see also Disease, pelvis, inflammatory) 614.9
- perivesical (see also Cystitis) 595.9
- petrous bone (acute) (chronic) 383.2
- pharynx (see also Pharyngitis) 462
- − follicular 472.1
- − granular 472.1
- pia mater - see Meningitis
- pleura - see Pleurisy
- postmastoidectomy cavity 383.3

Inflammation - *continued*
- prostate (see also Prostatitis) 601.9
- rectosigmoid - see Rectosigmoiditis
- rectum (see also Proctitis) 569.4
- respiratory, upper (see also Infection, respiratory, upper) 465.9
- − chronic, due to external agent - see condition, respiratory, chronic, due to
- − due to
- − − fumes or vapors (chemical) (inhalation) 506.2
- − − radiation 508.8
- retina (see also Chorioretinitis) 363.2
- retrocecal (see also Appendicitis) 541
- retroperitoneal (see also Peritonitis) 567.9
- salivary duct or gland (any) (suppurative) 527.2
- scorbutic, alveoli, teeth 267
- scrotum 608.4
- sigmoid - see Enteritis
- sinus (see also Sinusitis) 473.9
- Skene's duct or gland (see also Urethritis) 597.8
- skin 686.9
- spermatic cord 608.4
- sphenoidal (sinus) (see also Sinusitis, sphenoidal) 473.3
- spinal
- − cord (see also Encephalitis) 323.9
- − membrane - see Meningitis
- − nerve - see Disorder, nerve
- spine (see also Spondylitis) 720.9
- spleen (capsule) 289.5
- stomach - see Gastritis
- subcutaneous tissue NEC 686.9
- suprarenal (gland) 255.8
- synovial (fringe) (membrane) - see Bursitis
- tendon (sheath) NEC 727.9
- testis (see also Orchitis) 604.9
- thigh 686.9
- throat (see also Sore throat) 462
- thymus (gland) 254.8
- thyroid (gland) (see also Thyroiditis) 245.9
- tongue 529.0
- tonsil - see Tonsillitis
- trachea - see Tracheitis
- trochlear (nerve) 378.8
- tubal (see also Salpingo-oophoritis) 614.2
- tuberculous NEC (see also Tuberculosis) 011.9
- tubo-ovarian (see also Salpingo-oophoritis) 614.2
- tunica vaginalis 608.4
- tympanic membrane - see Tympanitis

Inflammation - *continued*
- umbilicus 686.9
- - newborn NEC 771.4
- uterine ligament (see also Disease, pelvis, inflammatory) 614.4
- uterus (catarrhal) (see also Endometritis) 615.9
- uveal tract (anterior) NEC - see also Iridocyclitis
- - posterior - see Chorioretinitis
- vagina (see also Vaginitis) 616.1
- vas deferens 608.4
- vein (see also Phlebitis) 451.9
- - thrombotic 451.9
- - - cerebral (see also Thrombosis, brain) 434.0
- - - leg 451.2
- - - - deep (vessels) 451.1
- - - - superficial (vessels) 451.0
- - - lower extremity 451.2
- - - - deep (vessels) 451.1
- - - - superficial (vessels) 451.0
- vocal cord 478.5
- vulva (see also Vulvitis) 616.1
Inflation, lung imperfect (newborn) 770.5
Influenza 487.1
- with
- - digestive manifestations 487.8
- - involvement of
- - - gastrointestinal tract 487.8
- - - nervous system 487.8
- - pneumonia (any form in 480-483, 485-486) 487.0
- - respiratory manifestations NEC 487.1
- Asian 487.1
- bronchial 487.1
- epidemic 487.1
- maternal affecting fetus or newborn 760.2
- respiratory (upper) 487.1
Influenza-like disease 487.1
Infraction, Freiberg's (metatarsal head) 732.5
Infusion complication, misadventure, or reaction - see Complications, infusion
Ingestion
- chemical - see Table of drugs and chemicals
- drug or medicament
- - correct substance properly administered 995.2
- - overdose or wrong substance given or taken 977.9
- - - specified drug - see Table of drugs and chemicals
- foreign body NEC (see also Foreign body) 938

Ingrowing
- hair 704.8
- nail (finger) (toe) 703.0
Inguinal - see also condition
- testicle 752.5
Inhalation
- carbon monoxide 986
- flame (asphyxia) 949.-
- food or foreign body (see also Asphyxia, food or foreign body) 933.1
- gas, fumes or vapor 987.9
- - specified agent - see Table of drugs and chemicals
- liquid or vomitus (see also Asphyxia, food or foreign body) 933.1
- meconium (fetus or newborn) 770.1
- mucus (see also Asphyxia, mucus) 933.1
- oil (causing suffocation) (see also Asphyxia, food or foreign body) 933.1
- smoke 987.9
- steam 987.9
- stomach contents or secretions 933.1
- - in labor and delivery 668.0
Inhibitor, systemic lupus erythematosus 286.5
Iniencephalus, iniencephaly 740.2
Injury 959.9
- abdomen, abdominal (viscera) 868.-
- - muscle or wall 959.1
- acoustic, resulting in deafness 951.5
- adenoid 959.0
- adrenal (gland) 868.-
- alveolar (process) 959.0
- ankle (and knee) (and leg, except thigh) (and foot) 959.7
- anterior chamber, eye 921.3
- anus 959.1
- aorta (thoracic) 901.0
- - abdominal 902.0
- appendix - see Injury, internal, appendix
- arm, upper (and shoulder) 959.2
- artery (complicating trauma) (see also Injury, blood vessel) 904.9
- - cerebral or meningeal (see also Hemorrhage, subdural, traumatic) 852.0
- auditory canal (external) (meatus) 959.0
- auricle, auris, ear 959.0
- axilla 959.2
- back 959.1
- bile duct 868.-
- birth - see also Birth injury
- - canal, nec, complicating delivery 665.9
- bladder 867.0
- - complicating abortion - see categories 634-639, fourth digit .2
- - obstetrical trauma 665.5

Injury - *continued*
- bladder - *continued*
- – sphincter - see Injury, internal, bladder
- blast (air) (hydraulic) (immersion) (underwater) NEC 869.0
- – with open wound into cavity NEC 869.1
- – abdomen or thorax - see Injury, internal, by site
- – brain 850
- – – with skull fracture - see Fracture, skull
- – ear (acoustic nerve trauma) 951.5
- – – with perforation of tympanic membrane - see Wound, open, ear
- blood vessel NEC 904.9
- – abdomen 902.9
- – – multiple 902.8
- – – specified NEC 902.8
- – arm NEC 903.9
- – axillary 903.0
- – azygos vein 901.8
- – basilic vein 903.1
- – brachial 903.1
- – carotid artery (common) (external) (internal) 900.0
- – celiac artery 902.2
- – cephalic vein (arm) 903.1
- – deep plantar 904.6
- – digital 903.5
- – due to accidental puncture or laceration during procedure 998.2
- – extremity
- – – lower 904.8
- – – – multiple 904.7
- – – – specified NEC 904.7
- – – upper 903.9
- – – – multiple 903.8
- – – – specified NEC 903.8
- – femoral
- – – artery (superficial) 904.1
- – – – common 904.0
- – – vein 904.2
- – gastric
- – – artery 902.2
- – – vein 902.3
- – head 900.9
- – – intracranial (see also Injury, intracranial) 854.0
- – – multiple 900.8
- – – specified NEC 900.8
- – hepatic
- – – artery 902.2
- – – vein 902.1
- – hypogastric 902.5
- – iliac 902.5
- – innominate

Injury - *continued*
- blood vessel NEC - *continued*
- – innominate - *continued*
- – – artery 901.1
- – – vein 901.3
- – intercostal (artery) (vein) 901.8
- – jugular vein (external) 900.8
- – – internal 900.1
- – leg NEC 904.9
- – mammary (artery) (vein) 901.8
- – mesenteric (inferior) (superior)
- – – artery 902.2
- – – vein 902.3
- – neck 900.9
- – – multiple 900.8
- – – specified NEC 900.8
- – ovarian 902.8
- – palmar artery 903.4
- – pelvis 902.9
- – – multiple 902.8
- – – specified NEC 902.8
- – popliteal 904.4
- – portal 902.3
- – pulmonary 901.4
- – radial 903.2
- – renal 902.4
- – saphenous
- – – artery 904.7
- – – vein (greater) (lesser) 904.3
- – specified NEC - see Injury, blood vessel, by site
- – splenic
- – – artery 902.2
- – – vein 902.3
- – subclavian
- – – artery 901.1
- – – vein 901.3
- – thoracic 901.9
- – – multiple 901.8
- – – specified NEC 901.8
- – tibial (anterior) (posterior) 904.5
- – ulnar 903.3
- – uterine 902.5
- – vena cava
- – – inferior 902.1
- – – superior 901.2
- brachial plexus 953.4
- – newborn 767.6
- brain NEC (see also Injury, intracranial) 854.0
- breast 959.1
- broad ligament - see Injury, internal, broad ligament
- bronchus, bronchi - see Injury, internal, bronchus
- brow 959.0
- buttock 959.1

Injury - *continued*
- canthus, eye 921.1
- cauda equina 952.4
- cavernous sinus (see also Injury, intracranial) 854.0
- cecum - see Injury, internal, cecum
- celiac ganglion or plexus 954.1

- cerebellum (see also Injury, intracranial) 854.0
- cervix (uteri) - see Injury, internal, cervix
- cheek 959.0
- chest - see also Injury, internal, chest
- – wall 959.1
- childbirth - see also Birth injury
- – maternal NEC 665.9
- chin 959.0
- choroid (eye) 921.3
- clitoris 959.1
- coccyx 959.1
- – complicating delivery 665.6
- coeliac ganglion or plexus 954.1

- colon - see Injury, internal, colon
- common duct 868.-
- conjunctiva 921.2
- – superficial 918.2
- cord
- – spermatic - see Injury, internal, spermatic cord
- – spinal - see Injury, spinal, by region
- cornea 921.3
- – abrasion 918.1
- – penetrating - see Injury, eyeball, penetrating
- – superficial 918.1
- cortex (cerebral) (see also Injury, intracranial) 854.0
- – visual 950.3
- costal region 959.1
- costochondral 959.1
- cranial
- – bones - see Fracture, skull
- – cavity (see also Injury, intracranial) 854.0
- – nerve - see Injury, nerve, cranial
- crushing - see Crush
- cutaneous sensory nerve
- – lower limb 956.4
- – upper limb 955.5
- delivery - see also Birth injury
- – maternal NEC 665.9
- Descemet's membrane - see Injury, eyeball, penetrating
- diaphragm - see Injury, internal, diaphragm
- duodenum - see Injury, internal, duodenum

Injury - *continued*
- ear (auricle) (external) (drum) (canal) 959.0
- elbow (and forearm) (and wrist) 959.3
- epididymis 959.1
- epigastric region 959.1
- epiglottis 959.0
- epiphyseal, current - see Fracture, by site
- esophagus - see Injury, internal, esophagus
- eustachian tube 959.0
- extremity (lower) (upper) NEC 959.8
- eye 921.9
- – penetrating eyeball - see Injury, eyeball, penetrating
- – superficial 918.9
- eyeball 921.3
- – penetrating 871.7
- – – with
- – – – partial loss (of intraocular tissue) 871.2
- – – – prolapse or exposure (of intraocular tissue) 871.1
- – – – foreign body (nonmagnetic) 871.6
- – – – – magnetic 871.5
- – – – without prolapse 871.0
- – superficial 918.9
- eyebrow 959.0
- eyelid(s) 921.1
- – laceration - see Laceration, eyelid
- – superficial 918.0
- face (and neck) 959.0
- fallopian tube - see Injury, internal, fallopian tube
- finger(s) (nail) 959.5
- flank 959.1
- foot (and knee) (and leg, except thigh) (and ankle) 959.7
- forceps NEC 767.9
- forearm (and elbow) (and wrist) 959.3
- forehead 959.0
- gallbladder 868.-
- gasserian ganglion 951.2
- gastro-intestinal tract - see Injury, internal, gastro-intestinal tract
- genital organ(s)
- – complicating
- – – abortion - see categories 634-639, fourth digit .2
- – – ectopic or molar pregnancy 639.2
- – external 959.1
- – internal - see Injury, internal, genital organs
- – obstetrical trauma NEC 665.9
- gland
- – lacrimal 921.1
- – – laceration 870.8

Injury - *continued*
- gland - *continued*
- – parathyroid 959.0
- – salivary 959.0
- – thyroid 959.0
- globe (eye) (see also Injury, eyeball) 921.3
- groin 959.1
- gum 959.0
- hand(s) (except fingers) 959.4

- head NEC (see also Injury, intracranial) 854.0
- heart 861.0
- – with open wound into thorax 861.1
- heel 959.7
- hip (and thigh) 959.6
- hymen 959.1
- ileum - see Injury, internal, ileum
- iliac region 959.1
- infrared rays NEC 990

- instrumental (during surgery) 998.2
- – birth injury - see Birth injury
- – nonsurgical (see also Injury, by site) 959.9
- – obstetrical 665.9
- – – bladder 665.5
- – – cervix 665.3
- – – high vaginal 665.4
- – – perineal NEC 664.9
- – – urethra 665.5
- – – uterus 665.5
- internal 869.-

Note – For injury of internal organ(s) by foreign body entering through a natural orifice (e.g. inhaled, ingested or swallowed) – *see* Foreign body, entering through orifice.

For internal injury of any of the following sites with internal injury of any other of the sites – *see* Injury, internal, multiple.

The following fourth-digit subdivisions are for use with categories 864–866 and 868–869:
    .0 *Without mention of open wound into cavity*
    .1 *With open wound into cavity.*

Injury - *continued*
- internal - *continued*
- – with fracture
- – – pelvis - see Fracture, pelvis
- – – specified site except pelvis - code by site under Injury, internal 869.-
- – abdomen, abdominal (viscera) NEC 868.-

Injury - *continued*
- internal - *continued*
- – abdomen - *continued*
- – – with fracture, pelvis - see Fracture, pelvis
- – adrenal (gland) 868.-
- – aorta (thoracic) 901.0
- – – abdominal 902.0
- – appendix 863.8
- – – with open wound into cavity 863.9
- – bile duct 868.-
- – bladder (sphincter) 867.0
- – – with abortion - see categories 634-639, fourth digit .2
- – – with open wound into cavity 867.1
- – – obstetrical trauma 665.5
- – blood vessel - see Injury, blood vessel
- – broad ligament 867.6
- – – with open wound into cavity 867.7
- – bronchus, bronchi 862.2
- – – with open wound into cavity 862.3
- – cecum 863.8
- – – with open wound into cavity 863.9
- – cervix (uteri) 867.4
- – – with abortion - see categories 634-639, fourth digit .2
- – – with open wound into cavity 867.5
- – – obstetrical trauma 665.3

- – chest (see also Injury, internal, intrathoracic) 862.8
- – – with open wound into cavity 862.9
- – colon 863.4
- – – with open wound into cavity 863.5
- – common duct 868.-
- – diaphragm 862.0
- – – with open wound into cavity 862.1
- – duodenum 863.2
- – – with open wound into cavity 863.3

- – esophagus (intrathoracic) 862.2
- – – with open wound into cavity 862.3
- – – cervical region 874.4
- – – – complicated 874.5
- – fallopian tube 867.6
- – – with open wound into cavity 867.7
- – gallbladder 868.-
- – gastrointestinal tract NEC 863.8
- – – with open wound into cavity 863.9
- – genital organ NEC 867.6
- – – with open wound into cavity 867.7
- – heart 861.0
- – – with open wound into thorax 861.1
- – ileum 863.2
- – – with open wound into cavity 863.3
- – intestine NEC 863.8
- – – with open wound into cavity 863.9
- – – large 863.4

Injury - *continued*
- internal - *continued*
- - intestine NEC - *continued*
- - - large - *continued*
- - - - with open wound into cavity
    863.5
- - - small 863.2
- - - - with open wound into cavity
    863.3
- - intra-abdominal (organs) (multiple)
    NEC 868.-
- - intrathoracic organs (multiple) 862.8
- - - with open wound into cavity 862.9
- - - diaphragm (only) - see Injury,
    internal, diaphragm
- - - heart (only) - see Injury, internal,
    heart
- - - lung (only) - see Injury, internal,
    lung
- - - specified NEC 862.2
- - - - with open wound into cavity
    862.3
- - intrauterine (see also Injury, internal,
    uterus 867.4
- - - with open wound into cavity 867.5
- - jejunum 863.2
- - - with open wound into cavity 863.3
- - kidney (subcapsular) 866.-
- - liver 864.-
- - lung 861.2
- - - with open wound into thorax 861.3
- - - hemopneumothorax - see
    Hemopneumothorax, traumatic
- - - hemothorax - see Hemothorax,
    traumatic
- - - pneumohemothorax - see
    Pneumohemothorax, traumatic
- - - pneumothorax - see Pneumothorax,
    traumatic
- - mediastinum 862.2
- - - with open wound into cavity 862.3
- - mesentery 863.8
- - - with open wound into cavity 863.9
- - mesosalpinx 867.6
- - - with open wound into cavity 867.7
- - multiple 869.-

Note – Multiple internal injuries of sites
classifiable to the same three- or four-digit
category should be classified to that category.
  Multiple injuries classifiable to different
fourth-digit subdivisions of 861.- (heart and
lung injuries) should be dealt with according
to the coding rules.
  Multiple injuries of sites classifiable to
different three-digit categories should be
coded according to the following list.

Injury - *continued*
- internal - *continued*
- - multiple - *continued*
- - - intra-abdominal organ (site
    classifiable to 863-868)
- - - - with
- - - - - intrathoracic organ(s) (site(s)
      classifiable to 861, 862) 869.-
- - - - - other intra-abdominal organ(s)
      (site(s) classifiable to 863-868,
      except where classifiable to the
      same three-digit category)
      868.-
- - - intrathoracic organ (site classifiable
    to 861, 862)
- - - - with
- - - - - intra-abdominal organ(s)
      (site(s) classifiable to 863-868)
      869.-
- - - - - other intrathoracic organ(s)
      (site(s) classifiable to 861, 862,
      except where classifiable to the
      same three-digit category)
      862.8
- - - - - - with open wound into cavity
        862.9

- - myocardium - see Injury, internal,
    heart
- - oesophagus (intrathoracic) 862.2

- - - with open wound into cavity 862.3
- - - cervical region 874.4
- - - - complicated 874.5
- - ovary 867.6
- - - with open wound into cavity 867.7
- - pancreas 863.8
- - - with open wound into cavity 863.9

- - pelvis, pelvic (organs) (viscera) 867.8
- - - with
- - - - fracture, pelvis - see Fracture,
      pelvis
- - - - open wound into cavity 867.9
- - - specified NEC 867.6
- - - - with open wound into cavity
      867.7
- - peritoneum 868.-
- - pleura 862.2
- - - with open wound into cavity 862.3
- - prostate 867.6
- - - with open wound into cavity 867.7
- - rectum 863.4
- - - with open wound into cavity 863.5

- - retroperitoneal 868.-
- - round ligament 867.6
- - - with open wound into cavity 867.7
- - seminal vesicle 867.6

Injury - *continued*
– internal - *continued*
– – seminal vesicle - *continued*
– – – with open wound into cavity 867.7
– – spermatic cord 867.6
– – – with open wound into cavity 867.7
– – – scrotal - see Wound, open,
    spermatic cord
– – spleen 865.-
– – stomach 863.0
– – – with open wound into cavity 863.1
– – suprarenal gland (multiple) 868.-
– – thorax, thoracic (cavity) (organs)
    (multiple) 862.8
– – – with open wound into cavity 862.9
– – thymus (gland) 862.2
– – – with open wound into cavity 862.3
– – trachea (intrathoracic) 862.2
– – – with open wound into cavity 862.3
– – – cervical region 874.0
– – – – complicated 874.1
– – ureter 867.2
– – – with open wound into cavity 867.3
– – urethra (sphincter) 867.0
– – – with open wound into cavity 867.1
– – – obstetrical trauma 665.5
– – uterus 867.4
– – – with open wound into cavity 867.5
– – – complication of abortion - see
    categories 634-639, fourth digit .2
– – – obstetrical trauma NEC 665.5
– – vas deferens 867.6
– – – with open wound into cavity 867.7
– – vesical (sphincter) 867.0
– – – with open wound into cavity 867.1
– – viscera (abdominal) (see also Injury,
    internal, multiple) 868.-
– – – with fracture, pelvis - see Fracture,
    pelvis
– – – thoracic NEC (see also Injury,
    internal, intrathoracic) 862.8
– – – – with open wound into cavity
    862.9
– interscapular region 959.1
– intervertebral disc 959.1
– intestine - see Injury, internal, intestine
– intra-abdominal (organs) NEC 868.-
– intracranial 854.0
– – with
– – – open intracranial wound 854.1
– – – skull fracture - see Fracture, skull
– intraocular - see Injury, eyeball,
    penetrating
– intrathoracic organs (multiple) - see
    Injury, internal, intrathoracic
– intrauterine - see Injury, internal,
    intrauterine

Injury - *continued*
– iris 921.3
– – penetrating - see Injury, eyeball,
    penetrating
– jaw 959.0
– jejunum - see Injury, internal, jejunum
– joint NEC 959.9
– – old or residual 718.8
– kidney 866.-
– knee (and leg, except thigh) (and ankle)
    (and foot) 959.7
– labium (majus) (minus) 959.1
– labyrinth, ear 959.0
– lacrimal apparatus or sac 870.2
– larynx 959.0
– leg except thigh (and knee) (and ankle)
    (and foot) 959.7
– – upper or thigh 959.6
– lens, eye 921.3
– – penetrating - see Injury, eyeball,
    penetrating
– lip 959.0
– liver 864.-
– lumbar (region) 959.1
– – plexus 953.5
– lumbosacral (region) 959.1
– – plexus 953.5
– lung - see Injury, internal, lung
– malar region 959.0
– mastoid region 959.0
– maternal, during pregnancy, affecting
    fetus or newborn 760.5
– maxilla 959.0
– mediastinum - see Injury, internal,
    mediastinum
– membrane
– – brain (see also Injury, intracranial)
    854.0
– – tympanic 959.0
– meningeal artery (see also Hemorrhage,
    subdural, traumatic) 852.0
– meninges (cerebral) (see also Injury,
    intracranial) 854.0
– mesenteric
– – artery (inferior) (superior) 902.2
– – plexus, inferior 954.1
– – vein (inferior) (superior) 902.3
– mesentery - see Injury, internal,
    mesentery
– mesosalpinx - see Injury, internal,
    mesosalpinx
– middle ear 959.0
– midthoracic region 959.1
– mouth 959.0
– multiple (not classifiable to the same
    four-digit category in 959.0-959.7) 959.8
– – extreme NEC 869.1

Injury - *continued*
- nerve - *continued*
- − tibial - *continued*
- − − lower leg 956.5
- − − posterior 956.2
- − − toe 956.9
- − trigeminal 951.2
- − trochlear 951.1
- − trunk, excluding shoulder and pelvic girdles 954.9
- − − specified NEC 954.8
- − − sympathetic NEC 954.1
- − ulnar 955.2
- − − forearm 955.2
- − − wrist (and hand) 955.2
- − upper limb 955.9
- − − multiple 955.8
- − − specified NEC 955.7
- − vagus 951.8
- − wrist and hand 955.9
- nervous system diffuse 957.8
- nose (septum) 959.0
- obstetrical NEC 665.9
- occipital (region) (scalp) 959.0
- − lobe (see also Injury, intracranial) 854.0
- oesophagus - see Injury, internal, oesophagus
- optic 950.9
- − chiasm 950.1
- − cortex 950.3
- − nerve 950.0
- − pathways 950.2
- orbit, orbital (region) 921.2
- − penetrating 870.3
- − − with foreign body 870.4
- ovary - see Injury, internal, ovary
- palate (soft) 959.0
- pancreas - see Injury, internal, pancreas
- parathyroid (gland) 959.0
- parietal (region) (scalp) 959.0
- − lobe (see also Injury, intracranial) 854.0
- pelvic
- − floor 959.1
- − − complicating delivery 664.1
- − joint or ligament, complicating delivery 665.6
- − organs - see Injury, internal, pelvis
- − − complication of abortion - see categories 634-639, fourth digit .2
- − − obstetrical trauma NEC 665.5
- pelvis 959.1
- penis 959.1
- perineum 959.1
- peritoneum 868.-
- periurethral tissue

Injury - *continued*
- periurethral tissue - *continued*
- − complicating
- − − abortion - see categories 634-639, fourth digit .2
- − − delivery 665.5
- phalanges
- − foot 959.7
- − hand 959.5
- pharynx 959.0
- pleura - see Injury, internal, pleura
- popliteal space 959.7
- prepuce 959.1
- prostate - see Injury, internal, prostate
- pubic region 959.1
- pudenda 959.1
- radiation NEC 990
- radioactive substance or radium NEC 990
- rectovaginal septum 959.1
- rectum - see Injury, internal, rectum
- retina 921.3
- − penetrating - see Injury, eyeball, penetrating
- retroperitoneal 868.-
- roentgen rays NEC 990
- round ligament - see Injury, internal, round ligament
- sacral (region) 959.1
- − plexus 953.5
- sacro-iliac ligament NEC 959.1
- sacrum 959.1
- salivary ducts or glands 959.0
- scalp 959.0
- − fetus or newborn 767.1
- scapular region 959.2
- sclera 921.3
- − penetrating - see Injury, eyeball, penetrating
- − superficial 918.2
- scrotum 959.1
- seminal vesicle - see Injury, internal, seminal vesicle
- shoulder (and upper arm) 959.2
- sinus
- − cavernous (see also Injury, intracranial) 854.0
- − nasal 959.0
- skeleton nec, birth injury 767.3
- skin NEC 959.9
- skull - see Fracture, skull
- soft tissue (severe) (of external sites) - see Wound, open
- specified site NEC 959.8
- spermatic cord - see Injury, internal, spermatic cord
- spinal (cord) 952.9
- − with

Injury - *continued*
- spinal - *continued*
- - with - *continued*
- - - fracture, vertebra (conditions in
        805-) - see Fracture, vertebra, by
        region, with spinal cord lesion
- - cervical 952.0
- - dorsal 952.1
- - lumbar 952.2
- - multiple sites 952.8
- - nerve (root) NEC - see Injury, nerve,
      spinal, root
- - plexus 953.9
- - - brachial 953.4
- - - lumbosacral 953.5
- - - multiple sites 953.8
- - sacral 952.3
- - thoracic 952.1
- spleen 865.-
- stellate ganglion 954.1
- sternal region 959.1
- stomach - see Injury, internal, stomach
- subconjunctival 921.2
- subcutaneous NEC 959.9
- submaxillary region 959.0
- submental region 959.0
- subungual
- - fingers 959.5
- - toes 959.7
- superficial 919.-

Note – The following fourth-digit subdivisions are for use with categories 910–917
and 919:
    *.0 Abrasion or friction burn without
        mention of infection*
    .1 Abrasion or friction burn, infected
    .2 Blister without mention of infection
    .3 Blister, infected
    *.4 Insect bite, nonvenomous, without
        mention of infection*
    .5 Insect bite, nonvenomous, infected
    *.6 Superficial foreign body (splinter)
        without major open wound and with-
        out mention of infection*
    *.7 Superficial foreign body (splinter)
        without major open wound, infected*
    *.8 Other and unspecified superficial in-
        jury without mention of infection*
    *.9 Other and unspecified superficial in-
        jury, infected.*

Injury - *continued*
- superficial - *continued*
- - abdomen, abdominal (muscle) (wall)
      (and other part(s) of trunk) 911.-

Injury - *continued*
- superficial - *continued*
- - ankle (and hip) (and thigh) (and leg)
      (and knee) 916.-
- - anus (and other part(s) of trunk) 911.-
- - arm 913.-
- - - upper (and shoulder) 912.-
- - auditory canal (external) (meatus)
      (and other part(s) of face, neck or
      scalp, except eye) 910.-
- - axilla (and upper arm) 912.-
- - back (and other part(s) of trunk) 911.-
- - breast (and other part(s) of trunk)
      911.-
- - brow (and other part(s) of face, neck,
      or scalp except eye) 910.-
- - buttock (and other part(s) of trunk)
      911.-
- - canthus, eye 918.0
- - cheek(s) (and other part(s) of face,
      neck, or scalp except eye) 910.-
- - chest wall (and other part(s) of trunk)
      911.-
- - chin (and other part(s) of face, neck, or
      scalp except eye) 910.-
- - clitoris (and other part(s) of trunk)
      911.-
- - conjunctiva 918.2
- - cornea 918.1
- - costal region (and other part(s) of
      trunk) 911.-
- - ear(s) (auricle) (canal) (drum)
      (external) (and other part(s) of face,
      neck, or scalp, except eye) 910.-
- - elbow (and forearm) (and wrist) 913.-
- - epididymis (and other part(s) of trunk)
      911.-
- - epigastric region (and other part(s) of
      trunk) 911.-
- - epiglottis (and other part(s) of face,
      neck, or scalp except eye) 910.-
- - eye(s) (and adnexa) NEC 918.9
- - eyelid(s) (and periocular area) 918.0
- - face (and neck or scalp) (any part(s),
      except eye) 910.-
- - finger(s) (nail) (any) 915.-
- - flank (and other part(s) of trunk) 911.-
- - foot (phalanges) (and toe(s)) 917.-
- - forearm (and elbow) (and wrist) 913.-
- - forehead (and other part(s) of face,
      neck, or scalp except eye) 910.-
- - globe (eye) 918.9
- - groin (and other part(s) of trunk) 911.-
- - gum(s) (and other part(s) of face, neck,
      or scalp except eye) 910.-
- - hand(s) (except fingers alone) 914.-

Injury - *continued*
− superficial - *continued*
− − head (and other part(s) of face, neck, or scalp except eye) 910.-
− − heel (and toe) (and foot) 917.-
− − hip (and thigh) (and leg) (and ankle) (and knee) 916.-
− − iliac region (and other part(s) of trunk) 911.-
− − interscapular region (and other part(s) of trunk) 911.-
− − knee (and hip) (and thigh) (and leg) (and ankle) 916.-
− − labium (majus) (minus) (and other part(s) of trunk) 911.-
− − lacrimal (apparatus) (gland) (sac) 918.0
− − leg (upper) (lower) (and hip) (and thigh) (and ankle) (and knee) 916.-
− − lip(s) (and other part(s) of face, neck, or scalp except eye) 910.-
− − lower extremity, except foot 916.-
− − lumbar region (and other part(s) of trunk) 911.-
− − malar region (and other part(s) of face, neck, or scalp except eye) 910.-
− − mastoid region (and other part(s) of face, neck, or scalp except eye) 910.-
− − midthoracic region (and other part(s) of trunk) 911.-
− − mouth (and other part(s) of face, neck, or scalp except eye) 910.-
− − multiple sites (not classifiable to the same three-digit category) 919.-
− − nasal (septum) (and other part(s) of face, neck, or scalp, except eye) 910.-
− − neck (and face or scalp) (and part(s), except eye) 910.-
− − nose (septum) (and other part(s) of face, neck, or scalp, except eye) 910.-
− − occipital region (and other part(s) of face, neck, or scalp except eye) 910.-
− − orbital region 918.0
− − palate (soft) (and other part(s) of face, neck, or scalp, except eye) 910.-
− − parietal region (and other part(s) of face, neck, or scalp except eye) 910.-
− − penis (and other part(s) of trunk) 911.-
− − perineum (and other part(s) of trunk) 911.-
− − periocular area 918.0
− − pharynx (and other part(s) of face, neck, or scalp except eye) 910.-
− − popliteal space (and ankle) (and hip) (and leg) (and thigh) 916.-
− − prepuce (and other part(s) of trunk) 911.-

Injury - *continued*
− superficial - *continued*
− − pubic region (and other part(s) of trunk) 911.-
− − pudenda (and other part(s) of trunk) 911.-
− − sacral region (and other part(s) of trunk) 911.-
− − salivary (ducts) (glands) (and other part(s) of face, neck, or scalp, except eye) 910.-
− − scalp (and other part(s) of face or neck except eye) 910.-
− − scapular region (and upper arm) 912.-
− − sclera 918.2
− − scrotum (and other part(s) of trunk) 911.-
− − shoulder (and upper arm) 912.-
− − skin NEC 919.-
− − specified site(s) NEC 919.-
− − sternal region (and other part(s) of trunk) 911.-
− − subconjunctival 918.2
− − subcutaneous NEC 919.-
− − submaxillary region (and other part(s) of face, neck, or scalp execpt eye) 910.-
− − submental region (and other part(s) of face, neck, or scalp except eye) 910.-
− − supraclavicular fossa 910.-
− − supraorbital 918.0
− − temple (and other part(s) of face, neck, or scalp except eye) 910.-
− − temporal region (and other part(s) of face, neck, or scalp except eye) 910.-
− − testis (and other part(s) of trunk) 911.-
− − thigh (and hip) (and leg) (and ankle) (and knee) 916.-
− − thorax, thoracic (external) (and other part(s) of trunk) 911.-
− − throat (and other part(s) of face, neck, or scalp except eye) 910.-
− − thumb(s) (nail) 915.-
− − toe(s) (nail) (subungual) (and foot) 917.-
− − tongue (and other part(s) of face, neck, or scalp except eye) 910.-
− − tooth, teeth 521.2
− − trunk (any part(s)) 911.-
− − tunica vaginalis (and other part(s) of trunk) 911.-
− − tympanum, tympanic membrane (and other part(s) of face, neck, or scalp except eye) 910.-
− − upper extremity NEC 913.-
− − uvula (and other part(s) of face, neck, or scalp except eye) 910.-

Insufficiency - *continued*
- arterial 447.1
- - basilar artery 435
- - carotid artery 435
- - cerebral 437.1
- - mesenteric 557.1
- - peripheral 443.9
- - pre-cerebral 435
- - vertebral artery 435
- arteriovenous 459.9
- biliary (see also Disease, biliary) 575.8
- cardiac (see also Insufficiency, myocardial) 428.0
- - complicating surgery 997.1
- - due to presence of (cardiac) prosthesis 429.4
- - postoperative 997.1
- - - long-term effect of cardiac surgery 429.4
- - specified during or due to a procedure 997.1
- - - long-term effect of cardiac surgery 429.4
- cardiorenal 404.9
- cardiovascular (see also Disease, cardiovascular) 429.2
- - renal 404.9
- cerebral (vascular) 437.9
- cerebrovascular 437.9
- - with transient focal neurological signs and symptoms 435
- - acute 437.1
- - - with transient focal neurological signs and symptoms 435
- circulatory NEC 459.9
- - fetus or newborn 779.8
- convergence 378.8
- coronary (acute or subacute) 411
- - chronic or with a stated duration of over 8 weeks 414.8
- cortico-adrenal 255.4
- dietary 269.9
- divergence 378.8
- food 994.2
- gastroesophageal 530.8
- gonadal
- - ovary 256.3
- - testis 257.2
- heart - see also Insufficiency, myocardial
- - fetus or newborn 779.8
- - valve (see also Endocarditis) 424.9
- - - congenital NEC 746.8
- hepatic 573.8
- idiopathic autonomic 333.0
- kidney (see also Disease, renal) 593.9
- lacrimal 375.1
- liver 573.8

Insufficiency - *continued*
- lung (see also Insufficiency, pulmonary) 518.8
- - following trauma, surgery or shock 518.5
- - newborn 770.8
- mental (congenital) (see also Retardation, mental) 319
- mitral 424.0
- - with
- - - aortic valve disease 396
- - - obstruction or stenosis 394.2
- - - - with aortic valve disease 396
- - congenital 746.6
- - rheumatic 394.1
- - - with
- - - - aortic valve disease 396
- - - - obstruction or stenosis 394.2
- - - - - with aortic valve disease 396
- - - active or acute 391.1
- - - - with chorea, rheumatic (Sydenham's) 392.0
- - specified cause, except rheumatic 424.0
- muscle
- - heart - see Insufficiency, myocardial
- - ocular NEC 378.9
- myocardial, myocardium 428.0
- - with
- - - rheumatic fever (conditions in 390)
- - - - active, acute or subacute 391.2
- - - - - with chorea 392.0
- - - - inactive or quiescent (with chorea) 398.0
- - congenital 746.8
- - fetus or newborn 779.8
- - hypertensive (see also Hypertension, heart) 402.9
- - rheumatic 398.0
- - - active, acute, or subacute 391.2
- - syphilitic 093.8
- nourishment 994.2
- organic 799.8
- ovary 256.3
- pancreatic 577.8
- parathyroid (gland) 252.1
- peripheral vascular 443.9
- pituitary 253.2
- placental - see Placenta, insufficiency
- progressive pluriglandular 258.9
- pulmonary 518.8
- - following
- - - shock 518.5
- - - surgery 518.5
- - - trauma 518.5
- - newborn 770.8

Insufficiency - *continued*
- pulmonary - *continued*
- - valve (see also Endocarditis,
     pulmonary) 424.3
- - - congenital 746.0
- pyloric 537.0
- renal (see also Disease, renal) 593.9
- - specified due to a procedure 997.5
- respiratory 786.0
- - newborn 770.8
- rotation - see Malrotation
- suprarenal 255.4
- tarso-orbital fascia, congenital 743.6
- testis 257.2
- thyroid (gland) (acquired) 244.9
- - congenital 243
- tricuspid (see also Endocarditis,
     tricuspid) 397.0
- - congenital 746.8
- urethral sphincter 788.3
- valve, valvular (heart) (see also
     Endocarditis) 424.9
- vascular 459.9
- - intestine NEC 557.9
- - mesenteric 557.1
- - peripheral 443.9
- - renal (see also Hypertension, kidney)
     403.9
- venous 459.9
- ventricular - see Insufficiency, myocardial
Insufflation, fallopian V26.2
Insular - see condition
Insulinoma (M8151/0)
- malignant (M8151/3)
- - pancreas 157.4
- - specified site NEC - see Neoplasm,
     malignant
- - unspecified site 157.4
- pancreas 211.7
- specified site NEC - see Neoplasm,
     benign
- unspecified site 211.7
Insuloma - see Insulinoma
Insult
- brain 437.9
- cerebral 437.9
- cerebrovascular 437.9
- vascular NEC 437.9
Intemperance - see Alcoholism
Interception of pregnancy V25.3
Intermenstrual - see condition
Intermittent - see condition
Internal - see condition
Interruption
- aortic arch 747.1
- bundle of His 426.5
- fallopian tube V25.2

Interruption - *continued*
- vas deferens V25.2
Interstitial - see condition
Intertrigo 695.8
Intervertebral disc - see condition
Intestine, intestinal - see condition
Intolerance
- disaccharide (hereditary) 271.3
- fat NEC 579.8
- foods NEC 579.8
- fructose (hereditary) 271.2
- glucose(-galactose) 271.3
- lactose (hereditary) (infantile) 271.3
- lysine 270.7
- milk NEC 579.8
- starch NEC 579.8
- sucrose(-isomaltose) 271.3
Intoxicated NEC 305.0
Intoxication
- acid 276.9
- alcoholic (acute) 305.0
- - hangover effects 305.0
- alimentary canal 558
- chemical - see also Table of drugs and
     chemicals
- - via placenta or breast milk - see
     Absorption, chemical, through
     placenta
- drug
- - correct substance properly
     administered (see also Allergy, drug)
     995.2
- - overdose or wrong substance given or
     taken - see Table of drugs and
     chemicals
- - pathologic 292.2
- - specific to newborn 779.4
- - via placenta or breast milk - see
     Absorption, chemical, through
     placenta
- enteric - see Intoxication, intestinal
- fetus or newborn, via placenta or breast
     milk - see Absorption, chemical, through
     placenta
- food - see Poisoning, food
- gastro-intestinal 558
- hallucinogenic (acute) 305.3
- intestinal 569.8
- - due to putrefaction of food 005.9
- methyl alcohol (see also Alcoholism)
     305.0
- pathologic 291.4
- - drug 292.2
- septic
- - with
- - - abortion see categories 634-639,
     fourth digit .0 639.0

Intoxication - *continued*
- septic - *continued*
- - with - *continued*
- - - ectopic gestation 639.0
- - during labor 659.3
- - general - see Septicemia
- - puerperal, postpartum, childbirth 670
- serum (prophylactic) (therapeutic) 999.5
- uremic - see Uremia
- water 276.6
Intracranial - see condition
Intrahepatic gallbladder 751.6
Intraligamentous - see also condition
- pregnancy - see Pregnancy, cornual
Intrathoracic - see also condition
- kidney 753.3
Intrauterine contraceptive device
- checking, re-insertion, removal V25.4
- in situ V45.5
- insertion V25.1
Intraventricular - see condition
Intrinsic deformity - see Deformity
Intumescence, lens (eye) NEC 366.9
Intussusception (colon) (intestine) (rectum) 560.0
- appendix 543
- congenital 751.5
- ureter (with obstruction) 593.4
Invagination, colon or intestine 560.0
Invalid (since birth) 799.8
Invalidism (chronic) 799.8
Inversion
- albumin-globulin (A-G) ratio 273.8
- bladder 596.8
- cecum (see also Intussusception) 560.0
- cervix 622.8
- nipple 611.7
- - congenital 757.6
- - puerperal, postpartum 676.3
- optic papilla 743.5
- organ or site, congenital NEC - see Anomaly, specified type NEC
- sleep rhythm 780.5
- - nonorganic origin 307.4
- testis (congenital) 752.5
- uterus 621.7
- - chronic 621.7
- - during delivery 665.2
- vagina - see Prolapse, vagina
Involuntary movement, abnormal 781.0
Involution, involutional - see also condition
- breast, cystic 610.1
- ovary, senile 620.3
Irideremia 743.4
Iridis rubeosis 364.4
Iridochoroiditis (panuveitis) 360.1
Iridocyclitis NEC 364.3

Iridocyclitis NEC - *continued*
- acute 364.0
- chronic 364.1
- due to allergy 364.0
- endogenous 364.0
- gonococcal 098.4 † 364.0*
- herpetic (simplex) 054.4 † 364.0*
- - zoster 053.2 † 364.0*
- hypopyon 364.0
- lens induced 364.2
- recurrent 364.0
- rheumatic 364.1
- subacute 364.0
- sympathetic 360.1
- tuberculous (chronic) 017.3 † 364.1*
Iridocyclochoroiditis (panuveitis) 360.1
Iridodialysis 364.7
Iridodonesis 364.8
Iridoplegia (complete) (partial) (reflex) 379.4
Iridoschisis 364.5
Iris - see condition
Iritis - see also Iridocyclitis
- diabetic 250.4 † 364.8*
- due to
- - herpes simplex 054.4 † 364.0*
- - leprosy 030.- † 364.1*
- gonococcal 098.4 † 364.0*
- gouty 274.8 † 364.1*
- papulosa 095 † 364.1*
- syphilitic (secondary) 091.5 † 364.1*
- - congenital 090.0 † 364.1*
- - late 095 † 364.1*
- tuberculous 017.3 † 364.1*
Iron - see condition
Iron-miner lung 503
Irradiated enamel (tooth, teeth) 521.8
Irradiation effects, adverse NEC 990
Irreducible, irreducibility - see condition
Irregular, irregularity
- action, heart 427.9
- alveolar process 525.8
- bleeding NEC 626.4
- breathing 786.0
- colon 569.8
- contour of cornea 743.4
- - acquired 371.7
- dentin in pulp 522.3
- menstruation (cause unknown) 626.4
- periods 626.4
- pupil 364.7
- respiratory 786.0
- septum (nasal) 470
- shape, organ or site, congenital NEC - see Distortion
- vertebra 733.9
Irritability

Irritability - *continued*
- bladder 596.8
- bowel (syndrome) 564.1
- bronchial (see also Bronchitis) 490
- cerebral, in newborn 779.1
- colon 564.1
- − psychogenic 306.4
- duodenum 564.8
- heart 306.2
- ileum 564.8
- jejunum 564.8
- myocardium 306.2
- rectum 564.8
- stomach 536.9
- − psychogenic 306.4
- sympathetic 337.9
- urethra 599.8
Irritable - see Irritability
Irritation
- anus 569.4
- bladder 596.8
- brachial plexus 353.0
- brain (traumatic) (see also Injury, intracranial) 854.0
- bronchial (see also Bronchitis) 490
- cerebral (traumatic) (see also Injury, intracranial) 854.0
- − nontraumatic - see Encephalitis
- cervix (see also Cervicitis) 616.0
- choroid, sympathetic 360.1
- cranial nerve - see Disorder, nerve, cranial
- digestive tract 536.9
- gastric 536.9
- − psychogenic 306.4
- gastro-intestinal (tract) (functional) 536.9
- − psychogenic 306.4
- globe, sympathetic 360.1
- intestinal 564.1
- labyrinth 386.5
- lumbosacral plexus 353.1
- meninges (traumatic) (see also Injury, intracranial) 854.0
- − nontraumatic - see Meningitis
- nerve - see Disorder, nerve
- nervous 799.2
- nose 478.1
- penis 607.8
- perineum NEC 709.9
- peripheral autonomic nervous system 337.9
- pharynx 478.2
- spinal (cord) (traumatic) - see also Injury, spinal, by region
- − nerve - see Disorder, nerve
- − − root NEC 724.9

Irritation - *continued*
- spinal - *continued*
- − nerve - *continued*
- − − traumatic - see Injury, nerve, spinal
- − − nontraumatic (see also Encephalitis) 323.9
- stomach 536.9
- − psychogenic 306.4
- sympathetic nerve NEC 337.9
- vagina 623.9
Ischemia, ischemic 459.9
- brain - see also Ischemia, cerebral
- − recurrent focal 435
- cardiac (see also Ischemia, heart) 414.9
- cerebral (chronic) (generalized) 437.1
- − arteriosclerotic 437.0
- − intermittent 435
- − puerperal, postpartum, childbirth 674.0
- − transient 435
- coronary (see also Ischemia, heart) 414.9
- heart (chronic or with a stated duration of over 8 weeks) 414.9
- − acute or with a stated duration of 8 weeks or less 410
- intestine 557.9
- myocardium, myocardial (chronic or with a stated duration of over 8 weeks) 414.8
- retina, retinal 362.8
- spinal cord 336.1
- subendocardial (see also Insufficiency, coronary) 411
Ischial spine - see condition
Ischialgia (see also Sciatica) 724.3
Ischiopagus 759.4
Ischium, ischial - see condition
Ischuria 788.5
Iselin's disease or osteochondrosis 732.5
Islands of
- parotid tissue in
- − lymph nodes 750.2
- − neck structures 750.2
- submaxillary glands in
- − fascia 750.2
- − lymph nodes 750.2
- − neck muscles 750.2
Islet cell tumor, pancreas (M8150/0) 211.7
Isoimmunization NEC (see also Incompatibility) 656.2
- fetus or newborn 773.2
Isolation V07.0
- social V62.4
Isosporosis 007.2
Issue of
- medical certificate NEC V68.0
- − cause of death V68.0
- − fitness V68.0

Issue of - *continued*
- medical certificate NEC - *continued*
- - incapacity V68.0
- repeat prescription NEC V68.1
- - appliance V68.1
- - contraceptive (pill) (device) V25.4
- - glasses V68.1
- - medicament V68.1
Itch (see also Pruritus) 698.9
- bakers' 692.8
- barbers' 110.0
- bricklayers' 692.8
- cheese 133.8
- clam diggers' 120.3
- coolie 126.9
- copra 133.8
- Cuban 050.1
- dew 126.9
- dhobie 110.3
- filarial (see also Infestation, filarial) 125.9
- grain 133.8
- grocers' 133.8

Itch - *continued*
- ground 126.9
- harvest 133.8
- jock 110.3
- Malabar 110.9
- - beard 110.0
- - foot 110.4
- - scalp 110.0
- meaning scabies 133.0
- Norwegian 133.0
- poultrymen's 133.8
- sarcoptic 133.0
- scrub 134.1
- seven-year V61.1
- straw 133.8
- swimmers' 120.3
- washerwomen's 692.4
- water 120.3
- winter 698.8
Itching (see also Pruritus) 698.9
Ixodes 134.8
Ixodiasis 134.8

J

Jaccoud's nodular fibrositis, chronic
 (Jaccoud's syndrome) 714.4
Jackson's
 − membrane 751.4
 − paralysis or syndrome 344.8
 − veil 751.4
Jacksonian
 − epilepsy 345.5
 − seizures (focal) 345.5
Jacquet's dermatitis 691.0
Jadassohn's
 − blue nevus (M8780/0) - see Neoplasm,
  skin, benign
 − intraepidermal epithelioma (M8096/0) -
  see Neoplasm, skin, benign
Jadassohn-Pellizari's disease 701.3
Jaffe-Lichtenstein syndrome 252.0

Jakob-Creutzfeldt disease or syndrome
 046.1 † 331.5*
 − with dementia 290.1
Jaksch-Luzet disease 285.8
Janet's disease 300.8
Janiceps 759.4
Jansky-Bielschowsky amaurotic familial
 idiocy 330.1

Jaundice (yellow) 782.4
 − acholuric (familial) (splenomegalic) (see
  also Spherocytosis) 282.0
 − − acquired 283.9
 − breast-milk 774.3
 − catarrhal (acute) 070.1 † 573.1*
 − − with hepatic coma 070.0 † 573.1*
 − − epidemic - see Jaundice, epidemic
 − chronic idiopathic 277.4
 − epidemic (catarrhal) 070.1 † 573.1*
 − − with hepatic coma 070.0 † 573.1*
 − − leptospiral 100.0
 − − spirochetal 100.0
 − febrile (acute) 070.1 † 573.1*
 − − with hepatic coma 070.0 † 573.1*
 − − leptospiral 100.0
 − − spirochetal 100.0
 − fetus or newborn 774.6
 − − due to or associated with
 − − − ABO
 − − − − antibodies 773.1
 − − − − incompatibility, maternal/fetal
    773.1
 − − − − isoimmunization 773.1

Jaundice - continued
 − fetus or newborn - continued
 − − due to or associated with - continued
 − − − absence or deficiency of enzyme
    system for bilirubin conjugation
    (congenital) 774.3
 − − − blood group incompatibility NEC
    773.2
 − − − breast milk inhibitors to conjugation
    774.3
 − − − bruising 774.1
 − − − Crigler-Najjar syndrome 277.4 †
    774.3*
 − − − delayed conjugation 774.3
 − − − − associated with preterm delivery
     774.2
 − − − drugs or toxins transmitted from
    mother 774.1
 − − − galactosemia 271.1 † 774.5*
 − − − Gilbert's syndrome 277.4 † 774.3*
 − − − G6PD deficiency 282.2 † 774.0*
 − − − hepatocellular damage 774.4
 − − − hereditary hemolytic anemia 282.- †
    774.0*
 − − − hypothyroidism, congenital 243 †
    774.3*
 − − − incompatibility, maternal/fetal NEC
    773.2
 − − − infection 774.1
 − − − inspissated bile syndrome 751.6 †
    774.5*
 − − − isoimmunization NEC 773.2
 − − − mucoviscidosis 277.0 † 774.5*
 − − − obliteration of bile duct, congenital
    751.6 † 774.5*
 − − − polycythemia 774.1
 − − − preterm delivery 774.2
 − − − red cell defect 282.- † 774.0*
 − − − Rh
 − − − − antibodies 773.0
 − − − − incompatibility, maternal/fetal
     773.0
 − − − − iso-immunisation 773.0
 − − − spherocytosis (congenital) 282.0 †
    774.0*
 − − − swallowed maternal blood 774.1
 − − physiological 774.6
 − from injection, inoculation, infusion or
  transfusion (blood) (plasma) (serum)
  (other substance) 070.3 † 573.1*

Jaundice - *continued*
- from injection - *continued*
- - with hepatic coma 070.2 † 573.1*
- hematogenous 283.9
- hemolytic (acquired) 283.9
- - congenital (see also Spherocytosis) 282.0
- hemorrhagic (acute) 100.0
- - leptospiral 100.0
- - spirochetal 100.0
- hepatocellular 573.8
- homologous (serum) 070.3 † 573.1*
- - with hepatic coma 070.2 † 573.1*
- idiopathic, chronic 277.4
- infectious (acute) (subacute) 070.1 † 573.1*
- - with hepatic coma 070.0 † 573.1*
- - leptospiral 100.0
- - spirochetal 100.0
- leptospiral 100.0
- malignant (see also Necrosis, liver) 570
- newborn (physiological) (see also Jaundice, fetus or newborn) 774.6
- nonhemolytic
- - congenital familial (Gilbert) 277.4
- nuclear, newborn (see also Kernicterus of newborn) 774.7
- obstructive (see also Obstruction, gallbladder) 576.8
- post-immunization 070.3 † 573.1*

Jaundice - *continued*
- post-immunization - *continued*
- - with hepatic coma 070.2 † 573.1*
- post-transfusion 070.3 † 573.1*
- - with hepatic coma 070.2 † 573.1*
- regurgitation (see also Obstruction, gallbladder) 576.8
- serum (homologous) (prophylactic) (therapeutic) 070.3 † 573.1*
- - with hepatic coma 070.2 † 573.1*
- spirochetal (hemorrhagic) 100.0
Jaw - see condition
Jaw-winking phenomenon 742.8
Jaybi's syndrome 759.8
Jealousy
- alcoholic 291.5
- childhood 313.3
- sibling 313.3
Jejunitis - see Enteritis
Jejunum, jejunal - see condition
Jensen's disease 363.0
Jerks, myoclonic 333.2
Jeune's disease 756.4
Jigger disease 134.1
Joint - see also condition
- mice 718.1
- - knee 717.6
- sinus to bone 730.9
Jungling's disease 135
Juvenile - see condition

K

Kahler's disease (M9730/3) 203.0
Kakergasia 300.9
Kakke 265.0
Kala-azar (Indian) (infantile)
  (Mediterranean) (Sudanese) 085.0
Kanner's syndrome 299.0
Kaposi's
 − disease 757.3
 − − meaning
 − − − lichen ruber moniliformis 697.8
 − − − xeroderma pigmentosum 757.3
 − sarcoma (M9140/3) - see Neoplasm, skin,
   malignant
 − varicelliform eruption 054.0
Kartagener syndrome or triad 759.3
Kaschin-Beck disease 716.0
Kast's syndrome 756.4
Katatonia 295.2
Katayama disease or fever 120.2
Kayser-Fleischer ring (cornea)
  (pseudosclerosis) 371.1
Kelis 701.4
Kelly-Patterson syndrome 280
Keloid, cheloid 701.4
 − Addison's 701.0
 − cornea 371.0
 − Hawkins' 701.4
 − scar 701.4
Keloma 701.4
Keratectasia 371.7
 − congenital 743.4
Keratitis (nonulcerative) NEC 370.9
 − with ulceration (central) (marginal)
   (perforated) (ring) 370.0
 − actinic 370.2
 − arborescens 054.4 † 370.1*
 − areolar 370.2
 − bullosa 370.8
 − deep 370.5
 − dendritic(a) 054.4 † 370.1*
 − disciform(is) 054.4 † 370.5*
 − − varicella 052 † 370.5*
 − exposure 370.3
 − filamentary 370.2
 − gonococcal (congenital or prenatal)
   098.4 † 370.4*
 − herpes, herpetic (simplex) NEC 054.4 †
   370.4*
 − − zoster 053.2 † 370.4*
 − hypopyon 370.0

Keratitis - *continued*
 − interstitial (nonsyphilitic) 370.5
 − − herpes, herpetic (simplex) 054.4 †
   370.5*
 − − − zoster 053.2 † 370.5*
 − − syphilitic (congenital) (hereditary)
   090.3 † 370.5*
 − − tuberculous 017.3 † 370.5*
 − lagophthalmic 370.4
 − neurotrophic 370.3
 − nummular 370.2
 − parenchymatous - see Keratitis,
   interstitial
 − petrificans 370.8
 − phlyctenular 370.3
 − punctata
 − − leprosa 030.- † 370.5*
 − − profunda 090.3 † 370.5*
 − purulent 370.8
 − pustuliformis profunda 090.3 † 370.5*
 − rosacea 695.3 † 370.4*
 − sclerosing 370.5
 − stellate 370.2
 − striate 370.2
 − superficial (punctate) 370.2
 − − with conjunctivitis 370.4
 − suppurative 370.8
 − syphilitic (congenital) (prenatal) 090.3 †
   370.5*
 − trachomatous 076.1 † 370.2*
 − tuberculous 017.3 † 370.3*
 − vesicular 370.8
 − xerotic 371.4
 − − vitamin A deficiency 264.4 † 371.4*
Keratoacanthoma 701.1
Keratocele 371.7
Keratoconjunctivitis (see also Keratitis)
  370.4
 − epidemic 077.1 † 370.4*
 − herpetic (simplex) 054.4 † 370.4*
 − − zoster 053.2 † 370.4*
 − infectious 077.1 † 370.4*
 − shipyard 077.1 † 370.4*
 − sicca 710.2 † 370.3*
 − tuberculous (phlyctenular) 017.3 † 370.3*
Keratoconus 371.6
 − congenital 743.4
Keratocyst 526.0
Keratoderma, keratodermia (congenital)
  (palmaris et plantaris) (symmetrical) 757.3

Keratoderma - *continued*
- acquired 701.1
- blenorrhagica 701.1
- - gonococcal 098.8 † 701.1*
- climactericum 701.1
- eccentrica 757.3
- gonorrheal 098.8 † 701.1*
- palmaris et plantaris 701.1
- punctata 701.1
- tylodes progressive 701.1
Keratodermatocele 371.7
Keratoglobus 371.7
- congenital 743.4
Keratohemia 371.1
Kerato-iritis (see also Iridocyclitis) 364.3
- syphilitic 090.3 † 370.5*
- tuberculous 017.3 † 370.3*
Keratolysis exfoliativa (congenital) 757.3
- acquired 695.8
- neonatorum 757.3
Keratoma 701.1
- congenital 757.1
- malignum congenitale 757.1
- palmaris and plantaris hereditarium 757.3
- senile 702
Keratomalacia 371.4
- vitamin A deficiency 264.4 † 371.4*
Keratomegaly 743.4
Keratomycosis 111.1
- nigricans (palmaris) 111.1
Keratopathy 371.4
- band (see also Keratitis) 371.4
- bullous (see also Keratitis) 371.2
Keratoscleritis, tuberculous 017.3 † 370.3*
Keratosis 701.1
- arsenical 692.4
- blenorrhagica 701.1
- - gonococcal 098.8 † 701.1*
- congenital (any type) 757.3
- female genital (external) 629.8
- follicularis 757.3
- - acquired 701.1
- - congenita (acneiformis) (Siemen's) 757.3
- - spinulosa (decalvans) 757.3
- - vitamin A deficiency 264.8 † 701.1*
- gonococcal 098.8 † 701.1*
- larynx 478.7
- male genital (external) 608.8
- nigricans 701.2
- - congenital 757.3
- obturans 380.2
- palmaris et plantaris (symmetrical) 757.3
- penile 607.8
- pharyngeus 478.2
- pilaris 757.3

Keratosis - *continued*
- pilaris - *continued*
- - acquired 701.1
- punctata (palmaris et plantaris) 701.1
- scrotal 608.8
- seborrheic 702
- senile 702
- suprafollicularis 757.3
- tonsillaris 478.2
- vegetans 757.3
- vitamin A deficiency 264.8 † 701.1*
Kerato-uveitis (see also Iridocyclitis) 364.3
Keraunoparalysis 994.0
Kerion (celsi) 110.0
Kernicterus of newborn (not due to isoimmunization) 774.7
- due to isoimmunization (conditions in 773.0-773.2) 773.4
Keto-acidosis 276.2
- diabetic 250.1
Ketonuria 791.6
Ketosis 276.2
- diabetic 250.1
Kidney - see condition
Kienbock's
- disease 732.3
- osteochondrosis 732.3
Kimmelstiel(-Wilson) disease or syndrome 250.3 † 581.8*
Kink
- appendix 543
- artery 447.1
- ileum or intestine (see also Obstruction, intestine) 560.9
- Lane's (see also Obstruction, intestine) 560.9
- organ or site, congenital NEC - see Anomaly, specified type NEC
- ureter (pelvic junction) 593.3
- - congenital 753.2
- vein(s) 459.9
- - caval 459.9
Kinking hair (acquired) 704.2
Klebs' disease (see also Nephritis) 583.9
Kleine-Levin syndrome 349.8
Kleine-Wardenburg syndrome 270.2
Kleptomania 312.2
Klinefelter's syndrome 758.7
Klippel's disease 723.8
Klippel-Feil deficiency or syndrome 756.1
Klippel-Trenaunay syndrome 759.8
Klumpke(-Dejerine) palsy, paralysis (birth) (newborn) 767.6
Knee - see condition
Knifegrinders' rot 011.4
Knock knee (acquired) 736.4
- congenital 755.6

L

La grippe - see Influenza
Labia, labium - see condition
Labile
– blood pressure 796.4
– vasomotor system 443.9
Labioglossal paralysis 335.2
Labium leporinum 749.1
– with cleft palate 749.2
Labor (see also Delivery)
– abnormal NEC 661.9
– – affecting fetus or newborn 763.7
– arrested active phase 661.1
– – fetus or newborn 763.7
– desultory 661.2
– – fetus or newborn 763.7
– dyscoordinate 661.4
– – fetus or newborn 763.7
– early onset (before 37 completed weeks'
    gestation) 644.1
– false 644.0
– forced or induced
– – affecting fetus or newborn 763.8
– hypertonic 661.4
– – fetus or newborn 763.7
– hypotonic 661.2
– – fetus or newborn 763.7
– – primary 661.0
– – secondary 661.1
– incoordinate 661.4
– – fetus or newborn 763.7
– irregular 661.2
– – fetus or newborn 763.7
– long - see Labor, prolonged
– missed 656.4
– obstructed NEC 660.9
– – affecting fetus or newborn 763.1
– precipitate 661.3
– – fetus or newborn 763.6
– premature 644.1
– prolonged or protracted 662.1
– – affecting fetus or newborn 763.9
– – first stage 662.0
– – second stage 662.2
Labored breathing (see also
    Hyperventilation) 786.0
Labyrinthitis (circumscribed) (destructive)
    (diffuse) (inner ear) (latent) (purulent)
    (suppurative) 386.3
– syphilitic 095
Laceration - see also Wound, open

Laceration - *continued*
– accidental, complicating surgery 998.2
– Achilles tendon 845.0
– – with open wound 892.2
– anus (sphincter) 863.8
– – complicating delivery 664.2
– – – with laceration anal or rectal mucosa
        664.3
– – nontraumatic, nonpuerperal 565.0
– bladder (urinary)
– – complicating abortion - see categories
        634-639, fourth digit .2
– – obstetrical trauma 665.5
– bowel
– – complicating abortion - see categories
        634-639, fourth digit .2
– – obstetrical trauma 665.5
– brain (any part) (cortex) (membrane)
    (see also Laceration, cerebral) 851.0
– – during birth 767.0
– broad ligament
– – complicating abortion - see categories
        634-639, fourth digit .2
– – obstetrical trauma 665.6
– capsule, joint - see Sprain

– causing eversion of cervix uteri (old)
    622.0
– central, complicating delivery 664.4
– cerebellum (see also Laceration,
    cerebral) 851.0
– cerebral 851.0
– – with
– – – open intracranial wound 851.1
– – – skull fracture - see Fracture, skull
– – during birth 767.0
– cervix (uteri)
– – complicating abortion - see categories
        634-639, fourth digit .2
– – nonpuerperal, nontraumatic 622.3
– – obstetrical trauma (current) 665.3
– – old (postpartal) 622.3
– – traumatic - see Injury, internal, cervix

– chordae heart 429.5
– cortex (cerebral) (see also Laceration,
    cerebral) 851.0
– eye(s) - see Laceration, ocular
– eyeball NEC 871.4
– – with prolapse or exposure of
        intraocular tissue 871.1

Laceration - *continued*
- uterus - *continued*
- - old (postpartal) 621.8
- vagina
- - with abortion - see categories 634-639, fourth digit .2
- - complicating delivery 665.4
- - - with perineum 664.0
- - - muscles 664.1
- - nonpuerperal, nontraumatic 623.4
- - old (postpartal) 623.4
- vulva
- - complicating delivery 664.0
- - nonpuerperal, nontraumatic 624.4
- - old (postpartal) 624.4
Lachrymal - see condition
Lachrymonasal duct - see condition
Lack of
- appetite (see also Anorexia) 783.0
- care
- - in home V60.4
- - of infant (at or after birth) 995.5
- coordination 781.3
- development - see also Hypoplasia
- - physiological 783.4
- financial resources V60.2
- food 994.2
- growth 783.4
- heating V60.1
- housing (permanent) (temporary) V60.0
- - adequate V60.1
- material resources V60.2
- memory (see also Amnesia) 780.9
- - mild, following organic brain damage 310.1
- ovulation 628.0
- person able to render necessary care V60.4
- shelter V60.0
- water 994.3
Lacrimal - see condition
Lacrimation, abnormal 375.2
Lacrimonasal duct - see condition
Lactation, lactating (breast) (puerperal, postpartum)
- defective 676.4
- disorder 676.9
- - specified NEC 676.8
- excessive 676.6
- failed 676.4
- mastitis NEC 675.2
- mother (care and/or examination) V24.1
- nonpuerperal 611.6
Lactosuria 271.3
Lacunar skull 756.0
Laennec's cirrhosis (alcoholic) 571.2
- nonalcoholic 571.5

Lafora's disease 333.2
Lag, lid (nervous) 374.4
Lagophthalmos (eyelid) (nervous) 374.2
- keratitis (see also Keratitis) 370.4
Lalling 307.9
Lambliasis 007.1
Lame back 724.5
Lancereaux's diabetes 250.7 † 261*
Landouzy-Dejerine dystrophy or fascioscapulohumeral atrophy 359.1
Landry's disease or paralysis 357.0
Lane's
- disease 569.8
- kink (see also Obstruction, intestine) 560.9
Langdon Down's syndrome 758.0
Large
- ear 744.2
- fetus - see Oversize fetus
- physiological cup 743.5
Large-for-dates (fetus or infant) 766.1
- affecting management of pregnancy 656.6
- exceptionally 766.0
- 4500g or more 766.0
Larsen's syndrome 755.8
Larsen-Johansson disease 732.4
Larva migrans
- cutaneous NEC 126.9
- - ancylostoma 126.9
- of diptera in vitreous 128.0
- visceral NEC 128.0
Laryngismus (stridulus) 478.7
- congenital 748.3
- diphtheritic 032.3
Laryngitis (acute) (edematous) (fibrinous) (gangrenous) (infective) (infiltrative) (malignant) (membranous) (phlegmonous) (pneumococcal) (pseudomembranous) (septic) (subglottic) (suppurative) (ulcerative) (viral) 464.0
- with
- - influenza, flu, or grippe 487.1
- - tracheitis (see also Laryngotracheitis) 464.2
- - - acute 464.2
- - - chronic 476.1
- atrophic 476.0
- Borrelia vincenti 101
- catarrhal 476.0
- chronic 476.0
- - with tracheitis (chronic) 476.1
- - due to external agent - see condition, respiratory, chronic, due to
- diphtheritic 032.3
- due to external agent - see Inflammation, respiratory, upper, due to

Laryngitis - *continued*
- H. influenzae 464.0
- hypertrophic 476.0
- influenzal 487.1
- pachydermic 478.7
- sicca 476.0
- spasmodic 478.7
- − acute 464.0
- streptococcal 034.0
- stridulous 478.7
- syphilitic 095
- − congenital 090.5
- tuberculous 012.3
- Vincent's 101
Laryngocele (congenital) (ventricular) 748.3
Laryngofissure 478.7
Laryngopharyngitis (acute) 465.0
- chronic 478.9
- − due to external agent - see condition, respiratory, chronic, due to
- due to external agent - see Inflammation, respiratory, upper, due to
Laryngoplegia 478.3
Laryngoptosis 478.7
Laryngospasm 478.7
- due to external agent - see condition, respiratory, acute, due to
Laryngostenosis 478.7
Laryngotracheitis (acute) (infectonal) 464.2
- atrophic 476.1
- Borrelia vincenti 101
- catarrhal 476.1
- chronic 476.1
- − due to external agent - see condition, respiratory, chronic, due to
- diphtheric 032.3
- diphtheritic 032.3
- due to external agent - see Inflammation, respiratory, upper, due to
- H. influenzae 464.2
- hypertrophic 476.1
- influenzal 487.1
- pachydermic 478.7
- sicca 476.1
- spasmodic 478.7
- − acute 464.2
- streptoccocal 034.0
- stridulous 478.7
- syphilitic 095
- − congenital 090.5
- tuberculous 012.3
- Vincent's 101
Laryngotracheobronchitis (see also Bronchitis) 490
- acute 466.0
- chronic 491.8

Laryngotracheobronchopneumonitis - see Pneumonia, broncho
Larynx, laryngeal - see condition
Lassitude - see Weakness
Lassa fever 078.8
Late
- effect(s) (of) - see also condition
- − abscess
- − − intracranial or intraspinal (conditions in 324) 326
- − amputation
- − − postoperative (late) 997.6
- − − traumatic (injury in 885-887 and 895-897) 905.9
- − burn (injury in 948-949) 906.9
- − − extremities NEC (injury in 943 or 945) 906.7
- − − − hand and wrist (injury in 944) 906.6
- − − eye (injury in 940) 906.5
- − − face, head and neck (injury in 941) 906.5
- − − specified site NEC (injury in 942 and 946-947) 906.8
- − cerebrovascular disease (conditions in 430-437) - see category 438
- − complication(s) of
- − − surgical and medical care (condition in 996-999) 909.3
- − − − trauma (condition in 958) 908.6
- − contusion (injury in 920-924) 906.3
- − crushing (injury in 925-929) 906.4
- − dislocation (injury in 830-839) 905.6
- − encephalitis or encephalomyelitis (conditions in 323) 326
- − − in infectious diseases 139.8
- − − − viral (conditions in 049.8, 049.9, 062-064) 139.0
- − external cause NEC (condition in 995) 909.9
- − − certain conditions classifiable to categories 991-994 909.4
- − foreign body in orifice (injury in 930-939) 908.5
- − fracture (multiple) (injury in 828-829) 905.5
- − − extremity
- − − − lower (injury in 821-827) 905.4
- − − − − neck of femur (injury in 820) 905.3
- − − − upper (injury in 810-819) 905.2
- − − face and skull (injury in 800-804) 905.0
- − − skull and face (injury in 800-804) 905.0
- − − spine and trunk (injury in 805 and 807-809) 905.1

Late - *continued*
− effect(s) - *continued*
− − fracture - *continued*
− − − spine and trunk - *continued*
− − − − with spinal cord lesion (injury in 806) 907.2
− − infection
− − − pyogenic, intracranial 326
− − infectious diseases (conditions in 001-136) NEC 139.8
− − injury (injury in 959) 908.9
− − − blood vessel 908.3
− − − − abdomen and pelvis (injury in 902) 908.4
− − − − extremity (injury in 903-904) 908.3
− − − − head and neck (injury in 900) 908.3
− − − − − intracranial (injury in 850-854) 907.0
− − − − − − with skull fracture 905.0
− − − − thorax (injury in 901) 908.4
− − − internal organ NEC (injury in 867 and 869) 908.2
− − − − abdomen (injury in 863-866 and 868) 908.1
− − − − thorax (injury in 860-862) 908.0
− − − intracranial (injury in 850-854) 907.0
− − − − with skull fracture (injury in 800-801 and 803-804) 905.0
− − − nerve NEC (injury in 957) 907.9
− − − − cranial (injury in 950-951) 907.1
−˙− − − peripheral NEC (injury in 957) 907.9
− − − − − lower limb and pelvic girdle (injury in 956) 907.5
− − − − − upper limb and shoulder girdle (injury in 955) 907.4
− − − − roots and plexus(es), spinal (injury in 953) 907.3
− − − − trunk (injury in 954) 907.3
− − − spinal
− − − − cord (injury in 806 and 952) 907.2
− − − − nerve root(s) and plexus(es) (injury in 953) 907.3
− − − superficial (injury in 910-919) 906.2
− − − tendon (tendon injury in 840-848, 880.2-884.2, and 890.2-894.2) 905.8
− − meningitis
− − − bacterial (conditions in 320) 326
− − − unspecified cause (conditions in 322) 326
− − myelitis (see also Late effects, encephalitis) 326

Late - *continued*
− effect(s) - *continued*
− − parasitic diseases (conditions in 001-136) NEC 139.8
− − phlebitis or thrombophlebitis of intracranial venous sinuses (conditions in 325) 326
− − poisoning due to drug, medicament or biological substance (condition in 960-979) 909.0
− − poliomyelitis, acute (conditions in 045-) 138
− − radiation (condition in 990) 909.2
− − rickets 268.1
− − sprain and strain without mention of tendon injury (injury in 840-848 except tendon injury) 905.7
− − − tendon involvement 905.8
− − toxic effect of
− − − drug, medicament or biological substance (condition in 960-979) 909.0
− − − nonmedical substance (condition in 980-989) 909.1
− − trachoma (conditions in 076-) 139.1
− − tuberculosis 137.0
− − − bones and joints (conditions in 015) 137.3
− − − central nervous system (conditions in 013) 137.1
− − − genitourinary (conditions in 016) 137.2
− − − pulmonary (conditions in 010-012) 137.0
− − − specified organs NEC (conditions in 017-018) 137.4
− − viral encephalitis (conditions in 049.8, 049.9, 062-064) 139.0
− − wound, open
− − − extremity (injury in 880-884 and 890-894 except .2) 906.1
− − − − tendon (injury in 880.2-884.2 and 890.2-894.2) 905.8
− − − head, neck and trunk (injury in 870-879) 906.0
Latent - see condition
Laterocession - see Lateroversion
Lateroflexion - see Lateroversion
Lateroversion
− cervix - see Lateroversion, uterus
− uterus, uterine (cervix) (postinfectional) (postpartal, old) 621.6
− − congenital 752.3
− − in pregnancy or childbirth 654.4
− − − fetus or newborn 763.8
Lathyrism 988.2
Launois' syndrome 253.0

Laurence-Moon(-Biedl) syndrome 759.8
Lax, laxity - see also Relaxation
− ligament 728.4
− skin (acquired) 701.8
− − congenital 757.3
Laxative habit 305.9
Lead miner's lung 503
Leakage
− amniotic fluid 658.1
− − with delayed delivery 658.2
− − affecting fetus or newborn 761.1
− blood (microscopic), fetal, into maternal
  circulation 656.0
− − affecting management of pregnancy or
  puerperium 656.0
− device, implant or graft - see
  Complications, mechanical
− spinal fluid at lumbar puncture site 997.0
Leaky heart - see Endocarditis
Learning defect, specific NEC 315.2
Leather bottle stomach (M8142/3) 151.9
Leber's
− congenital amaurosis 362.7
− optic atrophy (hereditary) 377.1
Lederer's anemia 283.1
Leeches (aquatic) (land) 134.2
Leg - see condition
Legg(-Calve)-Perthes disease, syndrome or
  osteochondrosis 732.1
Legionnaire's disease 482.8
Leigh's disease 330.8
Leiner's disease 695.8
Leiofibromyoma (M8890/0) - see also
  Leiomyoma
− uterus (cervix) (corpus) 218
Leiomyoblastoma (M8891/1) - see
  Neoplasm, connective tissue, uncertain
  behavior
Leiomyofibroma (M8890/0) - see also
  Neoplasm, connective tissue, benign
− uterus (cervix) (corpus) 218
Leiomyoma (M8890/0) - see also
  Neoplasm, connective tissue, benign
− bizarre (M8893/0) - see Neoplasm,
  connective tissue, benign
− cellular (M8892/1) - see Neoplasm,
  connective tissue, uncertain behavior
− epithelioid (M8891/1) - see Neoplasm,
  connective tissue, uncertain behavior
− uterus (cervix) (corpus) 218
− vascular (M8894/0) -see neoplasm,
  connective tissue, benign 215.9
Leiomyomatosis (intravascular) (M8890/1)
  - see Neoplasm, connective tissue,
  uncertain behavior
Leiomyosarcoma (M8890/3) - see also
  Neoplasm, connective tissue, malignant

Leiomyosarcoma - *continued*
− epithelioid (M8891/3) - see Neoplasm,
  connective tissue, malignant
Leishmaniasis 085.9
− American 085.5
− − cutaneous 085.4
− − mucocutaneous 085.5
− Asian Desert 085.2
− Brazilian 085.5
− cutaneous 085.9
− − acute necrotizing 085.2
− − American 085.4
− − Asian Desert 085.2
− − diffuse 085.3
− − dry form 085.1
− − Ethiopian 085.3
− − eyelid 085.- † 373.6*
− − late 085.1
− − lepromatous 085.3
− − recurrent 085.1
− − rural 085.2
− − ulcerating 085.1
− − urban 085.1
− − wet form 085.2
− − zoonotic form 085.2
− dermal - see also Leishmaniasis,
  cutaneous
− − post-kala-azar 085.0
− eyelid 085.- † 373.6*
− infantile 085.0
− Mediterranean 085.0
− mucocutaneous (American) 085.5
− naso-oral 085.5
− nasopharyngeal 085.5
− old world 085.1
− tegumentaria diffusa 085.4
− visceral (Indian) 085.0
Leishmanoid, dermal - see also
  Leishmaniasis, cutaneous
− post-kala-azar 085.0
Lengthening, leg 736.8
Lens - see condition
Lenticonus (anterior) (posterior)
  (congenital) 743.3
Lenticular degeneration, progressive 275.1
Lentiglobus (posterior) (congenital) 743.3
Lentigo (congenital) 709.0
− maligna (M8742/2) - see also Neoplasm,
  skin, in situ
− − melanoma (M8742/3) - see Melanoma
Leontiasis
− ossium 733.3
− syphilitic 095
− − congenital 090.5
Lepothrix 039.0
Lepra 030.9
− Willan's 696.1

Leprechaunism 259.8
Leprosy 030.9
- anesthetic 030.1
- borderline (infiltrated) (neuritic) (group
  B) 030.3
- cornea 030.- † 371.8*
- dimorphous (infiltrated) (lepromatous)
  (neuritic) (tuberculoid) (group B) 030.3
- eyelid 030.- † 373.4*
- indeterminate (macular) (neuritic) (group
  I) 030.2
- leonine 030.0
- lepromatous (diffuse) (infiltrated)
  (macular) (neuritic) (nodular) (type L)
  030.0
- macular (early) (neuritic) (simple) 030.2
- maculoanesthetic 030.1
- mixed 030.0
- neuro 030.1
- nodular 030.0
- primary neuritic 030.3
- specified type or group NEC 030.8
- tubercular 030.1
- tuberculoid (macular) (major) (minor)
  (neuritic) (maculoanesthetic) (type T)
  030.1
Leptocytosis, hereditary 282.4
Leptomeningitis (circumscribed) (chronic)
  (hemorrhagic) (nonsuppurative) (see also
  Meningitis) 322.9
- tuberculous 013.0 † 320.4*
Leptomeningopathy (see also Meningitis)
  322.9
Leptospiral - see condition
Leptospirochetal - see condition
Leptospirosis 100.9
- canicola 100.8
- grippotyphosa 100.8
- icterohemorrhagica 100.0
- pomona 100.8
Leptothricosis - see Actinomycosis
Leptothrix infestation - see Actinomycosis
Leri's pleonosteosis 756.8
Leriche's syndrome 444.0
Leri-Weill syndrome 756.5
Lermoyez's syndrome 386.0
Lesbianism 302.0
Lesch-Nyhan syndrome 277.2
Lesion
- alveolar process 525.8
- anorectal 569.4
- aortic (valve) - see Endocarditis, aortic
- auditory nerve 388.5
- basal ganglion 333.9
- bile duct (see also Disease, biliary) 576.8
- bone 733.9
- brachial plexus 353.0

Lesion - *continued*
- brain 348.8
- - congenital 742.9
- - vascular 437.9
- - - degenerative 437.1
- buccal 528.9
- calcified - see Calcification
- canthus 373.8
- carate - see Pinta, lesions
- cardia 537.8
- cardiac - see also Disease, heart
- - congenital 746.9
- - valvular - see Endocarditis
- cauda equina 344.6
- cecum 569.8
- cerebral - see Lesion, brain
- cerebrovascular (see also Disease,
  cerebrovascular NEC) 437.9
- - degenerative 437.1
- cervical root (nerve) NEC 353.2
- chiasmal 377.5
- chorda tympani 351.8
- coin, lung 793.1
- colon 569.8
- congenital - see Anomaly
- conjunctiva 372.9
- coronary artery (see also Ischemia, heart)
  414.9
- cystic - see Cyst
- degenerative - see Degeneration
- duodenum 537.8
- eyelid 373.9
- gasserian ganglion 350.8
- gastric 537.8
- gastroduodenal 537.8
- gastrointestinal 569.8
- heart (organic) - see Disease, heart
- helix (ear) 709.9
- hyperkeratotic (see also Hyperkeratosis)
  701.1
- hypopharynx 478.2
- hypothalamic 253.9
- ileocecal (coil) 569.8
- ileum 569.8
- in continuity - see Injury, nerve, by site
- inflammatory - see Inflammation
- intestine 569.8
- intracerebral - see Lesion, brain
- intrachiasmal (optic) 377.5
- intracranial, space-occupying NEC 784.2
- joint 719.9
- - sacroiliac (old) 724.6
- keratotic - see Keratosis
- kidney - see also Disease, renal
- laryngeal nerve (recurrent) 352.3
- lip 528.5
- liver 573.8

Lesion - *continued*
- lumbosacral
- − plexus 353.1
- − root (nerve) NEC 353.4
- lung (coin) 793.1
- mitral - see Endocarditis, mitral
- motor cortex 348.8
- nerve (see also Disorder, nerve) 355.9
- nervous system congenital 742.9
- nonallopathic NEC 739.9
- − in region (of)
- − − abdomen 739.9
- − − acromoclavicular 739.7
- − − cervical, cervicothoracic 739.1
- − − costochondral 739.8
- − − costovertebral 739.8
- − − extremity
- − − − lower 739.6
- − − − upper 739.7
- − − head 739.0
- − − hip 739.5
- − − lumbar, lumbosacral 739.3
- − − pelvic 739.5
- − − pubic 739.5
- − − rib cage 739.8
- − − sacral, sacrococcygeal, sacroiliac 739.4
- − − sternochondral 739.8
- − − sternoclavicular 739.7
- − − thoracic, thoracolumbar 739.2
- nose (internal) 478.1
- obstructive - see Obstruction
- organ or site NEC - see Disease, by site
- osteolytic 733.9
- peptic 537.8
- periodontal, due to traumatic occlusion 523.8
- perirectal 569.4
- pigmented (skin) 709.0
- pinta - see Pinta, lesions
- polypoid - see Polyp
- prechiasmal (optic) 377.5
- primary - see also Syphilis, primary
- − carate 103.0
- − pinta 103.0
- − yaws 102.0
- pulmonary 518.8
- − valve (see also Endocarditis, pulmonary) 424.3
- pylorus 537.8
- radiation NEC 990
- radium NEC 990
- rectosigmoid 569.8
- retina, retinal 362.9
- − vascular 362.1
- romanus 720.1
- sacro-iliac (joint) (old) 724.6

Lesion - *continued*
- salivary gland 527.8
- − benign lymphoepithelial 527.8
- secondary - see Syphilis, secondary
- sigmoid 569.8
- sinus (accessory) (nasal) (see also Sinusitis) 473.9
- skin 709.9
- − suppurative 686.0
- spinal cord 336.9
- − congenital 742.9
- − traumatic (complete) (incomplete) (transverse) - see also Injury, spinal, by region
- − − with
- − − − broken
- − − − − back - see Fracture, vertebra, by region, with spinal cord lesion
- − − − − neck (closed) 806.0
- − − − − − open 806.1
- − − − fracture, vertebra (conditions in 805-) - see Fracture, vertebra, by region, with spinal cord lesion
- spleen 289.5
- stomach 537.8
- syphilitic - see Syphilis
- tertiary - see Syphilis, tertiary
- thoracic root (nerve) 353.3
- tonsillar fossa 474.9
- tooth, teeth 525.8
- − white spot 521.0
- traumatic NEC (see also Nature and site of injury) 959.9
- tricuspid (valve) - see Endocarditis, tricuspid
- ulcerated or ulcerative - see Ulcer
- uterus NEC 621.9
- valvular - see Endocarditis
- vascular 459.9
- − affecting central nervous system (see also Lesion, cerebrovascular) 437.9
- − following trauma (see also Injury, blood vessel) 904.9
- − retina, retinal 362.1
- − umbilical cord 663.6
- − − affecting fetus or newborn 762.6
- warty - see Verruca
- X-ray NEC 990
Lethargic - see condition
Lethargy 780.7
- negro 086.5
Letterer-Siwe's disease (M9722/3) 202.5
Leuc(o)-for any term beginning thus - see Leuk(o)
Leucinosis 270.3
Leucosarcoma (M9850/3) 207.8

Leukasmus 270.2
Leukemia (congenital) (M9800/3) 208.9
– acute NEC (M9801/3) 208.0
– aleukemic NEC (M9804/3) 208.8
– basophilic (M9870/3) 205.1
– blast (cell) (M9801/3) 208.0
– blastic (M9801/3) 208.0
– – granulocytic (M9861/3) 205.0
– chronic NEC (M9803/3) 208.1
– compound (M9810/3) 207.8
– eosinophilic (M9880/3) 205.1
– giant cell (M9910/3) 207.2
– granulocytic (M9860/3) 205.9
– – acute (M9861/3) 205.0
– – aleukemic (M9864/3) 205.8
– – blastic (M9861/3) 205.0
– – chronic (M9863/3) 205.1
– – subacute (M9862/3) 205.2
– – subleukemic (M9864/3) 205.8
– hairy cell (M9940/3) 202.4
– hemoblastic (M9801/3) 208.0
– histiocytic (M9890/3) 206.9
– lymphatic (M9820/3) 204.9
– – acute (M9821/3) 204.0
– – aleukemic (M9824/3) 204.8
– – chronic (M9823/3) 204.1
– – subacute (M9822/3) 204.2
– – subleukemic (M9824/3) 204.8
– lymphoblastic (M9821/3) 204.0
– lymphocytic (M9820/3) 204.9
– – acute (M9821/3) 204.0
– – aleukemic (M9824/3) 204.8
– – chronic (M9823/3) 204.1
– – subacute (M9822/3) 204.2
– – subleukemic (M9824/3) 204.8
– lymphogenous (M9820/3) - see
Leukemia, lymphoid
– lymphoid (M9820/3) 204.9
– – acute (M9821/3) 204.0
– – aleukemic (M9824/3) 204.8
– – blastic (M9821/3) 204.0
– – chronic (M9823/3) 204.1
– – subacute (M9822/3) 204.2
– – subleukemic (M9824/3) 204.8
– lymphosarcoma cell (M9850/3) 207.8
– mast cell (M9900/3) 207.8
– megakaryocytic (M9910/3) 207.2
– megakaryocytoid (M9910/3) 207.2
– mixed (cell) (M9810/3) 207.8
– monoblastic (M9891/3) 206.0
– monocytic (Schilling-type) (M9890/3)
206.9
– – acute (M9891/3) 206.0
– – aleukemic (M9894/3) 206.8
– – chronic (M9893/3) 206.1
– – Naegeli-type (M9863/3) 205.1
– – subacute (M9892/3) 206.2

Leukemia - continued
– monocytic - continued
– – subleukemic (M9894/3) 206.8
– monocytoid (M9890/3) 206.9
– – acute (M9891/3) 206.0
– – aleukemic (M9894/3) 206.8
– – chronic (M9893/3) 206.1
– – myelogenous (M9863/3) 205.1
– – subacute (M9892/3) 206.2
– – subleukemic (M9894/3) 206.8
– monomyelocytic (M9860/3) - see
Leukemia, myelomonocytic
– myeloblastic (M9861/3) 205.0
– myelocytic (M9863/3) 205.1
– – acute (M9861/3) 205.0
– myelogenous (M9860/3) 205.9
– – acute (M9861/3) 205.0
– – aleukemic (M9864/3) 205.8
– – chronic (M9863/3) 205.1
– – monocytoid (M9863/3) 205.1
– – subacute (M9862/3) 205.2
– – subleukemic (M9864/3) 205.8
– myeloid (M9860/3) 205.9
– – acute (M9861/3) 205.0
– – aleukemic (M9864/3) 205.8
– – chronic (M9863/3) 205.1
– – subacute (M9862/3) 205.2
– – subleukemic (M9864/3) 205.8
– myelomonocytic (M9860/3) 205.9
– – acute (M9861/3) 205.0
– – chronic (M9863/3) 205.1
– Naegeli-type monocytic (M9863/3)
205.1
– neutrophilic (M9865/3) 205.1
– plasma cell (M9830/3) 203.1
– plasmacytic (M9830/3) 203.1
– prolymphocytic (M9825/3) 204.9
– promyelocytic, acute (M9866/3) 205.0
– Schilling-type monocytic (M9890/3) - see
Leukemia, monocytic
– stem cell (M9801/3) 208.0
– subacute NEC (M9802/3) 208.2
– subleukemic NEC (M9804/3) 208.8
– thrombocytic (M9910/3) 207.2
– undifferentiated (M9801/3) 208.0
Leukemoid reaction (lymphocytic)
(monocytic) (myelocytic) 288.8
Leukocytosis 288.8
Leukoderma 709.0
– syphilitic 091.3
– – late 095
Leukodermia (see also Leukoderma) 709.0
Leukodystrophy (cerebral) (globoid cell)
(metachromatic) (progressive)
(sudanophilic) 330.0
Leukoedema, mouth 528.7
Leukoencephalitis

Leukoencephalitis - *continued*
- acute hemorrhagic (postinfectious) NEC 136.9 † 323.6*
- - postimmunization or postvaccinal 323.5
- subacute sclerosing 046.2 † 323.1*
- van Bogaert's (sclerosing) 046.2 † 323.1*
Leukoencephalopathy (see also Encephalitis) 323.9
- acute necrotizing hemorrhagic (postinfectious) NEC 136.9 † 323.6*
- - postimmunization or postvaccinal 323.5
- metachromatic 330.0
- multifocal (progressive) 046.3 † 331.6*
Leukoerythroblastosis 289.0
Leukoerythrosis 289.0
Leukokeratosis 702
- nicotina palati 528.7
Leukokraurosis vulva(e) 624.0
Leukolymphosarcoma (M9850/3) 207.8
Leukoma (cornea) (adherent) 371.0
Leukomelanopathy, hereditary 288.2
Leukonychia (punctata) (striata) 703.8
- congenital 757.5
Leukopathia unguium 703.8
- congenital 757.5
Leukopenia (malignant) 288.0
Leukopenic - see condition
Leukoplakia 702
- anus 569.4
- bladder (postinfectional) 596.8
- buccal 528.6
- cervix (uteri) 622.2
- esophagus 530.8
- gingiva 528.6
- kidney (pelvis) (see also Lesion, kidney) 593.8
- larynx 478.7
- lip 528.6
- mouth 528.6
- oesophagus 530.8
- oral, including tongue (mucosa) (soft tissue) 528.6
- pelvis (kidney) 593.8
- penis (infectional) 607.0
- rectum 569.4
- syphilitic 095
- tongue 528.6
- ureter (postinfectional) 593.8
- urethra (postinfectional) 599.8
- uterus 621.8
- vagina 623.1
- vocal cords 478.5
- vulva 624.0
Leukopolioencephalopathy 330.0
Leukorrhea 623.5

Leukorrhea - *continued*
- due to Trichomonas (vaginalis) 131.0
- trichomonal 131.0
Leukosarcoma (M9850/3) 207.8
Leukosis (M9800/3) - see Leukemia
Levocardia (isolated) 746.8
- with situs inversus 759.3
Levulosuria 271.2
Lewandowsky's disease (primary) 017.0
Leyden-Moebius dystrophy 359.1
Leydig cell
- carcinoma (M8650/3)
- - specified site - see Neoplasm, malignant
- - unspecified site
- - - female 183.0
- - - male 186.9
- tumor (M8650/1)
- - benign (M8650/0)
- - - specified site - see Neoplasm, benign
- - - unspecified site
- - - - female 220
- - - - male 222.0
- - malignant (M8650/3)
- - - specified site - see Neoplasm, malignant
- - - unspecified site
- - - - female 183.0
- - - - male 186.9
- - specified site - see Neoplasm, uncertain behavior
- - unspecified site
- - - female 236.2
- - - male 236.4
Leydig-Sertoli cell tumor (M8631/0)
- specified site - see Neoplasm, benign
- unspecified site
- - female 220
- - male 222.0
Liar, pathologic 301.7
Libman-Sacks disease or endocarditis 710.0 † 424.9*
Lice (infestation) 132.9
- body (pediculus corporis) 132.1
- crab 132.2
- head (pediculus capitis) 132.0
- mixed (classifiable to more than one of the titles 132.0-132.2) 132.3
- pubic (phthirus pubis) 132.2
Lichen 697.9
- albus 701.0
- annularis 695.8
- atrophicus 701.0
- myxedematosus 701.8
- nitidus 697.1
- obtusus corneus 698.3
- pilaris 757.3

Lichen - *continued*
– pilaris - *continued*
– – acquired 701.1
– planus (chronicus) 697.0
– – sclerosus (et atrophicus) 701.0
– ruber 696.4
– – acuminatus 696.4
– – moniliforme 697.8
– – of Wilson 697.0
– – planus 697.0
– sclerosus (et atrophicus) 701.0
– scrofulosus (primary) 017.0
– simplex
– – chronicus 698.3
– – circumscriptus 698.3
– spinulosus 757.3
– – mycotic 117.9
– striata 697.8
– urticatus 698.2
Lichenification 698.3
Lichenoides tuberculosis (primary) 017.0
Lichtheim's disease or syndrome - see
  Degeneration, combined
Lien migrans 289.5
Lientery - see Diarrhea
Ligament - see condition
Light-for-dates (infant) 764.0
– with signs of fetal malnutrition 764.1
– affecting management of pregnancy
  656.5
Lightning (effects) (shock) (stroke) (struck
  by) 994.0
– burn - see Burn
Lignac(-de Toni-Fanconi-Debre) syndrome
  270.0
Lignac's disease 270.0
Lignac-Fanconi syndrome 270.0
Ligneous thyroiditis 245.3
Limb - see condition
Limitation motion, sacroiliac 724.6
Limited cardiac reserve - see Disease, heart
Lindau(-von Hippel) disease 759.6
Linea corneae senilis 371.4
Lines
– Beau's 703.8
– Harris' 733.9
Lingua
– geographica 529.1
– nigra (villosa) 529.3
– plicata 529.5
– – congenital 750.1
– tylosis 528.6
Lingual - see condition
Linitis (gastric) 535.4
– plastica (M8142/3) 151.9
Lip - see condition
Lipedema - see Edema

Lipemia - see also Hyperlipidemia
– retinal 272.3
Lipidosis 272.7
– cerebral (infantile) (juvenile) (late) 330.1
– cerebroretinal 330.1
– cerebroside 272.7
– cerebrospinal 272.7
– chemically-induced 272.7
– cholesterol 272.7
– glycolipid 272.7
– hereditary, dystopic 272.7
– sulfatide 330.0
Lipoadenoma (M8324/0) - see Neoplasm,
  benign
Lipoblastoma (M8881/0) 214
Lipoblastomatosis (M8881/0) 214
Lipochondrodystrophy 277.5
Lipodystrophy (progressive) 272.6
– insulin 272.6
– intestinal 040.2
Lipofibroma (M8851/0) 214
Lipoglycoproteinosis 272.8
Lipogranuloma, sclerosing 709.8
Lipogranulomatosis 272.8
Lipoid - see also condition
– histiocytosis 272.7
– – essential 272.7
– nephrosis (see also Nephrosis) 581.3
– proteinosis of Urbach 272.8
Lipoidemia (see also Hyperlipidemia) 272.4
Lipoidosis - see also Lipidosis
Lipoma (M8850/0) 214
– fetal (M8881/0) 214
– – fat cell (M8880/0) 214
– infiltrating (M8856/0) 214
– intramuscular (M8856/0) 214
– spindle cell (M8857/0) 214
Lipomatosis 272.8
– fetal (M8881/0) 214
– Launois-Bensaude 272.8
Lipomyohemangioma (M8860/0)
– specified site - see Neoplasm, connective
  tissue, benign
– unspecified site 223.0
Lipomyoma (M8860/0)
– specified site - see Neoplasm, connective
  tissue, benign
– unspecified site 223.0
Lipomyxoma (M8852/0) 214
Lipomyxosarcoma (M8852/3) - see
  Neoplasm, connective tissue, malignant
Lipoproteinemia (alpha) 272.4
– broad-beta 272.2
– floating-beta 272.2
– hyper-pre-beta 272.1
Liposarcoma (M8850/3) - see also
  Neoplasm, connective tissue, malignant

Loss - *continued*
- appetite - *continued*
- - psychogenic 307.5
- blood - see Hemorrhage
- control, sphincter, rectum 787.6
- - nonorganic origin 307.7
- extremity or member, traumatic, current - see Amputation, traumatic
- fluid (acute) 276.5
- - fetus or newborn 775.5
- hearing - see Deafness
- memory (see also Amnesia) 780.9
- - mild, following organic brain damage 310.1
- mind (see also Psychosis) 298.9
- organ or part - see Absence, by site, acquired
- sense of
- - smell (see also Disturbance, sensation) 781.1
- - taste (see also Disturbance, sensation) 781.1
- - touch (see also Disturbance, sensation) 782.0
- sight (acquired) (complete) (congenital) - see Blindness
- spinal fluid
- - headache 349.0
- substance of
- - bone 733.0
- - cartilage 733.9
- - - ear 380.3
- - vitreous (humor) 379.1
- tooth, teeth due to accident, extraction or local periodontal disease 525.1
- voice (see also Aphonia) 784.4
- weight (cause unknown) 783.2
Louis-Bar syndrome 334.8
Louping ill 063.1 † 323.3*
Lousiness - see Lice
Low
- basal metabolic rate 794.7
- birthweight 765.1
- - extreme (less than 1000 g) 765.0
- - for gestational age (see also Light-for-dates) 764.0
- blood pressure (see also Hypotension) 458.9
- - reading (incidental) (isolated) (nonspecific) 796.3
- cardiac reserve - see Disease, heart
- function - see also Hypofunction
- - kidney (see also Disease, renal) 593.9
- hemoglobin 285.9
- implantation, placenta - see Placenta, previa
- insertion, placenta - see Placenta, previa

Low - *continued*
- lying
- - kidney (see also Disease, renal) 593.9
- - organ or site, congenital - see Malposition, congenital
- - placenta - see Placenta, previa
- - platelets (blood) (see also Thrombocytopenia) 287.5
- reserve kidney (see also Disease, renal) 593.9
- salt syndrome (see also Disease, renal) 593.9
Lowe's syndrome 270.2
Lower extremity - see condition
Lown-Ganong-Levine syndrome 426.8
LSD reaction 305.3
L-shaped kidney 753.3
Ludwig's angina or disease 528.3
Lues (venerea), luetic - see Syphilis
Lumbago 724.2
- due to displacement, intervertebral disc 722.1
Lumbalgia 724.2
- due to displacement, intervertebral disc 722.1
Lumbar - see condition
Lumbarization, vertebra 756.1
Lump - see also Mass
- breast 611.7
- kidney 753.3
Lunacy (see also Psychosis) 298.9
Lung - see condition
Lupoid (miliary) of Boeck 135
Lupus (exedens) (Hillard's) (miliaris disseminatus faciei) (vulgaris) 017.0
- Cazenave's 695.4
- discoid (local) 695.4
- disseminated 710.0
- erythematodes (discoid) (local) 695.4
- erythematosus (discoid) (local) 695.4
- - disseminated 710.0
- - eyelid 373.3
- - systemic 710.0
- - - with lung involvement 710.0 † 517.8*
- - - inhibitor 286.6
- eyelid 017.0 † 373.4*
- hydralazine
- - correct substance properly administered 695.4
- - overdose or wrong substance given or taken 972.6
- nephritis 710.0 † 583.8*
- - chronic 710.0 † 582.8*
- nontuberculous, not disseminated 695.4
- pernio (Besnier) 135
- tuberculous 017.0

Lupus - *continued*
- tuberculous - *continued*
- - eyelid 017.0 † 373.4*
Luteinoma (M8610/0) 220
Lutembacher's disease or syndrome 745.5
Luteoma (M8610/0) 220
Lutz-Splendore-Almeida disease 116.1
Luxatio bulbi, birth injury 767.8
Luxation - see also Dislocation
- eyeball 360.8
- - birth injury 767.8
- genital organs (external) NEC - see
   Wound, open, genital organs
- globe 360.8
- lacrimal gland 375.1
- lens (old) (partial) (spontaneous) 379.3
- - congenital 743.3
- - - syphilitic 090.4 † 379.3*
- - in Marfan's disease 090.4 † 379.3*
- penis - see Wound, open, penis
- scrotum - see Wound, open, scrotum
- testis - see Wound, open, testis
L-xyloketosuria 271.8
Lycanthropy (see also Psychosis) 298.9
Lyell's syndrome 695.1
- due to drug
- - correct substance properly
   administered 695.1
- - overdose or wrong substance given or
   taken 977.9
- - - specified drug - see Table of drugs
   and chemicals
Lymph
- gland or node - see condition
- scrotum (see also Infestation, filarial)
   125.9
Lymphadenitis 289.3
- acute, unspecified site 683
- any site, except mesenteric 289.3
- - acute 683
- - chronic 289.1
- - subacute 289.1
- breast, puerperal, postpartum 675.2
- chancroidal (congenital) 099.0
- chronic 289.1
- - mesenteric 289.2
- dermatopathic 695.8
- due to
- - anthracosis 500
- - Brugia (Wuchereria) malayi 125.1
- - diphtheria (toxin) 032.8
- - lymphogranuloma venereum 099.1
- - Wuchereria bancrofti 125.0
- gonorrheal 098.8
- infectional 683
- mesenteric (acute) (chronic)
   (nonspecific) (subacute) 289.2

Lymphadenitis - *continued*
- mesenteric - *continued*
- - due to Bacillus typhi 002.0
- - tuberculous 014
- purulent 683
- pyogenic 683
- regional 078.3
- septic 683
- subacute, unspecified site 289.1
- suppurative 683
- syphilitic (early) (secondary) 091.4
- - late 095
- tuberculous - see Tuberculosis, lymph
   gland
- venereal 099.1
Lymphadenoid goiter 245.2
Lymphadenopathy (general) 785.6
- due to
- - toxoplasmosis (acquired) 130
- - - congenital (active) 771.2
Lymphadenosis 785.6
Lymphangiectasis 457.1
- conjunctiva 372.8
- postinfectional 457.1
- scrotum 457.1
Lymphangioendothelioma (M9170/0)
   228.1
- malignant (M9170/3) - see Neoplasm,
   connective tissue, malignant
Lymphangioma (M9170/0) 228.1
- capillary (M9171/0) 228.1
- cavernous (M9172/0) 228.1
- cystic (M9173/0) 228.1
- malignant (M9170/3) - see Neoplasm,
   connective tissue, malignant
Lymphangiomyoma (M9174/0) 228.1
Lymphangiomyomatosis (M9174/1) - see
   Neoplasm, connective tissue, uncertain
   behavior
Lymphangiosarcoma (M9170/3) - see
   Neoplasm, connective tissue, malignant
Lymphangitis 457.2
- with
- - abortion - see categories 634-639,
   fourth digit .0
- - abscess - code by site under Abscess
- - cellulitis - code by site under Cellulitis
- - ectopic gestation 639.0
- acute (with abscess or cellulitis) 682.9
- - specified site - code by site under
   Abscess
- breast, puerperal, postpartum 675.2
- chancroidal 099.0
- chronic (any site) 457.2
- due to
- - Brugia (Wuchereria) malayi 125.1
- - Wuchereria bancrofti 125.0

Lymphangitis - *continued*
- gangrenous 457.2
- penis
- - acute 607.2
- - gonococcal (acute) 098.0
- - - chronic or duration of 2 months or over 098.2
- puerperal, postpartum, childbirth 670
- strumous, tuberculous 017.2
- subacute (any site) 457.2
- tuberculous - see Tuberculosis, lymph gland
Lymphatic (vessel) - see condition
Lymphatism 254.8
Lymphectasia 457.1
Lymphedema (see also Elephantiasis) 457.1
- praecox 457.1
- secondary 457.1
- surgical NEC 997.9
- - postmastectomy (syndrome) 457.0
Lymph-hemangioma (M9120/0) 228.1
Lymphoblastic - see condition

Lymphoblastoma (diffuse) (M9630/3) 200.1
- giant follicular (M9690/3) 202.0
- macrofollicular (M9690/3) 202.0
Lymphocele 457.8
Lymphocytic
- chorioencephalitis (acute) (serous) 049.0 † 321.6*
- choriomeningitis (acute) (serous) 049.0 † 321.6*
Lymphocytoma (diffuse) (malignant) (M9620/3) 200.1
Lymphocytomatosis (M9620/3) 200.1

Lymphocytosis (symptomatic) 288.8
- infectious (acute) 078.8
Lymphoepithelioma (M8082/3) - see Neoplasm, malignant
Lymphogranuloma (malignant) (M9650/3) 201.9
- inguinale 099.1
- venereal (any site) 099.1
- - with stricture of rectum 099.1
- venereum 099.1
Lymphogranulomatosis (malignant) (M9650/3) 201.9
- benign (Boeck's sarcoid) (Schaumann's) 135
- Hodgkin's (M9650/3) 201.9
Lymphoid - see condition
Lympholeukoblastoma (M9850/3) 207.8
Lympholeukosarcoma (M9850/3) 207.8
Lymphoma (malignant) (M9590/3) 202.8
- benign (M9590/0) - see Neoplasm, benign

Lymphoma - *continued*
- Burkitt's type (lymphoblastic) (undifferentiated) (M9750/3) 200.2
- centroblastic type (diffuse) (M9632/3) 202.8
- - follicular (M9697/3) 202.0
- centroblastic-centrocytic
- - diffuse (M9614/3) 202.8
- - follicular (M9692/3) 202.0
- centrocytic (M9622/3) 202.8
- compound (M9613/3) 200.8
- convoluted cell type (lymphoblastic) (M9602/3) 202.8
- diffuse NEC (M9590/3) 202.8
- follicular (giant) (M9690/3) 202.0
- - center cell (diffuse) (M9615/3) 202.8
- - - cleaved (diffuse) (M9623/3) 202.8
- - - - follicular (M9695/3) 202.0
- - - non-cleaved (diffuse) (M9633/3) 202.8
- - - - follicular (M9698/3) 202.0
- - centroblastic type (M9697/3) 202.0
- - centroblastic-centrocytic (M9692/3) 202.0
- - lymphocytic
- - - intermediate differentiation (M9694/3) 202.0
- - - poorly differentiated (M9696/3) 202.0
- - mixed (cell type) (lymphocytic-histiocytic) (small cell and large cell) (M9691/3) 202.0
- germinocytic (M9622/3) 202.8

- giant, follicular or follicle (M9690/3) 202.0
- histiocytic (diffuse) (M9640/3) 200.0
- - nodular (M9642/3) 200.0
- - pleomorphic cell type (M9641/3) 200.0
- Hodgkin's (M9650/3) 201.9
- immunoblastic (type) (M9612/3) 200.8

- lymphoblastic (diffuse) (M9630/3) 200.1
- - Burkitt's type (M9750/3) 200.2
- - convoluted cell type (M9602/3) 202.8
- lymphocytic (cell type) (diffuse) (M9620/3) 200.1
- - with plasmacytoid differentiation, diffuse (M9611/3) 200.8
- - intermediate differentiation (diffuse) (M9621/3) 200.1
- - - follicular (M9694/3) 202.0
- - - nodular (M9694/3) 202.0
- - nodular (M9690/3) 202.0
- - poorly differentiated (diffuse) (M9630/3) 200.1
- - - follicular (M9696/3) 202.0

Lymphoma - *continued*
- lymphocytic - *continued*
- - well differentiated (diffuse) (M9620/3) 200.1
- - - follicular (M9693/3) 202.0
- - - nodular (M9693/3) 202.0
- lymphocytic-histiocytic, mixed (diffuse) (M9613/3) 200.8
- - follicular (M9691/3) 202.0
- - nodular (M9691/3) 202.0
- lymphoplasmacytoid type (M9611/3) 200.8
- lymphosarcoma type (M9610/3) 200.1
- macrofollicular (M9690/3) 202.0
- mixed cell type (diffuse) (M9613/3) 200.8
- - follicular (M9691/3) 202.0
- - nodular (M9691/3) 202.0
- nodular (M9690/3) 202.0
- - histiocytic (M9642/3) 200.0
- - lymphocytic (M9690/3) 202.0
- - - intermediate differentiation (M9694/3) 202.0
- - - poorly differentiated (M9696/3) 202.0
- - mixed (cell type) (lymphocytic-histiocytic) (small cell and large cell) (M9691/3) 202.0
- non-Hodgkin's type NEC (M9591/3) 202.8
- reticulum cell (type) (M9640/3) 200.0
- small cell and large cell, mixed (diffuse) (M9613/3) 200.8
- - follicular (M9691/3) 202.0
- - nodular (M9691/3) 202.0
- stem cell (type) (M9601/3) 202.8
- undifferentiated (cell type) (non-Burkitt's) (M9600/3) 202.8
- - Burkitt's type (M9750/3) 200.2
Lymphomatosis (M9590/3) - see Lymphoma
Lymphopathia
- venereum 099.1

Lymphopathia - *continued*
- veneris 099.1
Lymphopenia 288.8
- familial 279.2
Lymphoreticulosis, benign (of inoculation) 078.3
Lymphorrhea 457.8
Lymphosarcoma (M9610/3) 200.1
- diffuse (M9610/3) 200.1
- - with plasmacytoid differentiation (M9611/3) 200.8
- - lymphoplasmacytic (M9611/3) 200.8
- follicular (giant) (M9690/3) 202.0
- - lymphoblastic (M9696/3) 202.0
- - lymphocytic, intermediate differentiation (M9694/3) 202.0
- - mixed cell type (M9691/3) 202.0
- giant follicular (M9690/3) 202.0
- Hodgkin's (M9650/3) 201.9
- immunoblastic (M9612/3) 200.8
- lymphoblastic (diffuse) (M9630/3) 200.1
- - follicular (M9696/3) 202.0
- - nodular (M9696/3) 202.0
- lymphocytic (diffuse) (M9620/3) 200.1
- - intermediate differentiation (diffuse) (M9621/3) 200.1
- - - follicular (M9694/3) 202.0
- - - nodular (M9694/3) 202.0
- mixed cell type (diffuse) (M9613/3) 200.8
- - follicular (M9691/3) 202.0
- - nodular (M9691/3) 202.0
- nodular (M9690/3) 202.0
- - lymphoblastic (M9696/3) 202.0
- - lymphocytic, intermediate differentiation (M9694/3) 202.0
- - mixed cell type (M9691/3) 202.0
- prolymphocytic (M9631/3) 200.1
- reticulum cell (M9640/3) 200.0
Lymphostasis 457.8
Lypemania (see also Melancholia) 296.1
Lyssa 071

M

Macacus ear 744.2
Maceration
– fetus (cause not stated) 779.9
– wet feet, tropical (syndrome) 991.4
MacLeod's syndrome 492
Macrocephalia, macrocephaly 756.0
Macrocheilia (congenital) 744.8
Macrochilia (congenital) 744.8
Macrocolon 751.3
Macrocornea 743.2
Macrocytic - see condition
Macrocytosis 289.8
Macrodactylia, macrodactylism (fingers)
    (thumbs) 755.5
– toes 755.6
Macrodontia 520.2
Macrogenitosomia (praecox) (male) 255.2
Macroglobulinemia (idiopathic) (primary)
    273.3
– Waldenstrom's 273.3
Macroglossia (congenital) 750.1
– acquired 529.8
Macrognathia, macrognathism (congenital)
    (mandibular) (maxillary) 524.0
Macrogyria (congenital) 742.4
Macrohydrocephalus (see also
    ·Hydrocephalus) 331.4
Macromastia (see also Hypertrophy, breast)
    611.1
Macropsia 368.1
Macrosigmoid 564.7
– congenital 751.3
Macrostomia (congenital) 744.8
Macrotia (external ear) (congenital) 744.2
Macula
– cornea, corneal 371.0
– – due to infection 371.0
– degeneration (atrophic) (exudative)
    (senile) 362.5
– – hereditary 362.7
Maculae ceruleae 132.1
Maculopathy, toxic 362.5
Madarosis 374.5
Madelung's
– deformity (radius) 755.5
– disease 272.8
Madness (see also Psychosis) 298.9
Madura
– disease (actinomycotic) 039.9
– – mycotic 117.4

Madura - *continued*
– foot (actinomycotic) 039.4
– – mycotic 117.4
Maduromycosis (actinomycotic) 039.9
– mycotic 117.4
Maffucci's syndrome 756.4
Main en griffe (acquired) 736.0
– congenital 755.5
Maintenance
– chemotherapy V58.1
– external fixation NEC V54.8
– traction NEC V54.8
Majocchi's
– disease 709.1
– granuloma 110.6
Major - see condition
Mal de mer 994.6
Mal lie (see also Presentation, fetal) 763.1
Malabar itch 110.9
– beard 110.0
– foot 110.4
– scalp 110.0
Malabsorption 579.9
– calcium 579.8
– carbohydrate 579.8
– disaccharide 271.3
– fat 579.8
– galactose 271.1
– glucose(-galactose) 271.3
– intestinal 579.9
– isomaltose 271.3
– lactose (hereditary) 271.3
– monosaccharide 271.3
– protein 579.8
– sucrose 271.3
– syndrome 579.9
– – postsurgical 579.3
Malacia, bone 268.2
– juvenile (see also Rickets) 268.0
Malacoplakia
– bladder 596.8
– pelvis (kidney) 593.8
– ureter 593.8
– urethra 599.8
Malacosteon 268.2
– juvenile (see also Rickets) 268.0
Maladaptation - see Maladjustment
Maladjustment
– conjugal V61.1
– educational V62.3

Maladjustment - *continued*
- marital V61.1
- - involving divorce or estrangement V61.0
- occupational V62.2
- simple, adult (see also Reaction, adjustment) 309.9
- situational acute (see also Reaction, adjustment) 309.9
- social V62.4
Malaise 780.7
Malakoplakia - see Malacoplakia
Malaria, malarial (fever) 084.6
- algid 084.9
- any type, with
- - algid malaria 084.9
- - blackwater fever 084.8
- - fever
- - - blackwater 084.8
- - - hemoglobinuric (bilious) 084.8
- - hemoglobinuria 084.8
- - hepatitis 084.9 † 573.2*
- - nephrosis 084.9 † 581.8*
- - pernicious complication NEC 084.9
- - - cardiac 084.9
- - - cerebral 084.9
- cardiac 084.9
- cerebral 084.9
- complicating pregnancy, childbirth or puerperium 647.4
- congenital 771.2
- continued 084.0
- estivo-autumnal 084.0
- falciparum 084.0
- hemorrhagic 084.6
- induced (therapeutically) 084.7
- - accidental - code by type under Malaria 084.-
- liver 084.9
- malariae 084.2
- malignant (tertian) 084.0
- mixed infections (classifiable to more than one of the titles 084.0-084.4) 084.5
- monkey 084.4
- ovale 084.3
- pernicious, acute 084.0
- Plasmodium, P.
- - falciparum 084.0
- - malariae 084.2
- - ovale 084.3
- - vivax 084.1
- quartan 084.2
- quotidian 084.0
- recurrent 084.6
- - induced (therapeutically) 084.7
- - - accidental - code by type under Malaria 084.-

Malaria - *continued*
- remittent 084.6
- specified types NEC 084.4
- spleen 084.6
- subtertian 084.0
- tertian (benign) 084.1
- - malignant 084.0
- tropical 084.0
- typhoid 084.6
- vivax 084.1
Malassez's disease (cystic) 608.8
Malassimilation 579.9
Maldescent, testis 752.5

Maldevelopment - see also Anomaly
- brain 742.9
- colon 751.5
- hip 755.6
- - congenital dislocation 754.3
- mastoid process 756.0
- middle ear 744.0
- spine 756.1
- toe 755.6
Male type pelvis 755.6
- with disproportion 653.2
- - causing obstructed labor 660.1
- - fetus or newborn 763.1

Malformation (congenital) - see also Anomaly
- bone 756.9
- bursa 756.9
- circulatory system NEC 747.9
- digestive system NEC 751.9
- - lower 751.5
- - upper 750.9
- eye 743.9
- gum 750.9
- heart NEC 746.9
- - valve 746.9
- internal ear 744.0
- joint NEC 755.8
- muscle 756.9
- nervous system (central) 742.9
- pelvic organs or tissues
- - in pregnancy or childbirth NEC 654.9
- - - causing obstructed labor 660.2
- - - - fetus or newborn 763.1
- - - fetus or newborn 763.8
- placenta (see also Placenta, abnormal) 656.7
- respiratory organ NEC 748.9
- sense organs NEC 742.9
- skin NEC 757.9
- spinal cord 742.9
- tendon 756.9
- throat 750.9
- tooth, teeth NEC 520.9

Malformation - *continued*
- umbilical cord (complicating delivery) 663.9
- - affecting fetus or newborn 762.6
- umbilicus 759.9
- urinary system NEC 753.9

Malfunction - see also Dysfunction
- catheter device - see Complications, mechanical, catheter
- colostomy 569.6
- enteric stoma 569.6
- enterostomy 569.6
- gastroenteric 536.8
- pacemaker - see Complications, mechanical, pacemaker
- prosthetic device, internal - see Complications, mechanical
- tracheostomy 519.0

Malgaigne's fracture 808.4
- open 808.5

Malherbe's
- calcifying epithelioma (M8110/0) - see Neoplasm, skin, benign
- tumor (M8110/0) - see Neoplasm, skin, benign

Malibu disease 919.8
- infected 919.9

Malignancy (M8000/3) - see Neoplasm, malignant

Malignant - see condition

Malingerer, malingering V65.2

Mallet finger (acquired) 736.1
- congenital 755.5
- late effect of rickets 268.1

Malleus 024

Mallory's bodies 034.1

Mallory-Weiss syndrome 530.7

Malnutrition 263.9
- degree
- - first 263.1
- - mild 263.1
- - moderate 263.0
- - second 263.0
- - severe (protein-calorie) 262
- - third 262
- following gastrointestinal surgery 579.3
- intrauterine or fetal 764.2
- - fetus or infant light-for-dates 764.1
- lack of care, or neglect (child) (infant) 995.5
- malignant 260
- protein 260
- protein-calorie 263.9
- - specified NEC 263.8

Malocclusion (teeth) 524.4
- due to
- - abnormal swallowing 524.5

Malocclusion - *continued*
- due to - *continued*
- - missing teeth 524.3
- - mouth breathing 524.5
- - tongue, lip or finger habits 524.5
- temporomandibular (joint) 524.6

Malposition
- cervix - see Malposition, uterus
- congenital
- - adrenal (gland) 759.1
- - alimentary tract 751.8
- - - lower 751.5
- - - upper 750.8
- - aorta 747.2
- - appendix 751.5
- - arterial trunk 747.2
- - artery (peripheral) 747.6
- - - coronary 746.8
- - - pulmonary 747.3
- - auditory canal 744.2
- - - causing impairment of hearing 744.0
- - auricle (ear) 744.2
- - - causing impairment of hearing 744.0
- - - cervical 744.4
- - biliary duct or passage 751.6
- - bladder (mucosa) 753.8
- - - exteriorized or extroverted 753.5
- - brachial plexus 742.8
- - brain tissue 742.4
- - breast 757.6
- - bronchus 748.3
- - cecum 751.5
- - clavicle 755.5
- - colon 751.5
- - digestive organ or tract NEC 751.8
- - - lower 751.5
- - - upper 750.8
- - ear (auricle) (external) 744.2
- - - ossicles 744.0
- - endocrine (gland) NEC 759.2
- - epiglottis 748.3
- - eustachian tube 744.2
- - eye 743.8
- - facial features 744.8
- - fallopian tube 752.1
- - finger(s) 755.5
- - - supernumerary 755.0
- - foot 755.6
- - gallbladder 751.6
- - gastrointestinal tract 751.8
- - genitalia, genital organ(s) or tract
- - - female 752.8
- - - - external 752.4
- - - - internal NEC 752.8
- - - male 752.8
- - glottis 748.3
- - hand 755.5

Malposition - *continued*
- congenital - *continued*
- - heart 746.8
- - - dextrocardia 746.8
- - - - with complete transposition of
      viscera 759.3
- - hepatic duct 751.6
- - hip (joint) 754.3
- - intestine (large) (small) 751.5
- - - with anomalous adhesions, fixation
      or malrotation 751.4
- - joint NEC 755.8
- - kidney 753.3
- - larynx 748.3
- - limb 755.8
- - - lower 755.6
- - - upper 755.5
- - liver 751.6
- - lung (lobe) 748.6
- - nail(s) 757.5
- - nerve 742.8
- - nervous system NEC 742.8
- - nose, nasal (septum) 748.1
- - organ or site not listed - see Anomaly,
      specified type NEC
- - ovary 752.0
- - pancreas 751.7
- - parathyroid (gland) 759.2
- - patella 755.6
- - peripheral vascular system (any vessel)
      747.6
- - pituitary (gland) 759.2
- - respiratory organ or system NEC 748.9
- - rib (cage) 756.3
- - - supernumerary in cervical region
      756.2
- - scapula 755.5
- - shoulder 755.5
- - spinal cord 742.5
- - spine 756.1
- - spleen 759.0
- - sternum 756.3
- - stomach 750.7
- - symphysis pubis 755.6
- - testis (undescended) 752.5
- - thymus (gland) 759.2
- - thyroid (gland) (tissue) 759.2
- - - cartilage 748.3
- - toe(s) 755.6
- - - supernumerary 755.0
- - tongue 750.1
- - trachea 748.3
- - uterus 752.3
- - vein(s) (peripheral) 747.6
- - - great 747.4
- - - portal 747.4
- - - pulmonary 747.4

Malposition - *continued*
- congenital - *continued*
- - vena cava (inferior) (superior) 747.4
- device, implant or graft - see Listing
  under complications, mechanical
- fetus NEC (see also Presentation, fetal)
  652.9
- - with successful version 652.1
- - causing obstructed labor 660.0
- - in multiple gestation (one or more)
  652.6
- - - with locking 660.5
- - - causing obstructed labor 660.0
- gallbladder (see also Disease,
  gallbladder) 575.8
- gastrointestinal tract 569.8
- heart (see also Malposition, congenital,
  heart) 746.8
- intestine 569.8
- pelvic organs or tissues
- - in pregnancy or childbirth 654.4
- - - causing obstructed labor 660.2
- - - - fetus or newborn 763.1
- - - fetus or newborn 763.8
- placenta - see Placenta praevia
- stomach 537.8
- tooth, teeth (with impaction) 524.3
- uterus or cervix (acute) (acquired)
  (adherent) (any degree) (asymptomatic)
  (postinfectional) (postpartal, old) 621.6
- - anteflexion or anteversion (see also
    Anteversion, uterus) 621.6
- - flexion 621.6
- - - lateral (see also Lateroversion,
      uterus) 621.6
- - in pregnancy or childbirth 654.4
- - - causing obstructed labor 660.2
- - - - fetus or newborn 763.1
- - - fetus or newborn 763.8
- - inversion 621.6
- - lateral (flexion) (version) (see also
    Lateroversion, uterus) 621.6
- - retroflexion or retroversion (see also
    Retroversion, uterus) 621.6
Malposture 729.9
Malpresentation, fetus (see also
  Presentation, fetal) 652.9
Malrotation
- cecum 751.4
- colon 751.4
- intestine 751.4
- kidney 753.3
Maltreatment of child (emotional)
  (nutritional) 995.5
Maltworkers' lung 495.4
Malum coxae senilis 715.2
Malunion, fracture 733.8

Mammillitis (see also Mastitis) 611.0
- puerperal, postpartum 675.2
Mammitis (see also Mastitis) 611.0
- puerperal, postpartum 675.2
Mammoplasia 611.1
Management
- contraceptive V25.9
- - specified NEC V25.8
- procreative V26.9
- - specified NEC V26.8
Mangled NEC (see also Nature and site of injury) 959.9
Mania (monopolar) 296.0
- alcoholic (acute) (chronic) 291.9
- Bell's 296.0
- chronic 296.0
- delirious (acute) 296.0
- hysterical 300.1
- puerperal 296.0
- recurrent 296.0
- senile 290.8
- unproductive 296.6
Manic-depressive insanity, psychosis, reaction, or syndrome 296.6
- circular (alternating) 296.5
- - currently
- - - depressed 296.3
- - - manic 296.2
- - mixed 296.4
- depressed (type), depressive 296.1
- hypomanic 296.0
- manic 296.0
- mixed NEC 296.6
- stuporous 296.6
Manson's
- disease 120.1
- pyosis 684
- schistosomiasis 120.1
Mansonellosis 125.5
Manual - see condition
Maple syrup (urine) disease 270.3
Maple-bark strippers' lung 495.6
Marasmus 261
- brain 331.9
- due to malnutrition 261
- intestinal 569.8
- nutritional 261
- senile 797
- tuberculous NEC (see also Tuberculosis) 011.9
Marble
- bones 756.5
- skin 782.6
Marburg disease 078.8
March
- foot (closed) 825.2
- - open 825.3

March - continued
- hemoglobinuria 283.2
Marchand multiple nodular hyperplasia (liver) 571.5
Marchesani(-Weill) syndrome 759.8
Marchiafava(-Bignami) syndrome or disease 341.8
Marchiafava-Micheli syndrome 283.2
Marcus Gunn syndrome 742.8
Marfan's
- congenital syphilis 090.4
- disease 090.4
- syndrome 759.8
- - meaning congenital syphilis 090.4
- - - with luxation of lens 090.4 † 379.3*
Marginal
- implantation, placenta - see Placenta previa
- placenta - see Placenta, abnormal
- sinus (hemorrhage) (rupture) 641.2
- - fetus or newborn 762.1
Marie's
- cerebellar ataxia 334.2
- syndrome 253.0
Marie-Bamberger disease 731.2
Marie-Charcot-Tooth neuropathic atrophy muscle 356.1
Marie-Strumpell arthritis, disease or spondylitis 720.0
Marion's disease 596.0
Marital conflict V61.1
Mark
- port wine 757.3
- raspberry 757.3
- strawberry 757.3
- stretch 701.3
- tattoo 709.0
Maroteaux-Lamy syndrome 277.5
Marrow (bone)
- arrest 284.9
- megakaryocytic 287.3
- poor function 289.9
Marshall's (hidrotic) ectodermal dysplasia 757.3
Masculinization female with adrenal hyperplasia 255.2
Masculinovoblastoma (M8670/0) 220
Masochism 302.8
Masons' lung 502
Mass
- abdominal 789.3
- chest 786.6
- cystic - see Cyst
- head 784.2
- kidney 593.9
- malignant (M8000/3) - see Neoplasm, malignant

Maternal condition - *continued*
- toxemia (of pregnancy) 760.0
- toxoplasmosis (conditions in 130) 760.2
- - manifest toxoplasmosis in the infant or fetus 771.2
- transmission of chemical substance through the placenta 760.7
- uremia 760.1
- urinary tract conditions (conditions in 580-599) 760.1
- vomiting (pernicious) (persistent) (vicious) 761.8
Maternity - see Delivery
Mauclaire's disease or osteochondrosis 732.3
Maxilla, maxillary - see condition
May(-Hegglin) anomaly or syndrome 288.2
Mazoplasia 610.8
McArdle(-Schmid)(-Pearson) disease (glycogen storage) 271.0
Measles (black) (hemorrhagic) (suppressed) 055.9
- with pneumonia 055.1 † 484.0*
- complication 055.8
- - specified NEC 055.7
- French 056.9
- German 056.9
- liberty 056.9
- specified complications NEC 055.7
Meatitis, urethral (see also Urethritis) 597.8
Meatus, meatal - see condition
Meckel's
- diverticulitis 751.0
- diverticulum (displaced) (hypertrophic) 751.0
Meconium
- ileus, fetus or newborn 277.0 † 777.0*
- in liquor - see Distress, fetal
- obstruction, fetus or newborn 777.1
- - in mucoviscidosis 277.0 † 777.0*
- passage of - see Distress, fetal
- peritonitis 777.6
- plug syndrome (newborn) NEC 777.1
Median - see also condition
- bar (prostate) 600
- - vesical orifice 600
Mediastinitis (acute) (chronic) 519.2
- actinomycotic 039.8
- syphilitic 095
- tuberculous 012.8
Mediastinopericarditis (see also Pericarditis) 423.9
Mediastinum, mediastinal - see condition
Medical services provided for - see Health, services provided because (of)
Medicine poisoning (by overdose) (wrong substance given or taken in error) 977.9

Medicine poisoning - *continued*
- specified drug or substance - see Table of drugs and chemicals
Mediterranean
- disease or syndrome (hemipathic) 282.4
- fever (see also Brucellosis) 023.9
- - familial 277.3
- kala-azar 085.0
- leishmaniasis 085.0
Medulla - see condition
Medullated fibers
- optic (nerve) 743.5
- retina 743.5
Medulloblastoma (M9470/3)
- desmoplastic (M9471/3) 191.6
- specified site - see Neoplasm, malignant
- unspecified site 191.6
Medulloepithelioma (M9501/3) - see also Neoplasm, malignant
- teratoid (M9502/3) - see Neoplasm, malignant
Medullomyoblastoma (M9472/3)
- specified site - see Neoplasm, malignant
- unspecified site 191.6
Megacolon (acquired) (functional) (not Hirschsprung's disease) 564.7
- aganglionic 751.3
- congenital, congenitum 751.3
- Hirschsprung's (disease) 751.3
- toxic 556
Mega-esophagus (functional) 530.0
- congenital 750.4
Megalencephaly 742.4
Megalerythema 057.0
Megaloappendix 751.5
Megalocephalus, megalocephaly NEC 756.0
Megalocornea 743.2
Megalodactylia (fingers) (thumbs) 755.5
- toes 755.6
Megaloduodenum 751.5
Megaloesophagus (functional) 530.0
- congenital 750.4
Megalogastria (congenital) 750.7
Megalophthalmos 743.8
Megalopsia 368.1
Megalosplenia - see Splenomegaly
Megaloureter 593.8
- congenital 753.2
Megarectum 569.4
Megasigmoid 564.7
- congenital 751.3
Megaureter 593.8
- congenital 753.2
Megrim 346.9
Meibomian
- cyst infected 373.1
- gland - see condition

Meibomian - *continued*
- sty, stye 373.1
Meibomitis 373.1
Meige's disease 757.0
Melancholia 296.9
- climacteric 296.1
- hypochondriac 300.7
- intermittent 296.1
- involutional 296.1
- menopausal 296.1
- puerperal 296.1
- reactive (from emotional stress,
  psychological trauma) 298.0
- recurrent 296.1
- senile 290.2
- stuporous 296.1
Melanemia 275.0
Melanoameloblastoma (M9363/0) - see
  Neoplasm, bone, benign
Melanoblastoma (M8720/3) - see
  Melanoma
Melanocarcinoma (M8720/3) - see
  Melanoma
Melanocytoma, eyeball (M8726/0) 224.0
Melanoderma, melanodermia 709.0
Melanodontia, infantile 521.0
Melanoepithelioma (M8720/3) - see
  Melanoma
Melanoma (malignant) (M8720/3) 172.9

Note – Except where otherwise indicated,
the morphological varieties of melanoma in
the list below should be coded by site as for
"Melanoma (malignant)", i.e. according to
the list under "site classification" below. Internal sites should be coded to malignant
neoplasm of those sites.

Melanoma - *continued*
- amelanotic (M8730/3)
- balloon cell (M8722/3)
- benign (M8720/0) - see Neoplasm, skin,
  benign
- epithelioid cell (M8771/3)
- - and spindle cell, mixed (M8775/3)
- in
- - giant pigmented nevus (M8761/3)
- - Hutchinson's melanotic freckle
  (M8742/3)
- - junctional nevus (M8740/3)
- - precancerous melanosis (M8741/3)
- juvenile (M8770/0) - see Neoplasm, skin,
  benign
- metastatic
- - specified site - see Volume 1, page 728
- - unspecified site 172.9

Melanoma - *continued*
- nodular (M8721/3)
- spindle cell (M8772/3)
- - type A (M8773/3) 190.0
- - type B (M8774/3) 190.0
- superficial spreading (M8743/3)
- site classification
- - abdominal wall 172.5
- - ala nasi 172.3
- - ankle 172.7
- - anus, anal 154.3
- - arm 172.6
- - auditory canal (external) 172.2
- - auricle (ear) 172.2
- - auricular canal (external) 172.2
- - axilla 172.5
- - axillary fold 172.5
- - back 172.5
- - breast (female) (male) 172.5
- - brow 172.3
- - buttock 172.5
- - canthus (eye) 172.1
- - cheek (external) 172.3
- - chest wall 172.5
- - chin 172.3
- - choroid 190.6
- - conjuctiva 190.3
- - ear (external) 172.2
- - external meatus (ear) 172.2
- - eye 190.9
- - eyebrow 172.3
- - eyelid (lower) (upper) 172.1
- - face NEC 172.3
- - female genital organ (external) NEC
  184.4
- - finger 172.6
- - flank 172.5
- - foot 172.7
- - forearm 172.6
- - forehead 172.3
- - foreskin 187.1
- - glabella 172.3
- - gluteal region 172.5
- - groin 172.5
- - hand 172.6
- - heel 172.7
- - helix 172.2
- - hip 172.7
- - interscapular region 172.5
- - iris 190.0
- - jaw 172.3
- - knee 172.7
- - labia 184.4
- - - majora 184.1
- - - minora 184.2
- - labium 184.4
- - - majus 184.1

Melanoma - *continued*
- site classification - *continued*
- - labium - *continued*
- - - minus 184.2
- - lacrimal gland 190.2
- - leg 172.7
- - lip (lower) (upper) 172.0
- - liver 197.7
- - lower limb NEC 172.7
- - male genital organ (external) NEC 187.9
- - nail 172.9
- - - finger 172.6
- - - toe 172.7
- - nasolabial groove 172.3
- - nates 172.5
- - neck 172.4
- - nose (external) 172.3
- - orbit 190.1
- - palpebra 172.1
- - penis 187.4
- - perianal skin 172.5
- - perineum 172.5
- - pinna 172.2
- - popliteal fossa or space 172.7
- - prepuce 187.1
- - pubes 172.5
- - pudendum 184.4
- - retina 190.5
- - retrobulbar 190.1
- - scalp 172.4
- - scrotum 187.7
- - shoulder 172.6
- - skin 172.5
- - specified site NEC - see Neoplasm, malignant
- - submammary fold 172.5
- - temple 172.3
- - thigh 172.7
- - toe 172.7
- - trunk NEC 172.5
- - umbilicus 172.5
- - upper limb NEC 172.6
- - vulva 184.4
Melanoplakia 528.9
Melanosarcoma (M8720/3) - see also Melanoma
- epithelioid cell (M8771/3) - see Melanoma
Melanosis 709.0
- addisonian 255.4
- - tuberculous 017.6 † 255.4*
- adrenal 255.4
- colon 569.8
- conjunctiva 372.5
- - congenital 743.4
- cornea (presenile) (senile) 371.1

Melanosis - *continued*
- cornea - *continued*
- - congenital 743.4
- - prenatal 743.4
- eye 372.5
- - congenital 743.4
- lenticularis progressiva 757.3
- liver 573.8
- precancerous (M8741/2) - see also Neoplasm, skin, in situ
- - malignant melanoma in (M8741/3) - see Melanoma
- Riehl 709.0
- sclera 379.1
- - congenital 743.4
- suprarenal 255.4
- tar 709.0
- toxic 709.0
Melanuria 791.9
Melasma 709.0
- adrenal (gland) 255.4
- suprarenal (gland) 255.4
Melena 578.1
- with ulcer - code by site under Ulcer, with hemorrhage 533.4
- newborn 772.4
- - due to swallowed maternal blood 777.3
Meleney's
- gangrene (cutaneous) 686.0
- ulcer (chronic undermining) 686.0
Melioidosis 025
Melitensis, febris 023.0
Melitococcosis 023.0
Melkersson's syndrome 351.8
Mellitus, diabetes - see Diabetes
Melorheostosis (bone) (leri) 733.9
Melotia 744.2
Membrana
- capsularis lentis posterior 743.4
- epipapillaris 743.4
Membranacea placenta - see Placenta, abnormal
Membranaceous uterus 621.8
Membrane(s), membranous - see also condition
- folds, congenital - see Web
- Jackson's 751.4
- premature rupture - see Rupture, membranes, premature
- pupillary 364.7
- pupillary persistent 743.4
- retained (with hemorrhage) (complicating delivery) 666.2
- - without hemorrhage 667.1
- secondary (eye) 366.5
- unruptured (causing asphyxia) 768.9
Membranitis, fetal 658.4

Meningitis - *continued*
- nonspecific 322.9
- oidiomycosis 112.8 † 321.0*
- ossificans 349.2
- pneumococcal 320.1
- poliovirus 045.2 † 321.7*
- purulent 320.9
- – specified organism NEC 320.8
- pyogenic 320.9
- – specified organism NEC 320.8
- Salmonella 003.2 † 320.7*
- septic 320.9
- – specified organism NEC 320.8
- serosa circumscripta NEC 322.0
- serous NEC 047.9 † 321.7*
- – lymphocytic 049.0 † 321.6*
- specified organism NEC 320.8
- sporotrichosis 117.1 † 321.0*
- staphylococcal 320.3
- sterile 997.0
- streptococcal (acute) 320.2
- suppurative 320.9
- – specified organism NEC 320.8
- syphilitic 094.2 † 320.7*
- – acute 091.8 † 320.7*
- – congenital 090.4 † 320.7*
- – secondary 091.8 † 320.7*
- Torula 117.5 † 321.0*
- traumatic (complication of injury) 958.8
- trypanosomiasis 086.- † 321.8*
- tuberculous 013.0 † 320.4*
- typhoid 002.0 † 320.7*
- viral, virus NEC 047.9 † 321.7*
- Wallgren's 047.9 † 321.7*
Meningocele (spinal) 741.9
- with hydrocephalus 741.0
- cerebral 742.0
Meningocerebritis - see
  Meningo-encephalitis
Meningococcemia (acute) (chronic) 036.2
Meningococcus, meningococcal (see also
  Condition) 036.9
Meningo-encephalitis 323.9
- acute NEC 048 † 323.4*
- bacterial, purulent, pyogenic or septic -
  code as Meningitis 320.9
- chronic NEC 094.1
- diffuse NEC 094.1
- diphasic 063.2 † 323.3*
- due to
- – blastomycosis NEC 116.0 † 323.4*
- – free-living amebae 136.2 † 323.4*
- – mumps 072.2 † 323.4*
- – Naegleria (amebae) (organisms)
    (gruberi) 136.2 † 323.4*
- – toxoplasmosis (acquired) 130 † 323.4*
- – – congenital (active) 771.2 † 323.4*

Meningo-encephalitis - *continued*
- due to - *continued*
- – Trypanosoma 086.- † 323.4*
- epidemic 036.0 † 320.5*
- H. influenzae 320.0
- herpes 054.3 † 323.4*
- herpetic 054.3 † 323.4*
- infectious (acute) 048 † 323.4*
- influenzal 320.0
- Listeria monocytogenes 027.0 † 320.7*
- lymphocytic (serous) 049.0 † 321.6*
- mumps 072.2 † 323.4*
- parasitic NEC 123.9 † 323.4*
- pneumococcal 320.1
- primary amebic 136.2 † 323.4*
- serous 048 † 323.4*
- – lymphocytic 049.0 † 321.6*
- specific 094.2 † 320.7*
- specified organism NEC 323.8
- staphylococcal 320.3
- streptococcal 320.2
- syphilitic 094.2 † 320.7*
- toxic NEC 989.9 † 323.7*
- trypanosomic 086.- † 323.4*
- tuberculous 013.0 † 320.4*
- virus NEC 048 † 323.4*
Meningo-encephalocele 742.0
- syphilitic 094.8
- – congenital 090.4
Meningo-encephalomyelitis (see also
  Meningo-encephalitis) 323.9
- acute NEC 048 † 323.4*
- – disseminated (postinfectious) 136.9 †
    323.6*
- – – postimmunization or
      postvaccination 323.5
- due to
- – actinomycosis 039.8 † 320.8*
- – Torula 117.5 † 323.4*
- – toxoplasma or toxoplasmosis
    (acquired) 130 † 323.4*
- – – congenital (active) 771.2 † 323.4*
Meningo-encephalomyelopathy (see also
  Meningo-encephalomyelitis) 349.9
Meningo-encephalopathy (see also
  Meningo-encephalitis) 348.3
Meningo-encephalopoliomyelitis 045.0 †
  323.2*
Meningomyelitis (see also
  Meningo-encephalitis) 323.9
- blastomycotic NEC 116.0 † 323.4*
- due to
- – Torula 117.5 † 323.4*
- lethargic 049.8 † 323.4*
- meningococcal 036.0 † 320.5*
- syphilitic 094.2 † 320.7*
- tuberculous 013.0 † 320.4*

Meningomyelocele 741.9
– with hydrocephalus 741.0
– syphilitic 094.8
Meningomyeloneuritis - see
Meningo-encephalitis
Meningoradiculitis - see Meningitis
Meningovascular - see condition
Menke's syndrome - see Syndrome,
Menke's
Menometrorrhagia 626.2
Menopause, menopausal (symptoms)
(syndrome) 627.2
– arthritis (any site) NEC 716.3
– artificial 627.4
– crisis 627.2
– depression 296.1
– – agitated 296.1
– – psychotic 296.1
– melancholia 296.1
– paranoid state 297.2
– paraphrenia 297.2
– premature 256.3
– psychoneurosis, unspecified 627.2
– psychosis NEC 298.8
– surgical 627.4
– toxic polyarthritis NEC 716.3
Menorrhagia (primary) 626.2
– climacteric 627.0
– menopausal 627.0
– postclimacteric 627.1
– postmenopausal 627.1
– preclimacteric 627.0
– premenopausal 627.0
– puberty (menses retained) 626.3
Menses, retention 626.8
Menstrual - see also Menstruation
– cycle, irregular 626.4
– disorders NEC 626.9
– extraction V25.3
– period, normal V65.5
– regulation V25.3
Menstruation
– absent 626.0
– delayed 626.8
– disorder NEC 626.9
– – psychogenic 306.5
– during pregnancy 640.8
– excessive 626.2
– frequent 626.2
– infrequent 626.1
– irregular 626.4
– latent 626.8
– membranous 626.8
– painful (primary) (secondary) 625.3
– – psychogenic 306.5
– precocious 626.8
– protracted 626.8

Menstruation - *continued*
– retained 626.8
– retrograde 626.8
– scanty 626.1
– suppression 626.8
– vicarious (nasal) 625.8
Mentagra (see also Sycosis) 704.8
Mental - see also condition
– deficiency - see Retardation, mental
– deterioration (see also Psychosis) 298.9
– disorder (see also Disorder, mental)
300.9
– exhaustion 300.5
– insufficiency (congenital) (see also
Retardation, mental) 319
– observation without need for further
medical care V71.0
– retardation - see Retardation, mental
– subnormality (see also Retardation,
mental) 319
– – mild 317
– – moderate 318.0
– – profound 318.2
– – severe 318.1
– upset (see also Disorder, mental) 300.9
Meralgia paraesthetica 355.1
Mercurial - see condition
Mercurialism NEC 985.0
Merergasia 300.9
Merocele - see Hernia, femoral
Merzbacher-Pelizaeus disease 330.0
Mesaortitis - see Aortitis
Mesarteritis - see Arteritis

Mesencephalitis (see also Encephalitis)
323.9
Mesenchymoma (M8990/1) - see also
Neoplasm, connective tissue, uncertain
behavior
– benign (M8990/0) - see Neoplasm,
connective tissue, benign
– malignant (M8990/3) - see Neoplasm,
connective tissue, malignant
Mesentery, mesenteric - see condition

Mesiodens, mesiodentes 520.1
– causing crowding 524.3
Mesio-occlusion 524.2
Mesocardia (with asplenia) 746.8
Mesocolon - see condition
Mesonephroma (malignant) (M9110/3) -
see Neoplasm, malignant
– benign (M9110/0) - see Neoplasm,
benign
Mesophlebitis - see Phlebitis
Mesostromal dysgenesia 743.4
Mesothelioma (malignant) (M9050/3) - see
also Neoplasm, malignant

Mesothelioma - *continued*
- benign (M9050/0) - see Neoplasm, benign
- biphasic type (M9053/3) - see also Neoplasm, malignant
- - benign (M9053/0) - see Neoplasm, benign
- epithelioid (M9052/3) - see also Neoplasm, malignant
- - benign (M9052/0) - see Neoplasm, benign
- fibrous (M9051/3) - see also Neoplasm, malignant
- - benign (M9051/0) - see Neoplasm, benign
Metabolism disorders NEC 277.9
Metagonimiasis 121.5
Metagonimus infestation (small intestine) 121.5
Metal
- pigmentation 709.0
- polishers' disease 502
Metalliferous miners' lung 503
Metamorphopsia 368.1
Metaplasia
- cervix (squamous) 622.1
- endometrium (squamous) 621.8
- intestinal, of gastric mucosa 537.8
- kidney (pelvis) (squamous) (see also Disease, renal) 593.9
- myelogenous 289.8
- myeloid (agnogenic) (megakaryocytic) 289.8
- spleen 289.5
- squamous cell, bladder 596.8
Metastasis, metastatic
- abscess - see Abscess
- calcification 275.4
- cancer, neoplasm or disease
- - from specified site (M8000/3) - see Neoplasm, malignant, by site
- - of specified site - see Volume 1, page 728
- - to specified site (M8000/6) - see Secondary neoplasm, by site
- deposits (in) (M8000/6) - see Secondary neoplasm
- spread (to) (M8000/6) - see Secondary neoplasm
Metatarsalgia 726.7
- Morton's 355.6
Metatarsus, metatarsal - see also condition
- valgus (adductus) (congenital) 754.6
- varus (adductus) (congenital) 754.5
Methemoglobinemia 289.7
- acquired (with sulfhemoglobinemia) 289.7

Methemoglobinemia - *continued*
- congenital 289.7
- enzymatic 289.7
- Hb M disease 289.7
- hereditary 289.7
- toxic 289.7
Methemoglobinuria (see also Hemoglobinuria) 791.2
Methioninemia 270.4
Metritis (catarrhal) (septic) (suppurative) (see also Endometritis) 615.9
- cervical (see also Cervicitis) 616.0
- hemorrhagic 626.8
Metropathia hemorrhagica 626.8
Metroperitonitis (see also Peritonitis, pelvic, female) 614.5
Metrorrhagia 626.6
- arising during pregnancy - see Hemorrhage, pregnancy
- postpartum NEC 666.2
- primary 626.6
- psychogenic 306.5
Metrorrhexis - see Rupture, uterus
Metrosalpingitis (see also Salpingo-oophoritis) 614.2
Metrostaxis 626.6
Metrovaginitis (see also Endometritis) 615.9
Meyer-Schwickerath and Weyer's syndrome 759.8
Mibelli's disease 757.3
Mice, joint 718.1
- knee 717.6
Micrencephalon 742.1
Microaneurysm, retinal 362.1
- diabetic 250.4 † 362.0*
Microangiopathy, thrombotic 446.6
Microcephalus, microcephalic, microcephaly 742.1
- due to toxoplasmosis (congenital) 771.2
Microcheilia 744.8
Microcolon (congenital) 751.5
Microcornea (congenital) 743.4
Microcytic - see condition
Microdontia 520.2
Microdrepanocytosis 282.4
Microembolism, retinal 362.3
Microgastria (congenital) 750.7
Microgenia 524.0
Microgenitalia (congenital) 752.8
Microglioma (M9710/3)
- specified site - see Neoplasm, malignant
- unspecified site 191.9
Microglossia (congenital) 750.1
Micrognathia, micrognathism (congenital) (mandibular) (maxillary) 524.0
Microgyria (congenital) 742.2

Micro-infarct of heart (see also
  Insufficiency, coronary) 411
Microlithiasis, alveolar, pulmonary 516.2
Micromyelia (congenital) 742.5
Microphakia (congenital) 743.3
Microphthalmia (congenital) 743.1
Microphthalmos (congenital) 743.1
− due to toxoplasmosis (congenital) 771.2
Micropsia 368.1
Microsporon furfur infestation 111.0
Microsporosis (see also Dermatophytosis)
  110.9
− nigra 111.1
Microstomia (congenital) 744.8
Microtia (external ear) (congenital) 744.2
Microtropia 378.3
Micturition
− disorder NEC 788.6
− − psychogenic 306.5
− frequency (nocturnal) 788.4
− − psychogenic 306.5
− painful 788.1
− − psychogenic 306.5
Mid plane - see condition
Middle
− ear - see condition
− lobe syndrome 518.0
Miescher's disease 709.3
Mieten's syndrome 759.8
Migraine (idiopathic) 346.9
− with aura 346.0
− basilar 346.2
− classical 346.0
− common 346.1
− hemiplegic 346.8
− lower-half 346.2
− menstrual 625.4
− ophthalmoplegic 346.8
− retinal 346.2
− variant 346.2
Migratory, migrating - see condition
Mikulicz's disease or syndrome 527.1
Miliaria (crystallina) (rubra) (tropicalis)
  705.1
Miliary - see condition
Milium (see also Cyst, sebaceous) 706.2
− colloid 709.3
− eyelid 706.2
Milk
− crust 691.8
− excess secretion 676.6
− fever, female 672
− poisoning 988.8
− retention 676.2
− sickness 988.8
Milk-leg 451.1
− complicating pregnancy 671.3

Milk-leg - *continued*
− nonpuerperal 451.1
− puerperal, postpartum, childbirth 671.4
Milkman's disease or syndrome 268.2
Milky urine - see Chyluria
Mill's disease 335.2
Millar's asthma 478.7
Millard-Gubler syndrome 344.8

Millard-Gubler-Foville paralysis 344.8
Millstone makers'
− asthma 502
− lung 502
Milroy's disease 757.0
Miners'
− asthma 500
− elbow 727.2
− knee 727.2
− lung 500
− nystagmus 300.8
− phthisis 011.4
− tuberculosis 011.4
Minkowski-Chauffard syndrome (see also
  Spherocytosis) 282.0
Minor - see condition
Minor's disease 336.1
Minot's disease 776.0
Minot-von Willebrand-Jurgen disease 286.4
Minus (and plus) hand (intrinsic) 736.0
Miosis (pupil) 379.4
Mirror writing 315.0

Misadventure (prophylactic) (therapeutic)
  (see also Complications) 999.9
− administration of insulin 962.3
− infusion - see Complications, infusion
− local applications NEC (of fomentations,
  plasters, etc.) 999.9
− − burn or scald - see Burn
− medical care NEC (early) (late) 999.9
− − adverse effect of drugs or chemicals -
    see Table of drugs and chemicals
− − burn or scald - see Burn
− radiation NEC 990
− radiotherapy NEC 990
− surgical procedure (early) (late) - see
  Complications, surgical procedure
− transfusion - see Complications,
  transfusion
− vaccination or other immunilogical
  procedure - see Complications,
  vaccination
Misanthropy 301.7
Miscarriage - see Abortion, spontaneous
Mismanagement of feeding 783.3
Misplaced, misplacement
− kidney (see also Lesion, kidney) 593.0
− − congenital 753.3

Misplaced - *continued*
– organ or site, congenital NEC - see Malposition, congenital
Missed
– abortion 632
– delivery 656.4
– labor 656.4
Missing - see also Absence
– vertebrae (congenital) 756.1
Misuse of drugs NEC 305.9
Mitchell's disease 443.8
Mite(s)
– diarrhea 133.8
– grain (itch) 133.8
– hair follicle (itch) 133.8
– in sputum 133.8
Mitral - see condition
Mittelschmerz 625.2
Mixed - see condition
Mljet disease 757.3
Mobile, mobility
– cecum 751.4
– excessive - see Hypermobility
– gallbladder 751.6
– kidney 593.0
– organ or site, congenital NEC - see Malposition, congenital
Moebius
– disease 346.8
– syndrome
– – congenital oculofacial paralysis 352.6
– – ophthalmoplegic migraine 346.8
Moeller's
– disease 267
– glossitis 529.4
Mohr's syndrome (types I and II) 759.8
Mola destruens (M9100/1) 236.1
Molar pegnancy NEC 631
Molarisation, molarization of premolars 520.2
Mold(s) in vitreous 117.9
Molding, head (during birth) 767.3
Mole (pigmented) (M8720/0) - see also Neoplasm, skin, benign
– blood 631
– Breus' 631
– cancerous (M8720/3) - see Melanoma
– carneous 631
– destructive (M9100/1) 236.1
– ectopic - see Pregnancy, ectopic
– fleshy 631
– hemorrhagic 631
– hydatid, hydatidiform (benign) (complicating pregnancy) (delivered) (undelivered) 630
– – invasive (M9100/1) 236.1
– – malignant (M9100/1) 236.1

Mole - *continued*
– invasive (hydatidiform) (M9100/1) 236.1
– malignant
– – meaning
– – – malignant hydatidiform mole (M9100/1) 236.1
– – – melanoma (M8720/3) - see Melanoma
– nonpigmented (M8730/0) - see Neoplasm, skin, benign
– pregnancy NEC 631
– skin (M8720/0) - see Neoplasm, skin, benign
– tubal - see Pregnancy, tubal
– vesicular (see also Hydatidiform mole) 630
Molluscum
– contagiosum 078.0
– epitheliale 078.0
– fibrosum (M8851/0) 214
– pendulum (M8851/0) 214
Monckeberg's arteriosclerosis, degeneration, disease, or sclerosis 440.2
Mondor's disease 451.8
Mongolian, mongolianism, mongolism, mongoloid 758.0
– spot 757.3
Monilethrix (congenital) 757.4
Moniliasis - see also Candidiasis
– neonatal 771.7
Monoarthritis 716.6
Monoblastic - see condition
Monocytic - see condition
Monocytosis (symptomatic) 288.8
Monomania (see also Psychosis) 298.9
Mononeuritis 355.9
– cranial nerve - see Disorder, nerve, cranial
– femoral nerve 355.2
– lateral
– – cutaneous nerve of thigh 355.1
– – popliteal nerve 355.3
– lower limb 355.8
– – specified nerve NEC 355.7
– medial popliteal nerve 355.4
– median nerve 354.1
– multiplex 354.5
– plantar nerve 355.6
– posterior tibial nerve 355.5
– radial nerve 354.3
– sciatic nerve 355.0
– ulnar nerve 354.2
– upper limb 354.9
– – specified nerve NEC 354.8
Mononeuropathy (see also Mononeuritis) 355.9
– diabetic NEC 250.5 † 355.9*

Mononucleosis, infectious 075
Monoplegia 344.5
− brain (current episode) 437.8
− − fetus or newborn 767.8
− congenital or infantile (cerebral) (spastic)
  (spinal) 343.3
− embolic (current episode) (see also
  Embolism, brain) 434.1
− hysterical (transient) 300.1
− infantile (cerebral) (spastic) (spinal)
  343.3
− lower limb 344.3
− psychogenic 306.0
− − specified as conversion reaction 300.1
− thrombotic (current episode) (see also
  Thrombosis, brain) 434.0
− transient 781.4
− upper limb 344.4
Monorchism, monorchidism 752.8
Monster, monstrosity (single) 759.7
− acephalic 740.0
− composite 759.4
− compound 759.4
− double 759.4
− specified type NEC 759.8
− twin 759.4
Monteggia's fracture 813.0
− open 813.1
Moore's syndrome 345.5
Mooren's ulcer (cornea) 370.0
Mooser's bodies 081.0
Moral
− deficiency 301.7
− imbecility 301.7
Morax-Axenfeld conjunctivitis 372.0
Morbilli (see also Measles) 055.9
Morbus
− Beigel 111.2
− caducus (see also Epilepsy) 345.9
− caeruleus 746.8
− comitialis (see also Epilepsy) 345.9
− cordis - see also Disease, heart
− − valvulorum - see Endocarditis
− coxae 719.9
− − tuberculous 015.1
− hemorrhagicus neonatorum 776.0
− senilis 715.9
Morel-Kraepelin disease (see also
  Schizophrenia) 295.9
Morel-Moore syndrome 733.3
Morel-Morgagni syndrome 733.3
Morgagni
− cyst, organ, hydatid, or appendage 752.8
− syndrome 733.3
Morgagni-Stokes-Adams syndrome 426.9
Moria (see also Psychosis) 298.9
Moron 317

Morphea 701.0
Morphinism 304.0
Morphinomania 304.0
Morquio(-Ullrich) disease or syndrome
  277.5
Morquio-Brailsford (type) disease or
  kyphosis 277.5
Mortification (dry) (moist) (see also
  Gangrene) 785.4
Morton's
− disease 355.6
− foot 355.6
− metatarsalgia (syndrome) 355.6
− neuralgia 355.6
− neuroma 355.6
− toe 355.6
Morvan's disease 336.0
Mosaicism, mosaic (autosomal)
  (chromosomal) 758.9
− sex 758.8
Motion sickness (from travel, any vehicle)
  (from roundabouts or swings) 994.6
Mottled (enamel) teeth 520.3
Mottling enamel (teeth) 520.3
Mouchet's disease 732.5
Mould(s) (in vitreous) 117.9
Moulders'
− bronchitis 502
− tuberculosis 011.4
Mountain sickness 993.2
Mouse, joint 718.1
− knee 717.6
Mouth - see condition
Movable
− coccyx 724.7
− kidney (see also Lesion, kidney) 593.0
− − congenital 753.3
− organ or site, congenital NEC - see
  Malposition, congenital
− spleen 289.5
Movements, dystonic 781.0
Moyamoya disease 437.5
Mucinosis (cutaneous) (popular) 701.8
Mucocele
− appendix 543
− buccal cavity 528.9
− gallbladder (see also Disease,
  gallbladder) 575.3
− lacrimal sac 375.4
− salivary gland (any) 527.6
− sinus (accessory) (nasal) 478.1
− turbinate (bone) (middle) (nasal) 478.1
Mucoenteritis 564.1
Mucolipidosis I, II, III 272.7
Mucopolysaccharidosis (types 1-6) 277.5
− cardiopathy 277.5 † 425.7*
Mucormycosis (lung) 117.7

Mucositis necroticans agranulocytica 288.0
Mucous - see also condition
− patches (syphilitic) 091.3
− − congenital 090.0
Mucoviscidosis 277.0
− with meconium obstruction 277.0 †
  777.0*
Mucus
− asphyxia or suffocation (see also
  Asphyxia, mucus) 933.1
− − newborn 770.1
− in stool 792.1
− plug (see also Asphyxia, mucus) 933.1
− − aspiration newborn 770.1
− − tracheobronchial 934.8
− − − newborn 770.1
Muguet 112.0
Mulberry molars 090.5
Mullerian mixed tumor (M8950/3) - see
  Neoplasm, malignant
Multiparity V61.5
− affecting management of pregnancy
  V23.3
− fetus or newborn 763.8
− management of labor and delivery 659.4
− requiring contraceptive management
  V25.-
Multipartita placenta - see Placenta,
  abnormal
Multiple, multiplex - see also condition
− birth, fetus or newborn 761.5
− digits (congenital) 755.0
− organ or site not listed - see Accessory
Mumps 072.9
− complication 072.8
− − specified NEC 072.7
− encephalitis 072.2 † 323.4*
− meningitis (aseptic) 072.1 † 321.5*
− meningo-encephalitis 072.2 † 323.4*
− oophoritis 072.7
− orchitis 072.0 † 604.9*
− pancreatitis 072.3 † 577.0*
Mumu (see also Infestation, filarial) 125.9
Munchausen syndrome 301.5
Munchmeyer's disease 728.1
Mural - see condition
Murmur (cardiac) (heart) (innocent)
  (organic) 785.2
− aortic (valve) (see also Endocarditis,
  aortic) 424.1
− benign 785.2
− diastolic - see Endocarditis
− Flint (see also Endocarditis, aortic) 424.1
− functional 785.2
− Graham Steell (see also Endocarditis,
  pulmonary) 424.3
− mitral (valve) - see Insufficiency, mitral

Murmur - *continued*
− nonorganic 785.2
− presystolic, mitral - see Insufficiency,
  mitral
− pulmonic (valve) (see also Endocarditis,
  pulmonary) 424.3
− systolic (valvular) - see Endocarditis
− tricuspid (valve) - see Endocarditis,
  tricuspid
− valvular - see Endocarditis
Murri's disease 283.2
Muscle, muscular - see condition
Musculoneuralgia 729.1
Mushroom workers' lung 495.5
Mushrooming hip 718.9
Mutism (see also Aphasia) 784.3
− deaf (acquired) (congenital) NEC 389.7
− elective, adjustment reaction 309.8
− hysterical 300.1
Myalgia (intercostal) 729.1
− epidemic 074.1
− − cervical 078.8
− psychogenic 307.8
− traumatic NEC 959.9
Myasthenia, myasthenic 358.0
− cordis - see Failure, heart
− gravis 358.0
− − neonatal 775.2
− stomach 536.8
− − psychogenic 306.4
− syndrome
− − in
− − − diabetes mellitus 250.5 † 358.1*
− − − malignant neoplasm NEC
      (M8000/3) 199.1 † 358.1*
− − − thyrotoxicosis 242.- † 358.1*
Mycelium infection NEC 117.9
Mycetismus 988.1
Mycetoma (actinomycotic) 039.9
− bone 039.8
− − mycotic 117.4
− foot 039.4
− − mycotic 117.4
− madurae 039.9
− − mycotic 117.4
− maduromycotic 039.9
− − mycotic 117.4
− mycotic 117.4
− nocardial 039.9
Mycobacteriosis - see Mycobacterium
Mycobacterium, mycobacterial (infection)
  031.9
− acid-fast (bacilli) 031.9
− anonymous (see also Mycobacterium,
  atypical) 031.9
− atypical (acid-fast bacilli) 031.9
− − cutaneous 031.1

Mycobacterium - *continued*
- atypical - *continued*
- - pulmonary 031.0
- - - tuberculous (see also Tuberculosis, pulmonary) 011.9
- - specified site NEC 031.8
- avium 031.0
- balnei 031.1
- Battey 031.0
- cutaneous 031.1
- fortuitum 031.0
- intracellulare (Battey bacillus) 031.0
- kakerifu 031.8
- kansasii 031.0
- kasongo 031.8
- leprae - see Leprosy
- luciflavum 031.0
- marinum 031.1
- pulmonary 031.0
- - tuberculous (see also Tuberculosis, pulmonary) 011.9
- scrofulaceum 031.1
- tuberculosis (human, bovine) - see Tuberculosis
- - avian type 031.0
- ulcerans 031.1
- xenopi 031.0
Mycosis, mycotic 117.9
- cutaneous NEC 111.9
- ear 111.8
- fungoides (M9700/3) 202.1
- mouth 112.0
- pharynx 117.9
- skin NEC 111.9
- stomatitis 112.0
- systemic NEC 117.9
- tonsil 117.9
- vagina, vaginitis 112.1 † 616.1*
Mydriasis (pupil) 379.4
Myelatelia 742.5
Myelinoclasis, perivascular, acute (postinfectious) NEC 136.9 † 323.6*
- postimmunization or postvaccinal 323.5
Myelitis (acute) (ascending) (cerebellar) (childhood) (chronic) (descending) (diffuse) (disseminated) (pressure) (progressive) (disseminated) (pressure) (transverse) (see also Encephalitis) 323.9
- postvaccinal 323.5
- syphilitic (transverse) 094.8 † 323.4*
- tuberculous 013.8 † 323.4*
Myeloblastic - see condition
Myelocele 741.9
- with hydrocephalus 741.0
Myelocystocele 741.9
- with hydrocephalus 741.0
Myelocytic - see condition

Myelodysplasia (spinal cord) 742.5
Myeloencephalitis - see Encephalitis
Myelofibrosis (osteosclerosis) 289.8
Myelogenous - see condition
Myeloid - see condition
Myeloleukodystrophy 330.0
Myelolipoma (M8870/0) - see Neoplasm, benign
Myeloma (multiple) (plasma cell) (plasmacytic) (M9730/3) 203.0
- monostotic (M9731/1) 238.6
- solitary (M9731/1) 238.6
Myelomalacia 336.8
Myelomata, multiple (M9730/3) 203.0
Myelomatosis (M9730/3) 203.0
Myelomeningitis - see Meningoencephalitis
Myelomeningocele (spinal cord) 741.9
- with hydrocephalus 741.0
Myelopathic - see condition
Myelopathy (spinal cord) 336.9
- cervical 721.1 † 336.3*
- drug-induced 336.8
- due to or with
- - degeneration or displacement, intervertebral disc 722.7 † 336.3*
- - infection - see Encephalitis
- - intervertebral disc disorder 722.7 † 336.3*
- - neoplastic disease 239.9 † 336.3*
- - spondylosis 721.- † 336.3*
- lumbar, lumbosacral 721.4 † 336.3*
- necrotic (subacute) 336.1
- radiation-induced 336.8
- spondylogenic NEC 721.9 † 336.3*
- thoracic 721.4 † 336.3*
- toxic 989.9 † 323.7*
- transverse (see also Encephalitis) 323.9
- vascular 336.1
Myeloradiculitis (see also Polyneuropathy) 357.0
Myeloradiculodysplasia (spinal) 742.5
Myelosarcoma (M9930/3) 205.3
Myelosclerosis 289.8
- with myeloid metaplasia (M9961/1) 238.7
- disseminated, of nervous system 340
- megakaryocytic (M9961/1) 238.7
Myelosis (M9860/3) 205.9
- acute (M9861/3) 205.0
- aleukemic (M9864/3) 205.8
- chronic (M9863/3) 205.1
- erythremic (M9840/3) 207.0
- - acute (M9841/3) 207.0
- megakaryocytic (M9920/3) 207.2
- non-leukemic 288.8
- subacute (M9862/3) 205.2
Myesthenia - see Myasthenia

Myiasis (cavernous) 134.0
- orbit 134.0 † 376.1*
Myoadenoma, prostate 600
Myoblastoma
- granular cell (M9580/0) - see also
  Neoplasm, connective tissue, benign
- - malignant (M9580/3) - see Neoplasm,
  connective tissue, malignant
- tongue (M9580/0) 210.1
Myocardial - see condition
Myocardiopathy (see also Cardiomyopathy)
  425.4
Myocarditis (with arteriosclerosis) (chronic)
  (fibroid) (interstitial) (old) (progressive)
  (senile) 429.0
- with
- - rheumatic fever (conditions in 390)
    398.0
- - - active (see also Myocarditis, acute,
    rheumatic) 391.2
- - - inactive or quiescent (with chorea)
    398.0
- active 422.9
- - rheumatic 391.2
- - - with chorea (acute) (rheumatic)
    (Sydenham's) 392.0
- acute or subacute (interstitial) 422.9
- - rheumatic 391.2
- - - with chorea (acute) (rheumatic)
    (Sydenham's) 392.0
- arteriosclerotic (see also Disease,
  cardiovascular) 429.2
- aseptic of newborn 074.2 † 422.0*
- bacterial (acute) 422.9
- congenital 746.8
- Coxsackie (virus) 074.2 † 422.0*
- diphtheritic 032.8 † 422.0*
- due to or in
- - diphtheria 032.8 † 422.0*
- - epidemic louse-borne typhus 080 †
    422.0*
- - scarlet fever 034.1 † 422.0*
- - toxoplasmosis (acquired) 130 † 422.0*
- - typhoid 002.0 † 422.0*
- - typhus NEC 081.9 † 422.0*
- epidemic of newborn 074.2 † 422.0*
- Fiedler's (acute) (isolated) 422.9
- hypertensive (see also Hypertension,
  heart) 402.9
- idiopathic 422.9
- infective 422.9
- influenzal 487.8 † 422.0*
- isolated 422.9
- malignant 422.9
- rheumatic (chronic) (inactive) (with
  chorea) 398.0
- - active or acute 391.2

Myocarditis - continued
- rheumatic - continued
- - active or acute - continued
- - - with chorea (acute) (rheumatic)
    (Sydenham's) 392.0
- septic 422.9
- syphilitic (chronic) 093.8 † 422.0*
- toxic 422.9
- - rheumatic (see also Myocarditis, acute,
  rheumatic) 391.2
- tuberculous 017.8 † 422.0*
- typhoid 002.0 † 422.0*
- valvular - see Endocarditis
- virus, viral (except Coxsackie) 422.9
- - of newborn (Coxsackie) 074.2 † 422.0*
Myocardium, myocardial - see condition
Myocardosis (see also Cardiomyopathy)
  425.4
Myoclonia (essential) 333.2
- epileptica 333.2
- Friedrich's 333.2
- massive 333.2
Myoclonic jerks 333.2
Myoclonus (familial essential) (multifocal)
  (simplex) 333.2
- facial 351.8
- pharyngeal 478.2
Myodiastasis 728.9
Myoendocarditis - see Endocarditis
Myoepithelioma (M8982/0) - see
  Neoplasm, benign
Myofasciitis (acute) 729.1
- low back 724.2
Myofibroma (M8890/0) - see also
  Neoplasm, connective tissue, benign
- uterus (cervix) (corpus) 218
Myofibrosis 728.2
- heart (see also Myocarditis) 429.0
- humeroscapular region 726.2
- scapulohumeral 726.2
Myofibrositis 729.1
- scapulohumeral 726.2
Myogelosis (occupational) 728.8
Myoglobinuria 791.3
Myoglobulinuria, primary 791.3
Myokymia - see Myoclonus
Myolipoma (M8860/0)
- specified site - see Neoplasm, connective
  tissue, benign
- unspecified site 223.0
Myoma (M8895/0) - see also Neoplasm,
  connective tissue, benign
- malignant (M8895/3) - see Neoplasm,
  connective tissue, malignant
- prostate 600
- uterus (cervix) (corpus) 218
- - in pregnancy or childbirth 654.1

Myoma - *continued*
− uterus - *continued*
− − in pregnancy or childbirth - *continued*
− − − causing obstructed labor 660.2
− − − fetus or newborn 763.8
Myomalacia 728.9
− cordis, heart (see also Degeneration,
  myocardial) 429.1
Myometritis (see also Endometritis) 615.9
Myometrium - see condition
Myopathy 359.9
− alcoholic 359.4
− centronuclear 359.0
− congenital (benign) 359.0
− distal 359.1
− due to drugs 359.4
− endocrine NEC 259.9 † 359.5*
− extraocular muscles 376.8
− facioscapulohumeral 359.1
− in
− − Addison's disease 255.4 † 359.5*
− − amyloidosis 277.3 † 359.6*
− − cretinism 243 † 359.5*
− − Cushing's syndrome 255.0 † 359.5*
− − disseminated lupus erythematosus
    710.0 † 359.6*
− − giant-cell arteritis 446.5 † 359.6*
− − hyperadrenocorticism NEC 255.3 †
    359.5*
− − hyperparathyroidism 252.0 † 359.5*
− − hypopituitarism 253.2 † 359.5*
− − hypothyroidism 244.9 † 359.5*
− − malignant neoplasm NEC (M8000/3)
    199.1 † 359.6*
− − myxedema 244.9 † 359.5*
− − polyarteritis nodosa 446.0 † 359.6*
− − rheumatoid arthritis 714.0 † 359.6*
− − sarcoidosis 135 † 359.6*
− − scleroderma 710.1 † 359.6*
− − Sjogren's disease 710.2 † 359.6*
− − thyrotoxicosis NEC 242.9 † 359.5*
− inflammatory 359.8
− limb-girdle 359.1
− myotubular 359.0
− nemaline 359.0
− ocular 359.1
− oculopharyngeal 359.1
− primary 359.8
− progressive NEC 359.8
− rod 359.0
− scapulohumeral 359.1
− specified NEC 359.8
− toxic 359.4
Myopericarditis (see also Pericarditis) 423.9
Myopia (axial) (congenital) (increased
  curvature or refraction, nucleus of lens)
  (progressive) 367.1

Myopia - *continued*
− malignant 360.2
Myosarcoma (M8895/3) - see Neoplasm,
  connective tissue, malignant
Myosis 379.4
− stromal (endolymphatic) (M8931/1)
  236.0
Myositis 729.1
− clostridial 040.0
− due to posture 729.1
− epidemic 074.1
− fibrosa or fibrous (chronic) 728.2
− − Volkmann (complicating trauma)
    958.6
− infective 728.0
− interstitial 728.8
− multiple - see Polymyositis
− occupational 729.1
− orbital, chronic 376.1
− ossificans or ossifying (circumscribed)
  (progressive) (traumatic) 728.1
− purulent 728.0
− rheumatic 729.1
− rheumatoid 729.1
− suppurative 728.0
− traumatic (old) 729.1
Myotonia (acquisita) (intermittens) 728.8
− atrophica 359.2
− congenita 359.2
− dystrophica 359.2
Myotonic pupil 379.4
Myriapodiasis 134.1
Myringitis 384.8
− with otitis media - see Otitis, media
− acute 384.0
− bullous 384.0
− chronic 384.1
Mysophobia 300.2
Mytilotoxism 988.0

Myxadenitis labialis 528.5
Myxedema (infantile) 244.9
− circumscribed 244.9
− congenital 243
− cutis 701.8
− localized (pretibial) 244.9
− papular 701.8
− pituitary 244.8
− postpartum 674.8
− pretibial 244.9
− thyroid (gland) 244.9
Myxochondrosarcoma (M9220/3) - see
  Neoplasm, cartilage, malignant

Myxofibroma (M8811/0) - see Neoplasm,
  connective tissue, benign
− odontogenic (M9320/0) 213.1
− − upper jaw (bone) 213.0

Myxofibrosarcoma (M8811/3) - see
  Neoplasm, connective tissue, malignant
Myxolipoma (M8852/0) 214
Myxoliposarcoma (M8852/3) - see
  Neoplasm, connective tissue, malignant
Myxoma (M8840/0) - see also Neoplasm,
  connective tissue, benign

Myxoma - *continued*
– odontogenic (M9320/0) 213.1
– – upper jaw (bone) 213.0
Myxosarcoma (M8840/3) - see Neoplasm,
  connective tissue, malignant

N

Naegeli's
– disease 287.1
– leukemia, monocytic (M9863/3) 205.1
Naffziger's syndrome 353.0
Naga sore (see also Ulcer, skin) 707.9
Nagele's pelvis 738.6
– with disproportion 653.0
– – causing obstructed labor 660.1
– – fetus or newborn 763.1
Nail - see also condition
– biting 307.9
– patella syndrome 756.8
Nanism, nanosomia (see also Dwarfism)
  259.4
– pituitary 253.3
– renis, renalis 588.0
Nanukayami 100.8
Napkin rash 691.0
Narcissism 302.8
Narcolepsy 347
Narcosis
– carbon dioxide (respiratory) 786.0
– due to drug
– – correct substance properly
     administered 780.0
– – overdose or wrong substance given or
     taken 977.9
– – – specified drug - see Table of drugs
     and chemicals
Narcotism (chronic) (see also Dependence)
  304.9
– acute NEC
– – correct substance properly
     administered 349.8
– – overdose or wrong substance given or
     taken 965.8
– – – specified drug - see Table of drugs
     and chemicals
Narrow
– anterior chamber angle 365.0
– pelvis - see Contraction, pelvis
Narrowing
– artery NEC 447.1
– – auditory, internal 433.8
– – basilar 433.0
– – – with other precerebral artery 433.3
– – – bilateral 433.3
– – carotid 433.1
– – – with other precerebral artery 433.3
– – – bilateral 433.3

Narrowing - continued
– artery NEC - continued
– – cerebellar 433.8
– – choroidal 433.8
– – communicative posterior 433.8
– – coronary 414.0
– – – congenital 090.5
– – – due to syphilis 093.8
– – hypophyseal 433.8
– – pontine 433.8
– – precerebral NEC 433.9
– – – multiple or bilateral 433.3
– – vertebral 433.2
– – – with other precerebral artery 433.3
– – – bilateral 433.3
– auditory canal (external) 380.5
– cerebral arteries 437.0
– cicatricial - see Cicatrix
– eustachian tube 381.6
– eyelid 374.4
– intervertebral disc or space NEC - see
  Degeneration, intervertebral disc
– joint space, hip 719.8
– larynx 478.7
– mesenteric artery (with gangrene) 557.0
– palate 524.8
– palpebral fissure 374.4
– retinal artery 362.1
– ureter 593.3
– urethra (see also Stricture, urethra) 598.9
Narrowness, abnormal, eyelid 743.6
Nasal - see condition
Nasolachrymal, nasolacrimal - see condition
Nasopharyngeal - see also condition
– pituitary gland 759.2
Nasopharyngitis (acute) (infective)
  (subacute) 460
– chronic 472.2
– – due to external agent - see condition,
     respiratory, chronic, due to
– due to external agent - see condition,
  respiratory, due to
– septic 034.0
– streptococcal 034.0
– suppurative (chronic) 472.2
– ulcerative (chronic) 472.2
Nasopharynx, nasopharyngeal - see
  condition
Natal tooth, teeth 520.6
Nausea (see also Vomiting) 787.0

Nausea - *continued*
- epidemic 078.8
- gravidarum 643.0
- marina 994.6
Navel - see condition
Nearsightedness 367.1
Nebula, cornea 371.0
Necator americanus infestation 126.1
Necatoriasis 126.1
Neck - see condition
Necrencephalus (see also Softening, brain) 437.8
Necrobacillosis 040.3
Necrobiosis 799.8
- brain or cerebral (see also Softening, brain) 437.8
- lipoidica 709.3
- - diabeticorum 250.7 † 709.8*
Necrolysis, toxic epidermal 695.1
- due to drug
- - correct substance properly administered 695.1
- - overdose or wrong substance given or taken 977.9
- - - specified drug - see Table of drugs and chemicals
Necrophilia 302.8
Necrosis, necrotic (ischemic) (see also Gangrene) 785.4
- adrenal (capsule) (gland) 255.8
- antrum 478.1
- aorta (hyaline) (see also Aneurysm, aorta) 441.6
- - cystic medial 441.0
- - ruptured 441.5
- artery 447.5
- bladder (aseptic) (sphincter) 596.8
- bone 730.1
- - acute 730.0
- - aseptic or avascular 733.4
- - ethmoid 478.1
- - jaw 526.4
- - tuberculous - see Tuberculosis, bone
- brain (softening) (see also Softening, brain) 437.8
- breast (aseptic) (fat) (segmental) 611.3
- bronchi 519.1
- central nervous system NEC (see also Softening, brain) 437.8
- cerebellar (see also Softening, brain) 437.8
- cerebral (softening) (see also Softening, brain) 437.8
- cornea (see also Keratitis) 371.4
- cystic medial (aorta) 441.0
- dental 521.0
- esophagus 530.8

Necrosis - *continued*
- ethmoid (bone) 478.1
- eyelid 374.5
- fat (generalized) (see also Degeneration, fatty) 729.3
- - breast (aseptic) 611.3
- - localized - see Degeneration by site, fatty
- gallbladder (see also Cholecystitis, acute) 575.0
- gastric 537.8
- heart - see Infarct, myocardium
- hepatic (see also Necrosis, liver) 570
- hip (aseptic) (avascular) 733.4
- intestine (acute) (haemorrhagic) (massive) 557.0
- jaw 526.4
- kidney (bilateral) 583.9
- - acute 584.9
- - cortical 583.6
- - - acute 584.6
- - medullary (papillary) (see also Pyelitis) 590.8
- - - in
- - - - acute renal failure 584.7
- - - - nephritis, nephropathy 583.7
- - papillary - see Necrosis kidney, medullary
- - tubular 584.5
- - - with
- - - - abortion - see categories 634-639, fourth digit .3
- - - - ectopic or molar pregnancy 639.3
- - - complicating pregnancy 648.9
- - - - fetus or newborn 760.1
- - - following labor and delivery 669.3
- larynx 478.7
- liver (acute) (diffuse) (massive) (subacute) 570
- - complicating pregnancy 646.7
- - - fetus or newborn 760.8
- - puerperal, postpartum 674.8
- lung 513.0
- lymphatic gland 683
- mammary gland 611.3
- mastoid (chronic) 383.1
- mesentery 557.0
- - fat 567.8
- mitral valve - see Insufficiency, mitral
- myocardium, myocardial - see Infarct, myocardium
- nose 478.1
- oesophagus 530.8
- omentum 557.0
- - fat 567.8
- orbit, orbital 376.1
- ossicles, ear 385.2

	Malignant	Benign	In-situ	Un-certain be-haviour	Un-specified nature
Neoplasm, neoplastic	199.1	229.9	234.9	238.9	239.9

Notes

1. The list below gives the code numbers for neoplasms by anatomical site. For each site there are five possible code numbers according to whether the neoplasm in question is malignant, benign, in situ, of uncertain behaviour or of unspecified nature. The description of the neoplasm will often indicate which of the five columns is appropriate, e.g. *malignant* melanoma of skin, *benign* fibroadenoma of breast, carcinoma *in situ* of cervix uteri.

Where such descriptors are not present, the remainder of the Index should be consulted, where guidance is given to the appropriate column for each morphological (histological) variety listed, e.g. Mesonephroma – *see* Neoplasm, *malignant;* Embryoma – *see also* Neoplasm, *uncertain behaviour;* Disease, Bowen's – *see* Neoplasm, skin, *in situ.* However, the guidance in the Index can be overridden if one of the descriptors mentioned above is present, e.g. malignant adenoma of colon is coded to 153.9 and not to 211.3 as the adjective "malignant" overrides the Index entry "Adenoma – *see also* Neoplasm, benign".

2. The first of the five columns gives the code numbers for malignant neoplasms presumed or stated to be primary. For the code numbers of malignant neoplasms presumed or stated to be secondary, *see* "Secondary neoplasm".

3. Sites marked with the sign # (e.g. face NEC #) should be classified to malignant neoplasm of *skin* of these sites if the variety of neoplasm is a squamous cell carcinoma or an epidermoid carcinoma and to benign neoplasm of *skin* of these sites if the variety of neoplasm is a papilloma (any type).

4. Carcinomas and adenocarcinomas, of any type other than intraosseous or odontogenic, of sites marked with the sign ◊ (e.g. ischium ◊) should be considered as constituting metastatic spread from an unspecified primary site and coded to 198.5 for morbidity coding and to 199.1 for underlying cause of death coding.

	Malignant	Benign	In-situ	Uncertain behaviour	Unspecified nature
Neoplasm - *continued*					
– abdomen, abdominal	195.2	229.8	234.8	238.8	239.8
– – cavity	195.2	229.8	234.8	238.8	239.8
– – organ	195.2	229.8		238.8	239.8
– – viscera	195.2	229.8		238.8	239.8
– – wall	173.5	216.5	232.5	238.2	239.2
– abdominopelvic	195.8	229.8		238.8	239.8
– accessory sinus - see Neoplasm, sinus					
– acromion (process) ◊	170.4	213.4		238.0	239.2
– adenoid (tissue)	147.1	210.7	230.0	235.1	239.0
– adipose tissue - see Neoplasm, connective tissue					
– adnexa (uterine)	183.9	221.8	233.3	236.3	239.5
– adrenal (cortex) (gland) (medulla)	194.0	227.0	234.8	237.2	239.7
– ala nasi (external)	173.3	216.3	232.3	238.2	239.2
– alimentary canal or tract NEC	159.9	211.9	230.9	235.5	239.0
– alveolar					
– – mucosa	143.9	210.4	230.0	235.1	239.0
– – – lower	143.1	210.4	230.0	235.1	239.0
– – – upper	143.0	210.4	230.0	235.1	239.0
– – ridge or process ◊	170.1	213.1		238.0	239.2
– – – carcinoma	143.9				
– – – – lower	143.1				
– – – – upper	143.0				
– – – lower ◊	170.1	213.1		238.0	239.2
– – – mucosa	143.9	210.4	230.0	235.1	239.0
– – – – lower	143.1	210.4	230.0	235.1	239.0
– – – – upper	143.0	210.4	230.0	235.1	239.0
– – – upper ◊	170.0	213.0		238.0	239.2
– – sulcus	145.1	210.4	230.0	235.1	239.0
– alveolus	143.9	210.4	230.0	235.1	239.0
– – lower	143.1	210.4	230.0	235.1	239.0
– – upper	143.0	210.4	230.0	235.1	239.0
– ampulla of Vater	156.2	211.5	230.8	235.3	239.0
– ankle NEC #	195.5	229.8	232.7	238.8	239.8
– anorectum, anorectal (junction)	154.8	211.4	230.7	235.2	239.0
– antecubital fossa or space #	195.4	229.8	232.6	238.8	239.8
– antrum (Highmore) (maxillary)	160.2	212.0	231.8	235.9	239.1
– – pyloric	151.2	211.1	230.2	235.2	239.0
– – tympanicum	160.1	212.0	231.8	235.9	239.1
– anus, anal	154.3	211.4	230.6	235.5	239.0
– – canal	154.2	211.4	230.5	235.5	239.0
– – margin	173.5	216.5	232.5	238.2	239.2
– – skin	173.5	216.5	232.5	238.2	239.2

	Malignant	Benign	In-situ	Un-certain be-haviour	Un-specified nature
Neoplasm - *continued*					
− anus - *continued*					
− − sphincter	154.2	211.4	230.5	235.5	239.0
− aorta (thoracic)	171.4	215.4		238.1	239.2
− − abdominal	171.5	215.5		238.1	239.2
− aortic body	194.6	227.6		237.3	239.7
− aponeurosis	171.9	215.9		238.1	239.2
− − palmar	171.2	215.2		238.1	239.2
− − plantar	171.3	215.3		238.1	239.2
− appendix	153.5	211.3	230.3	235.2	239.0
− arachnoid (cerebral)	192.1	225.2		237.6	239.7
− − spinal	192.3	225.4		237.6	239.7
− areola (female)	174.0	217	233.0	238.3	239.3
− − male	175	217	233.0	238.3	239.3
− arm NEC #	195.4	229.8	232.6	238.8	239.8
− artery - see Neoplasm, connective tissue					
− ary-epiglottic fold	148.2	210.8	230.0	235.1	239.0
− − hypopharyngeal aspect	148.2	210.8	230.0	235.1	239.0
− − laryngeal aspect	161.1	212.1	231.0	235.6	239.1
− − marginal zone	148.2	210.8	230.0	235.1	239.0
− arytenoid (cartilage)	161.3	212.1	231.0	235.6	239.1
− − fold - see Neoplasm, ary-epiglottic					
− atlas ◊	170.2	213.2		238.0	239.2
− atrium, cardiac	164.1	212.7		238.8	239.8
− auditory					
− − canal (external)	173.2	216.2	232.2	238.2	239.2
− − − internal	160.1	212.0	231.8	235.9	239.1
− − nerve	192.0	225.1		237.9	239.7
− − tube	160.1	212.0	231.8	235.9	239.1
− − − opening	147.2	210.7	230.0	235.1	239.0
− auricle, ear	173.2	216.2	232.2	238.2	239.2
− − cartilage	171.0	215.0		238.1	239.2
− auricular canal (external)	173.2	216.2	232.2	238.2	239.2
− − internal	160.1	212.0	231.8	235.9	239.1
− autonomic nerve or nervous system NEC ...	171.9	215.9		238.1	239.2
− axilla, axillary	195.1	229.8	234.8	238.8	239.8
− − fold	173.5	216.5	232.5	238.2	239.2
− back NEC #	195.8	229.8	232.5	238.8	239.8
− Bartholin's gland	184.1	221.2	233.3	236.3	239.5
− basal ganglia	191.0	225.0		237.5	239.6
− basis pedunculi	191.7	225.0		237.5	239.6
− bile or biliary (tract)	156.9	211.5	230.8	235.3	239.0
− − canals, interlobular	155.1	211.5	230.8	235.3	239.0
− − duct or passage (common) (cystic)					
(extrahepatic)	156.1	211.5	230.8	235.3	239.0
− − − interlobular	155.1	211.5	230.8	235.3	239.0
− − − intrahepatic	155.1	211.5	230.8	235.3	239.0
− − − − and extrahepatic	156.9	211.5	230.8	235.3	239.0
− bladder (urinary)	188.9	223.3	233.7	236.7	239.4
− − dome	188.1	223.3	233.7	236.7	239.4
− − neck	188.5	223.3	233.7	236.7	239.4
− − orifice	188.9	223.3	233.7	236.7	239.4
− − − ureteric	188.6	223.3	233.7	236.7	239.4

	Malignant	Benign	In-situ	Un-certain be-haviour	Un-specified nature
Neoplasm - *continued*					
– bladder - *continued*					
– – orifice - *continued*					
– – – urethral	188.5	223.3	233.7	236.7	239.4
– – sphincter	188.8	223.3	233.7	236.7	239.4
– – trigone	188.0	223.3	233.7	236.7	239.4
– – urachus	188.7	223.3	233.7	236.7	239.4
– – wall	188.9	223.3	233.7	236.7	239.4
– – – anterior	188.3	223.3	233.7	236.7	239.4
– – – lateral	188.2	223.3	233.7	236.7	239.4
– – – posterior	188.4	223.3	233.7	236.7	239.4
– blood vessel - see Neoplasm, connective tissue					
– bone (periosteum) ◊	170.9	213.9		238.0	239.2

Note — Carcinomas and adenocarcinomas, of any type other than intraosseous or odontogenic, of the sites listed under "Neoplasm, bone" should be considered as constituting metastatic spread from an unspecified primary site and coded to 198.5 for morbidity coding and to 199.1 for underlying cause of death coding.

	Malignant	Benign	In-situ	Un-certain be-haviour	Un-specified nature
Neoplasm - *continued*					
– bone - *continued*					
– – acetabulum	170.6	213.6		238.0	239.2
– – acromion (process)	170.4	213.4		238.0	239.2
– – ankle	170.8	213.8		238.0	239.2
– – arm NEC	170.4	213.4		238.0	239.2
– – astragalus	170.8	213.8		238.0	239.2
– – atlas	170.2	213.2		238.0	239.2
– – axis	170.2	213.2		238.0	239.2
– – back NEC	170.2	213.2		238.0	239.2
– – calcaneus	170.8	213.8		238.0	239.2
– – calvarium	170.0	213.0		238.0	239.2
– – carpus (any)	170.5	213.5		238.0	239.2
– – cartilage NEC	170.9	213.9		238.0	239.2
– – clavicle	170.3	213.3		238.0	239.2
– – clivus	170.0	213.0		238.0	239.2
– – coccygeal vertebra	170.6	213.6		238.0	239.2
– – coccyx	170.6	213.6		238.0	239.2
– – costal cartilage	170.3	213.3		238.0	239.2
– – cranial	170.0	213.0		238.0	239.2
– – digital	170.9	213.9		238.0	239.2
– – – finger	170.5	213.5		238.0	239.2
– – – toe	170.8	213.8		238.0	239.2
– – elbow	170.4	213.4		238.0	239.2
– – ethmoid (labyrinth)	170.0	213.0		238.0	239.2
– – face	170.0	213.0		238.0	239.2
– – femur (any part)	170.7	213.7		238.0	239.2
– – fibula (any part)	170.7	213.7		238.0	239.2
– – finger (any)	170.5	213.5		238.0	239.2
– – foot	170.8	213.8		238.0	239.2
– – forearm	170.4	213.4		238.0	239.2
– – frontal	170.0	213.0		238.0	239.2

	Malignant	Benign	In-situ	Uncertain behaviour	Unspecified nature
Neoplasm - *continued*					
− bone - *continued*					
− − hand	170.5	213.5		238.0	239.2
− − heel	170.8	213.8		238.0	239.2
− − hip	170.6	213.6		238.0	239.2
− − humerus (any part)	170.4	213.4		238.0	239.2
− − hyoid	170.0	213.0		238.0	239.2
− − ilium	170.6	213.6		238.0	239.2
− − innominate	170.6	213.6		238.0	239.2
− − intervertebral cartilage or disc	170.2	213.2		238.0	239.2
− − ischium	170.6	213.6		238.0	239.2
− − jaw - see Neoplasm, jaw, bone					
− − knee	170.7	213.7		238.0	239.2
− − leg NEC	170.7	213.7		238.0	239.2
− − limb NEC	170.9	213.9		238.0	239.2
− − − lower (long bones)	170.7	213.7		238.0	239.2
− − − − short bones	170.8	213.8		238.0	239.2
− − − upper (long bones)	170.4	213.4		238.0	239.2
− − − − short bones	170.5	213.5		238.0	239.2
− − long	170.9	213.9		238.0	239.2
− − − lower limbs NEC	170.7	213.7		238.0	239.2
− − − upper limbs NEC	170.4	213.4		238.0	239.2
− − mandible	170.1	213.1		238.0	239.2
− − marrow NEC	202.9				
− − maxilla, maxillary (superior)	170.0	213.0		238.0	239.2
− − − inferior	170.1	213.1		238.0	239.2
− − metacarpus (any)	170.5	213.5		238.0	239.2
− − metatarsus (any)	170.8	213.8		238.0	239.2
− − nose, nasal	170.0	213.0		238.0	239.2
− − occipital	170.0	213.0		238.0	239.2
− − orbit	170.0	213.0		238.0	239.2
− − parietal	170.0	213.0		238.0	239.2
− − patella	170.8	213.8		238.0	239.2
− − pelvic	170.6	213.6		238.0	239.2
− − phalanges	170.9	213.9		238.0	239.2
− − − foot	170.8	213.8		238.0	239.2
− − − hand	170.5	213.5		238.0	239.2
− − pubic	170.6	213.6		238.0	239.2
− − radius (any part)	170.4	213.4		238.0	239.2
− − rib	170.3	213.3		238.0	239.2
− − sacral vertebra	170.6	213.6		238.0	239.2
− − sacrum	170.6	213.6		238.0	239.2
− − scapula (any part)	170.4	213.4		238.0	239.2
− − sella turcica	170.0	213.0		238.0	239.2
− − short	170.9	213.9		238.0	239.2
− − − lower limbs	170.8	213.8		238.0	239.2
− − − upper limbs	170.5	213.5		238.0	239.2
− − shoulder	170.4	213.4		238.0	239.2
− − skeleton, skeletal NEC	170.9	213.9		238.0	239.2
− − skull	170.0	213.0		238.0	239.2
− − sphenoid	170.0	213.0		238.0	239.2
− − spine, spinal (column)	170.2	213.2		238.0	239.2
− − − coccyx	170.6	213.6		238.0	239.2

	Malignant	Benign	In-situ	Un-certain be-haviour	Un-specified nature
Neoplasm - *continued*					
− bone - *continued*					
− − spine - *continued*					
− − − sacrum	170.6	213.6		238.0	239.2
− − sternum	170.3	213.3		238.0	239.2
− − tarsus (any)	170.8	213.8		238.0	239.2
− − temporal	170.0	213.0		238.0	239.2
− − thumb	170.5	213.5		238.0	239.2
− − tibia (any part)	170.7	213.7		238.0	239.2
− − toe (any)	170.8	213.8		238.0	239.2
− − turbinate	170.0	213.0		238.0	239.2
− − ulna (any part)	170.4	213.4		238.0	239.2
− − vertebra (column)	170.2	213.2		238.0	239.2
− − − coccyx	170.6	213.6		238.0	239.2
− − − sacrum	170.6	213.6		238.0	239.2
− − vomer	170.0	213.0		238.0	239.2
− − wrist	170.5	213.5		238.0	239.2
− − xiphoid process	170.3	213.3		238.0	239.2
− − zygomatic	170.0	213.0		238.0	239.2
− book leaf (mouth)	145.8	210.4	230.0	235.1	239.0
− bowel - see Neoplasm, intestine					
− brachial plexus	171.2	215.2		238.1	239.2
− brain NEC	191.9	225.0		237.5	239.6
− − meninges	192.1	225.2		237.6	239.7
− − stem	191.7	225.0		237.5	239.6
− branchial (cleft) (vestiges)	146.8	210.6	230.0	235.1	239.0
− breast (female) (connective tissue) (glandular tissue) (soft parts)	174.9	217	233.0	238.3	239.3
− − areola	174.0	217	233.0	238.3	239.3
− − axillary tail	174.6	217	233.0	238.3	239.3
− − central portion	174.1	217	233.0	238.3	239.3
− − ectopic site	174.8	217	233.0	238.3	239.3
− − inner	174.8	217	233.0	238.3	239.3
− − lower	174.8	217	233.0	238.3	239.3
− − lower-inner quadrant	174.3	217	233.0	238.3	239.3
− − lower-outer quadrant	174.5	217	233.0	238.3	239.3
− − male (any part)	175	217	233.0	238.3	239.3
− − midline	174.8	217	233.0	238.3	239.3
− − outer	174.8	217	233.0	238.3	239.3
− − skin	173.5	216.5	232.5	238.2	239.2
− − tail (axillary)	174.6	217	233.0	238.3	239.3
− − upper	174.8	217	233.0	238.3	239.3
− − upper-inner quadrant	174.2	217	233.0	238.3	239.3
− − upper-outer quadrant	174.4	217	233.0	238.3	239.3
− broad ligament	183.3	221.0		236.3	239.5
− bronchiogenic, bronchogenic (lung)	162.9	212.3	231.2	235.7	239.1
− bronchiole	162.9	212.3	231.2	235.7	239.1
− bronchus	162.9	212.3	231.2	235.7	239.1
− − carina	162.2	212.3	231.2	235.7	239.1
− − lower lobe of lung	162.5	212.3	231.2	235.7	239.1
− − main	162.2	212.3	231.2	235.7	239.1
− − middle lobe of lung	162.4	212.3	231.2	235.7	239.1
− − upper lobe of lung	162.3	212.3	231.2	235.7	239.1

	Malignant	Benign	In-situ	Uncertain behaviour	Unspecified nature
Neoplasm - *continued*					
– brow	173.3	216.3	232.3	238.2	239.2
– buccal (cavity)	145.9	210.4	230.0	235.1	239.0
– – mucosa	145.0	210.4	230.0	235.1	239.0
– – sulcus (lower) (upper)	145.1	210.4	230.0	235.1	239.0
– bulbo-urethral gland	189.3	223.8	233.9	236.9	239.5
– bursa - see Neoplasm, connective tissue					
– buttock NEC #	195.3	229.8	232.5	238.8	239.8
– caecum	153.4	211.3	230.3	235.2	239.0
– calf #	195.5	229.8	232.7	238.8	239.8
– calvarium ◊	170.0	213.0		238.0	239.2
– calyx, renal	189.1	223.1	233.9	236.9	239.5
– canal					
– – anal	154.2	211.4	230.5	235.5	239.0
– – auditory (external)	173.2	216.2	232.2	238.2	239.2
– – auricular (external)	173.2	216.2	232.2	238.2	239.2
– canaliculi					
– – biliferi	155.1	211.5	230.8	235.3	239.0
– – intrahepatic	155.1	211.5	230.8	235.3	239.0
– canthus (eye) (inner) (outer)	173.1	216.1	232.1	238.2	239.2
– capillary - see Neoplasm, connective tissue					
– capsule, internal	191.0	225.0		237.5	239.6
– cardia (gastric)	151.0	211.1	230.2	235.2	239.0
– cardiac orifice (stomach)	151.0	211.1	230.2	235.2	239.0
– cardio-esophageal junction	151.0	211.1	230.2	235.2	239.0
– cardio-esophagus	151.0	211.1	230.2	235.2	239.0
– carina (tracheal)	162.2	212.3	231.2	235.7	239.1
– carotid (artery)	171.0	215.0		238.1	239.2
– – body	194.5	227.5		237.3	239.7
– cartilage (articular) (joint) (see also Neoplasm, bone) NEC	170.9	213.9		238.0	239.2
– – arytenoid	161.3	212.1	231.0	235.6	239.1
– – auricular	171.0	215.0		238.1	239.2
– – bronchi	162.2	212.3		235.7	239.1
– – costal ◊	170.3	213.3		238.0	239.2
– – cricoid	161.3	212.1	231.0	235.6	239.1
– – cuneiform	161.3	212.1	231.0	235.6	239.1
– – ear (external)	171.0	215.0		238.1	239.2
– – epiglottis	161.1	212.1	231.0	235.6	239.1
– – eyelid	171.0	215.0		238.1	239.2
– – larynx, laryngeal	161.3	212.1	231.0	235.6	239.1
– – nose, nasal	160.0	212.0	231.8	235.9	239.1
– – rib ◊	170.3	213.3		238.0	239.2
– – semilunar (knee) ◊	170.7	213.7		238.0	239.2
– – thyroid	161.3	212.1	231.0	235.6	239.1
– – trachea	162.0	212.2		235.7	239.1
– cauda equina	192.2	225.3		237.5	239.7
– cavity					
– – buccal	145.9	210.4	230.0	235.1	239.0
– – nasal	160.0	212.0	231.8	235.9	239.1
– – oral	145.9	210.4	230.0	235.1	239.0
– – peritoneal	158.9	211.8		235.4	239.0
– – tympanic	160.1	212.0	231.8	235.9	239.1

	Malignant	Benign	In-situ	Un-certain be-haviour	Un-specified nature
Neoplasm - *continued*					
– cecum	153.4	211.3	230.3	235.2	239.0
– central					
– – nervous system - see Neoplasm, nervous system					
– – white matter	191.0	225.0		237.5	239.6
– cerebellopontine	191.6	225.0		237.5	239.6
– cerebellum, cerebellar	191.6	225.0		237.5	239.6
– cerebrum, cerebral (cortex) (hemisphere) (white matter)	191.0	225.0		237.5	239.6
– – meninges	192.1	225.2		237.6	239.7
– – peduncle	191.7	225.0		237.5	239.6
– – ventricle (any)	191.5	225.0		237.5	239.6
– cervical region	195.0	229.8	234.8	238.8	239.8
– cervix (uteri) (uterus)	180.9	219.0	233.1	236.0	239.5
– – canal	180.0	219.0	233.1	236.0	239.5
– – squamocolumnar junction	180.8	219.0	233.1	236.0	239.5
– – stump	180.8	219.0	233.1	236.0	239.5
– cheek	195.0	229.8	234.8	238.8	239.8
– – external	173.3	216.3	232.3	238.2	239.2
– – inner aspect	145.0	210.4	230.0	235.1	239.0
– – internal	145.0	210.4	230.0	235.1	239.0
– – mucosa	145.0	210.4	230.0	235.1	239.0
– chest (wall) NEC	195.1	229.8	234.8	238.8	239.8
– chiasma opticum	192.0	225.1		237.9	239.7
– chin	173.3	216.3	232.3	238.2	239.2
– choana	147.3	210.7	230.0	235.1	239.0
– cholangiole	155.1	211.5	230.8	235.3	239.0
– choledochal duct	156.1	211.5	230.8	235.3	239.0
– choroid	190.6	224.6	234.0	238.8	239.8
– – plexus	191.5	225.0		237.5	239.6
– ciliary body	190.0	224.0	234.0	238.8	239.8
– clavicle ◊	170.3	213.3		238.0	239.2
– clitoris	184.3	221.2	233.3	236.3	239.5
– clivus ◊	170.0	213.0		238.0	239.2
– cloacogenic zone	154.8	211.4	230.7	235.2	239.0
– coccygeal					
– – body or glomus	194.6	227.6		237.3	239.7
– – vertebra ◊	170.6	213.6		238.0	239.2
– coccyx ◊	170.6	213.6		238.0	239.2
– colon - see also Neoplasm, intestine, large					
– – and rectum	154.0	211.4	230.4	235.2	239.0
– column, spinal - see Neoplasm, spine					
– columnella	173.3	216.3	232.3	238.2	239.2
– commissure					
– – labial, lip	140.6	210.4	230.0	235.1	239.0
– – laryngeal	161.0	212.1	231.0	235.6	239.1
– common (bile) duct	156.1	211.5	230.8	235.3	239.0
– concha	173.2	216.2	232.2	238.2	239.2
– – nose	160.0	212.0	231.8	235.9	239.1
– conjunctiva	190.3	224.3	234.0	238.8	239.8
– connective tissue NEC	171.9	215.9		238.1	239.2

Note – For neoplasms of connective tissue (blood vessel, bursa, fascia, ligament, muscle, peripheral nerves, sympathetic and parasympathetic nerves and ganglia, synovia, tendon, etc) or of morphological types that indicate connective tissue, code according to the list under "Neoplasm, connective tissue"; for sites that do not appear in this list, code to neoplasm of that site, e.g.

> liposarcoma, shoulder 171.2
> leiomyosarcoma, stomach 151.9
> neurofibroma, chest wall 215.4

Morphological types that indicate connective tissue appear in their proper place in the alphabetic index with the instruction "*see* Neoplasm, connective tissue,...".

	Malignant	Benign	In-situ	Un-certain be-haviour	Un-specified nature
Neoplasm - *continued*					
– connective tissue NEC - *continued*					
– – abdomen	171.5	215.5		238.1	239.2
– – abdominal wall	171.5	215.5		238.1	239.2
– – ankle	171.3	215.3		238.1	239.2
– – antecubital fossa or space	171.2	215.2		238.1	239.2
– – arm	171.2	215.2		238.1	239.2
– – auricle (ear)	171.0	215.0		238.1	239.2
– – axilla	171.4	215.4		238.1	239.2
– – back	171.7	215.7		238.1	239.2
– – buttock	171.6	215.6		238.1	239.2
– – calf	171.3	215.3		238.1	239.2
– – cervical region	171.0	215.0		238.1	239.2
– – cheek	171.0	215.0		238.1	239.2
– – chest (wall)	171.4	215.4		238.1	239.2
– – chin	171.0	215.0		238.1	239.2
– – diaphragm	171.4	215.4		238.1	239.2
– – ear (external)	171.0	215.0		238.1	239.2
– – elbow	171.2	215.2		238.1	239.2
– – extrarectal	171.6	215.6		238.1	239.2
– – extremity	171.8	215.8		238.1	239.2
– – – lower	171.3	215.3		238.1	239.2
– – – upper	171.2	215.2		238.1	239.2
– – eyelid	171.0	215.0		238.1	239.2
– – face	171.0	215.0		238.1	239.2
– – finger	171.2	215.2		238.1	239.2
– – flank	171.7	215.7		238.1	239.2
– – foot	171.3	215.3		238.1	239.2
– – forearm	171.2	215.2		238.1	239.2
– – forehead	171.0	215.0		238.1	239.2
– – gluteal region	171.6	215.6		238.1	239.2
– – great vessels NEC	171.4	215.4		238.1	239.2
– – groin	171.6	215.6		238.1	239.2
– – hand	171.2	215.2		238.1	239.2
– – head	171.0	215.0		238.1	239.2
– – heel	171.3	215.3		238.1	239.2
– – hip	171.3	215.3		238.1	239.2
– – iliopsoas muscle	171.6	215.6		238.1	239.2
– – infraclavicular region	171.4	215.4		238.1	239.2
– – inguinal (canal) (region)	171.6	215.6		238.1	239.2
– – intrathoracic	171.4	215.4		238.1	239.2

	Malignant	Benign	In-situ	Un-certain be-haviour	Un-specified nature
Neoplasm - *continued*					
− connective tissue NEC - *continued*					
− − ischiorectal fossa	171.6	215.6		238.1	239.2
− − jaw...................................	143.9	210.4		235.1	239.0
− − knee	171.3	215.3		238.1	239.2
− − leg	171.3	215.3		238.1	239.2
− − limb NEC	171.9	215.9		238.1	239.2
− − − lower	171.3	215.3		238.1	239.2
− − − upper	171.2	215.2		238.1	239.2
− − nates	171.6	215.6		238.1	239.2
− − neck	171.0	215.0		238.1	239.2
− − orbit	190.1	224.1		238.8	239.8
− − pararectal	171.6	215.6		238.1	239.2
− − paraurethral	171.6	215.6		238.1	239.2
− − paravaginal	171.6	215.6		238.1	239.2
− − pelvis (floor)	171.6	215.6		238.1	239.2
− − pelvo-abdominal	171.8	215.8		238.1	239.2
− − perineum	171.6	215.6		238.1	239.2
− − perirectal (tissue)	171.6	215.6		238.1	239.2
− − periurethral (tissue)	171.6	215.6		238.1	239.2
− − popliteal fossa or space	171.3	215.3		238.1	239.2
− − presacral	171.6	215.6		238.1	239.2
− − psoas muscle	171.5	215.5		238.1	239.2
− − pterygoid fossa	171.0	215.0		238.1	239.2
− − rectovaginal septum or wall	171.6	215.6		238.1	239.2
− − rectovesical	171.6	215.6		238.1	239.2
− − retroperitoneal	158.0	211.8		235.4	239.0
− − sacrococcygeal region	171.6	215.6		238.1	239.2
− − scalp	171.0	215.0		238.1	239.2
− − scapular region	171.4	215.4		238.1	239.2
− − shoulder	171.2	215.2		238.1	239.2
− − submental	171.0	215.0		238.1	239.2
− − supraclavicular region	171.0	215.0		238.1	239.2
− − temple	171.0	215.0		238.1	239.2
− − temporal region	171.0	215.0		238.1	239.2
− − thigh	171.3	215.3		238.1	239.2
− − thoracic (duct) (wall)	171.4	215.4		238.1	239.2
− − thorax	171.4	215.4		238.1	239.2
− − thumb	171.2	215.2		238.1	239.2
− − toe	171.3	215.3		238.1	239.2
− − trunk	171.7	215.7		238.1	239.2
− − umbilicus	171.5	215.5		238.1	239.2
− − vesicorectal	171.6	215.6		238.1	239.2
− − wrist	171.2	215.2		238.1	239.2
− conus medullaris	192.2	225.3		237.5	239.7
− cord (true) (vocal)	161.0	212.1	231.0	235.6	239.1
− − false	161.1	212.1	231.0	235.6	239.1
− − spermatic	187.6	222.8	233.6	236.6	239.5
− − spinal (cervical) (lumbar) (thoracic)	192.2	225.3		237.5	239.7
− cornea (limbus)	190.4	224.4	234.0	238.8	239.8
− corpus					
− − callosum	191.8	225.0		237.5	239.6
− − cavernosum	187.3	222.1	233.5	236.6	239.5

	Malignant	Benign	In-situ	Un-certain be-haviour	Un-specified nature
Neoplasm - *continued*					
− corpus - *continued*					
− − gastric	151.4	211.1	230.2	235.2	239.0
− − penis	187.3	222.1	233.5	236.6	239.5
− − striatum	191.0	225.0		237.5	239.6
− − uteri	182.0	219.1	233.2	236.0	239.5
− − − isthmus	182.1	219.1	233.2	236.0	239.5
− cortex					
− − adrenal	194.0	227.0	234.8	237.2	239.7
− − cerebral	191.0	225.0		237.5	239.6
− costal cartilage ◊	170.3	213.3		238.0	239.2
− Cowper's gland	189.3	223.8	233.9	236.9	239.5
− cranial (fossa, any)	191.9	225.0		237.5	239.6
− − meninges	192.1	225.2		237.6	239.7
− − nerve (any)	192.0	225.1		237.9	239.7
− craniopharyngeal (duct) (pouch)	194.3	227.3	234.8	237.0	239.7
− cricoid	148.0	210.8	230.0	235.1	239.0
− − cartilage	161.3	212.1	231.0	235.6	239.1
− cricopharynx	148.0	210.8	230.0	235.1	239.0
− crypt of Morgagni	154.8	211.4	230.7	235.2	239.0
− cutaneous - see Neoplasm, skin					
− cutis - see Neoplasm, skin					
− cystic (bile) duct (common)	156.1	211.5	230.8	235.3	239.0
− dermis - see Neoplasm, skin					
− diaphragm	171.4	215.4		238.1	239.2
− digestive organs, system, tube, or tract NEC	159.9	211.9	230.9	235.5	239.0
− disc, intervertebral ◊	170.2	213.2		238.0	239.2
− disease, generalized	199.0				
− disseminated	199.0				
− Douglas' cul-de-sac or pouch	158.8	211.8		235.4	239.0
− duodenojejunal junction	152.8	211.2	230.7	235.2	239.0
− duodenum	152.0	211.2	230.7	235.2	239.0
− dura (mater) (cranial)	192.1	225.2		237.6	239.7
− − cerebral	192.1	225.2		237.6	239.7
− − spinal	192.3	225.4		237.6	239.7
− ear (external)	173.2	216.2	232.2	238.2	239.2
− − auricle	173.2	216.2	232.2	238.2	239.2
− − canal	173.2	216.2	232.2	238.2	239.2
− − cartilage	171.0	215.0		238.1	239.2
− − external meatus	173.2	216.2	232.2	238.2	239.2
− − inner	160.1	212.0	231.8	235.9	239.1
− − lobule	173.2	216.2	232.2	238.2	239.2
− − middle	160.1	212.0	231.8	235.9	239.1
− − skin	173.2	216.2	232.2	238.2	239.2
− earlobe	173.2	216.2	232.2	238.2	239.2
− ejaculatory duct	187.8	222.8	233.6	236.6	239.5
− elbow NEC #	195.4	229.8	232.6	238.8	239.8
− endocardium	164.1	212.7		238.8	239.8
− endocervix (canal) (gland)	180.0	219.0	233.1	236.0	239.5
− endocrine gland NEC	194.9	227.9		237.4	239.7
− − pluriglandular	194.8	227.8	234.8	237.4	239.7
− endometrium (gland) (stroma)	182.0	219.1	233.2	236.0	239.5
− enteric - see Neoplasm, intestine					

	Malignant	Benign	In-situ	Un-certain be-haviour	Un-specified nature
Neoplasm - *continued*					
− ependyma (brain)	191.5	225.0		237.5	239.6
− epicardium	164.1	212.7		238.8	239.8
− epididymis	187.5	222.3	233.6	236.6	239.5
− epidural	192.9	225.9		237.9	239.7
− epiglottis	161.1	212.1	231.0	235.6	239.1
− − anterior aspect or surface	146.4	210.6	230.0	235.1	239.0
− − cartilage	161.1	212.1	231.0	235.6	239.1
− − free border (margin)	146.4	210.6	230.0	235.1	239.0
− − posterior (laryngeal) surface	161.1	212.1	231.0	235.6	239.1
− − suprahyoid portion	161.1	212.1	231.0	235.6	239.1
− esophagogastric junction	151.0	211.1	230.2	235.2	239.0
− esophagus	150.9	211.0	230.1	235.5	239.0
− − abdominal	150.2	211.0	230.1	235.5	239.0
− − cervical	150.0	211.0	230.1	235.5	239.0
− − distal (third)	150.5	211.0	230.1	235.5	239.0
− − lower (third)	150.5	211.0	230.1	235.5	239.0
− − middle (third)	150.4	211.0	230.1	235.5	239.0
− − proximal (third)	150.3	211.0	230.1	235.5	239.0
− − thoracic	150.1	211.0	230.1	235.5	239.0
− − upper (third)	150.3	211.0	230.1	235.5	239.0
− ethmoid (sinus)	160.3	212.0	231.8	235.9	239.1
− − bone or labyrinth ◊	170.0	213.0		238.0	239.2
− eustachian tube	160.1	212.0	231.8	235.9	239.1
− exocervix	180.1	219.0	233.1	236.0	239.5
− external					
− − meatus (ear)	173.2	216.2	232.2	238.2	239.2
− − os uteri	180.1	219.0	233.1	236.0	239.5
− extradural	192.9	225.9		237.9	239.7
− extra-ocular muscle	190.1	224.1		238.8	239.8
− extrarectal	195.3	229.8		238.8	239.8
− extremity #	195.8	229.8	232.8	238.8	239.8
− − lower #	195.5	229.8	232.7	238.8	239.8
− − upper #	195.4	229.8	232.6	238.8	239.8
− eye NEC	190.9	224.9	234.0	238.8	239.8
− eyeball	190.0	224.0	234.0	238.8	239.8
− eyebrow	173.3	216.3	232.3	238.2	239.2
− eyelid (lower) (upper) (skin)	173.1	216.1	232.1	238.2	239.2
− − cartilage	171.0	215.0		238.1	239.2
− face NEC #	195.0	229.8	232.3	238.8	239.8
− fallopian tube	183.2	221.0	233.3	236.3	239.5
− falx (cerebelli) (cerebi)	192.1	225.2		237.6	239.7
− fascia - see also Neoplasm, connective tissue					
− − palmar	171.2	215.2		238.1	239.2
− − plantar	171.3	215.3		238.1	239.2
− fatty tissue - see Neoplasm, connective tissue					
− fauces, faucial NEC	146.9	210.6	230.0	235.1	239.0
− − pillars	146.2	210.6	230.0	235.1	239.0
− − tonsil	146.0	210.5	230.0	235.1	239.0
− femur (any part) ◊	170.7	213.7		238.0	239.2
− fetal membrane	181	219.8	233.2	236.1	239.5
− fibrous tissue - see Neoplasm, connective tissue					

	Malignant	Benign	In-situ	Un-certain be-haviour	Un-specified nature
Neoplasm - *continued*					
− fibula (any part) ◊	170.7	213.7		238.0	239.2
− filum terminale	192.2	225.3		237.5	239.7
− finger NEC #	195.4	229.8	232.6	238.8	239.8
− flank NEC #	195.8	229.8	232.5	238.8	239.8
− foot NEC #	195.5	229.8	232.7	238.8	239.8
− forearm NEC #	195.4	229.8	232.6	238.8	239.8
− forehead	173.3	216.3	232.3	238.2	239.2
− foreskin	187.1	222.1	233.5	236.6	239.5
− fornix					
− − pharyngeal	147.3	210.7	230.0	235.1	239.0
− − vagina	184.0	221.1	233.3	236.3	239.5
− fossa (of)					
− − anterior (cranial)	191.9	225.0		237.5	239.6
− − cranial	191.9	225.0		237.5	239.6
− − ischiorectal	195.3	229.8	234.8	238.8	239.8
− − middle (cranial)	191.9	225.0		237.5	239.6
− − pituitary	194.3	227.3	234.8	237.0	239.7
− − posterior (cranial)	191.9	225.0		237.5	239.6
− − pterygoid	171.0	215.0		238.1	239.2
− − pyriform	148.1	210.8	230.0	235.1	239.0
− − Rosenmuller	147.2	210.7	230.0	235.1	239.0
− − tonsillar	146.1	210.6	230.0	235.1	239.0
− fourchette	184.4	221.2	233.3	236.3	239.5
− frenulum					
− − labii - see Neoplasm, lip, internal					
− − linguae	141.3	210.1	230.0	235.1	239.0
− frontal					
− − bone ◊	170.0	213.0		238.0	239.2
− − lobe	191.1	225.0		237.5	239.6
− − pole	191.1	225.0		237.5	239.6
− − sinus	160.4	212.0	231.8	235.9	239.1
− fundus					
− − stomach	151.3	211.1	230.2	235.2	239.0
− − uterus	182.0	219.1	233.2	236.0	239.5
− gall duct (extrahepatic)	156.1	211.5	230.8	235.3	239.0
− − intrahepatic	155.1	211.5	230.8	235.3	239.0
− gallbladder	156.0	211.5	230.8	235.3	239.0
− ganglia - see also Neoplasm, connective tissue					
− − basal	191.0	225.0		237.5	239.6
− Gartner's duct	184.0	221.1	233.3	236.3	239.5
− gastric - see Neoplasm, stomach					
− gastroesophageal junction	151.0	211.1	230.2	235.2	239.0
− gastrointestinal (tract) NEC	159.9	211.9	230.9	235.5	239.0
− generalized	199.0				
− genital organ or tract					
− − female NEC	184.9	221.9	233.3	236.3	239.5
− − − specified site NEC	184.8	221.8	233.3	236.3	239.5
− − male NEC	187.9	222.9	233.6	236.6	239.5
− − − specified site NEC	187.8	222.8	233.6	236.6	239.5
− genitourinary tract					
− − female	184.9	221.9	233.3	236.3	239.5

	Malignant	Benign	In-situ	Un-certain be-haviour	Un-specified nature
Neoplasm - *continued*					
– genitourinary tract - *continued*					
– – male	187.9	222.9	233.6	236.6	239.5
– gingiva (alveolar) (marginal)	143.9	210.4	230.0	235.1	239.0
– – lower	143.1	210.4	230.0	235.1	239.0
– – mandibular	143.1	210.4	230.0	235.1	239.0
– – maxillary	143.0	210.4	230.0	235.1	239.0
– – upper	143.0	210.4	230.0	235.1	239.0
– gland, glandular (lymphatic) (system) - see also Neoplasm, lymph gland					
– – endocrine NEC	194.9	227.9		237.4	239.7
– – salivary - see Neoplasm, salivary gland					
– glans penis	187.2	222.1	233.5	236.6	239.5
– globus pallidus	191.0	225.0		237.5	239.6
– glomus					
– – coccygeal	194.6	227.6		237.3	239.7
– – jugularis	194.6	227.6		237.3	239.7
– glosso-epiglottic fold(s)	146.4	210.6	230.0	235.1	239.0
– glossopalatine fold	146.2	210.6	230.0	235.1	239.0
– glossopharyngeal sulcus	146.1	210.6	230.0	235.1	239.0
– glottis	161.0	212.1	231.0	235.6	239.1
– gluteal region #	195.3	229.8	232.5	238.8	239.8
– great vessels NEC	171.4	215.4		238.1	239.2
– groin NEC #	195.3	229.8	232.5	238.8	239.8
– gum	143.9	210.4	230.0	235.1	239.0
– – lower	143.1	210.4	230.0	235.1	239.0
– – upper	143.0	210.4	230.0	235.1	239.0
– hand NEC #	195.4	229.8	232.6	238.8	239.8
– head NEC #	195.0	229.8	232.4	238.8	239.8
– heart	164.1	212.7		238.8	239.8
– heel NEC #	195.5	229.8	232.7	238.8	239.8
– helix	173.2	216.2	232.2	238.2	239.2
– hematopoietic, hemopoietic tissue NEC	202.8				
– hemisphere, cerebral	191.0	225.0		237.5	239.6
– hemorrhoidal zone	154.2	211.4	230.5	235.5	239.0
– hepatic	155.2	211.5	230.8	235.3	239.0
– – duct (bile)	156.1	211.5	230.8	235.3	239.0
– – flexure (colon)	153.0	211.3	230.3	235.2	239.0
– – primary	155.0				
– hilus of lung	162.2	212.3	231.2	235.7	239.1
– hip NEC #	195.5	229.8	232.7	238.8	239.8
– hippocampus	191.2	225.0		237.5	239.6
– humerus (any part) ◊	170.4	213.4		238.0	239.2
– hymen	184.0	221.1	233.3	236.3	239.5
– hypopharynx, hypopharyngeal NEC	148.9	210.8	230.0	235.1	239.0
– – posterior wall	148.3	210.8	230.0	235.1	239.0
– hypophysis	194.3	227.3	234.8	237.0	239.7
– hypothalamus	191.0	225.0		237.5	239.6
– ileocecum, ileocecal (coil) (junction) (valve)	153.4	211.3	230.3	235.2	239.0
– ileum	152.2	211.2	230.7	235.2	239.0
– ilium ◊	170.6	213.6		238.0	239.2
– immunoproliferative NEC	203.8				
– infraclavicular (region) #	195.1	229.8	232.5	238.8	239.8

	Malignant	Benign	In-situ	Un-certain be-haviour	Un-specified nature
Neoplasm - *continued*					
– inguinal (region) #	195.3	229.8	232.5	238.8	239.8
– insula	191.0	225.0		237.5	239.6
– insular tissue (pancreas)	157.4	211.7	230.9	235.5	239.0
– – brain	191.0	225.0		237.5	239.6
– interarytenoid fold	148.2	210.8	230.0	235.1	239.0
– – hypopharyngeal aspect	148.2	210.8	230.0	235.1	239.0
– – laryngeal aspect	161.1	212.1	231.0	235.6	239.1
– – marginal zone	148.2	210.8	230.0	235.1	239.0
– internal					
– – capsule	191.0	225.0		237.5	239.6
– – os	180.0	219.0	233.1	236.0	239.5
– intervertebral cartilage or disc ◊	170.2	213.2		238.0	239.2
– intestine, intestinal	159.0	211.9	230.7	235.2	239.0
– – large	153.9	211.3	230.3	235.2	239.0
– – – appendix	153.5	211.3	230.3	235.2	239.0
– – – cecum	153.4	211.3	230.3	235.2	239.0
– – – colon	153.9	211.3	230.3	235.2	239.0
– – – – and rectum	154.0	211.4	230.4	235.2	239.0
– – – – ascending	153.6	211.3	230.3	235.2	239.0
– – – – caput	153.4	211.3	230.3	235.2	239.0
– – – – descending	153.2	211.3	230.3	235.2	239.0
– – – – distal	153.3	211.3	230.3	235.2	239.0
– – – – left	153.2	211.3	230.3	235.2	239.0
– – – – pelvic	153.3	211.3	230.3	235.2	239.0
– – – – right	153.6	211.3	230.3	235.2	239.0
– – – – sigmoid (flexure)	153.3	211.3	230.3	235.2	239.0
– – – – transverse	153.1	211.3	230.3	235.2	239.0
– – – hepatic flexure	153.0	211.3	230.3	235.2	239.0
– – – ileocecum	153.4	211.3	230.3	235.2	239.0
– – – sigmoid flexure	153.3	211.3	230.3	235.2	239.0
– – – splenic flexure	153.7	211.3	230.3	235.2	239.0
– – small	152.9	211.2	230.7	235.2	239.0
– – – duodenum	152.0	211.2	230.7	235.2	239.0
– – – ileum	152.2	211.2	230.7	235.2	239.0
– – – jejunum	152.1	211.2	230.7	235.2	239.0
– – tract NEC	159.0	211.9	230.7	235.2	239.0
– intra-abdominal	195.2	229.8		238.8	239.8
– intracranial NEC	191.9	225.0		237.5	239.6
– intraocular	190.0	224.0	234.0	238.8	239.8
– intraorbital	190.1	224.1	234.0	238.8	239.8
– intrasellar	194.3	227.3		237.0	239.7
– intrathoracic (cavity) (organs NEC)	195.1	229.8		238.8	239.8
– iris	190.0	224.0	234.0	238.8	239.8
– ischiorectal (fossa)	195.3	229.8		238.8	239.8
– ischium ◊	170.6	213.6		238.0	239.2
– island of Reil	191.0	225.0		237.5	239.6
– islands or islets of Langerhans	157.4	211.7	230.9	235.5	239.0
– isthmus uteri	182.1	219.1	233.2	236.0	239.5
– jaw	195.0	229.8	234.8	238.8	239.8
– – bone	170.1	213.1		238.0	239.2
– – – carcinoma	143.9				
– – – – lower	143.1				

	Malignant	Benign	In-situ	Un-certain be-haviour	Un-specified nature
Neoplasm - *continued*					
− jaw - *continued*					
− − bone - *continued*					
− − − carcinoma - *continued*					
− − − − upper	143.0				
− − − lower	170.1	213.1		238.0	239.2
− − − upper	170.0	213.0		238.0	239.2
− − carcinoma (any type) (lower) (upper)	195.0				
− − skin	173.3	216.3	232.3	238.2	239.2
− − soft tissues	143.9	210.4		235.1	239.0
− − − lower	143.1	210.4		235.1	239.0
− − − upper	143.0	210.4		235.1	239.0
− jejunum	152.1	211.2	230.7	235.2	239.0
− joint NEC (see also Neoplasm, bone) ◊	170.9	213.9		238.0	239.2
− − acromioclavicular ◊	170.4	213.4		238.0	239.2
− − bursa or synovial membrane - see Neoplasm, connective tissue					
− − costovertebral ◊	170.3	213.3		238.0	239.2
− − sternocostal ◊	170.3	213.3		238.0	239.2
− − temporomandibular ◊	170.1	213.1		238.0	239.2
− junction					
− − anorectal	154.8	211.4	230.7	235.2	239.0
− − cardioesophageal	151.0	211.1	230.2	235.2	239.0
− − esophagogastric	151.0	211.1	230.2	235.2	239.0
− − gastroesophageal	151.0	211.1	230.2	235.2	239.0
− − hard and soft palate	145.5	210.4	230.0	235.1	239.0
− − ileocecal	153.4	211.3	230.3	235.2	239.0
− − pelvirectal	154.0	211.4	230.4	235.2	239.0
− − pelviureteric	189.1	223.1	233.9	236.9	239.5
− − rectosigmoid	154.0	211.4	230.4	235.2	239.0
− − squamocolumnar of cervix	180.8	219.0	233.1	236.0	239.5
− kidney (parenchyma)	189.0	223.0	233.9	236.9	239.5
− − calyx	189.1	223.1	233.9	236.9	239.5
− − hilus	189.1	223.1	233.9	236.9	239.5
− − pelvis	189.1	223.1	233.9	236.9	239.5
− knee NEC #	195.5	229.8	232.7	238.8	239.8
− labia (skin)	184.4	221.2	233.3	236.3	239.5
− − majora	184.1	221.2	233.3	236.3	239.5
− − minora	184.2	221.2	233.3	236.3	239.5
− labial - see also Neoplasm, lip					
− − sulcus (lower) (upper)	145.1	210.4	230.0	235.1	239.0
− labium (skin)	184.4	221.2	233.3	236.3	239.5
− − majus	184.1	221.2	233.3	236.3	239.5
− − minus	184.2	221.2	233.3	236.3	239.5
− lacrimal					
− − canaliculi	190.7	224.7	234.0	238.8	239.8
− − duct (nasal)	190.7	224.7	234.0	238.8	239.8
− − gland	190.2	224.2	234.0	238.8	239.8
− − punctum	190.7	224.7	234.0	238.8	239.8
− − sac	190.7	224.7	234.0	238.8	239.8
− Langerhans, islands or islets	157.4	211.7	230.9	235.5	239.0
− laryngopharynx	148.9	210.8	230.0	235.1	239.0
− larynx NEC	161.9	212.1	231.0	235.6	239.1

	Malignant	Benign	In-situ	Un-certain be-haviour	Un-specified nature
Neoplasm - *continued*					
– lobe - *continued*					
– – temporal	191.2	225.0		237.5	239.6
– – upper	162.3	212.3	231.2	235.7	239.1
– lumbosacral plexus	171.6	215.6		238.1	239.2
– lung	162.9	212.3	231.2	235.7	239.1
– – azygos lobe	162.3	212.3	231.2	235.7	239.1
– – carina	162.2	212.3	231.2	235.7	239.1
– – hilus	162.2	212.3	231.2	235.7	239.1
– – lingula	162.3	212.3	231.2	235.7	239.1
– – lower lobe	162.5	212.3	231.2	235.7	239.1
– – main bronchus	162.2	212.3	231.2	235.7	239.1
– – middle lobe	162.4	212.3	231.2	235.7	239.1
– – upper lobe	162.3	212.3	231.2	235.7	239.1
– lymph, lymphatic					
– – channel NEC (see also Neoplasm, connective tissue)	171.9	215.9		238.1	239.2
– – gland (secondary)	196.9	229.0		238.8	239.8
– – – abdominal	196.2	229.0		238.8	239.8
– – – aortic	196.2	229.0		238.8	239.8
– – – arm	196.3	229.0		238.8	239.8
– – – auricular (anterior) (posterior)	196.0	229.0		238.8	239.8
– – – axilla, axillary	196.3	229.0		238.8	239.8
– – – brachial	196.3	229.0		238.8	239.8
– – – bronchial	196.1	229.0		238.8	239.8
– – – bronchopulmonary	196.1	229.0		238.8	239.8
– – – celiac	196.2	229.0		238.8	239.8
– – – cervical	196.0	229.0		238.8	239.8
– – – cervicofacial	196.0	229.0		238.8	239.8
– – – Cloquet	196.5	229.0		238.8	239.8
– – – colic	196.2	229.0		238.8	239.8
– – – common duct	196.2	229.0		238.8	239.8
– – – cubital	196.3	229.0		238.8	239.8
– – – diaphragmatic	196.1	229.0		238.8	239.8
– – – epigastric, inferior	196.6	229.0		238.8	239.8
– – – epitrochlear	196.3	229.0		238.8	239.8
– – – esophageal	196.1	229.0		238.8	239.8
– – – face	196.0	229.0		238.8	239.8
– – – femoral	196.5	229.0		238.8	239.8
– – – gastric	196.2	229.0		238.8	239.8
– – – groin	196.5	229.0		238.8	239.8
– – – head	196.0	229.0		238.8	239.8
– – – hepatic	196.2	229.0		238.8	239.8
– – – hilar (pulmonary)	196.1	229.0		238.8	239.8
– – – – splenic	196.2	229.0		238.8	239.8
– – – hypogastric	196.6	229.0		238.8	239.8
– – – ileocolic	196.2	229.0		238.8	239.8
– – – iliac	196.6	229.0		238.8	239.8
– – – infraclavicular	196.3	229.0		238.8	239.8
– – – inguina, inguinal	196.5	229.0		238.8	239.8
– – – innominate	196.1	229.0		238.8	239.8
– – – intercostal	196.1	229.0		238.8	239.8
– – – intestinal	196.2	229.0		238.8	239.8

	Malignant	Benign	In-situ	Un-certain be-haviour	Un-specified nature

Neoplasm - *continued*
- lymph - *continued*
- - gland - *continued*

	Malignant	Benign	In-situ	Un-certain be-haviour	Un-specified nature
Neoplasm - *continued*					
- lymph - *continued*					
- - gland - *continued*					
- - - subscapular	196.3	229.0		238.8	239.8
- - - supraclavicular	196.0	229.0		238.8	239.8
- - - thoracic	196.1	229.0		238.8	239.8
- - - tibial	196.5	229.0		238.8	239.8
- - - tracheal	196.1	229.0		238.8	239.8
- - - tracheobronchial	196.1	229.0		238.8	239.8
- - - upper limb	196.3	229.0		238.8	239.8
- - - Virchow's	196.0	229.0		238.8	239.8
- - node - see also Neoplasm, lymph gland					
- - - primary NEC	202.9				
- - vessel (see also Neoplasm, connective					
tissue)	171.9	215.9		238.1	239.2
- mammary gland - see Neoplasm, breast					
- mandible	170.1	213.1		238.0	239.2
- - alveolar					
- - - mucosa	143.1	210.4	230.0	235.1	239.0
- - - ridge or process	170.1	213.1		238.0	239.2
- - - - carcinoma	143.1				
- - carcinoma	143.1				
- marrow (bone)	202.9				
- mastoid (antrum) (cavity) (air cell)	160.1	212.0	231.8	235.9	239.1
- - bone or process ◊	170.0	213.0		238.0	239.2
- maxilla, maxillary (superior)	170.0	213.0		238.0	239.2
- - alveolar					
- - - mucosa	143.0	210.4	230.0	235.1	239.0
- - - ridge or process	170.0	213.0		238.0	239.2
- - - - carcinoma	143.0				
- - antrum	160.2	212.0	231.8	235.9	239.1
- - carcinoma	143.0				
- - inferior - see Neoplasm, mandible					
- - sinus	160.2	212.0	231.8	235.9	239.1
- meatus					
- - external (ear)	173.2	216.2	232.2	238.2	239.2
- Meckel's diverticulum	152.3	211.2	230.7	235.2	239.0
- mediastinum, mediastinal	164.9	212.5		235.8	239.8
- - anterior	164.2	212.5		235.8	239.8
- - posterior	164.3	212.5		235.8	239.8
- medulla					
- - adrenal	194.0	227.0	234.8	237.2	239.7
- - oblongata	191.7	225.0		237.5	239.6
- meibomian gland	173.1	216.1	232.1	238.2	239.2
- meninges (brain) (cerebreal) (cranial)					
(intracranial)	192.1	225.2		237.6	239.7
- - spinal (cord)	192.3	225.4		237.6	239.7
- meniscus, knee joint (lateral) (medial) ◊	170.7	213.7		238.0	239.2
- mesentery, mesenteric	158.8	211.8		235.4	239.0
- mesoappendix	158.8	211.8		235.4	239.0
- mesocolon	158.8	211.8		235.4	239.0
- mesopharynx - see Neoplasm, oropharynx					
- mesosalpinx	183.3	221.0		236.3	239.5

	Malignant	Benign	In-situ	Un-certain be-haviour	Un-specified nature
Neoplasm - *continued*					
– mesovarium	183.3	221.0	233.3	236.3	239.5
– metacarpus (any bone) ◊	170.5	213.5		238.0	239.2
– metastatic NEC (see also Volume 1, page					
728)	199.1				199.1
– metatarsus (any bone) ◊	170.8	213.8		238.0	239.2
– midbrain	191.7	225.0		237.5	239.6
– mons					
– – pubis	184.4	221.2	233.3	236.3	239.5
– – veneris	184.4	221.2	233.3	236.3	239.5
– mouth	145.9	210.4	230.0	235.1	239.0
– – floor	144.9	210.3	230.0	235.1	239.0
– – – anterior	144.0	210.3	230.0	235.1	239.0
– – – lateral	144.1	210.3	230.0	235.1	239.0
– – roof	145.5	210.4	230.0	235.1	239.0
– – specified part NEC	145.8	210.4	230.0	235.1	239.0
– – vestibule	145.1	210.4	230.0	235.1	239.0
– mucosa					
– – alveolar (ridge or process)	143.9	210.4	230.0	235.1	239.0
– – – lower	143.1	210.4	230.0	235.1	239.0
– – – upper	143.0	210.4	230.0	235.1	239.0
– – buccal	145.0	210.4	230.0	235.1	239.0
– – cheek	145.0	210.4	230.0	235.1	239.0
– – lip - see Neoplasm, lip, internal					
– – nasal	160.0	212.0	231.8	235.9	239.1
– – oral NEC	145.9	210.4	230.0	235.1	239.0
– mullerian duct					
– – female	184.8	221.8	233.3	236.3	239.5
– – male	187.8	222.8	233.6	236.6	239.5
– multiple NEC	199.0	229.9	234.9	238.9	239.9
– muscle - see also Neoplasm, connective					
tissue					
– – extra-ocular	190.1	224.1	234.0	238.8	239.8
– myocardium	164.1	212.7		238.8	239.8
– myometrium	182.0	219.1		236.0	239.5
– Nabothian gland (follicle)	180.0	219.0	233.1	236.0	239.5
– nail	173.9	216.9	232.9	238.2	239.2
– – finger	173.6	216.6	232.6	238.2	239.2
– – toe	173.7	216.7	232.7	238.2	239.2
– nares, naris (anterior) (posterior)	160.0	212.0	231.8	235.9	239.1
– nasal - see Neoplasm, nose					
– nasolabial groove	173.3	216.3	232.3	238.2	239.2
– nasolacrimal duct	190.7	224.7	234.0	238.8	239.8
– nasopharynx	147.9	210.7	230.0	235.1	239.0
– – floor	147.3	210.7	230.0	235.1	239.0
– – roof	147.0	210.7	230.0	235.1	239.0
– – wall	147.9	210.7	230.0	235.1	239.0
– – – anterior	147.3	210.7	230.0	235.1	239.0
– – – lateral	147.2	210.7	230.0	235.1	239.0
– – – posterior	147.1	210.7	230.0	235.1	239.0
– – – superior	147.0	210.7	230.0	235.1	239.0
– neck NEC #	195.0	229.8	234.8	238.8	239.8

	Malignant	Benign	In-situ	Un-certain be-haviour	Un-specified nature

Neoplasm - *continued*
- nerve (autonomic) (ganglion)
  (parasympathetic) (peripheral) (sympathetic)
  - see also Neoplasm, connective tissue

	Malignant	Benign	In-situ	Un-certain be-haviour	Un-specified nature
− − abducens	192.0	225.1		237.9	239.7
− − accessory (spinal)	192.0	225.1		237.9	239.7
− − acoustic	192.0	225.1		237.9	239.7
− − auditory	192.0	225.1		237.9	239.7
− − brachial	171.2	215.2		238.1	239.2
− − cranial (any)	192.0	225.1		237.9	239.7
− − facial	192.0	225.1		237.9	239.7
− − femoral	171.3	215.3		238.1	239.2
− − glossopharyngeal	192.0	225.1		237.9	239.7
− − hypoglossal	192.0	225.1		237.9	239.7
− − intercostal	171.4	215.4		238.1	239.2
− − lumbar	171.7	215.7		238.1	239.2
− − median	171.2	215.2		238.1	239.2
− − obturator	171.3	215.3		238.1	239.2
− − oculomotor	192.0	225.1		237.9	239.7
− − olfactory	192.0	225.1		237.9	239.7
− − optic	192.0	225.1		237.9	239.7
− − peripheral NEC	171.9	215.9		238.1	239.2
− − radial	171.2	215.2		238.1	239.2
− − sacral	171.6	215.6		238.1	239.2
− − sciatic	171.3	215.3		238.1	239.2
− − spinal NEC	171.9	215.9		238.1	239.2
− − trigeminal	192.0	225.1		237.9	239.7
− − trochlear	192.0	225.1		237.9	239.7
− − ulnar	171.2	215.2		238.1	239.2
− − vagus	192.0	225.1		237.9	239.7
− nervous system (central) NEC	192.9	225.9		237.9	239.7
− − autonomic NEC	171.9	215.9		238.1	239.2
− − parasympathetic NEC	171.9	215.9		238.1	239.2
− − sympathetic NEC	171.9	215.9		238.1	239.2
− nipple (female)	174.0	217	233.0	238.3	239.3
− − male	175	217	233.0	238.3	239.3
− nose, nasal	195.0	229.8	232.3	238.8	239.8
− − ala (external)	173.3	216.3	232.3	238.2	239.2
− − bone ◊	170.0	213.0		238.0	239.2
− − cartilage	160.0	212.0	231.8	235.9	239.1
− − cavity	160.0	212.0	231.8	235.9	239.1
− − choana	147.3	210.7	230.0	235.1	239.0
− − external (skin)	173.3	216.3	232.3	238.2	239.2
− − fossa	160.0	212.0	231.8	235.9	239.1
− − internal	160.0	212.0	231.8	235.9	239.1
− − mucosa	160.0	212.0	231.8	235.9	239.1
− − septum	160.0	212.0	231.8	235.9	239.1
− − − posterior margin	147.3	210.7	230.0	235.1	239.0
− − sinus - see Neoplasm, sinus					
− − skin	173.3	216.3	232.3	238.2	239.2
− − turbinate (mucosa)	160.0	212.0	231.8	235.9	239.1
− − − bone ◊	170.0	213.0		238.0	239.2
− − vestibule	160.0	212.0	231.8	235.9	239.1

	Malignant	Benign	In-situ	Un-certain be-haviour	Un-specified nature
Neoplasm - *continued*					
− paravaginal	195.3	229.8		238.8	239.8
− parenchyma, kidney	189.0	223.0	233.9	236.9	239.5
− parietal lobe	191.3	225.0		237.5	239.6
− parotid (duct) (gland)	142.0	210.2	230.0	235.0	239.0
− parovarium	183.3	221.0	233.3	236.3	239.5
− patella ◊	170.8	213.8		238.0	239.2
− peduncle, cerebral	191.7	225.0		237.5	239.6
− pelvirectal junction	154.0	211.4	230.4	235.2	239.0
− pelvis, pelvic	195.3	229.8	234.8	238.8	239.8
− − bone ◊	170.6	213.6		238.0	239.2
− − floor	195.3	229.8	234.8	238.8	239.8
− − renal	189.1	223.1	233.9	236.9	239.5
− − viscera	195.3	229.8		238.8	239.8
− − wall	195.3	229.8	234.8	238.8	239.8
− pelvo-abdominal	195.8	229.8	234.8	238.8	239.8
− penis	187.4	222.1	233.5	236.6	239.5
− − body	187.3	222.1	233.5	236.6	239.5
− − corpus (cavernosum)	187.3	222.1	233.5	236.6	239.5
− − glans	187.2	222.1	233.5	236.6	239.5
− − skin NEC	187.4	222.1	233.5	236.6	239.5
− periadrenal	158.0	211.8		235.4	239.0
− perianal (skin)	173.5	216.5	232.5	238.2	239.2
− pericardium	164.1	212.7		238.8	239.8
− perinephric	158.0	211.8		235.4	239.0
− perineum	195.3	229.8	234.8	238.8	239.8
− periodontal tissue NEC	143.9	210.4	230.0	235.1	239.0
− periosteum - see Neoplasm, bone					
− peripancreatic	158.0	211.8		235.4	239.0
− peripheral nerve NEC	171.9	215.9		238.1	239.2
− perirectal (tissue)	195.3	229.8		238.8	239.8
− perirenal (tissue)	158.0	211.8		235.4	239.0
− peritoneal cavity	158.9	211.8		235.4	239.0
− peritoneum	158.9	211.8		235.4	239.0
− − parietal	158.8	211.8		235.4	239.0
− − pelvic	158.8	211.8		235.4	239.0
− − specified part NEC	158.8	211.8		235.4	239.0
− periurethral tissue	195.3	229.8		238.8	239.8
− phalanges ◊	170.9	213.9		238.0	239.2
− − foot ◊	170.8	213.8		238.0	239.2
− − hand ◊	170.5	213.5		238.0	239.2
− pharynx, pharyngeal	149.0	210.9	230.0	235.1	239.0
− − fornix	147.3	210.7	230.0	235.1	239.0
− − recess	147.2	210.7	230.0	235.1	239.0
− − region	149.0	210.9	230.0	235.1	239.0
− − tonsil	147.1	210.7	230.0	235.1	239.0
− − wall (lateral) (posterior)	149.0	210.9	230.0	235.1	239.0
− pia mater (cerebral) (cranial)	192.1	225.2		237.6	239.7
− − spinal	192.3	225.4		237.6	239.7
− pillars of fauces	146.2	210.6	230.0	235.1	239.0
− pineal (body) (gland)	194.4	227.4	234.8	237.1	239.7
− pinna (ear) NEC	173.2	216.2	232.2	238.2	239.2
− piriform fossa or sinus	148.1	210.8	230.0	235.1	239.0

	Malignant	Benign	In-situ	Un-certain be-haviour	Un-specified nature
Neoplasm - *continued*					
– retrobulbar	190.1	224.1		238.8	239.8
– retrocecal	158.0	211.8		235.4	239.0
– retromolar (area) (triangle) (trigone)	145.6	210.4	230.0	235.1	239.0
– retroperitoneal (space) (tissue)	158.0	211.8		235.4	239.0
– retroperitoneum	158.0	211.8		235.4	239.0
– retropharyngeal	149.0	210.9	230.0	235.1	239.0
– retrovesical	195.3	229.8		238.8	239.8
– rhinencephalon	191.0	225.0		237.5	239.6
– rib ◊	170.3	213.3		238.0	239.2
– Rosenmuller's fossa	147.2	210.7	230.0	235.1	239.0
– round ligament	183.5	221.0		236.3	239.5
– sacrococcyx, sacrococcygeal ◊	170.6	213.6		238.0	239.2
– – region	195.3	229.8	234.8	238.8	239.8
– sacro-uterine ligament	183.4	221.0		236.3	239.5
– sacrum, sacral (vertebra) ◊	170.6	213.6		238.0	239.2
– salivary gland or duct (major)	142.9	210.2	230.0	235.0	239.0
– – minor NEC	145.9	210.4	230.0	235.1	239.0
– – parotid	142.0	210.2	230.0	235.0	239.0
– – sublingual	142.2	210.2	230.0	235.0	239.0
– – submandibular	142.1	210.2	230.0	235.0	239.0
– – submaxillary	142.1	210.2	230.0	235.0	239.0
– salpinx	183.2	221.0	233.3	236.3	239.5
– Santorini's duct	157.3	211.6	230.9	235.5	239.0
– scalp	173.4	216.4	232.4	238.2	239.2
– scapula (any part) ◊	170.4	213.4		238.0	239.2
– scapular region #	195.1	229.8	232.5	238.8	239.8
– sclera	190.0	224.0	234.0	238.8	239.8
– scrotum	187.7	222.4	233.6	236.6	239.5
– sebaceous gland - see Neoplasm, skin					
– secondary - see Secondary neoplasm					
– sella turcica	194.3	227.3		237.0	239.7
– – bone ◊	170.0	213.0		238.0	239.2
– seminal vesicle	187.8	222.8	233.6	236.6	239.5
– septum					
– – nasal	160.0	212.0	231.8	235.9	239.1
– – – posterior margin	147.3	210.7	230.0	235.1	239.0
– – rectovaginal	195.3	229.8	234.8	238.8	239.8
– – rectovesical	195.3	229.8	234.8	238.8	239.8
– – urethrovaginal	184.9	221.9	233.3	236.3	239.5
– – vesicovaginal	184.9	221.9	233.3	236.3	239.5
– shoulder NEC #	195.4	229.8	232.6	238.8	239.8
– sigmoid (flexure)	153.3	211.3	230.3	235.2	239.0
– sinus (accessory)	160.9	212.0	231.8	235.9	239.1
– – bone (any) ◊	170.0	213.0		238.0	239.2
– – ethmoidal	160.3	212.0	231.8	235.9	239.1
– – frontal	160.4	212.0	231.8	235.9	239.1
– – maxillary	160.2	212.0	231.8	235.9	239.1
– – nasal, paranasal NEC	160.9	212.0	231.8	235.9	239.1
– – pyriform	148.1	210.8	230.0	235.1	239.0
– – sphenoidal	160.5	212.0	231.8	235.9	239.1
– skeleton, skeletal NEC ◊	170.9	213.9		238.0	239.2
– Skene's gland	189.4	223.8	233.9	236.9	239.5

	Malignant	Benign	In-situ	Un-certain be-haviour	Un-specified nature
Neoplasm - *continued*					
– skin NEC - *continued*					
– – knee	173.7	216.7	232.7	238.2	239.2
– – labia	184.4	221.2	233.3	236.3	239.5
– – – majora	184.1	221.2	233.3	236.3	239.5
– – – minora	184.2	221.2	233.3	236.3	239.5
– – leg	173.7	216.7	232.7	238.2	239.2
– – lid (lower) (upper)	173.1	216.1	232.1	238.2	239.2
– – limb NEC	173.9	216.9	232.9	238.2	239.2
– – – lower	173.7	216.7	232.7	238.2	239.2
– – – upper	173.6	216.6	232.6	238.2	239.2
– – lip (lower) (upper)	173.0	216.0	232.0	238.2	239.2
– – male genital organ	187.9	222.9	233.6	236.6	239.5
– – – penis NEC	187.4	222.1	233.5	236.6	239.5
– – – prepuce	187.1	222.1	233.5	236.6	239.5
– – – scrotum	187.7	222.4	233.6	236.6	239.5
– – nates	173.5	216.5	232.5	238.2	239.2
– – neck	173.4	216.4	232.4	238.2	239.2
– – nose (external)	173.3	216.3	232.3	238.2	239.2
– – palm	173.6	216.6	232.6	238.2	239.2
– – palpebra	173.1	216.1	232.1	238.2	239.2
– – penis NEC	187.4	222.1	233.5	236.6	239.5
– – perianal	173.5	216.5	232.5	238.2	239.2
– – perineum	173.5	216.5	232.5	238.2	239.2
– – pinna	173.2	216.2	232.2	238.2	239.2
– – plantar	173.7	216.7	232.7	238.2	239.2
– – popliteal fossa or space	173.7	216.7	232.7	238.2	239.2
– – prepuce	187.1	222.1	233.5	236.6	239.5
– – pubes	173.5	216.5	232.5	238.2	239.2
– – sacrococcygeal region	173.5	216.5	232.5	238.2	239.2
– – scalp	173.4	216.4	232.4	238.2	239.2
– – scapular region	173.5	216.5	232.5	238.2	239.2
– – scrotum	187.7	222.4	233.6	236.6	239.5
– – shoulder	173.6	216.6	232.6	238.2	239.2
– – sole (foot)	173.7	216.7	232.7	238.2	239.2
– – submammary fold	173.5	216.5	232.5	238.2	239.2
– – supraclavicular region	173.4	216.4	232.4	238.2	239.2
– – temple	173.3	216.3	232.3	238.2	239.2
– – thigh	173.7	216.7	232.7	238.2	239.2
– – thoracic wall	173.5	216.5	232.5	238.2	239.2
– – thumb	173.6	216.6	232.6	238.2	239.2
– – toe	173.7	216.7	232.7	238.2	239.2
– – tragus	173.2	216.2	232.2	238.2	239.2
– – trunk	173.5	216.5	232.5	238.2	239.2
– – umbilicus	173.5	216.5	232.5	238.2	239.2
– – vulva	184.4	221.2	233.3	236.3	239.5
– – wrist	173.6	216.6	232.6	238.2	239.2
– skull ◊	170.0	213.0		238.0	239.2
– soft parts or tissues - see Neoplasm, connective tissue					
– specified site NEC	195.8	229.8	234.8	238.8	239.8
– spermatic cord	187.6	222.8	233.6	236.6	239.5
– sphenoid	160.5	212.0	231.8	235.9	239.1

	Malignant	Benign	In-situ	Un-certain be-haviour	Un-specified nature
Neoplasm - *continued*					
− suprasellar (region)	191.9	225.0		237.5	239.6
− sweat gland (apocrine) (eccrine), site unspecified	173.9	216.9	232.9	238.2	239.2
− sympathetic nerve or nervous system NEC ..	171.9	215.9		238.1	239.2
− symphysis pubis	170.6	213.6		238.0	239.2
− synovial membrane - see Neoplasm, connective tissue					
− tapetum	191.8	225.0		237.5	239.6
− tarsus (any bone) ◊	170.8	213.8		238.0	239.2
− temple	173.3	216.3	232.3	238.2	239.2
− temporal					
− − pole or lobe	191.2	225.0		237.5	239.6
− − region	195.0	229.8	234.8	238.8	239.8
− tendon (sheath) - see Neoplasm, connective tissue					
− tentorium (cerebelli)	192.1	225.2		237.6	239.7
− testis (descended) (scrotal)	186.9	222.0	233.6	236.4	239.5
− − ectopic	186.0	222.0	233.6	236.4	239.5
− − retained	186.0	222.0	233.6	236.4	239.5
− − undescended	186.0	222.0	233.6	236.4	239.5
− thalamus	191.0	225.0		237.5	239.6
− thigh NEC #	195.5	229.8	232.7	238.8	239.8
− thorax, thoracic (cavity) (organs NEC)	195.1	229.8	234.8	238.8	239.8
− − duct	171.4	215.4		238.1	239.2
− − wall NEC	195.1	229.8	234.8	238.8	239.8
− throat	149.0	210.9	230.0	235.1	239.0
− thumb NEC #	195.4	229.8	232.6	238.8	239.8
− thymus (gland)	164.0	212.6		235.8	239.8
− thyroglossal duct	193	226	234.8	237.4	239.7
− thyroid (gland)	193	226	234.8	237.4	239.7
− − cartilage	161.3	212.1	231.0	235.6	239.1
− tibia (any part) ◊	170.7	213.7		238.0	239.2
− toe NEC #	195.5	229.8	232.7	238.8	239.8
− tongue	141.9	210.1	230.0	235.1	239.0
− − anterior (two-thirds) NEC	141.4	210.1	230.0	235.1	239.0
− − − dorsal surface	141.1	210.1	230.0	235.1	239.0
− − − ventral surface	141.3	210.1	230.0	235.1	239.0
− − base (dorsal surface)	141.0	210.1	230.0	235.1	239.0
− − border (lateral)	141.2	210.1	230.0	235.1	239.0
− − fixed part	141.0	210.1	230.0	235.1	239.0
− − frenulum	141.3	210.1	230.0	235.1	239.0
− − junctional zone	141.5	210.1	230.0	235.1	239.0
− − margin (lateral)	141.2	210.1	230.0	235.1	239.0
− − midline NEC	141.1	210.1	230.0	235.1	239.0
− − mobile part NEC	141.4	210.1	230.0	235.1	239.0
− − posterior (third)	141.0	210.1	230.0	235.1	239.0
− − root	141.0	210.1	230.0	235.1	239.0
− − surface (dorsal)	141.1	210.1	230.0	235.1	239.0
− − − base	141.0	210.1	230.0	235.1	239.0
− − − ventral	141.3	210.1	230.0	235.1	239.0
− − tip	141.2	210.1	230.0	235.1	239.0
− − tonsil	141.6	210.1	230.0	235.1	239.0

	Malignant	Benign	In-situ	Un-certain be-haviour	Un-specified nature
Neoplasm - *continued*					
− tonsil	146.0	210.5	230.0	235.1	239.0
− − fauces, faucial	146.0	210.5	230.0	235.1	239.0
− − lingual	141.6	210.1	230.0	235.1	239.0
− − palatine	146.0	210.5	230.0	235.1	239.0
− − pharyngeal	147.1	210.7	230.0	235.1	239.0
− − pillar (anterior) (posterior)	146.2	210.6	230.0	235.1	239.0
− tonsillar fossa	146.1	210.6	230.0	235.1	239.0
− tooth socket NEC	143.9	210.4	230.0	235.1	239.0
− trachea (cartilage) (mucosa)	162.0	212.2	231.1	235.7	239.1
− tracheobronchial	162.8	212.2	231.1	235.7	239.1
− tragus	173.2	216.2	232.2	238.2	239.2
− trunk NEC #	195.8	229.8	232.5	238.8	239.8
− tubo-ovarian	183.8	221.8	233.3	236.3	239.5
− tunica vaginalis	187.8	222.8		236.6	239.5
− turbinate (bone) ◊	170.0	213.0		238.0	239.2
− − nasal	160.0	212.0	231.8	235.9	239.1
− tympanic cavity	160.1	212.0	231.8	235.9	239.1
− ulna (any part) ◊	170.4	213.4		238.0	239.2
− umbilicus, umbilical	173.5	216.5	232.5	238.2	239.2
− uncus	191.2	225.0		237.5	239.6
− urachus	188.7	223.3	233.7	236.7	239.4
− ureter	189.2	223.2	233.9	236.9	239.5
− − orifice	188.6	223.3	233.7	236.7	239.4
− urethra, urethral (gland)	189.3	223.8	233.9	236.9	239.5
− − orifice, internal	188.5	223.3	233.7	236.7	239.4
− urethrovaginal (septum)	184.9	221.9	233.3	236.3	239.5
− urinary organ or system NEC	189.9	223.9	233.9	236.9	239.5
− − bladder - see Neoplasm, bladder					
− utero-ovarian	183.8	221.8		236.3	239.5
− − ligament	183.3	221.0		236.3	239.5
− uterosacral ligament	183.4	221.0		236.3	239.5
− uterus, uteri, uterine	179	219.9	233.2	236.0	239.5
− − adnexa	183.9	221.8	233.3	236.3	239.5
− − body	182.0	219.1	233.2	236.0	239.5
− − cervix	180.9	219.0	233.1	236.0	239.5
− − cornu	182.0	219.1	233.2	236.0	239.5
− − corpus	182.0	219.1	233.2	236.0	239.5
− − endocervix (canal) (gland)	180.0	219.0	233.1	236.0	239.5
− − exocervix	180.1	219.0	233.1	236.0	239.5
− − external os	180.1	219.0	233.1	236.0	239.5
− − fundus	182.0	219.1	233.2	236.0	239.5
− − internal os	180.0	219.0	233.1	236.0	239.5
− − isthmus	182.1	219.1	233.2	236.0	239.5
− − ligament	183.4	221.0		236.3	239.5
− − − broad	183.3	221.0	233.3	236.3	239.5
− − − round	183.5	221.0		236.3	239.5
− − lower segment	182.1	219.1	233.2	236.0	239.5
− − squamocolumnar junction	180.8	219.0	233.1	236.0	239.5
− − tube	183.2	221.0	233.3	236.3	239.5
− utricle, prostatic	189.3	223.8	233.9	236.9	239.5
− uveal tract	190.0	224.0	234.0	238.8	239.8
− uvula	145.4	210.4	230.0	235.1	239.0

	Malignant	Benign	In-situ	Un- certain be- haviour	Un- specified nature
Neoplasm - *continued*					
– vagina, vaginal (fornix) (vault) (wall)	184.0	221.1	233.3	236.3	239.5
– vaginovesical	184.9	221.9	233.3	236.3	239.5
– – septum	184.9	221.9	233.3	236.3	239.5
– vallecula (epiglottis)	146.3	210.6	230.0	235.1	239.0
– vas deferens	187.6	222.8	233.6	236.6	239.5
– vascular - see Neoplasm, connective tissue					
– vein, venous - see Neoplasm, connective tissue					
– vena cava (abdominal) (inferior)	171.5	215.5		238.1	239.2
– – superior	171.4	215.4		238.1	239.2
– ventricle (cerebral) (floor) (fourth) (lateral) (third)	191.5	225.0		237.5	239.6
– – cardiac (left) (right)	164.1	212.7		238.8	239.8
– ventricular band of larynx	161.1	212.1	231.0	235.6	239.1
– ventriculus - see Neoplasm, stomach					
– vermilion border - see Neoplasm, lip					
– vermis, cerebellum	191.6	225.0		237.5	239.6
– vertebra (column) ◊	170.2	213.2		238.0	239.2
– – coccyx ◊	170.6	213.6		238.0	239.2
– – sacrum ◊	170.6	213.6		238.0	239.2
– vesical - see Neoplasm, bladder					
– vesicle, seminal	187.8	222.8	233.6	236.6	239.5
– vesicocervical tissue	184.9	221.9	233.3	236.3	239.5
– vesicorectal	195.3	229.8	234.8	238.8	239.8
– vesicovaginal	184.9	221.9	233.3	236.3	239.5
– – septum	184.9	221.9	233.3	236.3	239.5
– vessel (blood) - see Neoplasm, connective tissue					
– vestibular gland, greater	184.1	221.2	233.3	236.3	239.5
– vestibule					
– – mouth	145.1	210.4	230.0	235.1	239.0
– – nose	160.0	212.0	231.8	235.9	239.1
– Virchow's gland	196.0	229.0		238.8	239.8
– viscera NEC	195.8	229.8		238.8	239.8
– vocal cords (true)	161.0	212.1	231.0	235.6	239.1
– – false	161.1	212.1	231.0	235.6	239.1
– vulva	184.4	221.2	233.3	236.3	239.5
– vulvovaginal gland	184.4	221.2	233.3	236.3	239.5
– Waldeyer's ring	149.1	210.9	230.0	235.1	239.0
– Wharton's duct	142.1	210.2	230.0	235.0	239.0
– white matter (central) (cerebral)	191.0	225.0		237.5	239.6
– windpipe	162.0	212.2	231.1	235.7	239.1
– Wirsung's duct	157.3	211.6	230.9	235.5	239.0
– Wolffian (body) (duct)					
– – female	184.8	221.8	233.3	236.3	239.5
– – male	187.8	222.8	233.6	236.6	239.5
– womb - see Neoplasm, uterus					
– wrist NEC #	195.4	229.8	232.6	238.8	239.8
– xiphoid process ◊	170.3	213.3		238.0	239.2
– Zuckerkandl's organ	194.6	227.6		237.3	239.7

Neovascularization
- ciliary body 364.4
- cornea 370.6
- iris 364.4
- retina 362.1

Nephralgia 788.0

Nephritis, nephritic (albuminuric)
(azotemic) (congenital) (degenerative)
(diffuse) (disseminated) (epithelial)
(exudative) (familial) (focal) (granular)
(granulomatous) (hemorrhagic) (infantile)
(nonsuppurative excretory) (uremic) 583.9
- with
- - edema - see Nephrosis
- - lesion of
- - - glomerulonephritis
- - - - hypocomplementemic persistent
    583.2
- - - - - chronic 582.2
- - - - lobular 583.2
- - - - - chronic 582.2
- - - - membranoproliferative 583.2
- - - - - chronic 582.2
- - - - membranous 583.1
- - - - - chronic 582.1
- - - - mesangiocapillary 583.2
- - - - - chronic 582.2
- - - - mixed membranous and
    proliferative 583.2
- - - - - chronic 582.2
- - - - proliferative 583.0
- - - - - acute 580.0
- - - - - chronic 582.0
- - - - rapidly progressive 583.4
- - - - - acute 580.4
- - -.- - - chronic 582.4
- - - interstitial nephritis 583.8
- - - necrotizing glomerulitis 583.4
- - - - acute 580.4
- - - - chronic 582.4
- - - renal necrosis
- - - - cortical 583.6
- - - - medullary 583.7
- - - specified pathology NEC 583.8
- - - - acute 580.8
- - - - chronic 582.8
- - necrosis, renal 583.9
- - - cortical 583.6
- - - medullary (papillary) 583.7
- acute NEC 580.9
- - hypertensive (see also Hypertension,
    kidney) 403.9
- amyloid 277.3 † 583.8*
- - chronic 277.3 † 583.8*
- arteriolar (see also Hypertension, kidney)
    403.9

Nephritis - *continued*
- arteriosclerotic (see also Hypertension,
    kidney) 403.9
- ascending (see also Pyelitis) 590.8
- calculous, calculus 592.0
- cardiac 403.9
- cardiovascular 403.9
- chronic NEC 582.9
- - arteriosclerotic (see also Hypertension,
    kidney) 403.9
- - hypertensive (see also Hypertension,
    kidney) 403.9
- cirrhotic (see also Sclerosis, renal) 587
- complicating pregnancy, childbirth or
    puerperium 648.9
- - with hypertension 642.1
- - - fetus or newborn 760.0
- - fetus or newborn 760.1
- desquamative - see Nephrosis
- due to
- - diabetes mellitus 250.3 † 583.8*
- - specified kidney pathology NEC 583.8
- - - acute 580.8
- - - chronic 582.8
- - systemic lupus erythematosus 710.0 †
    583.8*
- - - chronic 710.0 † 582.8*
- gonococcal (acute) 098.1 † 583.8*
- - chronic or duration of 2 months or over
    098.3 † 583.8*
- gouty 274.1 † 583.8*
- hereditary 753.3
- hydremic - see Nephrosis
- hypertensive (see also Hypertension,
    kidney) 403.9
- hypocomplementemic persistent 583.2
- - chronic 582.2
- infective (see also Pyelitis) 590.8
- interstitial 583.8
- latent or quiescent - see Nephritis,
    chronic
- lead 984.-
- - specified type of lead - see Table of
    drugs and chemicals
- lobular 583.2
- - chronic 582.2
- membranoproliferative 583.2
- - chronic 582.2
- membranous 583.1
- - chronic 582.1
- mesangiocapillary 583.2
- - chronic 582.2
- mixed membranous and proliferative
    583.2
- - chronic 582.2
- necrotic, necrotizing 583.4
- - acute 580.4

Nephritis - *continued*
- necrotic - *continued*
- - chronic 582.4
- nephrotic - see Nephrosis
- old - see Nephritis, chronic
- parenchymatous 581.8
- polycystic 753.1
- pregnancy - see Nephritis complicating pregnancy
- proliferative 583.0
- - acute 580.0
- - chronic 582.0
- purulent (see also Pyelitis) 590.8
- rapidly progressive 583.4
- - acute 580.4
- - chronic 582.4
- salt losing or wasting (see also Disease, renal) 593.9
- saturnine 984.-
- - specified type of lead - see Table of drugs and chemicals
- septic (see also Pyelitis) 590.8
- streptotrichosis 039.8 † 583.8*
- subacute (see also Nephrosis) 581.9
- - hypertensive (see also Hypertension, kidney) 403.9
- suppurative (see also Pyelitis) 590.8
- syphilitic (late) 095 † 583.8*
- - congenital 090.5 † 583.8*
- - early 091.6 † 583.8*
- toxic - see Nephritis, acute
- tubal, tubular - see Nephrosis
- tuberculous 016.0 † 583.8*
- type II (Ellis) - see Nephrosis
- vascular - see Hypertension, kidney
Nephroblastoma (M8960/3) 189.0
- epithelial (M8961/3) 189.0
- mesenchymal (M8962/3) 189.0
Nephrocalcinosis 275.4
Nephrocystitis, pustular (see also Pyelitis) 590.8
Nephrolithiasis (congenital) (pelvis) (recurrent) 592.0
- uric acid 274.1 † 592.0*
Nephroma (M8960/3) 189.0
- mesoblastic (M8960/1) 236.9
Nephronephritis (see also Nephrosis) 581.9
Nephropathy (see also Nephritis) 583.9
- analgesic 583.8
- - with medullary necrosis, acute 584.7
- complicating pregnancy 646.2
- diabetic 250.3 † 583.8*
- hypertensive (see also Hypertension, kidney) 403.9
- obstructive 593.8
- - congenital 753.2
- proliferative 583.0

Nephropathy - *continued*
- sickle cell (see also Disease, sickle cell) 282.6 † 583.8*
Nephroptosis (see also Disease, renal) 593.0
- congenital 753.3
Nephropyosis (see also Abscess, kidney) 590.2
Nephrorrhagia 593.8
Nephrosclerosis (arteriolar) (arteriosclerotic) (chronic) (hyaline) (see also Hypertension, kidney) 403.9
- gouty 274.1 † 583.8*
- hyperplastic (see also Hypertension, kidney) 403.9
- senile (see also Sclerosis, renal) 587
Nephrosis, nephrotic (Epstein's) (syndrome) 581.9
- with
- - lesion of
- - - glomerulonephritis
- - - - hypocomplementemic persistent 581.2
- - - - lobular 581.2
- - - - membranoproliferative 581.2
- - - - membranous 581.1
- - - - mesangiocapillary 581.2
- - - - minimal change 581.3
- - - - mixed membranous and proliferative 581.2
- - - - proliferative 581.0
- - - specified pathology NEC 581.8
- acute - see Nephrosis, tubular
- anoxic - see Nephrosis, tubular
- chemical - see Nephrosis, tubular
- complicating pregnancy, childbirth or puerperium - see Nephritis, complicating pregnancy
- diabetic 250.3 † 581.8*
- hemoglobinuric - see Nephrosis, tubular
- in
- - amyloidosis 277.3 † 581.8*
- - diabetes mellitus 250.3 † 581.8*
- - epidemic hemorrhagic fever 078.6 † 581.8*
- - malaria 084.9 † 581.8*
- - systemic lupus erythematosus 710.0 † 581.8*
- ischemic - see Nephrosis, tubular
- lipoid 581.3
- lower nephron - see Nephrosis, tubular
- malarial 084.9 † 581.8*
- minimal change 581.3
- necrotizing - see Nephrosis, tubular
- radiation 581.9
- syphilitic 095 † 583.8*
- toxic - see Nephrosis, tubular
- tubular (acute) 584.5

Nephrosis - *continued*
- tubular - *continued*
- - radiation 581.9
- - specified due to a procedure 997.5
Nephroso-nephritis hemorrhagic (endemic)
  078.6 † 581.8*
Nerve - see condition
Nerves 799.2
Nervous (see also Condition) 799.2
- heart 306.2
- stomach 306.4
- tension 799.2
Nervousness 799.2
Nesidioblastoma (M8150/0)
- pancreas 211.7
- specified site NEC - see Neoplasm,
  benign
- unspecified site 211.7
Nettle rash 708.8
Nettleship's disease 757.3
Neumann's disease 694.4
Neuralgia, neuralgic (acute) (see also
  Neuritis) 729.2
- ciliary 346.2
- cranial nerve - see also Disorder, nerve,
  cranial
- - fifth or trigeminal (see also Neuralgia,
    trigeminal) 350.1
- ear 388.7
- facial 351.8
- Fothergill's (see also Neuralgia,
  trigeminal) 350.1
- glossopharyngeal (nerve) 352.1
- Hunt's 053.1 † 351.1*
- hypoglossal (nerve) 352.5
- infra-orbital (see also Neuralgia,
  trigeminal) 350.1
- malarial (see also Malaria) 084.6
- migrainous 346.2
- Morton's 355.6
- nerve, cranial - see Disorder, nerve,
  cranial
- pleura 511.0
- postherpetic NEC 053.1 † 357.4*
- - trigeminal 053.1 † 350.0*
- specified nerve NEC - see Disorder,
  nerve
- trifacial (see also Neuralgia, trigeminal)
  350.1
- trigeminal 350.1
- - postherpetic 053.1 † 350.0*
- writers' 300.8
- - organic 333.8
Neurapraxia - see Injury, nerve, by site
Neurasthenia 300.5
- cardiac 306.2
- gastric 306.4

Neurasthenia - *continued*
- heart 306.2
Neurilemmoma (M9560/0) - see also
  Neoplasm, connective tissue, benign
- acoustic (nerve) 225.1
- malignant (M9560/3) - see also
  Neoplasm, connective tissue, malignant
- - acoustic (nerve) 192.0

Neurilemmosarcoma (M9560/3) - see
  Neoplasm, connective tissue, malignant
Neurinoma (M9560/0) - see
  Neurilemmoma
Neurinomatosis (M9560/1) - see Neoplasm,
  connective tissue, uncertain behavior

Neuritis (see also Neuralgia) 729.2
- abducens (nerve) 378.8
- acoustic (nerve) 388.5
- - syphilitic 094.8 † 388.5*
- amyloid, any site 277.3
- arising during pregnancy 646.4
- auditory (nerve) 388.5
- brachial 723.4
- - due to displacement, intervertebral
    disc 722.0
- cranial nerve
- - eighth or acoustic 388.5
- - fourth or trochlear 378.8
- - second or optic 377.3
- - seventh or facial
- - - newborn 767.5
- - sixth or abducens 378.8
- - third or oculomotor 378.8
- Dejerine-Sottas 356.0
- diabetic 250.5 † 357.2*
- diphtheritic 032.8
- due to
- - beriberi 265.0 † 357.4*
- - displacement, prolapse, protrusion or
    rupture, intervertebral disc 722.2
- - - cervical 722.0
- - - lumbar, lumbosacral 722.1
- - - thoracic, thoracolumbar 722.1
- - herniation, nucleus pulposus 722.2
- - - cervical 722.0
- - - lumbar, lumbosacral 722.1
- - - thoracic, thoracolumbar 722.1
- endemic 265.0 † 357.4*
- facial 351.8
- - newborn 767.5
- general - see Polyneuropathy
- geniculate ganglion 351.1
- - due to herpes (zoster) 053.1 † 351.1*
- gouty 274.8 † 357.4*
- in disease classified elsewhere - see
  Polyneuropathy in
- infectious (multiple) NEC 357.0

Neuritis - *continued*
- interstitial hypertrophic progressive NEC 356.9
- lumbosacral nos 724.4
- multiple (acute) (infective) 356.9
- - endemic 265.0 † 357.4*
- multiplex endemica 265.0 † 357.4*
- nerve root (see also Radiculitis) 729.2
- oculomotor (nerve) 378.8
- olfactory nerve 352.0
- optic (nerve) (hereditary) (sympathetic) 377.3
- - in myelitis 341.0
- - meningococcal 036.8 † 377.3*
- peripheral (nerve) - see also Neuropathy, peripheral
- - complicating pregnancy or puerperium 646.4
- - specified nerve - see Mononeuritis
- post-herpetic 053.1
- progressive hypertrophic interstitial NEC 356.9
- puerperal, postpartum 646.4
- retrobulbar 377.3
- - syphilitic 094.8 † 377.3*
- rheumatic (chronic) 729.2
- sciatic (nerve) 724.3
- - due to displacement of intervebral disc 722.1
- serum 999.5
- specified nerve NEC - see Disorder, nerve
- spinal (nerve) root (see also Radiculitis) 729.2
- syphilitic 095
- thoracic nos 724.4
- toxic NEC 357.7
- trochlear (nerve) 378.8
Neuroastrocytoma (M9505/1) - see Neoplasm, uncertain behavior
Neuro-avitaminosis 269.2

Neuroblastoma (M9500/3)
- olfactory (M9522/3) 160.0
- specified site - see Neoplasm, malignant
- unspecified site 194.0
Neurochorioretinitis (see also Chorioretinitis) 363.2
Neurocirculatory asthenia 306.2

Neurocytoma (M9506/0) - see Neoplasm, benign
Neurodermatitis (circumscribed) (circumscripta) (local) 698.3
- atopic 691.8
- diffuse (Brocq) 691.8
- disseminated 691.8
Neuro-encephalomyelopathy, optic 341.0

Neuroepithelioma (M9503/3) - see also Neoplasm, malignant
- olfactory (M9523/3) 160.0
Neurofibroma (M9540/0) - see also Neoplasm, connective tissue, benign
- melanotic (M9541/0) - see Neoplasm, connective tissue, benign
- multiple (M9540/1) 237.7
- plexiform (M9550/0) - see Neoplasm, connective tissue, benign
Neurofibromatosis (multiple) (M9540/1) 237.7
- malignant (M9540/3) - see Neoplasm, connective tissue, malignant
Neurofibrosarcoma (M9540/3) - see Neoplasm, connective tissue, malignant

Neurogenic - see also condition
- bladder 344.6
- heart 306.2
Neuroglioma (M9505/1) - see Neoplasm, uncertain behavior
Neurolathyrism 988.2
Neuroleprosy 030.1
Neuroma (M9570/0) - see also Neoplasm, connective tissue, benign
- acoustic (nerve) (M9560/0) 225.1
- amputation (traumatic) - see also Injury, nerve, by site
- - surgical complication (late) 997.6
- digital 355.6
- interdigital 355.6
- intermetatarsal 355.6
- Morton's 355.6
- optic (nerve) 225.1
- plexiform (M9550/0) - see Neoplasm, connective tissue, benign
- traumatic - see Injury nerve, by site
Neuromyalgia 729.1
Neuromyasthenia (epidemic) 049.8 † 323.4*
Neuromyelitis 341.8
- ascending 357.0
- optica 341.0
Neuromyopathy NEC 358.9
Neuromyositis 729.1
Neuronevus (M8725/0) - see Neoplasm, skin, benign
Neuronitis 357.0
- ascending (acute) 355.2
- vestibular 386.1
Neuroparalytic - see condition

Neuropathy, neuropathic (see also Disorder, nerve) 355.9
- autonomic (peripheral) - see Neuropathy, peripheral, autonomic
- brachial plexus 353.0
- chronic

Neuropathy - *continued*
- chronic - *continued*
- - progressive segmentally demyelinating 357.8
- - relapsing demyelinating 357.8
- Dejerine-Sottas 356.0
- diabetic 250.5 † 357.2*
- entrapment 355.9
- - lateral cutaneous nerve of thigh 355.1
- - median nerve 354.0
- - peroneal nerve 355.3
- - posterior tibial nerve 355.5
- - ulnar nerve 354.2
- facial nerve 351.9
- hereditary 356.9
- - peripheral 356.0
- - sensory 356.2
- hypertrophic
- - Charcot-Marie-Tooth 356.1
- - Dejerine-Sottas 356.0
- - interstitial 356.9
- - Refsum 356.3
- ischemic - see Disorder, nerve
- Jamaica (ginger) 357.7
- lumbar plexus 353.1
- multiple (acute) (chronic) 356.9
- peripheral (nerve) (see also Polyneuropathy) 356.9
- - autonomic 337.9
- - - idiopathic 337.0
- - - in
- - - - amyloidosis 277.3 † 337.1*
- - - - diabetes mellitus 250.5 † 337.1*
- - - - gout 274.8 † 337.1*
- - - - hyperthyroidism 242.9 † 337.1*
- - hereditary 356.0
- - idiopathic 356.9
- - - progressive 356.4
- - - specified NEC 356.8
- radicular NEC 729.2
- - brachial 723.4
- - cervical NEC 723.4
- - hereditary sensory 356.2
- - lumbar 724.4
- - lumbosacral 724.4
- - thoracic NEC 724.4
- sacral plexus 353.1
- sciatic 355.0
- toxic 357.7
- uremic 585 † 357.4*
- vitamin B12 266.2 † 357.4*
- - with anemia (pernicious) 281.0 † 357.4*
- - - due to dietary deficiency 281.1 † 357.4*
Neurophthisis - see also Disorder, nerve
- peripheral, diabetic 250.5 † 357.2*

Neuroretinitis 363.2
Neurosarcoma (M9540/3) - see Neoplasm, connective tissue, malignant
Neurosclerosis - see Disorder, nerve
Neurosis, neurotic 300.9
- anancastic 300.3
- anankastic 300.3
- anxiety (state) 300.0
- asthenic 300.5
- bladder 306.5
- cardiac (reflex) 306.2
- cardiovascular 306.2
- climacteric, unspecified type 627.2
- colon 306.4
- compensation 300.1
- compulsive, compulsion 300.3
- conversion 300.1
- craft 300.8
- cutaneous 306.3
- depressive (reaction) (type) 300.4
- environmental 300.8
- fatigue 300.5
- functional (see also Disorder, psychogenic) 306.9
- gastric 306.4
- gastrointestinal 306.4
- heart 306.2
- hypochondriacal 300.7
- hysterical 300.1
- impulsive 300.3
- incoordination 306.0
- - larynx 306.1
- - vocal cord 306.1
- intestine 306.4
- larynx 306.1
- - hysterical 300.1
- - sensory 306.1
- menopause, unspecified type 627.2
- mixed NEC 300.8
- musculoskeletal 306.0
- obsessional 300.3
- - phobia 300.3
- obsessive-compulsive 300.3
- occupational 300.8
- ocular 306.7
- organ (see also Disorder, psychogenic) 306.9
- pharynx 306.1
- phobic 300.2
- psychasthenic (type) 300.8
- railroad 300.1
- rectum 306.4
- respiratory 306.1
- rumination 306.4
- senile 300.8
- sexual 302.9
- situational 300.8

Neurosis - *continued*
- specified type NEC 300.8
- state 300.9
- - with depersonalization episode 300.6
- stomach 306.4
- vasomotor 306.2
- visceral 306.4
- war 300.1
Neurosyphilis (arrested) (early) (late)
  (latent) (inactive) (recurrent) 094.9
- with ataxia (cerebellar) (locomotor)
  (spastic) (spinal) 094.0
- acute meningitis 094.2 † 320.7*
- aneurysm 094.8
- arachnoid (adhesive) 094.2 † 320.7*
- arteritis (any artery) 094.8
- asymptomatic 094.3
- congenital 090.4
- dura (mater) 094.8
- general paresis 094.1
- gumma 094.9
- hemorrhagic 094.9
- juvenile (asymptomatic) (meningeal)
  090.4
- leptomeninges (aseptic) 094.2 † 320.7*
- meningeal 094.2 † 320.7*
- meninges (adhesive) 094.2 † 320.7*
- meningovascular (diffuse) 094.2 † 320.7*
- optic atrophy 094.8 † 377.1*
- parenchymatous (degenerative) 094.1
- paresis (see also Paresis, general) 094.1
- paretic (see also Paresis, general) 094.1
- relapse 094.9
- remission in (sustained) 094.9
- serological 094.3
- specified nature or site NEC 094.8
- tabes (dorsalis) 094.0
- - juvenile 090.4
- tabetic 094.0
- - juvenile 090.4
- taboparesis 094.1
- - juvenile 090.4
- thrombosis 094.8
- vascular 094.8
Neurotic (see also Neurosis) 300.9
- excoriation 698.4
- - psychogenic 306.3
Neurotmesis - see Injury, nerve, by site
Neurotoxemia - see Toxemia
Neutropenia, neutropenic (chronic)
  (cyclical) (drug induced) (genetic)
  (infantile) (malignant) (periodic)
  (pernicious) (primary) (splenic) (toxic)
  288.0
- neonatal, transitory (isoimmune)
  (maternal transfer) 776.7
Nevocarcinoma (M8720/3) - see Melanoma

Nevus (M8720/0) - see also Neoplasm, skin,
  benign

Note – Except where otherwise indicated,
the varieties of nevus in the list below that
are followed by a morphology code number
(M----/O) should be coded by site as for
"Neoplasm, skin, benign".

Nevus - *continued*
- acanthotic 702
- achromic (M8730/0)
- amelanotic (M8730/0)
- anemic, anemicus 709.0
- angiomatous (M9120/0) 228.0
- araneus 448.1
- avasculosus 709.0
- balloon cell (M8722/0)
- bathing trunk (M8761/1) 238.2
- blue (M8780/0)
- - cellular (M8790/0)
- - giant (M8790/0)
- - Jadassohn's (M8780/0)
- - malignant (M8780/3) - see Melanoma
- capillary (M9131/0) 228.0
- cavernous (M9121/0) 228.0
- cellular (M8720/0)
- - blue (M8790/0)
- comedonicus 757.3
- compound (M8760/0)
- conjunctiva (M8720/0) 224.3
- dermal (M8750/0)
- - and epidermal (M8760/0)
- epitheloid cell (and spindle cell)
  (M8770/0)
- flammeus 757.3
- hairy (M8720/0)
- halo (M8723/0)
- hemangiomatous (M9120/0) 228.0
- intradermal (M8750/0)
- intraepidermal (M8740/0)
- involuting (M8724/0)
- Jadassohn's (blue) (M8780/0)
- junction, junctional (M8740/0)
- - malignant melanoma in (M8740/3) -
  see Melanoma
- juvenile (M8770/0)
- lymphatic (M9170/0) 228.1
- magnocellular (M8726/0)
- - specified site - see Neoplasm, benign
- - unspecified site 224.0
- malignant (M8720/3) - see Melanoma
- meaning hemangioma (M9120/0) 228.0
- melanotic (pigmented) (M8720/0)
- non-neoplastic 448.1
- nonpigmented (M8730/0)

Nevus - *continued*
- nonvascular (M8720/0)
- oral mucosa
- - white sponge 750.2
- papillaris (M8720/0)
- papillomatosus (M8720/0)
- pigmented (M8720/0)
- - giant (M8761/1) - see also Neoplasm, skin, uncertain behavior
- - - malignant melanoma in (M8761/3) - see Melanoma
- pilosus (M8720/0)
- port wine 757.3
- sanguineous 757.3
- sebaceous (senile) 702
- senile 448.1
- spider 448.1
- spindle cell (and epithelioid cell) (M8770/0)
- stellar 448.1
- strawberry 757.3
- syringocystadenomatous papilliferus (M8406/0)
- unius lateris 757.3
- Unna's 757.3
- vascular 757.3
- verrucous 757.3
Newcastle's conjunctivitis or disease 077.8 † 372.0*
Nezelof's syndrome 279.1
Niacin(amide) deficiency 265.2
Nicholas-Durand-Favre disease 099.1
Nicholas-Favre disease 099.1
Nicotinic acid deficiency 265.2
Niemann-Pick disease, splenomegaly or syndrome 272.7
Night
- blindness 368.6
- - congenital 368.6
- - vitamin A deficiency 264.5 † 368.6*
- sweats 780.8
- terrors (child) 307.4
Nightmare 307.4
Nipple - see condition
Nisbet's chancre 099.0
Nitritoid crisis or reaction - see Crisis, nitritoid
Nitrosohemoglobinemia 289.8
Njovera 104.0
No
- diagnosis 799.9
- disease (found) V71.9
Nocardiasis - see Nocardiosis
Nocardiosis 039.9
- lung 039.1 † 484.8*
- pneumonia 039.1 † 484.8*
- specified type NEC 039.8

Nocturia 788.4
- psychogenic 306.5
Nocturnal - see condition
Nodal rhythm 426.0
Node(s) (see also Nodule)
- Heberden's 715.0
- larynx 478.7
- lymph - see condition
- milkers' 051.1
- Osler's 421.0
- rheumatic 729.8
- Schmorl's 722.3
- singers' 478.5
- tuberculous - see Tuberculosis, lymph gland
- vocal cords 478.5
Nodosities, Haygarth's 715.0
Nodule(s), nodular
- actinomycotic (see also Actinomycosis) 039.9
- arthritic - see Arthritis, nodosa
- cutaneous 782.2
- Haygarth's 715.0
- inflammatory - see Inflammation
- juxta-articular 102.7
- - syphilitic 095
- - yaws 102.7
- larynx 478.7
- milkers' 051.1
- prostate 600
- rheumatoid - see Arthritis, rheumatoid
- scrotum (inflammatory) 608.4
- singers' 478.5
- solitary, lung 518.8
- subcutaneous 782.2
- thyroid (gland) 241.0
- - toxic or with hyperthyroidism 242.1
- vocal cords 478.5
Noma (gangrenous) (hospital) (infective) 528.1
- auricle (see also Gangrene) 785.4
- mouth 528.1
- pudendi (see also Vulvitis) 616.1
- vulvae (see also Vulvitis) 616.1
Nomad V60.0
Non-autoimmune hemolytic anemia 283.1
Nonclosure - see also Imperfect closure
- ductus
- - arteriosus 747.0
- - botalli 747.0
- eustachian valve 746.8
- foramen
- - botalli 745.5
- - ovale 745.5
Nondescent (congenital) - see also Malposition, congenital
- cecum 751.4

Nondescent - *continued*
- colon 751.4
- testicle 752.5
Nondevelopment (newborn)
- brain 742.1
- - part of 742.2
- heart 746.8
- organ or site, congenital NEC - see
  Hypoplasia
Nonengagement
- head NEC 652.5
- - in labor 660.1
- - - fetus or newborn 763.0
Nonexpansion lung (newborn) 770.4
Nonfunctioning
- cystic duct (see also Disease, gallbladder)
  575.8
- gallbladder (see also Disease,
  gallbladder) 575.8
- kidney (see also Disease, renal) 593.9
- labyrinth 386.5
Nonhealing stump (surgical) 997.6
Nonimplantation, ovum 628.3
Noninsufflation, fallopian tube 628.2
Nonovulation 628.0
Nonpatent fallopian tube 628.2
Nonpneumatization, lung NEC 770.4
Nonretention food 787.0
Nonrotation - see Malrotation
Nonsecretion urine (see also Anuria) 788.5
- newborn 753.3
Nonunion
- fracture 733.8
- organ or site, congenital NEC - see
  Imperfect closure
- symphysis pubis, congenital 755.6
- top sacrum, congenital 756.1
Nonviability 765.0
Nonvisualization gallbladder 793.3
Nonvitalized tooth 522.9

Normal
- delivery - see Note at category 650
- state (feared complaint unfounded)
  V65.5
North American blastomycosis 116.0
Nose, nasal - see condition
Nosebleed 784.7
Nosomania 298.9
Nosophobia 300.2
Nostalgia 309.8
Notch of iris 743.4
Notching nose, congenital (tip) 748.1
Nothnagel's
- syndrome 378.5
- vasomotor acroparesthesia 443.8
Novy's relapsing fever (American) 087.1
Nuchal hitch (arm) 652.8
Nucleus pulposus - see condition
Numbness (see also Disturbance, sensation)
  782.0
Nuns' knee 727.2
Nutmeg liver 573.8
Nutrition deficient or insufficient (particular
  kind of food) 263.9
- due to
- - insufficient food 994.2
- - lack of
- - - care 995.5
- - - food 994.2
Nyctalopia (night blindness) 368.6
- vitamin A deficiency 264.5 † 368.6*
Nycturia 788.4
- psychogenic 306.5
Nymphomania 302.8
Nystagmus (congenital) (deprivation)
  (dissociated) (latent) 379.5
- benign paroxysmal 386.1
- central positional 386.2
- miner's 300.8

O

Obstruction - *continued*
- airway - *continued*
- − − chronic 496
- alimentary canal (see also Obstruction, intestine) 560.9
- aortic (heart) (valve) (see also Stenosis, aortic) 424.1
- − − rheumatic (see also, stenosis, aortic, rheumatic) 395.0
- aqueduct of Sylvius 331.4
- − − congenital 742.3
- − − − with spina bifida 741.0
- − Arnold-Chiari 741.0
- artery (see also Embolism, artery) 444.9
- − − basilar (complete) (partial) (see also Occlusion, artery, basilar) 433.0
- − − carotid (complete) (partial) (see also Occlusion, artery, carotid) 433.1
- − − precerebral NEC - see Occlusion, artery, precerebral NEC
- − − retinal (central) 362.3
- − − vertebral (complete) (partial) (see also Occlusion, artery, vertebral) 433.2
- bile duct or passage (see also Obstruction, biliary) 576.2
- − − congenital 751.6
- − − − jaundice from 751.6 † 774.5*
- − biliary (duct) (tract) 576.2
- − − with calculus - see Choledocholithiasis
- − − congenital 751.6
- − − − jaundice from 751.6 † 774.5*
- − bladder neck (acquired) 596.0
- − − congenital 753.6
- − bowel (see also Obstruction, intestine) 560.9
- − bronchus 519.1
- − canal, ear 380.5
- − cardia 537.8
- − caval veins (inferior) (superior) 459.2
- − cecum (see also Obstruction, intestine) 560.9
- − circulatory 459.9
- − colon (see also Obstruction, intestine) 560.9
- − common duct (see also Obstruction, biliary) 576.2
- − coronary (artery) (heart) 414.0
- − cystic duct (see also Obstruction, gallbladder) 575.2
- − device, implant or graft - see also Complications, mechanical
- − − due to infection 996.6
- − due to foreign body accidentally left in operation wound 998.4
- − duodenum 537.3
- − ejaculatory duct 608.8
- − esophagus 530.3

Obstruction - *continued*
- − eustachian tube (complete) (partial) 381.6
- − fallopian tube (bilateral) 628.2
- − fecal 560.3
- − − with hernia - see also Hernia, by site with obstruction
- − − − gangrenous - see Hernia, by site, gangrenous
- − foramen of Monro (congenital) 742.3
- − − with spina bifida 741.0
- − foreign body - see Foreign body
- − gallbladder or duct 575.2
- − − with calculus, cholelithiasis, stones - see Cholelithiasis
- − − congenital 751.6 † 774.5*
- − gastric outlet 537.0
- − gastrointestinal (see also Obstruction, intestine) 560.9
- − hepatic 573.8
- − − duct (see also Obstruction, biliary) 576.2
- − icterus (see also Obstruction, gallbladder) 576.8
- − ileocecal coil (see also Obstruction, intestine) 560.9
- − ileum (see also Obstruction, intestine) 560.9
- − intestine (mechanical) (neurogenic) (paroxysmal) (postinfectional) (reflex) 560.9
- − − with
- − − − adhesions (intestinal) (peritoneal) 560.8
- − − adynamic (see also Ileus) 560.1
- − − by gallstone 560.3
- − − congenital or infantile (small) 751.1
- − − − large 751.2
- − − newborn
- − − − due to
- − − − − fecaliths 777.1
- − − − − inspissated milk 777.2
- − − − − meconium (plug) 777.1
- − − − − − in mucoviscidosis 277.0 † 777.0*
- − − specified due to a procedure 997.4
- − − − involving urinary tract 997.5
- − − volvulus 560.2
- − jaundice (see also Obstruction, gallbladder) 576.8
- − jejunum (see also Obstruction, intestine) 560.9
- − kidney 593.8
- − labor 660.9
- − − by
- − − − bony pelvis (conditions in 653.-) 660.1

Occlusion - *continued*
- artery - *continued*
- - cerebellar (anterior inferior) (posterior inferior) (superior) 433.8
- - choroidal (anterior) 433.8
- - communicating posterior 433.8
- - hypophyseal 433.8
- - pontine 433.8
- - precerebral NEC 433.9
- - - multiple or bilateral 433.3
- - - puerperal, postpartum, childbirth 674.0
- - vertebral 433.2
- - - with other precerebral artery 433.3
- - - bilateral 433.3
- basilar artery - see Occlusion, artery, basilar
- bile duct (see also Obstruction, biliary) 576.2
- bowel (see also Obstruction, intestine) 560.9
- brain 435.9
- carotid (artery) (common) (internal) - see Occlusion, artery, carotid
- cerebellar (artery) 433.8
- cerebral (see also Infarct, brain) 434.9
- cerebrovascular (see also Infarct, brain) 434.9
- - diffuse 437.0
- cervical canal (see also Stricture, cervix) 622.4
- - by falciparum malaria 084.0
- cervix (uteri) (see also Stricture, cervix) 622.4
- colon (see also Obstruction, intestine) 560.9
- coronary (artery) (thrombotic) (see also Infarct, myocardium) 410
- cystic duct (see also Obstruction, gallbladder) 575.2
- embolic - see Embolism
- fallopian tube 628.2
- - congenital 752.1
- gallbladder (see also Obstruction, gallbladder) 575.2
- - congenital 751.6
- - - jaundice from 751.6 † 774.3*
- gingiva, traumatic 523.8
- hymen 623.3
- - congenital 752.4
- intestine (see also Obstruction, intestine) 560.9
- kidney 593.8
- lacrimal apparatus 375.5
- lung 518.8
- lymph or lymphatic channel 457.1
- mammary duct 611.8

Occlusion - *continued*
- mesenteric artery (embolic) (thrombotic) (with gangrene) 557.0
- nose 478.1
- - congenital 748.0
- organ or site, congenital NEC - see Atresia
- oviduct 628.2
- - congenital 752.1
- periodontal, traumatic 523.8
- peripheral arteries 444.2
- posterior lingual, of mandibular teeth 524.2
- precerebral artery - see Occlusion, artery, precerebral NEC
- puncta lacrimalia 375.5
- pupil 364.7
- pylorus (see also Stricture, pylorus) 537.0
- renal artery 593.8
- retinal (artery) (branch) (central) (tributary) (partial) (total) (transient) (vein) 362.3
- thoracic duct 457.1
- tubal 628.2
- ureter (complete) (partial) 593.4
- - congenital 753.2
- urethra (see also Stricture, urethra) 598.9
- - congenital 753.6
- uterus 621.8
- vagina 623.2
- vascular NEC 459.9
- vein - see Thrombosis
- vena cava 453.2
- ventricle (brain) NEC 331.4
- vertebral (artery) - see Occlusion, artery, vertebral
- vessel (blood) 459.9
- vulva 624.8
Occupational
- problems NEC V62.2
- therapy V57.2
Ochlophobia 300.2
Ochronosis (endogenous) 270.2
- with chloasma of eyelid 270.2
Ocular muscle - see condition
Oculogyric crisis or disturbance 378.8
- psychogenic 306.7
Oculomotor syndrome 378.8
Odontalgia 525.9
Odontoameloblastoma (M9311/0) 213.1
- upper jaw (bone) 213.0
Odontoclasia 521.0
- complicated 873.7
Odontodysplasia, regional 520.4
Odontogenesis imperfecta 520.5
Odontoma (M9280/0) 213.1
- ameloblastic (M9311/0) 213.1

Odontoma - *continued*
- ameloblastic - *continued*
- - upper jaw (bone) 213.0
- calcified (M9280/0) 213.1
- - upper jaw (bone) 213.0
- complex (M9282/0) 213.1
- - upper jaw (bone) 213.0
- compound (M9281/0) 213.1
- - upper jaw (bone 213.0
- fibroameloblastic (M9290/0) 213.1
- - upper jaw (bone) 213.0
- follicular 526.0
- upper jaw (bone) 213.0
Odontomyelitis (closed) (open) 522.0
Odontonecrosis 521.0
Odontorrhagia 525.8
Odontosarcoma, ameloblastic (M9290/3)
   170.1
- upper jaw (bone) 170.0
Oedema, oedematous - see Edema
Oesophagectasis 530.8
Oesophagismus 530.5
Oesophagitis - see Esophagitis
Oesophagomalacia 530.8
Oesophagostomiasis 127.7
Oesophagotracheal - see condition
Oesophagus - see condition
Oestriasis 134.0
Oguchi's disease 368.6
Ohara's disease 021
Oidiomycosis (see also Candidiasis) 112.9
Old age 797
- dementia 290.0
Olfactory - see condition
Oligemia 285.9
Oligergasia (see also Retardation, mental)
   319
Oligoastrocytoma, mixed (M9382/3)
- specified site - see Neoplasm, malignant
- unqpecified site 191.9
Oligocythemia 285.9
Oligodendroblastoma (M9460/3)
- specified site - see Neoplasm, malignant
- unspecified site 191.9
Oligodendroglioma (M9450/3)
- anaplastic type (M9451/3)
- - specified site - see Neoplasm,
     malignant
- - unspecified site 191.9
- specified site - see Neoplasm, malignant
- unspecified site 191.9
Oligodontia (see also Anodontia) 520.0
Oligohydramnios 658.0
- due to premature rupture of membranes
   658.1
- fetus or newborn 761.2
Oligohydrosis 705.0

Oligomenorrhea 626.1
Oligophrenia (see also Retardation, mental)
   319
- phenylpyruvic 270.1
Oligospermia 606
Oligotrichia 704.0
- congenita 757.4
Oliguria 788.5
- complicating
- - abortion - see categories 634-639,
     fourth digit .3
- - ectopic or molar pregnancy 639.3
- following labor and delivery 669.3
- specified due to a procedure 997.5
Ollier's disease 756.4
Omentitis (see also Peritonitis) 567.9
Omentocele - see Hernia, abdominal
Omentum, omental - see condition
Omphalitis (congenital) (newborn) 771.4
- not of newborn 686.9
- tetanus 771.3
Omphalocele - see Hernia, umbilicus
Omphalomesenteric duct persistent 751.0
Omphalorrhagia, newborn 772.3
Onanism 307.9
Onchocerciasis 125.3
- eye 125.3 † 360.1*
- eyelid 125.3 † 373.6*
Onchocercosis - see Onchocerciasis
Oncocytoma (M8290/0) - see Neoplasm,
   benign
Oneirophrenia 295.4
Onychauxis 703.8
- congenital 757.5
Onychia (with lymphangitis) 681.9
- dermatophytic 110.1
- finger 681.0
- toe 681.1
Onychitis (with lymphangitis) 681.9
- finger 681.0
- toe 681.1
Onychocryptosis 703.8
Onychodystrophy 703.8
- congenital 757.5
Onychogryphosis 703.8
Onychogryposis 703.8
Onycholysis 703.8
Onychomadesis 703.8
Onychomalacia 703.8
Onychomycosis 110.1
- finger 110.1
- toe 110.1
Onychophagy 307.9
Onychoptosis 703.8
Onychorrhexis 703.8
- congenital 757.5
Onychoschizia 703.8

Onychotrophia (see also Atrophy, nail)
   703.8
Onyxis (finger) (toe) 703.0
Onyxitis (with lymphangitis) 681.9
− finger 681.0
− toe 681.1
Oophoritis (cystic) (infectional) (interstitial)
   (see also Salpingo-oophoritis) 614.2
− fetal (acute) 752.0
Opacities enamel (teeth) (fluoride)
   (nonfluoride) 520.3
Opacity
− cornea NEC 371.0
− − congenital 743.4
− − degenerative 371.4
− − hereditary 371.5
− − inflammatory - see Keratitis
− lens (see also Cataract) 366.9
− vitreous (humor) 379.2
− − congenital 743.5
Opalescent dentin 520.5
Open, opening
− abnormal, organ or site, congenital - see
   Imperfect closure
− angle with
− − borderline intraocular pressure 365.0
− − cupping of discs 365.0
− false - see Imperfect closure
− wound - see Wound, open

Openbite (anterior) (posterior) 524.2
Operation NEC 799.9
− causing multilation of fetus 763.8
− for delivery
− − fetus or newborn 763.8
− maternal, unrelated to current delivery,
   affecting fetus or newborn 760.6
Operational fatigue 300.8
Operative - see condition
Ophiasis 704.0

Ophthalmia (catarrhal) (purulent) 372.0
− actinic rays 370.2
− allergic (acute) 372.0
− blennorrhagic (neonatorum) 098.4 †
   372.0*
− diphtheritic 032.8 † 372.0*
− Egyptian 076.1
− electrica 370.2
− gonococcal (neonatorum) 098.4 † 372.0*
− metastatic 360.0
− neonatorum, newborn 771.6
− − gonococcal 098.4 † 372.0*
− nodosa 360.1
− sympathetic 360.1
Ophthalmitis - see Ophthalmia
Ophthalmocele (congenital) 743.0
Ophthalmoneuromyelitis 341.0

Ophthalmoplegia (see also Strabismus)
   378.9
− diabetic 250.4 † 378.8*
− exophthalmic 242.0
− internal (complete) (total) 367.5
− internuclear 378.8
− migraine 346.8
− Parinaud's 378.5
− progressive external 378.7
− supranuclear, progressive 333.0
− total (external) 378.5
Opisthognathism 524.0
Opisthorchiasis (felineus) (tenuicollis)
   (viverrini) 121.0
Opitz's disease 289.5
Opiumism 304.0
Oppenheim's disease 358.8
Oppenheim-Urbach disease 250.7 † 709.8*
Optic nerve - see condition
Orbit - see condition
Orchioblastoma (M9071/3) 186.9
Orchitis (gangrenous) (nonspecific) (septic)
   (suppurative) 604.9
− with abscess 604.0
− blennorrhagic (acute) 098.1 † 604.9*
− − chronic or duration of 2 months or over
   098.3 † 604.9*
− gonococcal (acute) 098.1 † 604.9*
− − chronic or duration of 2 months or over
   098.3 † 604.9*
− mumps 072.0 † 604.9*
− parotidea 072.0 † 604.9*
− syphilitic 095
− tuberculous 016.3 † 608.8*
Orf 051.2
Organ of Morgagni (persistence of) 752.8
Organic - see also condition
− heart - see Disease, heart
− insufficiency 799.8
Orifice - see condition
Origin of both great vessels from right
   ventricle 745.1
Ormond's disease 593.4
Ornithosis 073
− with pneumonia 073 † 484.2*
Orotaciduria, oroticaciduria (congenital)
   (hereditary) (pyrimidine deficiency) 281.4
Orthodontics V58.5
− adjustment V53.4
− fitting V53.4
Orthopnea 786.0
Orthoptic training V57.4
Os, uterus - see condition
Osgood-Schlatter disease or
   osteochondrosis 732.4
Osler's nodes 421.0
Osler-Rendu disease 448.0

Osler-Vaquez disease (M9950/1) 238.4
Osmidrosis 705.8
Osseous - see condition
Ossification
- artery - see Arteriosclerosis
- auricle (ear) 380.3
- bronchi 519.1
- cardiac (see also Degeneration, myocardial) 429.1
- cartilage (senile) 733.9
- coronary (artery) 414.0
- diaphragm 728.1
- ear 380.3
- falx cerebri 349.2
- fascia 728.1
- fontanel
- - defective or delayed 756.0
- - premature 756.0
- heart (see also Degeneration, myocardial) 429.1
- - valve - see Endocarditis
- larynx 478.7
- ligament
- - posterior longitudinal 724.8
- - - cervical 723.7
- meninges (cerebral) 349.2
- - spinal 336.8
- multiple, eccentric centers 733.9
- muscle 728.1
- myocardium, myocardial (see also Degeneration, myocardial) 429.1
- penis 607.8
- periarticular 728.8
- sclera 379.1
- tendon 727.8
- trachea 519.1
- tympanic membrane 384.8
- vitreous (humor) 360.4
Osteitis (see also Osteomyelitis) 730.2
- alveolar 526.5
- condensans (ilii) 733.5
- deformans 731.0
- due to yaws 102.6
- fibrosa NEC 733.2
- - cystica (generalisata) 252.0
- - disseminata 756.5
- - osteoplastica 252.0
- fragilitans 756.5
- Garre's (sclerosing) 730.1
- jaw (acute) (chronic) (lower) (neonatal) (suppurative) (upper) 526.4
- parathyroid 252.0
- petrous bone (acute) (chronic) 383.2
- sclerotic, nonsuppurative 730.1
- tuberculosa
- - cystica (of Jungling) 135
- - multiplex cystoides 135

Osteoarthritis (see also Osteoarthrosis) 715.9
- distal interphalangeal 715.3
- spine, spinal NEC'721.9
Osteoarthropathy (see also Osteoarthrosis) 715.9
- hypertrophic pulmonary 715.9
- secondary, hypertrophic 715.9
Osteoarthrosis (degenerative) (hypertrophic) (rheumatoid) 715.9
- deformans alkaptonurica 270.2
- generalized 715.0
- localized 715.3
- - primary 715.1
- - secondary 715.2
- more than one site, but not specified as generalized 715.8
- polyarticular 715.0
- spine (see also Spondylosis) 721.9
Osteoblastoma (M9200/0) - see Neoplasm, bone, benign
Osteochondritis (see also Osteochondrosis) 732.9
- dissecans 732.7
- multiple 756.5
- syphilitic (congenital) 090.0
Osteochondrodermodysplasia 756.5
Osteochondrodystrophy 277.5
- deformans 277.5
- familial 277.5
- fetalis 756.4
Osteochondroma (M9210/0) - see Neoplasm, bone, benign
- multiple, congenital 756.4
Osteochondromatosis (M9210/1) 238.0
- synovial 727.8
Osteochondromyxosarcoma (M9180/3) - see Neoplasm, bone, malignant
Osteochondropathy NEC 732.9
Osteochondrosarcoma (M9180/3) - see Neoplasm, bone, malignant
Osteochondrosis 732.9
- acetabulum (juvenile) 732.1
- adult, any site 732.8
- astragalus (juvenile) 732.5
- Blount's 732.4
- Buchanan's 732.1
- Buchman's 732.1
- Burn's 732.3
- calcaneus (juvenile) 732.5
- capitular epiphysis (femur) (juvenile) 732.1
- carpal scaphoid (juvenile) 732.3
- coxae juvenilis 732.1
- deformans juvenilis (coxae) 732.1
- Diaz's 732.5
- dissecans (knee) (shoulder) 732.7

Osteochondrosis - *continued*
- femoral capital epiphysis (juvenile) 732.1
- femur (head) (juvenile) 732.1
- foot (juvenile) 732.5
- Freiberg's 732.5
- Haglund's 732.5
- Hass's 732.3
- hip (juvenile) 732.1
- humerus (juvenile) 732.3
- ilium, iliac crest (juvenile) 732.1

- ischiopubic synchondrosis 732.1
- Iselin's 732.5
- juvenile, juvenilis 732.6
- − arm 732.3
- − capitular epiphysis 732.1
- − clavicle, sternal epiphysis 732.6
- − coxae 732.1
- − deformans 732.1
- − foot 732.5
- − hand 732.3
- − hip and pelvis 732.1
- − lower extremity, except foot 732.4
- − medial cuneiform bone 732.5
- − specified site NEC 732.6
- − spine 732.0
- − upper extremity 732.3
- − vertebra (body) (of calve) 732.0
- − − epiphyseal plates (of Schuermann) 732.0
- Kienbock's 732.3
- Kohler's
- − patellar 732.4
- − tarsal navicular 732.5
- Legg-Perthes(-Calve) 732.1
- lower extremity (juvenile) 732.4
- lunate bone (juvenile) 732.3
- Mauclaire's 732.3
- metacarpal (head) (juvenile) 732.3

- metatarsal (fifth) (head) (second) 732.5
- navicular (juvenile) 732.5
- os
- − calcis (juvenile) 732.5
- − tibiale externum (juvenile) 732.5
- Osgood-Schlatter 732.4
- Panner's 732.3
- patellar center (primary) (secondary) 732.4
- pelvis (juvenile) 732.1
- Pierson's 732.1
- Scheuermann's 732.0
- Sever's 732.5
- Sinding-Larsen 732.4
- spine (juvenile) 732.0
- − adult 732.8
- symphysis pubis (juvenile) 732.1
- syphilitic (congenital) 090.0

Osteochondrosis - *continued*
- tarsal (scaphoid) (navicular) (juvenile) 732.5
- tibia (proximal) (tubercle) (juvenile) 732.4
- tuberculous - see Tuberculosis, bone
- ulna (juvenile) 732.3
- upper extremity (juvenile) 732.3
- van Neck's 732.1
- vertebral (juvenile) 732.0
- − adult 732.8
Osteoclastoma (M9250/1) 238.0
- malignant (M9250/3) - see Neoplasm, bone, malignant
Osteocopic pain 733.9
Osteodynia 733.9
Osteodystrophy
- azotemic 588.0
- congenital 756.5
- parathyroid 252.0
- renal 588.0
Osteofibroma (M9262/0) - see Neoplasm, bone, benign
Osteofibrosarcoma (M9182/3) - see Neoplasm, bone, malignant
Osteogenesis imperfecta 756.5
Osteogenic - see condition
Osteoma (M9180/0) - see also Neoplasm, bone, benign
- osteoid (M9191/0) - see also Neoplasm, bone, benign
- − giant (M9200/0) - see Neoplasm, bone, benign
Osteomalacia 268.2
- infantile (see also Rickets) 268.0
- juvenile (see also Rickets) 268.0
- pelvis 268.2
- vitamin D resistant 275.3
Osteomalacosis 268.2
Osteomyelitis (general) (infective) (localized) (neonatal) (purulent) (pyogenic) (septic) (staphylococcal) (streptococcal) (suppurative) (with periostitis) 730.2
- acute or subacute 730.0
- chronic or old 730.1
- Garre's 730.1
- jaw (acute) (chronic) (lower) (neonatal) (suppurative) (upper) 526.4
- nonsuppurating 730.1
- orbit 376.0
- petrous bone 383.2
- salmonella 003.2 † 730.2*
- sclerosing, nonsuppurative 730.1
- syphilitic 095 † 730.8*
- − congenital 090.0 † 730.8*
- tuberculous - see Tuberculosis, bone

Osteomyelitis - *continued*
– typhoid 002.0 † 730.2*
Osteomyelofibrosis 289.8
Osteomyelosclerosis 289.8
Osteonecrosis 730.1
Osteopathia
– condensans disseminata 756.5
– hyperostotica multiplex infantilis 756.5
Osteopecilia 756.5
Osteoperiostitis (see also Osteomyelitis) 730.2
Osteopetrosis (familial) 756.5
Osteophyte - see Exostosis
Osteopoikilosis 756.5
Osteoporosis 733.0
– posttraumatic 733.7
– senilis 733.0
Osteopsathyrosis 756.5
Osteoradionecrosis, jaw 526.8
Osteosarcoma (M9180/3) - see also
Neoplasm, bone, malignant
– chondroblastic (M9181/3) - see
Neoplasm, bone, malignant
– fibroblastic (M9182/3) - see Neoplasm,
bone, malignant
– in Paget's disease of bone (M9184/3) -
see Neoplasm, bone, malignant
– juxtacortical (M9190/3) - see Neoplasm,
bone, malignant
– parosteal (M9190/3) - see Neoplasm,
bone, malignant
– telangiectatic (M9183/3) - see Neoplasm,
bone, malignant
Osteosclerosis 756.5
– fragilis (generalisata) 756.5
– myelofibrosis 289.8
Osteosclerotic anemia 289.8
Osteosis cutis 709.3
Osterreicher-Turner syndrome 756.8
Ostium
– atrioventriculare commune 745.6
– primum (arteriosum) (defect) (persistent)
745.6
– secundum (arteriosum) (defect) (patent)
(persistent) 745.5
Ostrum-Furst syndrome 756.5
Otalgia 388.7
Othematoma (pinna) 380.3
Otitis 382.9
– acute 382.9
– adhesive 385.1
– chronic 382.9
– diffuse parasitic 136.8
– externa (acute) (diffuse) (hemorrhagica)
(malignant) 380.1
– – tropical 111.8
– interna 386.3

Otitis - *continued*
– media 382.9
– – with effusion 381.4
– – acute 382.9
– – – with effusion 381.0
– – – allergic 381.0
– – – catarrhal 381.0
– – – exudative 381.0
– – – mucoid 381.0
– – – necrotizing 382.0
– – – – in
– – – – – influenza 487.8 † 382.0*
– – – – – measles 055.2 † 382.0*
– – – – – scarlet fever 034.1 † 382.0*
– – – nonsuppurative 381.0
– – – purulent 382.0
– – – secretory 381.0
– – – seromucinous 381.0
– – – serous 381.0
– – – suppurative 382.0
– – – transudative 381.0
– – allergic 381.4
– – catarrhal 381.4
– – chronic 382.9
– – – with effusion 381.3
– – – allergic 381.3
– – – catarrhal 381.1
– – – exudative 381.3
– – – mucinous 381.2
– – – mucoid 381.2
– – – purulent 382.3
– – – secretory 381.3
– – – seromucinous 381.3
– – – serous 381.1
– – – suppurative 382.3
– – – – atticoantral 382.2
– – – – benign 382.1
– – – – tubotympanic 382.1
– – – transudative 381.3
– – exudative 381.4
– – mucoid 381.4
– – nonsuppurative 381.4
– – purulent 382.4
– – secretory 381.4
– – seromucinous 381.4
– – serous 381.4
– – suppurative 382.4
– – transudative 381.4
– – tuberculous 017.4 † 382.3*
– postmeasles 055.2 † 382.0*
Otolith syndrome 386.1
Otomycosis (diffuse) NEC 111.9 † 380.1*
– in
– – aspergillosis 117.3 † 380.1*
– – moniliasis 112.8 † 380.1*
Otoporosis - see Otosclerosis
Otorrhagia 388.6

Otorrhagia - *continued*
- traumatic - code by type of injury
Otorrhea 388.6
- cerebrospinal 388.6
Otosclerosis 387.9
- cochlear 387.2
- involving
- - optic capsule 387.2
- - oval window
- - - nonobliterative 387.0
- - - obliterative 387.1
- - round window 387.2
- nonobliterative 387.0
- obliterative 387.1
- specific type 387.8
Otospongiosis - see Otosclerosis
Otto's disease or pelvis 715.3
Outburst, aggressive 312.0
- in children and adolescents 313.9
Outcome of delivery
- multiple births NEC V27.9
- - all liveborn V27.5
- - all stillborn V27.7
- - some liveborn V27.6
- - unspecified V27.9
- single NEC V27.9
- - live birth V27.0
- - stillborn V27.1
- twins NEC V27.9
- - both live born V27.2
- - both stillborn V27.4
- - one liveborn, one stillborn V27.3
Outlet - see condition
Outstanding ears (bilateral) 744.2
Ovalocytosis (congenital) (hereditary) (see
   also Elliptocytosis) 282.1
Ovaritis (cystic) (see also Salpingo-
   oophoritis) 614.2
Ovary, ovarian - see condition
Overactive
- hypothalmus 253.8
- thyroid (see also Hyperthyroidism) 242.9
Overbite (deep) (excessive) (horizontal)
   (vertical) 524.2
Overbreathing (see also Hyperventilation)
   786.0
Overdevelopment - see also Hypertrophy
- breast 611.1
- congenital, prostate 752.8
- nasal bones 738.0
Overdistension - see Distension
Overdose, overdosage (drug) 977.9
- specified drug or substance - see Table of
   drugs and chemicals

Overeating 783.6
- nonorganic origin 307.5
Overexertion (effects) (exhaustion) 994.5
Overexposure (effects) 994.9
- exhaustion 994.4
Overfeeding 783.6
Overgrowth, bone NEC 733.9
Overheated (places) (effects) - see Heat
Overjet 524.2
Overlaid, overlying (suffocation) 994.7
Overlapping toe (acquired) 735.8
- congenital (fifth toe) 755.6
Overload
- fluid 276.6
- potassium 276.7
- sodium 276.0
Overnutrition (see also Hyperalimentation)
   783.6
Overproduction - see Hypersecretion
Overriding
- aorta 747.2
- finger (acquired) 736.2
- - congenital 755.5
- toe (acquired) 735.8
- - congenital 755.6
Oversize
- fetus 766.0
- - affecting management of pregnancy
   656.6
- - causing disproportion 653.5
- - - with obstructed labor 660.1
- - - fetus or newborn 763.1
Overstrained 780.7
- heart - see Hypertrophy, cardiac
Overweight (see also Obesity) 278.0
Overwork 780.7
Oviduct - see condition
Ovotestis 752.7
Ovulation (cycle)
- failure or lack of 628.0
- pain 625.2
Owren's disease (see also Defect,
   coagulation) 286.3
Ox heart - see Hypertrophy, cardiac
Oxalosis 271.8
Oxaluria 271.8
Oxycephaly, oxycephalic 756.0
- syphilitic, congenital 090.0
Oxyuriasis 127.4
Oxyuris vermicularis (infestation) 127.4
Ozena 472.0

P

P U O (see also Pyrexia) 780.6
Pachyderma, pachydermia 701.8
– laryngis 478.7
– larynx (verrucosa) 478.7
Pachydermatocele (congenital) 757.3
– acquired 701.8
Pachydermatosis 701.8
Pachymeningitis (adhesive) (basal) (brain)
  (cerebral) (cervical) (chronic)
  (circumscribed) (external) (fibrous)
  (hemorrhagic) (hypertrophic) (internal)
  (purulent) (spinal) (suppurative) (see also
  Meningitis) 322.9
Pachyonychia (congenital) 757.5
Pacinian tumor (M9507/0) -see neoplasm,
  skin, benign 216.9
Pad, knuckle or Garrod's 728.7
Paget's disease 731.0
– with infiltrating duct carcinoma of the
  breast (M8541/3) - see Neoplasm, breast,
  malignant
– bone 731.0
– – osteosarcoma in (M9184/3) - see
    Neoplasm, bone, malignant
– breast (M8540/3) 174.0
– extramammary (M8542/3) - see also
  Neoplasm, skin, malignant
– – anus 154.3
– – – skin 173.5
– malignant (M8540/3)
– – breast 174.0
– – specified site NEC (M8542/3) - see
  Neoplasm, skin, malignant
– – unspecified site 174.0
– mammary (M8540/3) 174.0
– nipple (M8540/3) 174.0
– osteitis deformans 731.0
Pain(s)
– abdominal 789.0
– alimentary due to vascular insufficiency
  557.9
– anginoid (see also Pain, precordial) 786.5
– anus 569.4
– arch 729.5
– arm 729.5
– back (postural) 724.5
– – low 724.2
– – psychogenic 307.8
– bladder 788.9
– bone 733.9

Pain(s) - *continued*
– breast 611.7
– – psychogenic 307.8
– cecum 789.0
– cervicobrachial 723.6
– chest 786.5
– – wall, anterior 786.5
– coccyx 724.7
– colon 789.0
– coronary - see Angina
– due to (presence of) any device, implant
  or graft classifiable to 996.0 - 996.5 996.7
– ear 388.7
– epigastric 789.0
– epigastrium 789.0
– extremity (lower) (upper) 729.5
– eye 379.8
– face, facial 784.0
– – atypical 350.2
– – nerve 351.8
– false (labor) 644.0
– female genital organs NEC 625.9
– finger 729.5
– flank 789.0
– foot 729.5
– gas (intestinal) 787.3
– gastric 536.8
– generalized 780.9
– genital organ
– – female 625.9
– – male 608.9
– – psychogenic 307.8
– groin 789.0
– hand 729.5
– head (see also Headache) 784.0
– heart (see also Pain, precordial) 786.5
– infra-orbital (see also Neuralgia,
  trigeminal) 350.1
– intermenstrual 625.2
– jaw 526.9
– joint 719.4
– – psychogenic 307.8
– kidney 788.0
– labor, false or spurious 644.0
– leg 729.5
– limb 729.5
– low back 724.2
– lumbar region 724.2
– mastoid 388.7
– maxilla 526.9

Pain(s) - *continued*
- metacarpophalangeal (joint) 719.4
- metatarsophalangeal (joint) 719.4
- mouth 528.9
- muscle 729.1
- nasal 478.1
- nasopharynx 478.2
- neck NEC 723.1
- - psychogenic 307.8
- nerve NEC 729.2
- neuromuscular 729.1
- nose 478.1
- ophthalmic 379.8
- orbital region 379.8
- osteocopic 733.9
- ovary 625.9
- over heart (see also Pain, precordial) 786.5
- ovulation 625.2
- penis 607.9
- - psychogenic 307.8
- pericardial (see also Pain, precordial) 786.5
- pharynx 478.2
- pleura, pleural, pleuritic 786.5
- preauricular 388.7
- precordial (region) 786.5
- - psychogenic 307.8
- psychogenic 307.8
- - cardiovascular system 307.8
- - gastrointestinal system 307.8
- - genitourinary system 307.8
- - heart 307.8
- - musculoskeletal system 307.8
- - respiratory system 307.8
- - skin 306.3
- radicular (spinal) (see also Radiculitis) 729.2
- rectum 569.4
- rheumatic, muscular 729.1
- rib 786.5
- root (spinal) (see also Radiculitis) 729.2
- sacroiliac 724.6
- sciatic 724.3
- scrotum 608.9
- - psychogenic 307.8
- seminal vesicle 608.9
- spermatic cord 608.9
- spinal root (see also Radiculitis) 729.2
- stomach 536.8
- - psychogenic 307.8
- temporomandibular (joint) 524.6
- temporomaxillary joint 524.6
- testis 608.9
- - psychogenic 307.8
- thoracic spine 724.1
- - with radicular and visceral pain 724.4

Pain(s) - *continued*
- throat 784.1
- tibia 733.9
- toe 729.5
- tongue 529.6
- tooth 525.9
- trigeminal (see also Neuralgia, trigeminal) 350.1
- ureter 788.0
- urinary (organ) (system) 788.0
- uterus 625.9
- - psychogenic 307.8
- vertebrogenic (syndrome) 724.5
- vesical 788.9
Painful - see also Pain
- coitus
- - female 625.0
- - male 608.8
- - psychogenic 302.7
- ejaculation (semen) 608.8
- - psychogenic 302.7
- erection 607.3
- menstruation 625.3
- - psychogenic 306.5
- respiration 786.5
- scar 709.2
- wire sutures 998.8
Painter's colic 984.-
- specified type of lead - see Table of drugs and chemicals
Palate - see condition
Palatoplegia 528.9
Palatoschisis 749.0
- with cleft lip 749.2
Palilalia 784.6
Pallor 782.6
Palmar - see also condition
- fascia - see condition
Palpable
- cecum 569.8
- kidney 593.8
- liver 573.9
- ovary 620.8
- spleen - see Splenomegaly
Palpitation (heart) 785.1
- psychogenic 306.2
Palsy (see also Paralysis) 344.9
- atrophic diffuse 335.2
- Bell's (see also Palsy, facial) 351.0
- brachial plexus 353.0
- - fetus or newborn 767.6
- brain - see Palsy, cerebral
- bulbar (progressive) (chronic) 335.2
- - pseudo NEC 335.2
- - supranuclear NEC 344.8
- cerebral (congenital) (infantile) (spastic) 343.9

Palsy - *continued*
- cerebral - *continued*
- - athetoid 333.7
- - diplegic 343.0
- - hemiplegic 343.1
- - monoplegic 343.3
- - not congenital or infantile 437.8
- - paraplegic 343.0
- - quadriplegic 343.2
- - spastic, not congenital or infantile 344.8
- - syphilitic 094.8
- - - congenital 090.4
- - tetraplegic 343.2
- cranial nerve - see also Disorder, nerve, cranial
- - multiple 352.6
- creeping 335.2
- divers' 993.3
- Erb's 767.6
- facial 351.0
- - newborn 767.5
- glossopharyngeal 352.2
- Klumpke(-Dejerine) 767.6
- lead 984.-
- - specified type of lead - see Table of drugs and chemicals
- median nerve (tardy) 354.1
- peroneal nerve (acute) (tardy) 355.3
- pseudobulbar NEC 335.2
- radial nerve (acute) 354.3
- seventh nerve (see also Palsy, facial) 351.0
- shaking (see also Parkinsonism) 332.0
- specified nerve not listed - see Disorder, nerve
- ulnar nerve (tardy) 354.2
- wasting 335.2
Paludism - see Malaria
Panaris (with lymphangitis) 681.9
- finger 681.0
- toe 681.1
Panaritium (with lymphangitis) 681.9
- finger 681.0
- toe 681.1
Panarteritis (nodosa) 446.0
- brain or cerebral 437.4
Pancarditis (acute) (chronic) 429.8
Pancoast's syndrome or tumor (M8010/3) 162.3
Pancreas, pancreatic - see condition
Pancreatitis 577.0
- acute (edematous) (hemorrhagic) (recurrent) 577.0
- annular 577.0
- apoplectic 577.0
- chronic (infectious) 577.1

Pancreatitis - *continued*
- chronic - *continued*
- - recurrent 577.1
- cystic 577.2
- fibrous 577.8
- gangrenous 577.0
- hemorrhagic (acute) 577.0
- interstitial (chronic) 577.1
- - acute 577.0
- malignant 577.0
- mumps 072.3 † 577.0*
- recurrent 577.1
- relapsing 577.1
- subacute 577.0
- suppurative 577.0
- syphilitic 095
Pancreolithiasis 577.8
Pancytolysis 289.9
Pancytopenia (acquired) 284.8
- with malformations 284.0
- congenital 284.0
Panencephalitis, subacute, sclerosing 046.2 † 323.1*
Panhematopenia 284.8
- constitutional 284.0
- splenic, primary 289.4
Panhemocytopenia 284.8
- constitutional 284.0
Panhypogonadism 257.2
Panhypopituitarism 253.2
- prepubertal 253.2
Panic (attack) (state) 300.0
- reaction to exceptional stress (transient) 308.0
Panmyelophthisis 284.9
Panmyelosis (acute) (M9951/1) 238.7
Panner's disease 732.3
Panneuritis endemica 265.0 † 357.4*
Panniculitis 729.3
- back 724.8
- neck 723.6
- nodular, nonsuppurative 729.3
- sacral 724.8
Panniculus adiposus (abdominal) 278.1
Pannus 370.6
- allergic eczematous (see also Keratitis) 370.6
- degenerativus 370.6
- keratic 370.6
- trachomatosus, trachomatous (active) 076.1 † 370.6*
Panophthalmitis 360.0
Panotitis - see Otitis media
Pansinusitis (chronic) (hyperplastic) (nonpurulent) (purulent) 473.8
- acute 461.8
- due to fungus NEC 117.9

Pansinusitis - *continued*
- tuberculous 012.8
Panuveitis (sympathetic) 360.1
Panvalvular disease - see Endocarditis,
mitral
Papanicolaou smear, cervix V76.2
- for suspected malignant neoplasm V76.2
- - no disease found V71.1
- routine V76.2
Papilledema 377.0
- choked disc 377.0
- infectional 377.0
Papillitis 377.3
- anus 569.4
- necrotizing, kidney 584.7
- optic 377.3
- rectum 569.4
- renal, necrotizing 584.7
- tongue 529.0
Papilloma (M8050/0) - see also Neoplasm,
benign

Note – Except where otherwise indicated,
the morphological varieties of papilloma in
the list below should be coded by site as for
"Neoplasm, benign".

Papilloma - *continued*
- acuminatum (female) (male) 078.1
- bladder (urinary) (transitional cell)
(M8120/1) 236.7
- - benign (M8120/0) 223.3
- choroid plexus (M9390/0) 225.0
- - anaplastic type (M9390/3) 191.5
- - malignant (M9390/3) 191.5
- ductal (M8503/0)
- dyskeratotic (M8052/0)
- epidermoid (M8052/0)
- hyperkeratotic (M8052/0)
- intracystic (M8504/0)
- intraductal (M8503/0)
- inverted (M8053/0)
- keratotic (M8052/0)
- parakeratotic (M8052/0)
- renal pelvis (transitional cell) (M8120/1)
236.9
- - benign (M8120/0) 223.1
- Schneiderian (M8121/0)
- - specified site - see Neoplasm, benign
- - unspecified site 212.0
- serous surface (M8461/0)
- - borderline malignancy (M8461/1)
- - - specified site - see Neoplasm,
uncertain behavior
- - - unspecified site 236.2
- - specified site - see Neoplasm, benign

Papilloma - *continued*
- serous surface - *continued*
- - unspecified site 220
- squamous (cell) (M8052/0)
- transitional (cell) (M8120/0)
- - bladder (urinary) (M8120/1) 236.7
- - inverted type (M8121/1) - see
Neoplasm, uncertain behavior
- - renal pelvis (M8120/1) 236.9
- - ureter (M8120/1) 236.9
- ureter (transitional cell) (M8120/1)
236.9
- - benign (M8120/0) 223.2
- urothelial (M8120/1) - see Neoplasm,
uncertain behavior
- verrucous (M8051/0)
- villous (M8261/1) - see Neoplasm,
uncertain behavior
- yaws, plantar or palmar 102.1
Papillomata, multiple, of yaws 102.1
Papillomatosis (M8060/0) - see also
Neoplasm, benign
- confluent and reticulate 701.8
- ductal, breast 610.1
- intraductal (diffuse) (M8505/0) - see
Neoplasm, benign
- subareolar duct (M8506/0) 217
Papillon-Leage and Psaume syndrome
759.8
Papule 709.8
- carate (primary) 103.0
- fibrous, of nose (M8724/0) 216.3
- pinta (primary) 103.0
Papyraceous fetus 779.8
- complicating pregnancy 646.0
Paracephalus 759.7
Paracoccidioidomycosis 116.1
- mucocutaneous-lymphangitic 116.1
- pulmonary 116.1
- visceral 116.1
Paradentosis 523.5
Paraffinoma 999.9
Paraganglioma (M8680/1)
- adrenal (M8700/0) 227.0
- - malignant (M8700/3) 194.0
- aortic body (M8691/1) 237.3
- - malignant (M8691/3) 194.6
- carotid body (M8692/1) 237.3
- - malignant (M8692/3) 194.5
- chromaffin (M8700/0) - see also
Neoplasm, benign
- - malignant (M8700/3) - see Neoplasm,
malignant
- extra-adrenal (M8693/1)
- - malignant (M8693/3)
- - - specified site - see Neoplasm,
malignant

Paraganglioma - *continued*
- extra-adrenal - *continued*
- - malignant - *continued*
- - - unspecified site 194.6
- - specified site - see Neoplasm, uncertain
    behavior
- - unspecified site 237.3
- glomus jugulare (M8690/1) 237.3
- - malignant (M8690/3) 194.6
- jugular (M8690/1) 237.3
- malignant (M8680/3)
- - specified site - see Neoplasm,
    malignant
- - unspecified site 194.6
- nonchromaffin (M8693/1)
- - malignant (M8693/3)
- - - specified site - see Neoplasm,
      malignant
- - - unspecified site 194.6
- - specified site - see Neoplasm, uncertain
    behavior
- - unspecified site 237.3
- parasympathetic (M8682/1)
- - specified site - see Neoplasm, uncertain
    behavior
- - unspecified site 237.3
- specified site - see Neoplasm, uncertain
    behavior
- sympathetic (M8681/1)
- - specified site - see Neoplasm, uncertain
    behavior
- - unspecified site 237.3
- unspecified site 237.3
Parageusia 781.1
- psychogenic 306.7
Paragonimiasis 121.2
Paragranuloma, Hodgkin's (M9660/3)
  201.0
Parahemophilia (see also Defect,
  coagulation) 286.3
Parakeratosis 690
- variegata 696.2
Paralysis, paralytic (complete) (incomplete)
  344.9
- with
- - broken
- - - back - see Fracture, vertebra, by
      region, with spinal cord lesion
- - - neck (closed) 806.0
- - - - open 806.1
- - fracture, vertebra - see Fracture,
    vertebra, by region, with spinal cord
    lesion
- - syphilis 094.8
- abducens (nerve) 378.5
- accommodation 367.5
- - hysterical 300.1

Paralysis - *continued*
- acoustic nerve 388.5
- agitans 332.0
- - arteriosclerotic 332.0
- alternating 344.8
- - oculomotor 344.8
- amyotrophic 335.2
- anus (sphincter) 569.4
- apoplectic (current episode) (see also
    Disease, cerebrovascular, acute) 436
- arm 344.4
- - both 344.2
- - hysterical 300.1
- - psychogenic 306.0
- - transient 781.4
- - - traumatic NEC (see also Injury,
      nerve, upper limb) 955.9
- arteriosclerotic (current episode) (see
    also Ischemia, cerebral, arteriosclerotic)
    437.8
- ascending (spinal), acute 357.0
- associated, nuclear 344.8
- ataxic NEC 334.9
- - general 094.1
- atrophic 356.9
- - infantile, acute 045.1 † 323.2*
- - progressive 335.2
- - spinal (acute) 045.1 † 323.2*
- attack (see also Disease, cerebrovascular,
    acute) 436
- axillary 353.0
- Bell's 351.0
- - newborn 767.5
- Benedikt's 344.8
- birth 767.7
- - intracranial 767.0
- bladder (sphincter) 596.5
- - neurogenic 344.6
- - puerperal, postpartum, childbirth
    665.5
- bowel, colon or intestine (see also Ileus)
    560.1
- brachial plexus 353.0
- - birth injury 767.6
- - newborn 767.6
- bronchi 519.1
- Brown-Sequard 344.8
- bulbar (progressive) (chronic) 335.2
- - infantile 045.0 † 323.2*
- - poliomyelitic 045.0 † 323.2*
- - pseudo 344.8
- - supranuclear 344.8
- cardiac - see also Failure, heart
- cerebral
- - current episode 437.8
- - spastic infantile - see Palsy, cerebral
- cerebrocerebellar 437.8

Paralysis - *continued*
- cerebrocerebellar - *continued*
- − diplegic infantile 343.0
- cervical sympathetic NEC 337.9
- Cestan-Chenais 344.8
- Charcot-Marie-Tooth type 356.1
- childhood - see Palsy, cerebral
- Clark's 343.9
- colon NEC 560.1
- compressed air 993.3
- congenital (cerebral) (spastic) (spinal) 343.9
- conjugate movement (of eye) 378.8
- − cortical (nuclear) (supranuclear) 378.8
- convergence 378.8
- cordis (see also Failure, heart) 428.9
- creeping 335.2
- crossed leg 344.8
- crutch 953.4
- deglutition 784.9
- − hysterical 300.1
- dementia 094.1
- descending (spinal) NEC 335.9
- diaphragm (flaccid) 519.4
- − due to accidental section of phrenic nerve during procedure 998.2
- digestive organs NEC 564.8
- diplegic - see Diplegia
- divergence (nuclear) 378.8
- divers' 993.3
- Duchenne's 335.2
- due to intracranial or spinal birth injury - see Palsy, cereral
- embolic (current episode) (see also Embolism, brain) 434.1
- Erb(-Duchenne) (birth) (newborn) 767.6
- Erb's syphilitic spastic spinal 094.8
- esophagus 530.8
- extremity, transient (cause unknown) 781.4
- eye muscle (extrinsic) 378.5
- − intrinsic 367.5
- facial (nerve) 351.0
- − birth injury 767.5
- − following operation NEC 998.2
- − newborn 767.5
- familial 359.3
- − periodic 359.3
- − spastic 334.1
- fauces 478.2
- gait 781.2
- gaze 378.8
- general 094.1
- − ataxic 094.1
- − insane 094.1
- − juvenile 090.4
- − progressive 094.1

Paralysis - *continued*
- general - *continued*
- − tabetic 094.1
- glottis 478.3
- gluteal 353.4
- Gubler-Millard 344.8
- hand
- − hysterical 300.1
- − psychogenic 306.0
- heart (see also Failure, heart) 428.9
- hemiplegic - see Hemiplegia
- hypertensive (current episode) 437.8
- hysterical 300.1
- ileus (see also Ileus) 560.1
- infantile (see also Poliomyelitis) 045.9 † 323.2*
- − atrophic acute 045.1 † 323.2*
- − bulbar 045.0 † 323.2*
- − cerebral - see Palsy, cerebral
- − paralytic 045.1 † 323.2*
- − progressive acute 045.9 † 323.2*
- − spastic - see Palsy, cerebral
- − spinal 045.9 † 323.2*
- infective 045.9 † 323.2*
- inferior nuclear 344.9
- insane, general or progressive 094.1
- internuclear 378.8
- intestine NEC 560.1
- iris 379.4
- − due to diphtheria (toxin) 032.8 † 379.4*
- ischemic, Volkmann's (complicating trauma) 958.6
- Jackson's 344.8
- jake 989.8
- Jamaica ginger 357.7
- juvenile general 090.4
- Klumpke(-Dejerine) (birth) (newborn) 767.6
- labioglossal (laryngeal) (pharyngeal) 335.2
- Landry's 357.0
- laryngeal nerve (bilateral) (recurrent) (superior) (unilateral) 478.3
- larynx 478.3
- − due to diphtheria (toxin) 032.3
- lateral 335.2
- lead 984.-
- − specified type of lead - see Table of drugs and chemicals
- left side - see Hemiplegia
- leg 344.3
- − both (see also Paraplegia) 344.1
- − crossed 344.3
- − hysterical 300.1
- − psychogenic 306.0
- − transient or transitory 781.4

Paralysis - *continued*
- leg - *continued*
- − − transient or transitory - *continued*
- − − − traumatic NEC (see also Injury,
  nerve, lower limb) 956.9
- levator palpebrae superioris 374.3
- limb NEC 344.5
- − all four (see also Quadriplegia) 344.0
- lip 528.5
- Lissauer's 094.1
- lower limb 344.3
- − both (see also Paraplegia) 344.1
- lung 518.8
- medullary (tegmental) 344.8
- mesencephalic NEC 344.8
- − tegmental 344.8
- middle alternating 344.8
- Millard-Gubler-Foville 344.8
- monoplegic - see Monoplegia
- motor NEC 344.9
- muscle (flaccid) 359.9
- − due to nerve lesion NEC 355.9
- − eye (extrinsic) 378.5
- − − intrinsic 367.5
- − − oblique 378.5
- − ischemic (Volkmann's) (complicating
  trauma) 958.6
- − pseudohypertrophic 359.1
- muscular 359.9
- − progressive 335.2
- nerve - see also Disorder, nerve
- − auditory 388.5
- − birth injury 767.7
- − cranial or cerebral - see also Disorder,
  nerve, cranial
- − facial 351.0
- − − birth injury 767.5
- − − newborn 767.5
- − fourth or trochlear 378.5
- − newborn 767.7
- − radial
- − − birth injury 767.6
- − − newborn 767.6
- − seventh (see also Paralysis, nerve,
  facial) 351.0
- − seventh or facial 351.0
- − − due to
- − − − injection NEC 999.9
- − − − − operation NEC 997.0
- − − − newborn 767.5
- − sixth or abducens 378.5
- − syphilitic 094.8
- − third or oculomotor 378.5
- − traumatic NEC (see also Injury, nerve)
  957.9
- newborn NEC 767.0
- ocular 378.8

Paralysis - *continued*
- oculofacial, congenital 352.6
- oculomotor (nerve) 378.5
- − external bilateral 378.5
- oesophagus 530.8
- palate 528.9
- periodic (familial) (hypokalemic) 359.3
- peripheral autonomic nervous system -
  see Neuropathy, peripheral, autonomic
- peroneal (nerve) 355.3
- pharynx 478.2
- poliomyelitis (current) 045.1 † 323.2*
- − bulbar 045.0 † 323.2*
- progressive 335.2
- − atrophic 335.2
- − general 094.1
- − infantile acute 045.9 † 323.2*
- − multiple 335.2
- pseudobulbar 344.8
- pseudohypertrophic 359.1
- − muscle 359.1
- psychogenic 306.0
- quadriplegic (see also Quadriplegia)
  344.0
- radial nerve
- − birth injury 767.6
- rectus muscle (eye) 378.5
- respiratory (muscle) (system) (tract)
  786.0
- − center NEC 344.8
- − − fetus or newborn 770.8
- − congenital 768.9
- − newborn 768.9
- right side - see Hemiplegia
- saturnine 984.-
- − specified type of lead - see Table of
  drugs and chemicals
- seizure (current episode) (see also
  Disease, cerebrovascular, acute) 436
- senile NEC 344.9
- shaking (see also Parkinsonism) 332.0
- soft palate 528.9
- spastic 344.9
- − cerebral infantile - see Palsy, cerebral
- − congenital (cerebral) - see Palsy,
  cerebral
- − familial 334.1
- − hereditary 334.1
- − not infantile or congenital, cerebral
  344.9
- − syphilitic 094.0
- − − spinal 094.8
- sphincter, bladder (see also Paralysis,
  bladder) 596.5
- spinal (cord) NEC 344.1
- − acute 045.9 † 323.2*
- − ascending acute 357.0

Paralysis - *continued*
- spinal - *continued*
- - atrophic (acute) 045.1 † 323.2*
- - - spastic, syphilitic 094.8
- - congenital NEC 343.9
- - infantile 045.9 † 323.2*
- - progressive 335.1
- - spastic NEC 343.9
- sternomastoid 352.4
- stomach 536.8
- stroke (current episode) (see also Disease, cerebrovascular, acute) 436
- superior nuclear NEC 344.9
- supranuclear 356.8
- sympathetic
- - cervical NEC 337.9
- - nervous system - see Neuropathy, peripheral, autonomic
- syndrome NEC 344.9
- syphilitic spastic spinal (Erb's) 094.8
- tabetic general 094.1
- throat 478.2
- - diphtheritic 032.0
- - muscle 478.2
- thrombotic (current episode) (see also Thrombosis, brain) 434.0
- tick 989.5
- Todd's 344.8
- tongue 529.8
- transient
- - arm or leg NEC 781.4
- - traumatic NEC (see also Injury, nerve) 957.9
- trapezius 352.4
- traumatic, transient NEC (see also Injury, nerve) 957.9
- trembling (see also Parkinsonism) 332.0
- trochlear (nerve) 378.5
- upper limb 344.4
- - both (see also Diplegia) 344.2
- uremic - see Uremia
- uveoparotitic 135
- uvula 528.9
- - postdiphtheritic 032.0
- vasomotor NEC 337.9
- velum palati 528.9
- vesical (see also Paralysis, bladder) 596.5
- vestibular nerve 388.5
- vocal cords 478.3
- Volkmann's (complicating trauma) 958.6
- wasting 335.2
- Weber's 344.8
Paramedial orifice urethrovesical 753.8
Paramenia 626.9
Parametritis (see also Disease, pelvis, inflammatory) 614.4
Parametrium, parametric - see condition

Paramnesia (see also Amnesia) 780.9
Paramolar 520.1
- causing crowding 524.3
Paramyloidosis 277.3
Paramyoclonus multiplex 333.2
Paramyotonia 359.2
- congenita 359.2
Parangi (see also Yaws) 102.9
Paranoia 297.1
- alcoholic 291.5
- drug-induced 292.1
- querulans 297.8
- senile 290.2
Paranoid
- dementia 295.3
- - praecox (acute) 295.3
- - senile 290.2
- personality 301.0
- psychosis 297.9
- - alcoholic 291.5
- - climacteric 297.2
- - involutional 297.2
- - menopausal 297.2
- - protracted reactive 298.4
- - psychogenic 298.4
- - - acute 298.3
- - senile 290.2
- reaction (chronic) 297.9
- - acute 298.3
- schizophrenia (acute) 295.3
- state 297.9
- - climacteric 297.2
- - induced by drug 292.1
- - involution 297.2
- - menopausal 297.2
- - senile 290.2
- - simple 297.0
- - specified NEC 297.8
- tendencies 301.0
- traits 301.0
- trends 301.0
- type, psychopathic personality 301.0
Paraparesis (see also Paralysis) 344.9
Paraphasia 784.3
Paraphimosis (congenital) 605
- chancroidal 099.0
Paraphrenia, paraphrenic (late) 297.2
- climacteric 297.2
- dementia 295.3
- involutional 297.2
- menopausal 297.2
- schizophrenia (acute) 295.3
Paraplegia 344.1
- with
- - broken
- - - back - see Fracture, vertebra, by region, with spinal cord lesion

Paraplegia - *continued*
- with - *continued*
- - fracture, vertebra - see Fracture,
    vertebra, by region, with spinal cord
    lesion
- ataxic - see Degeneration, combined,
    spinal cord
- congenital or infantile (cerebral) (spastic)
    (spinal) 343.0
- functional (hysterical) 300.1
- hysterical 300.1
- Pott's 015.0 † 730.4*
- psychogenic 306.0
- spastic
- - Erb's spinal 094.8
- - hereditary 334.1
- spinal (cord)
- - traumatic - see Injury, spinal, by region
- syphilitic (spastic) 094.8
- traumatic NEC - see Injury, spinal, by
    region
Paraproteinemia 273.2
- benign (familial) 273.1
- monoclonal 273.1
- secondary to malignant or inflammatory
    disease 273.1
Parapsoriasis 696.2
- en plaques 696.2
- guttata 696.2
- retiformis 696.2
- varioliformis (acuta) 696.2
Parascarlatina 057.8
Parasitic - see also condition
- twin 759.4
Parasitism NEC 136.9
- intestinal NEC 129
- skin NEC 134.9
- specified - see Infestation
Parasitophobia 300.2
Paraspadias 752.8
Paraspasm facialis 351.8
Parathyroid gland - see condition
Parathyroiditis (autoimmune) 252.1
Parathyroprivic tetany 252.1
Paratrachoma 077.0 † 372.0*
Paratyphlitis (see also Appendicitis) 541
Paratyphoid (fever) - see Fever,
 paratyphoid
Paratyphus - see Fever, paratyphoid
Paraurethral duct 753.8
Paraurethritis 597.8
- gonococcal (acute) 098.0
- - chronic or duration of 2 months or over
    098.2
Paravaccinia NEC 051.9
- milker's node 051.1
Paravaginitis (see also Vaginitis) 616.1

Parencephalitis (see also Encephalitis)
 323.9
Parergasia 298.9
Paresis (see also Paralysis) 344.9
- bladder (sphincter) (see also Paralysis,
    bladder) 596.5
- - tabetic 094.0
- bowel, colon or intestine (see also Ileus)
    560.1
- extrinsic muscle, eye 378.5
- general 094.1
- - arrested 094.1
- - brain 094.1
- - cerebral 094.1
- - insane 094.1
- - juvenile 090.4
- - - remission 090.4
- - progressive 094.1
- - remission (sustained) 094.1
- - tabetic 094.1
- heart (see also Failure, heart) 428.9
- insane 094.1
- juvenile 090.4
- peripheral progressive 356.9
- pseudohypertrophic 359.1
- stomach 536.8
- syphilitic (general) 094.1
- - congenital 090.4
- vesical NEC 596.5
Paresthesia (see also Disturbance,
 sensation) 782.0
- Berger's 782.0
- Bernhardt 355.1
Paretic - see condition
Parinaud's
- conjunctivitis 372.0
- oculoglandular syndrome 372.0
- ophthalmoplegia 378.5
- syndrome 378.8
Parkinson's disease, syndrome or tremor -
 see Parkinsonism
Parkinsonism (arteriosclerotic) (idiopathic)
 (primary) 332.0
- associated with orthostatic hypotension
    (idiopathic) (symptomatic) 333.0
- due to drugs 332.1
- secondary 332.1
- syphilitic 094.8 † 332.1*
Parodontitis 523.4
Parodontosis 523.5
Paronychia (with lymphangitis) 681.9
- candidal 112.3
- chronic 681.9
- - candidal 112.3
- - finger 681.0
- - toe 681.1
- finger 681.0

Paronychia - *continued*
- toe 681.1
- tuberculous (primary) 017.0
Parorexia NEC 307.5
- hysterical 300.1
Parosmia 781.1
- psychogenic 306.7
Parotid gland - see condition
Parotiditis (see also Parotitis) 527.2
Parotitis 527.2
- chronic 527.2
- epidemic (see also Mumps) 072.9
- infectious (see also Mumps) 072.9
- nonspecific toxic 527.2
- not mumps 527.2
- postoperative 527.2
- purulent 527.2
- septic 527.2
- suppurative (acute) 527.2
- surgical 527.2
Parrot fever 073
Parrot's disease 090.0
Parry's disease 242.0
Parry-Romberg syndrome 349.8
Pars planitis 363.2
Parson's disease 242.0
Parsonage-Aldren-Turner syndrome 353.5
Particolored infant 757.3
Parturition - see Delivery
Passage
- false, urethra 599.4
- of sounds or bougies - see Attention to
  artificial opening
Passive - see condition
Pasteurella septica 027.2
Pasteurellosis (see also Infection,
  Pasteurella) 027.2
Patau's syndrome 758.1
Patches
- mucous (syphilitic) 091.3
- - congenital 090.0
- smokers' (mouth) 528.6
Patellar - see condition
Patent - see also Imperfect closure
- atrioventricular ostium 745.6
- canal of Nuck 752.4
- cervix 622.5
- - complicating pregnancy 654.5
- - - fetus or newborn 761.0
- ductus arteriosus or botalli 747.0
- eustachian valve 746.8
- foramen
- - botalli 745.5
- - ovale 745.5
- interauricular septum 745.5
- interventricular septum 745.4
- omphalomesenteric duct 751.0

Patent - *continued*
- os (uteri) - see Patent, cervix
- ostium secundum 745.5
- urachus 753.7
- vitelline duct 751.0
Paterson(-Brown)-Kelly syndrome 280
Pathologic, pathological - see condition
Pathology (of) - see Disease
Patulous - see also Patent
- anus 569.4
- eustachian tube 381.7
Pavy's disease 593.6
Paxton's disease 111.2
Pearls, enamel 520.2
Pearl-worker's disease 730.1
Pectenosis 569.4
Pectoral - see condition
Pectus
- carinatum (congenital) 754.8
- - acquired 738.3
- - rachitic - see Rickets
- excavatum (congenital) 754.8
- - acquired 738.3
- - rachitic - see Rickets
Pederosis 302.2
Pediculosis (infestation) 132.9
- capitis (head louse) (any site) 132.0
- corporis (body louse) (any site) 132.1
- mixed (classifiable to more than one of
  the titles 132.0-132.2) 132.3
- pubis (pubic louse) (any site) 132.2
- vestimenti 132.1
- vulvae 132.2
Pediculus (infestation) - see Pediculosis
  (infestation)
Pedophilia 302.2
Peg shaped teeth 520.2
Pel's crisis 094.0
Pelade (see also Alopecia) 704.0
Pelger-Huet anomaly or syndrome 288.2
Peliosis (rheumatica) 287.0
Pelizaeus-Merzbacher disease 330.0
Pellagra 265.2
- alcoholic or with alcoholism 265.2
Pellegrini-Stieda disease or syndrome 726.6
Pellizzi's syndrome 259.8
Pelvic - see also condition
- kidney 753.3
Pelviolithiasis 592.0
Pelviperitonitis
- female (see also Peritonitis, pelvic,
  female) 614.5
- male (see also Peritonitis) 567.2
Pelvis - see condition or type
Pemphigoid 694.5
- benign, mucous membrane 694.6
- bullous 694.5

Perforation - *continued*
- jejunum - *continued*
- - ulcer - see Ulcer, gastrojejunal, with perforation
- mastoid (antrum) (cell) 383.8
- membrana tympani - see Perforation, tympanum
- nasal
- - septum 478.1
- - - congenital 748.1
- - - syphilitic 095
- - sinus (see also Sinusitis) 473.9
- - - congenital 748.1
- oesophagus 530.4
- palate (hard) 526.8
- - soft 528.9
- - - syphilitic 095
- - syphilitic 095
- palatine vault 526.8
- - syphilitic 095
- - - congenital 090.5
- pelvic
- - floor
- - - complicating abortion - see categories 634-639, fourth digit .2
- - - obstetrical trauma 664.1
- - organ
- - - complicating abortion - see categories 634-639, fourth digit .2
- - - obstetrical trauma 665.5
- perineum - see Laceration, perineum
- periurethral tissue
- - complicating abortion - see categories 634-639, fourth digit .2
- pharynx 478.2
- pylorus, pyloric (ulcer) - see Ulcer, stomach, with perforation
- rectum 569.4
- sigmoid 569.8
- sinus (accessory) (chronic) (nasal) (see also Sinusitis) 473.9
- stomach (due to ulcer) - see Ulcer, stomach, with perforation
- surgical (accidental) (by instrument) (blood vessel) (nerve) (organ) 998.2
- traumatic
- - external - see Wound, open
- - eye (see also Penetrating wound, ocular) 871.7
- - internal organ - see Injury, internal, by site
- tympanum (membrane) (persistent post-traumatic) (postinflammatory) 384.2
- - traumatic - see Wound, open, ear
- - - complicated 872.7
- typhoid, gastro-intestinal 002.0

Perforation - *continued*
- ulcer - see Ulcer, by site, with perforation
- ureter 593.8
- urethra
- - complicating abortion - see categories 634-639, fourth digit .2
- - obstetrical trauma 665.5
- uterus - see also Injury, internal, uterus
- - by intrauterine contraceptive device 996.3
- - complicating abortion - see categories 634-639, fourth digit .2
- - obstetrical trauma - see Injury, internal uterus, obstetrical trauma
- uvula 528.9
- - syphilitic 095
- vagina - see Laceration, vagina
- viscus NEC 799.8
Periadenitis mucosa necrotica recurrens 528.2
Periappendicitis (see also Appendicitis) 541
Periarteritis (disseminated) (infectious) (necrotising) (nodosa) 446.0
Periarthritis (joint) 726.9
- Duplay's 726.2
- gonococcal 098.5 † 726.8*
- humeroscapularis 726.2
- scapulohumeral 726.2
- shoulder 726.2
- wrist 726.4
Periarthrosis (angioneural) - see Periarthritis
Peribronchitis 491.9
- tuberculous 011.3
Pericapsulitis, adhesive (shoulder) 726.0
Pericarditis (granula) (with decompensation) (with effusion) 423.9
- with
- - rheumatic fever (conditions in 390)
- - - active (see also Pericarditis, rheumatic) 391.0
- - - inactive or quiescent 393
- acute (nonrheumatic) 420.9
- - with chorea (acute) (rheumatic) (Sydenham's) 392.0
- - benign 420.9
- - nonspecific 420.9
- - rheumatic 391.0
- adhesive or adherent 423.1
- - acute - see Pericarditis, acute
- - rheumatic 393
- bacterial (acute) (subacute) (with serous or seropurulent effusion) 420.9
- calcareous 423.2
- chronic (nonrheumatic) 423.8
- - rheumatic 393
- constrictive 423.2

Periostitis - *continued*
- tuberculous (see also Tuberculosis, bone) 015.9 † 730.6*
- yaws (hypertrophic) (early) (late) 102.6
Periostosis 733.9
- with osteomyelitis 730.2
- - acute or subacute 730.0
- - chronic or old 730.1
- hyperplastic 733.9
Periphlebitis (see also Phlebitis) 451.9
- retina 362.1
- tuberculous 017.8
- - retina 017.3 † 362.1*
Peripneumonia - see Pneumonia
Periproctitis 569.4
Periprostatitis (see also Prostatitis) 601.9
Perirectal - see condition
Perirenal - see condition
Perisalpingitis (see also Salpingo-oophoritis) 614.2
Perisigmoiditis 569.8
Perisplenitis (infectional) 289.5
Perispondylitis - see Spondylitis
Peristalsis visible or reversed 787.4
Peritendinitis (see also Tenosynovitis) 726.9
- adhesive (shoulder) 726.0
Perithelioma (M9150/1) - see Pericytoma
Peritoneum, peritoneal - see condition
Peritonitis (acute) (adhesive) (fibrinous) (fibrous) (focal) (hemorrhagic) (idiopathic) (localized) (perforative) 567.9 (primary) (with adhesions) (with effusion)
- with or following
- - abscess 567.2
- - appendicitis 540.0
- aseptic 998.7
- bile,biliary 567.8
- chemical 998.7
- complicating
- - abortion - see categories 634-639, fourth digit .0
- - ectopic gestation 639.0
- congenital NEC 777.6
- diaphragmatic 567.2
- diffuse NEC 567.2
- diphtheritic 032.8 † 567.0*
- disseminated NEC 567.2
- due to foreign substance accidentally left during a procedure (chemical) (powder) (talc) 998.7
- fibrocaseous 014 † 567.0*
- fibropurulent 567.2
- general(ized) 567.2
- gonococcal 098.8 † 567.0*
- meconium (newborn) 777.6
- pancreatic 577.8
- paroxysmal, benign 277.3

Peritonitis - *continued*
- pelvic
- - female 614.5
- - - acute 614.5
- - - chronic 614.7
- - - - with adhesions 614.6
- - male 567.2
- periodic 277.3
- pneumococcal 567.1
- proliferative, chronic 567.8
- puerperal, postpartum, childbirth 670
- purulent 567.2
- septic 567.2
- subdiaphragmatic 567.2
- subphrenic 567.2
- suppurative 567.2
- syphilitic 095 † 567.0*
- - congenital 090.0 † 567.0*
- tuberculous 014 † 567.0*
- urine 567.8
Peritonsillar - see condition
Peritonsillitis 475
Perityphlitis (see also Appendicitis) 541
Periureteritis 593.8
Periurethral - see condition
Periurethritis (gangrenous) 597.8
Periuterine - see condition
Perivaginitis (see also Vaginitis) 616.1
Perivasculitis, retinal 362.1
Perivasitis (chronic) 608.4
Perivesiculitis (seminal) (see also Vesiculitis) 608.0
Perleche 686.8
- due to
- - moniliasis 112.0
- - riboflavin deficiency 266.0
Pernicious - see condition
Pernio 991.5
Persecution
- delusion 297.9
- social V62.4
Perseveration (tonic) 784.6
Persistence, persistent (congenital) 759.8
- anal membrane 751.2
- arteria stapedia 744.0
- atrioventricular canal 745.6
- branchial cleft 744.4
- bulbus cordis in left ventricle 745.8
- canal of Cloquet 743.5
- capsule (opaque) 743.3
- cilioretinal artery or vein 743.5
- cloaca 751.5
- communication - see Fistula, congenital
- convolutions
- - aortic arch 747.2
- - fallopian tube 752.1
- - oviduct 752.1

Persistence - *continued*
- convolutions - *continued*
- - uterine tube 752.1
- double aortic arch 747.2
- ductus
- - arteriosus 747.0
- - botalli 747.0
- fetal
- - circulation 747.9
- - form of cervix (uteri) 752.4
- - hemoglobin, hereditary 282.7
- foramen
- - botalli 745.5
- - ovale 745.5
- Gartner's duct 752.1
- hemoglobin, fetal (hereditary) 282.7
- hyaloid
- - artery (generally incomplete) 743.5
- - system 743.5
- hymen
- - in pregnancy or childbirth 654.8
- lanugo 757.4
- left
- - posterior cardinal vein 747.4
- - root with right arch of aorta 747.2
- - superior vena cava 747.4
- Meckel's diverticulum 751.0
- nail(s), anomalous 757.5
- occiput anterior or posterior 660.3
- - fetus or newborn 763.1
- omphalomesenteric duct 751.0
- organ or site not listed - see Anomaly, specified type NEC
- ostium
- - atrioventriculare commune 745.6
- - primum 745.6
- - secundum 745.5
- ovarian rests in fallopian tube 752.1
- pancreatic tissue in intestinal tract 751.5
- primary (deciduous)
- - teeth 520.6
- - vitreous hyperplasia 743.5
- pupillary membrane 743.4
- - iris 743.4
- right aortic arch 747.2
- sinus
- - urogenitalis 752.8
- - venosus with imperfect incorporation in right auricle 747.4
- thymus (gland) 254.8
- - hyperplasia of 254.0
- thyroglossal duct 759.2
- thyrolingual duct 759.2
- truncus arteriosus or communis 745.0
- tunica vasculosa lentis 743.5
- urachus 753.7
- vitelline duct 751.0

Personality
- affective 301.1
- aggressive 301.3
- amoral 301.7
- anancastic 301.4
- anankastic 301.4
- antisocial 301.7
- asocial 301.7
- asthenic 301.6
- change, disorder, disturbance NEC 301.9
- - with sociopathic disturbance 301.7
- compulsive 301.4
- cycloid 301.1
- cyclothymic 301.1
- dependent 301.6
- depressive 301.1
- dual 300.1
- dyssocial 301.7
- eccentric 301.8
- - haltlose type 301.8
- emotionally unstable 301.5
- explosive 301.3
- fanatic 301.0
- histrionic 301.5
- hyperthymic 301.1
- hypothymic 301.1
- hysterical 301.5
- immature 301.8
- inadequate 301.6
- labile 301.5
- morally defective 301.7
- multiple 300.1
- obsessional 301.4
- obsessive(-compulsive) 301.4
- paranoid 301.0
- passive(-dependent) 301.6
- passive-agressive 301.8
- pathologic NEC 301.9
- pattern defect or disturbance 301.9
- psychoinfantile 301.5
- psychoneurotic NEC 301.8
- psychopathic 301.9
- - with
- - - amoral trend 301.7
- - - antisocial trend 301.7
- - - asocial trend 301.7
- - mixed types 301.9
- schizoid 301.2
- sociopathic 301.7
- - antisocial 301.7
- - dyssocial 301.7
- unstable (emotional) 301.5
Perthes' disease 732.1
Pertussis (see also Whooping cough) 033.9
Perversion, perverted
- appetite 307.5
- - hysterical 300.1

Perversion - *continued*
- sense of smell or taste 781.1
- - psychogenic 306.7
- sexual (see also Deviation, sexual) 302.9
Pervious, congenital - see also Imperfect
closure
- ductus arteriosus 747.0
Pes (congenital) (see also Talipes) 754.7
- acquired (any type except planus) 736.7
- adductus 754.7
- cavus 754.7
- planus (acquired) (any degree) 734
- - congenital 754.6
- - rachitic 268.1
- valgus 754.6
Pest (see also Plague) 020.9
Pestis (see also Plague) 020.9
- bubonica 020.0
- fulminans 020.0
- minor 020.8
- pneumonica - see Plague, pneumonic
Petechia, petechiae 782.7
- fetus or newborn 772.6
Petges-Clejat or Petjes-Clegat syndrome
710.3
Petit mal (idiopathic) 345.0
- status 345.2
Petit's disease (see also Hernia, diaphragm)
553.3
Petrellidosis 117.6
Petrositis 383.2
Peutz-Jeghers disease or syndrome 759.6
Peyronie's disease 607.8
Pfeiffer's disease 075
Phaeohyphomycosis 117.8
Phagedena (dry) (moist) (see also
Gangrene) 785.4
- geometric 686.0
- penis 607.8
- tropical (see also Ulcer, skin) 707.9
- vulva 616.5
Phagedenic - see condition
Phakoma 362.8
Phantom limb (syndrome) 353.6
Pharyngitis (acute) (catarrhal) (gangrenous)
(infective) (malignant) (membranous)
(phlegmonous) (pneumococcal)
pseudomembranous) (simple)
(staphylococcal) (subacute) (suppurative)
(ulcerative) (viral) 462
- with influenza, flu, or grippe 487.1
- aphthous 074.0
- atrophic 472.1
- chronic 472.1
- Coxsackie virus 074.0
- diphtheritic 032.0
- follicular 472.1

Pharyngitis - *continued*
- fusospirochetal 101
- gonococcal 098.6
- granular (chronic) 472.1
- herpetic 054.7
- hypertrophic 472.1
- influenzal 487.1
- lymphonodular, acute 074.8
- septic 034.0
- streptococcal 034.0
- tuberculous 012.8
- vesicular 074.0
Pharyngoconjunctivitis, viral 077.2 † 372.0*

Pharyngolaryngitis (acute) 465.0
- chronic 478.9
- septic 034.0
Pharyngoplegia 478.2
Pharyngotracheitis (acute) 465.8
- chronic 478.9
Pharynx, pharyngeal - see condition
Phenomenon
- Arthus' - see Arthus' phenomenon
- jaw-winking 742.8
- L. E. cell 710.0
- lupus erythematosus cell 710.0
- Raynaud's (secondary) 443.0
- vasomotor 780.2
- vasospastic 443.9
- vasovagal 780.2
- Wenckebach's 426.1
Phenylketonuria 270.1

Pheochromoblastoma (M8700/3)
- specified site - see Neoplasm, malignant
- unspecified site 194.0
Pheochromocytoma (M8700/0)
- malignant (M8700/3)
- - specified site - see Neoplasm,
malignant
- - unspecified site 194.0
- specified site - see Neoplasm, benign
- unspecified site 227.0
Phimosis (congenital) 605
- chancroidal 099.0
- due to infection 605
Phlebectasia (see also Varicose vein) 454.9
- congenital 747.6
Phlebitis (infective) (pyemic) (septic)
(suppurative) 451.9
- breast, superficial 451.8
- cavernous (venous) sinus - see Phlebitis,
intracranial (venous) sinus
- cerebral (venous) sinus - see Phlebitis,
intracranial (venous) sinus
- chest wall, superficial 451.8
- complicating pregnancy 671.9
- - fetus or newborn 760.3

Phlebitis - *continued*
- cranial (venous) sinus - see Phlebitis, intracranial (venous) sinus
- due to implanted device 996.7
- during or resulting from a procedure 997.2
- femoral 451.1
- following infusion, perfusion or transfusion 999.2
- gouty 274.8 † 451.9*
- hepatic veins 451.8
- ilio-femoral 451.1
- intracranial (venous) sinus (any) 325
- - nonpyogenic 437.6
- lateral (venous) sinus - see Phlebitis, intracranial (venous) sinus
- leg 451.2
- - deep (vessels) 451.1
- - superficial (vessels) 451.0
- longitudinal sinus - see Phlebitis, intracranial (venous) sinus
- lower extremity 451.2
- - deep (vessels) 451.1
- - superficial (vessels) 451.0

- migrans, migrating (superficial) 453.1
- pelvic
- - with
- - - abortion - see categories 634-639, fourth digit .0
- - - ectopic gestation 639.0
- - puerperal, postpartum 671.4
- portal 572.1
- postoperative 997.2
- pregnancy 671.9
- - deep 671.3
- - specified NEC 671.5
- - superficial 671.2

- puerperal, postpartum, childbirth 671.9
- - deep 671.4
- - pelvis 671.4
- - specified NEC 671.5
- - superficial 671.2
- retina 362.1
- saphenous 451.0
- sinus (meninges) - see Phlebitis, intracranial (venous) sinus
- specified site NEC 451.8
- syphilitic 093.8
- ulcerative 451.9
- - leg 451.2
- - - deep (vessels) 451.1
- - - superficial (vessels) 451.0
- - lower extremity 451.2
- - - deep (vessels) 451.1
- - - superficial (vessels) 451.0
- umbilicus 451.8

Phlebitis - *continued*
- uterus (septic) (see also Endometritis) 615.9
- varicose (leg) (lower extremity) (see also Varicose vein) 454.1
Phleboliths 459.8
Phlebosclerosis 459.8
Phlebothrombosis - see Thrombosis
Phlegmasia
- alba dolens 451.1
- - complicating pregnancy 671.3
- - nonpuerperal 451.1
- - puerperal, postpartum, childbirth 671.4
- cerulea dolens 451.1
Phlegmon - see Abscess
Phlegmonous - see condition
Phlyctenulosis (allergic) (keratoconjunctivitis) (nontuberculous) 370.3
- cornea 370.3
- tuberculous 017.3 † 370.3*
Phobia, phobic 300.2
- animal 300.2
- obsessional 300.3
- reaction 300.2
- state 300.2
Phocas' disease 610.1
Phocomelia 755.4
- lower limb 755.3
- upper limb 755.2
Phoria 378.4
Phosphate-losing tabular disorder 588.0
Phosphatemia 275.3
Phosphaturia 275.3
Photodermatitis (sun) 692.7
- light other than sun 692.8
Photokeratitis 370.2
Photophobia 368.1
Photophthalmia 370.2
Photopsia 368.1
Photoretinitis 363.3
Photosensitiveness (sun) 692.7
- light other than sun 692.8
Photosensitization (sun) skin 692.7
- light other than sun 692.8
Phrenitis 323.9
Phrynoderma 264.8
Phthiriasis (pubis) (any site) 132.2
- with any infestation classifiable to 132.0 and 132.1 132.3
Phthirus infestation - see Phthiriasis
Phthisis (see also Tuberculosis) 011.9
- bulbi (infectional) 360.4
- colliers' 011.4
- eyeball (due to infection) 360.4
- millstone makers' 011.4
- miners' 011.4

Phthisis - *continued*
– potters' 011.4
– sandblasters' 011.4
– stonemasons' 011.4
Phycomycosis 117.7
Physalopteriasis 127.7
Physical therapy NEC V57.1
Physiological cup, large, optic disc 377.1
Phytobezoar 938
– intestine 936
– stomach 935.2
Pian (see also Yaws) 102.9
Pianoma 102.1
Piarhemia, bilharziasis 120.9
Pica 307.5
– hysterical 300.1
Pick's
– disease (brain) 331.1
– – dementia in 290.1
– – liver 423.2
– syndrome
– – heart 423.2
– – liver 423.2
– tubular adenoma (M8640/0)
– – specified site - see Neoplasm, benign
– – unspecified site
– – – female 220
– – – male 222.0
Pick-Niemann disease 272.7
Pickwickian syndrome 278.8
Piebaldism, classic 709.0
Piedra 111.2
– beard 111.2
– – black 111.3
– – white 111.2
– black 111.3
– scalp 111.3
– – black 111.3
– – white 111.2
– white 111.2
Pierre Robin deformity or syndrome 756.0
Pierson's disease or osteochondrosis 732.1
Pigeon
– breast or chest (acquired) 738.3
– – congenital 754.8
– – rachitic - see Rickets
– breeders' disease or lung 495.2
– fanciers' disease or lung 495.2
– toe 735.8
Pigmentation (abnormal) 709.0
– anomalies NEC 709.0
– conjunctiva 372.5
– cornea 371.1
– lids, congenital 757.3
– limbus corneae 371.1
– metals 709.0
– optic papilla, congenital 743.5

Pigmentation - *continued*
– retina (congenital) (grouped) (nevoid)
  743.5
– scrotum, congenital 757.3
Piles - see Hemorrhoids
Pili annulati or torti (congenital) 757.4
Pill roller hand (intrinsic) 736.0
Pilomatrixoma (M8110/0) - see Neoplasm,
  skin, benign
Pilonidal - see condition
Pimple 709.8
Pinched nerve - see Neuropathy,
  entrapment
Pineal body or gland - see condition
Pinealoblastoma (M9362/3) 194.4
Pinealoma (M9360/1) 237.1
– malignant (M9360/3) 194.4
Pineoblastoma (M9362/3) 194.4
Pineocytoma (M9361/1) 237.1
Pinguecula 372.5
Pinhole meatus (see also Stricture, urethra)
  598.9
Pink
– disease 985.0
– eye 372.0
Pinkus' disease 697.1
Pinpoint
– meatus (see also Stricture, urethra) 598.9
– os (uteri) (see also Stricture, cervix)
  622.4
Pinta 103.9
– cardiovascular lesions 103.2
– chancre (primary) 103.0
– erythematous plaques 103.1
– hyperchromic lesions 103.1
– hyperkeratosis 103.1
– lesions 103.9
– – cardiovascular 103.2
– – hyperchromic 103.1
– – intermediate 103.1
– – late 103.2
– – mixed 103.3
– – primary 103.0
– – skin (achromic) (cicatricial)
    (dyschromic) 103.2
– – – hyperchromic 103.1
– – – mixed (achromic and hyperchromic)
      103.3
– papule (primary) 103.0
– skin lesions (achromic) (cicatricial)
    (dyschromic) 103.2
– – hyperchromic 103.1
– – mixed (achromic and hyperchromic)
    103.3
– vitiligo 103.2
Pintid 103.0

Pinworms (disease) (infection) (infestation) 127.4
Pistol wound - see Gunshot wound
Pithecoid pelvis 755.6
 - with disproportion 653.2
 - - causing obstructed labor 660.1
 - - fetus or newborn 763.1
Pithiatism 300.1
Pitted - see also Pitting
 - teeth 520.4
Pitting - see also Edema
 - lip 782.3
 - nail 703.8
 - - congenital 757.5
Pituitary gland - see condition
Pituitary-snuff-takers' disease 495.8
Pityriasis 696.5
 - alba 696.5
 - capitis 690
 - circinata (et maculata) 696.3
 - Hebra's 695.8
 - lichenoides et varioliformis 696.2
 - maculata (et circinata) 696.3
 - pilaris 757.3
 - - acquired 701.1
 - rosea 696.3
 - rotunda 696.3
 - rubra (Hebra's) 695.8
 - - pilaris 696.4
 - simplex 690
 - streptogenes 696.5
 - versicolor 111.0
 - - scrotal 111.0
Placenta, placental
 - ablatio 641.2
 - - fetus or newborn 762.1
 - abnormal, abnormality 656.7
 - - with hemorrhage 641.8
 - - - fetus or newborn 762.1
 - - fetus or newborn 762.2
 - abruptio 641.2
 - - fetus or newborn 762.1
 - accreta (without hemorrhage) 667.0
 - - with hemorrhage 666.0
 - adherent (without hemorrhage) 667.0
 - - with hemorrhage 666.0
 - apoplexy - see Placenta, separation
 - battledore - see Placenta, abnormal
 - bipartita - see Placenta, abnormal
 - centralis - see Placenta, previa
 - circumvallata - see Placenta, abnormal
 - cyst (amniotic) - see Placenta, abnormal
 - deficiency - see Placenta, insufficiency
 - degeneration - see Placenta, insufficiency
 - detachment (partial) (premature) (with hemorrhage) 641.2
 - - fetus or newborn 762.1

Placenta - *continued*
 - dimidiata - see Placenta, abnormal
 - disease 656.7
 - - fetus or newborn 762.2
 - duplex - see Placenta, abnormal
 - dysfunction - see Placenta, insufficiency
 - fenestrata - see Placenta, abnormal
 - fibrosis - see Placenta, abnormal
 - hematoma - see Placenta, abnormal
 - hemorrhage NEC - see also Placenta, separation
 - hyperplasia - see Placenta, abnormal
 - increta (without hemorrhage) 667.0
 - - with hemorrhage 666.0
 - infarction 656.7
 - - fetus or newborn 762.2
 - insertion, vicious - see Placenta, previa
 - insufficiency
 - - affecting management of pregnancy 656.5
 - - fetus or newborn 762.2
 - lateral - see Placenta, previa
 - low implantation or insertion - see Placenta, previa
 - low-lying - see Placenta, previa
 - malformation - see Placenta, abnormal
 - malposition - see Placenta, previa
 - marginal sinus (hemorrhage) (rupture) 641.2
 - - fetus or newborn 762.1
 - marginalis, marginata - see Placenta, abnormal
 - membranacea - see Placenta, abnormal
 - multilobed - see Placenta, abnormal
 - multipartita - see Placenta, abnormal
 - necrosis - see Placenta, abnormal
 - percreta (without hemorrhage) 667.0
 - - with hemorrhage 666.0
 - polyp 674.4
 - previa (central) (centralis) (complete) (lateral) (marginal) (marginalis) (partial) (partialis) (total) (with hemorrhage) 641.1
 - - fetus or newborn 762.0
 - - noted
 - - - before labor, delivered by cesarean section, without hemorrhage 641.0
 - - - during pregnancy (without hemorrhage) 641.0
 - - without hemorrhage 641.0
 - retention (with hemorrhage) 666.0
 - - fragments, complicating puerperium (delayed hemorrhage) 666.2
 - - - without hemorrhage 667.1
 - - without hemorrhage 667.0
 - separation (normally implanted) (partial) (premature) (with hemorrhage) 641.2

Placenta - *continued*
- separation - *continued*
- - fetus or newborn 762.1
- septuplex - see Placenta, abnormal
- small - see Placenta, insufficiency
- softening (premature) - see Placenta, abnormal
- spuria - see Placenta, abnormal
- succenturiata - see Placenta, abnormal
- syphilitic 095
- transmission of chemical substance - see Absorption, chemical, through placenta
- trapped (with hemorrhage) 666.0
- - without hemorrhage 667.0
- tripartita - see Placenta, abnormal
- triplex - see Placenta, abnormal
- varicose vessel - see Placenta, abnormal
- vicious insertion - see Placenta, previa
Placentitis
- complicating pregnancy 658.4
- fetus or newborn 762.7

Plagiocephaly (skull) 754.0
Plague 020.9
- abortine 020.8
- ambulatory 020.8
- bubonic 020.0
- cellulocutaneous 020.1
- lymphatic gland 020.0
- pneumonic 020.5
- - primary 020.3
- - secondary 020.4
- pulmonary - see Plague, pneumonic
- pulmonic - see Plague, pneumonic
- septicemic 020.2
- tonsillar 020.9
- - septicemic 020.2
Plaque
- artery, arterial - see Arteriosclerosis
- calcareous - see Calcification
- tongue 528.6
Plasmacytoma (solitary) (M9731/1) 238.6
- benign (M9731/0) - see Neoplasm, benign
- malignant (M9731/3) 203.8
Plasmacytosis 288.8
Plaster ulcer 707.0
Platybasia 756.0
Platyonychia (congenital) 757.5
- acquired 703.8

Platypelloid pelvis 738.6
- with disproportion 653.2
- - causing obstructed labor 660.1
- - fetus or newborn 763.1
- congenital 755.6
Pleura, pleural - see condition
Pleuralgia 786.5

Pleurisy (acute) (adhesive) (chronic) (costal) (diaphragmatic) (double) (dry) (fetid) (fibrinous) (fibrous) (interlobar) (latent) (lung) (old) (plastic) (residual) (sicca) (sterile) (subacute) (unresolved) (with adherent pleura) 511.03.9
- with
- - effusion (without mention of cause) 511.9
- - - bacterial, nontuberculous 511.1
- - - nontuberculous NEC 511.9
- - - pneumococcal 511.1
- - - staphylococcal 511.1
- - - streptococcal 511.1
- - - tuberculous 012.0
- - - - primary, progressive 010.1
- - influenza, flu, or grippe 487.1
- - tuberculosis - see Pleurisy, tuberculous
- encysted 511.8
- exudative (see also Pleurisy with effusion) 511.9
- - bacterial, nontuberculous 511.1
- fibrinopurulent 510.9
- - with fistula 510.0
- fibropurulent 510.9
- - with fistula 510.0
- hemorrhagic 511.8
- influenzal 487.1
- pneumococcal 511.0
- - with effusion 511.1
- purulent 510.9
- - with fistula 510.0
- septic 510.9
- - with fistula 510.0
- serofibrinous (see also Pleurisy with effusion) 511.9
- - bacterial, nontuberculous 511.1
- seropurulent 510.9
- - with fistula 510.0
- serous (see also Pleurisy with effusion) 511.9
- - bacterial, nontuberculous 511.1
- staphylococcal 511.0
- - with effusion 511.1
- streptococcal 511.0
- - with effusion 511.1
- suppurative 510.9
- - with fistula 510.0
- traumatic (post) (current) 862.2
- - with open wound into cavity 862.3
- tuberculous (with effusion) 012.0
- - primary, progressive 010.1
Pleuritis sicca - see Pleurisy
Pleurobronchopneumonia - see Pneumonia, broncho
Pleurodynia 786.5
- epidemic 074.1

Pneumonia - *continued*
- bacterial - *continued*
- - specified NEC 482.8
- basal, basic, basilar - see Pneumonia, lobar
- broncho, bronchial (confluent) (croupous) (diffuse) (disseminated) (involving lobes) (lobar) 485
- - with influenza 487.0
- - allergic 518.3
- - aspiration (see also Pneumonia, aspiration) 507.0
- - bacterial 482.9
- - - specified NEC 482.8
- - capillary 466.1
- - - with bronchospasm or obstruction 466.1
- - chronic (see also Fibrosis, lung) 515
- - diplococcal 481
- - Eaton's agent 483
- - Escherichia coli (E. coli) 482.8
- - Friedlander's bacillus 482.0
- - Hemophilus influenzae 482.2
- - hiberno-vernal 083.0 † 484.8*
- - hypostatic 514
- - influenzal 487.0
- - inhalation (see also Pneumonia, aspiration) 507.0
- - - due to fumes or vapors (chemical) 506.0
- - Klebsiella 482.0
- - lipid 507.1
- - - endogenous 516.8
- - mycoplasma (pneumoniae) 483
- - pleuropneumonia-like organisms (PPLO) 483
- - pneumococcal 481
- - proteus 482.8
- - pseudomonas 482.1
- - specified organism NEC 483
- - staphylococcal 482.4
- - streptococcal 482.3
- - typhoid 002.0 † 484.8*
- - viral, virus (see also Pneumonia, viral) 480.9
- candida 112.4 † 484.7*
- capillary 466.1
- - with bronchospasm or obstruction 466.1
- caseous 011.6
- central - see Pneumonia, lobar
- cholesterol 516.8
- chronic (see also Fibrosis, lung) 515
- cirrhotic (chronic) (see also Fibrosis, lung) 515
- confluent - see Pneumonia, broncho
- congenital (infective) 770.0

Pneumonia - *continued*
- congenital - *continued*
- - aspiration 770.1
- croupous - see Pneumonia, lobar
- cytomegalic inclusion 078.5 † 484.1*
- deglutition 507.0
- diffuse - see Pneumonia, broncho
- diplococcal, diplococcus (broncho) (lobar) 481
- disseminated (focal) - see Pneumonia, broncho
- due to
- - adenovirus 480.0
- - Diplococcus (pneumoniae) 481
- - Eaton's agent 483
- - Escherichia coli (E. coli) 482.8
- - Friedlander's bacillus 482.0
- - fumes or vapors (chemical) (inhalation) 506.0
- - Hemophilus influenzae (H. influenzae) 482.2
- - influenza 487.0
- - Klebsiella pneumoniae 482.0
- - Mycoplasma (pneumoniae) 483
- - parainfluenza virus 480.2
- - pleuropneumonia-like organisms (PPLO) 483
- - pneumococcus 481
- - Proteus 482.8
- - Pseudomonas 482.1
- - respiratory syncytial virus 480.1
- - specified
- - - bacteria NEC 482.8
- - - organism NEC 483
- - - virus NEC 480.8
- - Staphylococcus 482.4
- - Streptococcus 482.3
- - virus (see also Pneumonia, viral) 480.9
- Eaton's agent 483
- embolic, embolism (see also Embolism, pulmonary) 415.1
- eosinophilic 518.3
- Escherichia coli (E. coli) 482.8
- fibrinous - see Pneumonia, lobar
- fibroid (chronic) (see also Fibrosis, lung) 515
- fibrous (see also Fibrosis, lung) 515
- Friedlander's bacillus 482.0
- gangrenous 513.0
- giant cell (see also Pneumonia, viral) 480.9
- grippal 487.0
- Hemophilus influenzae (broncho) (lobar) 482.2
- hypostatic (broncho) (lobar) 514
- in
- - actinomycosis 039.1 † 484.8*

Pneumonitis - *continued*
- due to - *continued*
- - inhalation - *continued*
- - - food (regurgitated), milk, vomit 507.0
- - - oils, essences 507.1
- - - solids, liquids NEC 507.8
- - toxoplasmosis (acquired) 130 † 484.8*
- - - congenital (active) 771.2 † 484.8*
- eosinophilic 518.3
- fetal aspiration 770.1
- hypersensitivity 495.9
- meconium 770.1
- postanesthetic
- - correct substance properly administered 507.0
- - obstetric 668.0
- - overdose or wrong substance given 968.-
- - - specified anesthetic - see Table of drugs and chemicals
- postoperative 997.3
- - obstetric 668.0
- radiation 508.0
- rubella, congenital 771.0
- ventilation 495.7
Pneumonoconiosis - see Pneumoconiosis
Pneumopathy NEC 518.8
- alveolar NEC 516.9
- due to dust NEC 504
- parietoalveolar NEC 516.9
- - specified condition NEC 516.8
Pneumopericarditis (see also Pericarditis) 423.9
Pneumopericardium - see also Pericarditis
- congenital 770.2
- fetus or newborn 770.2
- traumatic (post) (see also Pneumothorax, traumatic) 860.0
- - with open wound into thorax 860.1
Pneumophagia (psychogenic) 306.4
Pneumopleurisy, pneumopleuritis (see also Pneumonia) 486
Pneumopyopericardium 420.9
Pneumopyothorax (see also Pyopneumothorax) 510.9
Pneumorrhagia 786.3
- newborn 770.3
- tuberculous (see also Tuberculosis, pulmonary) 011.9
Pneumosiderosis 503
Pneumothorax 512
- acute 512
- chronic 512
- congenital 770.2
- due to operative injury of chest wall or lung 997.3

Pneumothorax - *continued*
- due to operative injury of chest wall or *continued*
- - accidental puncture or laceration 998.2
- fetus or newborn 770.2
- spontaneous 512
- - fetus or newborn 770.2
- sucking 512
- tense valvular, infectional 512
- tension 512
- traumatic 860.0
- - with
- - - hemothorax 860.4
- - - - with open wound into thorax 860.5
- - - open wound into thorax 860.1
- tuberculous 011.7
Podagra 274.9
Podencephalus 759.8
Poikilocytosis 790.0
Poikiloderma 709.0
- Civatte's 709.0
- congenital 757.3
- vasculare atrophicans 696.2
Poikilodermatomyositis 710.3
Pointed ear 744.2
Poise imperfect 729.9
Poison ivy, oak, sumac or other plant dermatitis 692.6
Poisoning (acute) - see also Table of drugs and chemicals
- Bacillus, B.
- - aertrycke (see also Infection, salmonella) 003.9
- - botulinus 005.1
- - choleraesuis (see also Infection, salmonella) 003.9
- - suipestifer (see also Infection, salmonella) 003.9
- bacterial toxins NEC 005.9
- berries, noxious 988.2
- blood (general) - see Septicemia
- botulism 005.1
- bread, moldy, mouldy - see Poisoning, food
- damaged meat - see Poisoning, food
- decomposed food - see Poisoning, food
- diseased food - see Poisoning, food
- drug - see Table of drugs and chemicals
- epidemic, fish, meat, or other food - see Poisoning, food
- fava bean 282.2
- fish (bacterial) - see also Poisoning, food
- - noxious 988.0
- food (acute) (bacterial) (diseased) (infected) NEC 005.9
- - due to

Polyarthritis - *continued*
- due to or associated with other specified conditions - see Arthritis
- inflammatory 714.9
- juvenile, chronic 714.3
- migratory - see Fever, rheumatic
- rheumatic 714.0
- - fever (acute) - see Fever, rheumatic
Polycarential syndrome of infancy 260

Polychondritis (atrophic) (chronic) (relapsing) 733.9
Polycoria 743.4
Polycystic (disease) 759.8
- degeneration, kidney 753.1
- kidney 753.1
- liver 751.6
- lung 518.8
- - congenital 748.4
- ovary, ovaries 256.4
- spleen 759.0
Polycythemia (primary) (rubra) (vera) (M9950/1) 238.4
- acquired 289.0
- due to
- - fall in plasma volume 289.0
- - high altitude 289.0
- emotional 289.0
- erythropoietin 289.0
- familial (benign) 289.6
- hypertonica 289.0
- hypoxemic 289.0
- neonatorum 776.4
- nephrogenous 289.0
- relative 289.0
- secondary 289.0
- stress 289.0
Polycytosis cryptogenica 289.0

Polydactylism, polydactyly 755.0
Polydipsia 783.5
Polyembryoma (M9072/3) - see Neoplasm, malignant
Polyglandular
- deficiency 258.9
- dyscrasia 258.9
- dysfunction 258.9
Polyhydramnios (see also Hydramnios) 657
Polymastia 757.6
Polymenorrhea 626.2
Polymyalgia 725
- arteritica 446.5
- rheumatica 725
Polymyositis (acute) (chronic) (hemorrhagic) 710.4
- with involvement of
- - lung 710.4 † 517.8*
- - skin 710.3

Polymyositis - *continued*
- ossificans (generalisata) (progressiva) 728.1
Polyneuritis, polyneuritic (see also Polyneuropathy) 357.9
- diabetic 250.2 † 357.2*
- due to lack of vitamin NEC 269.2 † 357.4*
- endemic 265.0 † 357.4*
- erythredema 985.0
- febrile 357.0
- infective (acute) 357.0
- nutritional 269.9 † 357.4*
Polyneuropathy (peripheral) 356.9
- alcoholic 357.5
- arsenical 357.7
- due to
- - antitetanus serum 357.6
- - arsenic 357.7
- - drug or medicament 357.6
- - - correct substance properly administered 357.6
- - - overdose or wrong substance given or taken 977.9
- - - - specified drug - see Table of drugs and chemicals
- - lack of vitamin NEC 269.2 † 357.4*
- - lead 357.7
- - organophosphate compounds 357.7
- - serum 357.6
- - toxic agent NEC 357.7
- - triorthocresylphosphate 357.7
- hereditary 356.0
- idiopathic progressive 356.4
- in
- - amyloidosis 277.3 † 357.4*
- - avitaminosis NEC 269.2 † 357.4*
- - beriberi 265.0 † 357.4*
- - collagen vascular disease NEC 710.9 † 357.1*
- - deficiency of B vitamins 266.- † 357.4*
- - diabetes 250.5 † 357.2*
- - diphtheria 032.- † 357.4*
- - disseminated lupus erythematosus 710.0 † 357.1*
- - herpes zoster 053.1 † 357.4*
- - hypoglycemia 251.2 † 357.4*
- - malignant neoplasm NEC (M8000/3) 199.1 † 357.3*
- - mumps 072.7 † 357.4*
- - pellagra 265.2 † 357.4*
- - polyarteritis nodosa 446.0 † 357.1*
- - porphyria 277.1 † 357.4*
- - rheumatoid arthritis 714.0 † 357.1*
- - sarcoidosis 135 † 357.4*
- - uremia 585 † 357.4*
- nutritional NEC 269.9 † 357.4*

Polyneuropathy - *continued*
- postherpetic 053.1 † 357.4*
- sensory 356.2
Polyopia 368.3
Polyorchism, polyorchidism 752.8
Polyorrhomenitis (peritoneal) 568.8
- pleural - see Pleurisy
Polyorrhymenitis (see also Polyserositis) 568.8
Polyostotic fibrous dysplasia 756.5
Polyotia 744.1
Polyp, polypus

Note — Polyps of organs or sites that do not appear in the list below should be coded to the residual category for diseases of the organ or site concerned.

Polyp - *continued*
- accessory sinus 471.8
- adenoid tissue 471.0
- adenomatous (M8210/0) - see also Neoplasm, benign
- - adenocarcinoma in (M8210/3) - see Neoplasm, malignant
- - carcinoma in (M8210/3) - see Neoplasm, malignant
- - multiple (M8221/0) - see Neoplasm, benign
- antrum 471.8
- anus, anal (canal) 569.0
- bladder (M8120/1) 236.7
- cervix (uteri) 622.7
- - in pregnancy or childbirth 654.6
- - - causing obstructed labor 660.2
- - - fetus or newborn 763.8
- - mucous 622.7
- choanal 471.0
- colon (M8210/0) (see also Polyp, adenomatous) 211.3
- corpus uteri 621.0
- dental 522.0
- ear (middle) 385.3
- endometrium 621.0
- ethmoidal (sinus) 471.8
- fallopian tube 620.8
- frontal (sinus) 471.8
- gingiva 523.8
- gum 523.8
- labia 624.6
- larynx (mucous) 478.4
- malignant (M8000/3) - see Neoplasm, malignant
- maxillary (sinus) 471.8
- middle ear 385.3
- nasal (mucous) 471.9

Polyp - *continued*
- nasal - *continued*
- - cavity 471.0
- nasopharyngeal 471.0
- neoplastic (M8210/0) - see Neoplasm, benign
- nose (mucous) 471.9
- oviduct 620.8
- pharynx 478.2
- - congenital 750.2
- placenta 674.4
- pudenda 624.6
- pulpal 522.0
- rectum 569.0
- septum (nasal) 471.9
- sinus (accessory) (ethmoidal) (frontal) (maxillary) (sphenoidal) 471.8
- sphenoidal (sinus) 471.8
- stomach (M8210/0) 211.1
- tube, fallopian 620.8
- turbinate, mucous membrane 471.8
- ureter 593.8
- urethra 599.3
- uterus (body) (corpus) (mucous) 621.0
- - in pregnancy or childbirth 654.1
- - - causing obstructed labor 660.2
- - - - fetus or newborn 763.8
- vagina 623.7
- vocal cord (mucous) 478.4
- vulva 624.6
Polyphagia 783.6
Polypoid - see condition
Polyposis - see also Polyp
- coli (adenomatous) (M8220/0) 211.3
- - adenocarcinoma in (M8220/3) 153.9
- - carcinoma in (M8220/3) 153.9
- familial (M8220/0) 211.3
- intestinal (adenomatous) (M8220/0) 211.3
- multiple (M8221/0) - see also Neoplasm, benign
Polyradiculitis (acute) 357.0
Polyradiculoneuropathy (acute) (segmentally demyelinating) 357.0
Polysarcia 278.0
Polyserositis (peritoneal) 568.8
- periodic 277.3
- pleural - see Pleurisy
- tuberculous (see also Tubeculosis, polyserositis) 018.9
Polytrichia (see also Hypertrichosis) 704.1
Polyunguia 757.5
- acquired 703.8
Polyuria (nocturnal) 788.4
Pompe's disease (glycogen storage) 271.0
Pompholyx 705.8
Poncet's disease 015.9

Pond fracture 800.-
Ponos 085.0
Pons, pontine - see condition
Poor
 - contractions, labor 661.2
 - - fetus or newborn 763.7
 - fetal growth NEC 764.9
 - - affecting management of pregnancy
   656.5
 - vision NEC 369.9
Poradenitis, nostras 099.1
Porencephaly (congenital) (developmental)
 742.4
 - acquired 348.0
 - nondevelopmental 348.0
 - traumatic (post) 310.2
Porocephaliasis 134.1
Porokeratosis 757.3
Poroma, eccrine (M8402/0) - see
 Neoplasm, skin, benign
Porphyria (acute) (congenital)
 (erythropoietic) (familial) (hepatic)
 (intermittent) (latent) (Swedish) (South
 African) 277.1
 - acquired 277.1
 - cutanea tarda
 - - hereditaria 277.1
 - - symptomatica 277.1
 - due to drugs
 - - correct substance properly
   administered 277.1
 - - overdose or wrong substance given or
   taken 977.9
 - - - specified drug - see Table of drugs
   and chemicals
 - secondary 277.1
 - toxic NEC 277.1
 - variegata 277.1
Porphyrinuria (congenital) 277.1
 - acquired 277.1
Porphyruria (congenital) 277.1
 - acquired 277.1
Portal - see condition
Posadas-Wernicke disease 114
Position
 - fetus, abnormal (see also Presentation,
   fetal) 652.9
 - teeth, faulty 524.3
Positive
 - culture (nonspecific) 795.3
 - - nose 795.3
 - - sputum 795.3
 - - throat 795.3
 - - wound 795.3
 - serology 097.1
 - - with signs or symptoms - code by site
   and stage under Syphilis 097.9

Positive - *continued*
 - serology - *continued*
 - - false 795.6
 - VDRL 097.1
 - - with signs or symptoms - code by site
   and stage under Syphilis 097.9
 - - false 795.6
Postcardiotomy syndrome 429.4
Postcaval
 - ureter 753.4
Postcholecystectomy syndrome 576.0
Postcommissurotomy syndrome 429.4
Postconcussional syndrome 310.2
Postcontusional syndrome 310.2
Postcricoid region - see condition
Post-dates (pregnancy) 645
Postencephalitic syndrome 310.8
Posterior - see condition
Posterolateral sclerosis (spinal cord) - see
 Degeneration, combined
Postexanthematous - see condition
Postfebrile - see condition
Postgastrectomy dumping syndrome 564.2
Postherpetic neuralgia (zoster) 053.1
 - trigeminal 053.1 † 350.0*
Posthitis 607.1
Postimmunization complication or reaction
 - see Complications, vaccination
Postinfectious - see condition
Postlaminectomy syndrome 722.8
Postleukotomy syndrome 310.0
Postmastectomy lymphedema (syndrome)
 457.0
Postmaturity, postmature (fetus or
 newborn) 766.2
 - affecting management of pregnancy 645
Postmeasles (see also Condition)
 - complication 055.8
 - - specified NEC 055.7
Postmenopausal endometrium (atrophic)
 627.8
 - suppurative (see also Endometritis) 615.9
Postnatal - see condition
Postoperative NEC V45.8
Postpartum - see condition
Postpoliomyelitic - see condition
Postsurgery status NEC (see also Status
 (post)) V45.8
Post-term (pregnancy) 645
 - infant 766.2
Post-traumatic brain syndrome,
 nonpsychotic 310.2
Postures, hysterical 300.1
Postvaccinal reaction or complication - see
 Complications, vaccination
Postvalvulotomy syndrome 429.4
Pott's

Pott's - *continued*
- curvature (spinal) 015.0 † 737.4*
- disease or paraplegia 015.0 † 730.4*
- fracture 824.4
- - open 824.5
- spinal curvature 015.0 † 737.4*
- tumor, puffy (see also Osteomyelitis) 730.2
Potter's
- asthma 502
- facies 754.0
- lung 502
- syndrome (with renal agenesis) 753.0
Pouch
- bronchus 748.3
- Douglas' - see condition
- esophagus, esophageal 750.4
- - acquired 530.6
- gastric 537.1
- oesophagus, oesophageal 750.4
- pharynx 750.2
Poulet's disease 714.2
Poultrymen's itch 133.8
Poverty V60.2
Preauricular appendage 744.1
Prebetalipidproteinemia
- familial 272.1
Precipitate labor or delivery 661.3
- fetus or newborn 763.6
Precocious
- menstruation 626.8
- puberty 259.1
Precocity sexual (female) (male) (constitutional) (cryptogenic) (idiopathic) NEC 259.1
- with adrenal hyperplasia 255.2
Precordial pain 786.5
- psychogenic 307.8
Prediabetes, prediabetic 790.2
- complicating pregnancy, childbirth or puerperium 648.8
- - fetus or newborn 775.8
Predislocation
- status of hip at birth 754.3
Pre-eclampsia (mild) 642.4
- with preexisting hypertension 642.7
- fetus or newborn 760.0
- severe 642.5
Pre-excitation atrioventricular conduction 426.7
Pregnancy (single) (uterine)
- abdominal (ectopic) 633.0
- - fetus or newborn 761.4
- abnormal NEC 646.9
- ampullar - see Pregnancy, tubal
- broad ligament - see Pregnancy, cornual
- cervical - see Pregnancy, cornual

Pregnancy - *continued*
- complicated by
- - abnormal, abnormality NEC 646.9
- - - cervix 654.6
- - - cord (umbilical) 663.9
- - - glucose tolerance NEC 648.8
- - - pelvic organs or tissues NEC 654.9
- - - pelvis (bony) (major) NEC 653.0
- - - perineum or vulva 654.8
- - - placenta, placental (vessel) 656.7
- - - position
- - - - cervix 654.4
- - - - placenta 641.1
- - - - - without hemorrhage 641.0
- - - - uterus 654.4
- - - size, fetus 653.5
- - - uterus (congenital) 654.0
- - abscess or cellulitis
- - - bladder 646.6
- - - genital organ or tract 646.6
- - - kidney 646.6
- - - urinary tract NEC 646.6
- - albuminuria 646.2
- - - with hypertension - see Toxemia, of pregnancy
- - amnionitis 658.4
- - anemia (conditions in 280-285) 648.2
- - asymptomatic bacteriuria 646.5
- - atrophy, yellow (acute) (liver) (subacute) 648.9
- - bicornis or bicornuate uterus 654.0
- - bone and joint disorders of back, pelvis and lower limbs 648.7
- - breech presentation 652.2
- - - with successful version 652.1
- - cardiovascular diseases (conditions in 390-398, 410-429, 435, 440-459) 648.6
- - - congenital (conditions in 745-747) 648.5
- - cerebrovascular disorders (conditions in 430-434, 436-437) 674.0
- - cervicitis (conditions in 616.0) 646.6
- - chloasma (gravidarum) 646.8
- - chorea (gravidarum) - see Eclampsia, pregnancy
- - conditions in
- - - 001-139, NEC 647.8
- - - 010-018 647.3
- - - 050-079, except 056 647.6
- - - 056 647.5
- - - 084 647.4
- - - 090-097 647.0
- - - 098 647.1
- - - 099 647.2
- - - 240-246 648.1
- - - 250 648.0

Pregnancy - *continued*
- complicated by - *continued*
- - conditions in - *continued*
- - - 260-269 648.9
- - - 280-285 648.2
- - - 290-303, 305-316, 317-319 648.4
- - - 304 648.3
- - - 390-398, 410-429, 435, 440-459 648.6
- - - 401.0, 402-404 642.2
- - - 401.1, 401.9 642.0
- - - 405 642.1
- - - 430-434, 436-437 674.0
- - - 570 646.7
- - - 580-589 648.9
- - - 590, 595, 597, 599.0 646.6
- - - 614-616 646.6
- - - 711-719, 725-738 affecting lower limbs 648.7
- - - 720-724 648.7
- - - 745-747 648.5
- - - 790.2 648.8
- - contraction, pelvis (general) 653.1
- - - inlet 653.2
- - - outlet 653.3
- - convulsions (eclamptic) (uremic) 642.6
- - - with pre-existing hypertension 642.7
- - cystitis 646.6
- - cystocele 654.4
- - death of fetus (near term) 656.4
- - - early pregnancy 632
- - deciduitis 658.4
- - diabetes (mellitus) 648.0
- - disorders of liver 646.7
- - displacement, uterus NEC 654.4
- - disproportion - see Disproportion
- - drug dependence (conditions in 304.-) 648.3
- - early onset of delivery (spontaneous) 644.1
- - eclampsia, eclamptic (coma) (convulsions) (delirium) (nephritis) (uremia) 642.6
- - - with pre-existing hypertension 642.7
- - edema 646.1
- - - with hypertension - see Toxemia, of pregnancy
- - effusion, amniotic fluid 658.1
- - - delayed delivery following 658.2
- - embolism
- - - air 673.0
- - - amniotic fluid 673.1
- - - blood-clot 673.2
- - - pulmonary NEC 673.2
- - - pyemic 673.3
- - - septic 673.3

Pregnancy - *continued*
- complicated by - *continued*
- - emesis (gravidarum) - see Pregnancy, complicated by vomiting
- - endometritis 646.6
- - - decidual 658.4
- - excessive weight gain NEC 646.1
- - face presentation 652.4
- - failure, fetal head to enter pelvic brim 652.5
- - false labor (pains) 644.0
- - fatigue 646.8
- - fatty metamorphosis of liver 646.7
- - fetal deformity 653.7
- - fibroid (tumor) (uterus) 654.1
- - gonococcal infection 647.1
- - hemorrhage 641.9
- - - accidental 641.2
- - - before 22 completed weeks' gestation NEC 640.9
- - - due to
- - - - afibrinogenemia or other coagulation defect (conditions in category 286) 641.3
- - - - marginal sinus (rupture) 641.2
- - - - premature separation, placenta 641.2
- - - threatened abortion 640.0
- - - unavoidable 641.1
- - hepatitis acute, subacute, or malignant 646.7
- - herniation of uterus 654.3
- - high head at term 652.5
- - hydatidiform mole 630
- - hydramnios 657
- - hydrocephalic fetus 653.6
- - hydrops amnii 657
- - hydrorrhea 658.1
- - hyperemesis (gravidarum) - see Hyperemesis, gravidarum
- - hypertension - see Hypertension, complicating pregnancy
- - hypertensive
- - - heart and renal disease 642.2
- - - heart disease 642.2
- - - renal disease 642.2
- - hysteralgia 646.8
- - icterus gravis 646.7
- - incarceration, uterus 654.3
- - incompetent cervix 654.5
- - infection 647.9
- - - amniotic fluid 658.4
- - - bladder 646.6
- - - conditions in 134.9, 136.9 647.9
- - - genital organ or tract (conditions in categories 614-616) 646.6
- - - kidney (conditions in 590.-) 646.6

Pregnancy - *continued*
- complicated by - *continued*
- - threatened
- - - abortion 640.0
- - - premature delivery 644.1
- - thrombophlebitis (superficial) 671.2
- - - deep 671.3
- - thrombosis 671.9
- - - venous (superficial) 671.2
- - - - deep 671.3
- - thyroid dysfunction (conditions in 240-246) 648.1
- - torsion of uterus 654.4
- - toxemia - see Toxemia, of pregnancy
- - transverse lie or presentation 652.3
- - - with successful version 652.1
- - tuberculosis (conditions in 010-018) 647.3
- - tumor
- - - ovary 654.4
- - - pelvic organs or tissues NEC 654.4
- - - uterus (body) 654.1
- - - - cervix 654.6
- - unstable lie 652.0
- - uremia - see also Pregnancy, complicated by renal disease
- - urethritis 646.6
- - vaginitis or vulvitis (conditions in category 616.1) 646.6
- - varicose
- - - placental vessels 656.7
- - - veins (legs) 671.0
- - varicosity, labia or vulva 671.1
- - venereal disease NEC (conditions in 099) 647.2
- - viral diseases (conditions in 050-079, except 056) 647.6
- - vomiting 643.9
- - - due to organic disease or other cause 643.8
- - - early - see Hyperemesis, gravidarum
- - - late 643.2
- complications NEC 646.9
- cornual 633.8
- - fetus or newborn 761.4
- death from NEC 646.9
- delivered - see Delivery
- ectopic (ruptured) NEC 633.9
- - combined - see Pregnancy, cornual
- - fetus or newborn 761.4
- extra-uterine - see Pregnancy, ectopic
- fallopian - see Pregnancy, tubal
- false 300.1
- illegitimate V61.6
- in double uterus 654.0
- incidental finding V22.2
- interstitial - see Pregnancy, cornual

Pregnancy - *continued*
- intraligamentous - see Pregnancy, cornual
- intramural - see Pregnancy, cornual
- intraperitoneal - see Pregnancy, abdominal
- isthmian - see Pregnancy, tubal
- management affected by
- - abnormal, abnormality
- - - fetus (suspected) 655.9
- - - - specified NEC 655.8
- - - placenta 656.7
- - antibodies (maternal)
- - - anti-D 656.1
- - - blood group (ABO) 656.2
- - - - Rh(esus) 656.1
- - elderly primigravidity 659.5
- - fetal (suspected)
- - - abnormality 655.9
- - - - acid-base balance 656.3
- - - - heart rate or rhythm 656.3
- - - - specified NEC 655.8
- - - acidemia 656.3
- - - anencephaly 655.0
- - - bradycardia 656.3
- - - central nervous system malformation 655.0
- - - chromosal abnormality (conditions in 758) 655.1
- - - damage from
- - - - drugs 655.5
- - - - - obstetric, anesthetic or sedator 655.5
- - - - intrauterine contraceptive device 655.8
- - - - maternal
- - - - - alcohol addiction 655.4
- - - - - disease NEC 655.4
- - - - - drug use 655.5
- - - - - listeriosis 655.4
- - - - - rubella 655.3
- - - - - toxoplasmosis 655.4
- - - - - viral infection 655.3
- - - - radiation 655.6
- - - distress 656.3
- - - excessive growth 656.6
- - - growth retardation 656.5
- - - hereditary disease 655.2
- - - hydrocephalus 655.0
- - - intrauterine death 656.4
- - - poor growth 656.5
- - - spina bifida 655.0
- - feto-maternal hemorrage 656.0
- - hereditary disease in family (possibly) affecting fetus 655.2
- - incompatibility, blood groups (ABO) 656.2
- - - Rh(esus) 656.1

Prepuce - see condition
Presbycardia 797
Presbycusis 388.0
Presbyophrenia 310.1
Presbyopia 367.4
Prescription of contraceptives V25.0
 - repeat V25.4
Presenile - see also condition
 - aging 259.8
 - dementia 290.1
Presenility 259.8
Presentation, fetal
 - abnormal 652.9
 - - with successful version 652.1
 - - before labor, affecting fetus or
       newborn 761.7
 - - causing obstructed labor 660.0
 - - - affecting fetus or newborn, any,
          except breech 763.1
 - - in multiple gestation (one or more)
       652.6
 - - specified NEC 652.8
 - arm 652.7
 - - causing obstructed labor 660.0
 - breech 652.2
 - - with successful version 652.1
 - - - before labor, affecting fetus or
          newborn 761.4
 - - before labor, affecting fetus or
       newborn 761.7
 - - causing obstructed labor 660.0
 - - - fetus or newborn 763.0
 - brow 652.4
 - - causing obstructed labor 660.0
 - chin 652.4
 - - causing obstructed labor 660.0
 - compound 652.8
 - - causing obstructed labor 660.0
 - cord 663.0
 - extended head 652.4
 - - causing obstructed labor 660.0
 - face 652.4
 - - causing obstructed labor 660.0
 - - to pubes 652.8
 - - - causing obstructed labor 660.3
 - hand, leg or foot, NEC 652.8
 - - causing obstructed labor 660.0
 - mentum 652.4
 - - causing obstructed labor 660.0
 - oblique 652.3
 - - with successful version 652.1
 - - causing obstructed labor 660.0
 - shoulder 652.8
 - - causing obstructed labor 660.0
 - transverse 652.3
 - - with successful version 652.1
 - - causing obstructed labor 660.0

Presentation - *continued*
 - umbilical cord 663.0
 - unstable 652.0
Prespondylolisthesis (congenital) 756.1
Pressure
 - area, skin ulcer 707.0
 - atrophy, spine 733.9
 - birth, fetus or newborn, NEC 767.9
 - brachial plexus 353.0
 - brain 348.4
 - - injury at birth 767.8
 - cerebral - see Pressure, brain
 - cone, tentorial 348.8
 - - injury at birth 767.8
 - funis - see Compression, umbilical cord
 - hyposystolic (see also Hypotension)
     458.9
 - increased
 - - intracranial
 - - - injury at birth 767.8
 - - intracranial NEC 348.2
 - - intraocular 365.0
 - lumbosacral plexus 353.1
 - mediastinum 519.3
 - necrosis (chronic) (skin) 707.0
 - sore (chronic) 707.0
 - spinal cord 336.9
 - ulcer (chronic) 707.0
 - umbilical cord - see Compression,
     umbilical cord
 - venous, increased 459.8
Priapism 607.3
Prickling sensation (see also Disturbance,
   sensation) 782.0
Prickly heat 705.1
Primary - see condition
Primigravida, elderly
 - affecting
 - - fetus or newborn 763.8
 - - management of pregnancy, labor and
       delivery 659.5
Primipara, old
 - affecting
 - - fetus or newborn 763.8
 - - management of pregnancy, labor and
       delivery 659.5
Primus varus (bilateral) - see Talipes, varus
Pringle's disease 759.5
Prizefighter ear 738.7
Problem (with) V49.9
 - adopted child V61.2
 - aged
 - - in-law V61.3
 - - parent V61.3
 - - person NEC V61.8
 - alcoholism in family V61.4
 - behavioral V40.9

Procidentia - *continued*
- stomach 537.8
- uteri 618.3
Proctalgia 569.4
- fugax 564.6
- spasmodic 564.6
- - psychogenic 307.8
Proctitis 569.4
- amebic 006.8
- gonococcal 098.7
- tuberculous 014
- ulcerative (chronic) 556
Proctocele
- female 618.0
- male 569.1
Proctoptosis 569.1
Proctosigmoiditis 569.8
- ulcerative (chronic) 556
Proctospasm 564.6
- psychogenic 306.4
Profichet's syndrome 729.9
Progeria 259.8
Prognathism (mandibular) (maxillary) 524.1
Progonoma (melanotic) (M9363/0) - see Neoplasm, benign
Progressive - see condition
Prolapse, prolapsed
- anus, anal (canal) (sphincter) 569.1
- arm or hand 652.7
- - causing obstructed labor 660.0
- - fetus or newborn 763.1
- bladder (mucosa) (sphincter) (acquired)
- - congenital (female) (male) 753.8
- - female 618.0
- - male 596.8
- cecostomy 569.6
- cecum 569.8
- cervix, cervical (stump) (hypertrophied) 618.1
- - anterior lip, obstructing labor 660.2
- - - fetus or newborn 763.1
- - congenital 752.4
- - postpartal, old 618.1
- ciliary body 871.1
- colon (pedunculated) 569.8
- colostomy 569.6
- cord - see Prolapse, umbilical cord
- disc (intervertebral) - see Displacement, intervertebral disc
- eye implant 996.5
- fallopian tube 620.4
- fetal extremity 652.8
- - causing obstructed labor 660.0
- - fetus or newborn 763.1
- funis - see Prolapse, umbilical cord
- gastric (mucosa) 537.8

Prolapse - *continued*
- genital, female 618.9
- globe 360.8
- ileostomy bud 569.6
- intervertebral disc - see Displacement, intervertebral disc
- intestine (small) 569.8
- iris 871.1
- - nontraumatic 364.8
- kidney (see also Lesion, kidney) 593.0
- - congenital 753.3
- laryngeal muscles or ventricle 478.7
- leg 652.8
- - causing obstructed labor 660.0
- - fetus or newborn 763.1
- liver 573.8
- meatus urinarius 599.5
- organ or site, congenital NEC - see Malposition, congenital
- ovary 620.4
- pelvic (floor), female 618.8
- perineum female 618.8
- rectum (mucosa) (sphincter) 569.1
- spleen 289.5
- stomach 537.8
- umbilical cord
- - complicating delivery 663.0
- - fetus or newborn 762.4
- ureter 593.8
- - with obstruction 593.4
- ureterovesical orifice 593.8
- urethra (acquired) (infected) (mucosa) 599.5
- - congenital 753.8
- uterovaginal 618.4
- - complete 618.3
- - incomplete 618.2
- - specified NEC 618.8
- uterus
- - with mention of vaginal wall prolapse - see Prolapse, uterovaginal
- - congenital 752.3
- - in pregnancy or childbirth 654.4
- - postpartal (old) 618.1
- - pregnant, affecting fetus or newborn 763.8
- - without mention of vaginal wall prolapse 618.1
- uveal 871.1
- vagina (anterior) (posterior) (wall) 618.0
- - with mention of uterine prolapse - see Prolapse, uterovaginal
- - posthysterectomy 618.5
- vitreous (humor), in wound 871.1
- womb - see Prolapse, uterus
Prolapsus, female (see also Prolapse, uterus) 618.9

Proliferative - see condition
Prolongation of bleeding, coagulation or
prothrombin time (see also Defect,
coagulation) 286.9
Prolonged
− labor 662.1
− − fetus or newborn 763.8
− − first stage 662.0
− − second stage 662.2
− uterine contractions in labor 661.4
− − fetus or newborn 763.7
Prominauris 744.2
Prominence of auricle (congenital) (ear)
744.2
Prominent ischial spine or sacral
promontory
− with disproportion 653.3
− − causing obstructed labor 660.1
− − fetus or newborn 763.1
Pronation
− ankle 736.7
− foot 736.7
− − congenital 755.6
Prophylactic
− administration of
− − antibiotics V07.3
− − immune sera (gamma globulin) V07.2
− chemotherapy V07.3
− immunotherapy V07.2
− measure V07.9
− − specified NEC V07.8
− sterilization V25.2
Proptosis (ocular) 376.3
− thyroid 242.0
Prosecution, anxiety concerning V62.5
Prostate, prostatic - see condition
Prostatism 600
Prostatitis (congestive) (suppurative) 601.9
− acute 601.0
− chronic 601.1
− due to Trichomonas (vaginalis) 131.0 †
601.4*
− fibrous 600
− gonococcal (acute) 098.1 † 601.4*
− − chronic or duration of 2 months or over
098.3 † 601.4*
− granulomatous 601.8
− hypertrophic 600
− specified type NEC 601.8
− subacute 601.1
− trichomonal 131.0 † 601.4*
− tuberculous 016.3 † 601.4*
Prostatocystitis 601.3
Prostatorrhea 602.8
Prostration 780.7
− heat - see Heat, exhaustion
− nervous 300.5

Prostration - *continued*
− senile 797
Protanomaly 368.5
Protanopia (anomalous trichromat)
(complete) (incomplete) 368.5
Protein
− deficiency 260
− malnutrition 260
− sickness (prophylactic) (therapeutic)
999.5
Proteinemia 790.9
Proteinosis
− alveolar, lung or pulmonary 516.0
− lipid 272.8
− lipoid (of Urbach) 272.8
Proteinuria (see also Albuminuria) 791.0
− Bence Jones NEC 791.0
− gestational 646.2
− − with hypertension - see Toxemia, of
pregnancy
− postural 593.6
Protrusio acetabuli 718.6
Protrusion
− acetabulum (into pelvis) 718.6
− device, implant or graft - see
Complications, mechanical
− intervertebral disc - see Displacement,
intervertebral disc
− nucleus pulposus - see Displacement,
intervertebral disc
Prune belly (syndrome) 756.7
Prurigo 698.2
− Besnier's 691.8
− estivalis 692.7
− Hebra's 698.2
− mitis 698.2
− nodularis 698.3
− psychogenic 306.3
Pruritus, pruritic 698.9
− ani 698.0
− − psychogenic 306.3
− conditions NEC 698.9
− − psychogenic 306.3
− ear 698.9
− genital organ(s) 698.1
− − psychogenic 306.3
− gravidarum 646.8
− neurogenic (any site) 306.3
− psychogenic (any site) 306.3
− scrotum 698.1
− − psychogenic 306.3
− senile 698.8
− Trichomonas 131.9
− vulva, vulvae 698.1
− − psychogenic 306.3
Psammocarcinoma (M8140/3) - see
Neoplasm, malignant

Pseudarthrosis, pseudoarthrosis (bone) 733.8
– joint following fusion 718.5
Pseudo-aneurysm - see Aneurysm
Pseudo-angina (pectoris) - see Angina
Pseudo-angioma 452
Pseudo-arteriosus 747.8
Pseudoarthrosis - see Pseudarthrosis
Pseudocholera 025
Pseudochromhidosis 705.8
Pseudocirrhosis, liver, pericardial 423.2
Pseudocowpox 051.1
Pseudocroup 478.7
Pseudocyesis 300.1
Pseudocyst
– lung 518.8
– pancreas 577.2
– retina 361.1
Pseudoexfoliation, capsule (lens) 366.1
Pseudoglanders 025
Pseudoglioma 360.4
Pseudohemophilia (Bernuth's) (hereditary) (type B) 286.4
– A 287.8
– vascular 287.8
Pseudohermaphroditism 752.7
– with chromosomal anomaly - see Anomaly, chromosomal
– adrenal 255.2
– female 752.7
– – with adrenocortical disorder 255.2
– – adrenal 255.2
– – without adrenocortical disorder 752.7
– male 752.7
– – with
– – – adrenocortical disorder 255.2
– – – cleft scrotum 752.7
– – – feminizing testis 257.8
– – – gonadal disorder 257.9
– – adrenal 255.2
– – without gonadal disorder 752.7
Pseudohydrocephalus 348.2
Pseudohypoparathyroidism 275.4
Pseudo-influenza 487.1
Pseudoleukemia 288.8
– infantile 285.8
Pseudomembranous - see condition
Pseudomenstruation 626.8
Pseudomucinous peritoneum 568.8
Pseudomyxoma peritonei (M8480/6) 197.6
Pseudoneuritis optic (nerve) (disc) (congenital) 743.5
Pseudoneuroma - see Injury, nerve, by site
Pseudopapilledema (congenital) 743.5
Pseudoparalysis
– arm or leg 781.4
– atonic, congenital 358.8

Pseudopelade (see also Alopecia) 704.0
Pseudophakia V43.1
Pseudopolycythemia 289.0
Pseudopolyposis of colon 556
Pseudo-pseudohypoparathyroidism 275.4
Pseudopterygium 372.5
Pseudoptosis (eyelid) 374.3
Pseudorickets 588.0
Pseudorubella 057.8
Pseudoscarlatina 057.8
Pseudosclerema 778.1
Pseudosclerosis (brain)
– of Westphal 275.1
– spastic 046.1 † 331.5*
– – with dementia 290.1
Pseudotetanus (see also Convulsions) 780.3
Pseudotetany 781.7
– hysterical 300.1
Pseudothalassemia 285.0
Pseudotrichinosis 710.3
Pseudotruncus arteriosus 747.2
Pseudotuberculosis, Pasteurella (infection) 027.2
Pseudotumor
– cerebri 348.2
– orbital 376.1
Pseudoturner's syndrome 759.8
Pseudoxanthoma elasticum 757.3
Psilosis 579.1
– monilia 112.8
– not sprue 704.0
Psittacosis 073
Psoitis 728.8
Psora NEC 696.1
Psoriasis 696.1
– any type, except arthropathic 696.1
– arthropathic 696.0 † 713.3*
– buccal 528.6
– guttate 696.1
– mouth 528.6
– pustular 696.1
Psorospermiasis 136.4
Psorospermosis 136.4
– follicularis 757.3
Psychalgia 307.8
Psychasthenia 300.8
– compulsive 300.3
– mixed compulsive states 300.3
– obsession 300.3
Psychiatric disorder or problem NEC 300.9
Psychogenic - see also condition
– factors associated with physical conditions 316
Psychoneurosis, psychoneurotic (see also Neurosis) 300.9
– anxiety (state) 300.0
– climacteric, unspecified type 627.2

Psychosis - *continued*
- organic NEC - *continued*
- - due to or associated with - *continued*
- - - conditions - *continued*
- - - - in 303 - see psychosis, alcoholic
  291.0
- - - dependence
- - - - alcohol (see also Psychosis,
  alcoholic) 291.9
- - - - drug 292.9
- - - disease
- - - - brain
- - - - - arteriosclerotic 290.4
- - - - cerebrovascular
- - - - - acute (psychosis) 293.0
- - - - - arteriosclerotic 290.4
- - - - endocrine or metabolic 293.9
- - - - - acute (psychosis) 293.0
- - - - - subacute (psychosis) 293.1
- - - - Jakob-Creutzfeldt 290.1
- - - - liver
- - - - - alcoholic (see also Psychosis,
  alcoholic) 291.9
- - - disorder
- - - - cerebrovascular
- - - - - acute (psychosis) 293.0
- - - - endocrine or metabolic 293.9
- - - - - acute (psychosis) 293.0
- - - - - subacute (psychosis) 293.1
- - - epilepsy 294.1
- - - - transient (acute) 293.0
- - - Huntington's chorea 294.1
- - - infection
- - - - brain 293.9
- - - - - acute (psychosis) 293.0
- - - - - chronic (psychosis) 294.8
- - - - - subacute (psychosis) 293.1
- - - - intracranial NEC 293.9
- - - - - acute (psychosis) 293.0
- - - - - chronic (psychosis) 294.8
- - - - - subacute (psychosis) 293.1
- - - intoxication
- - - - alcoholic (acute) (see also
  Psychosis, alcoholic) 291.9
- - - - drug (see also Psychosis, drug)
  292.9
- - - ischemia
- - - - cerebrovascular (generalized)
  290.4
- - - Jakob-Creutzfeldt's disease or
  syndrome 290.1
- - - multiple sclerosis 294.1
- - - presenility 290.1
- - - puerperium - see Psychosis,
  puerperal
- - - sclerosis, multiple 294.1
- - - senility 290.2

Psychosis - *continued*
- organic NEC - *continued*
- - due to or associated with - *continued*
- - - trauma
- - - - brain (birth) (from electric
  current) (surgical) 293.9
- - - - - acute (psychosis) 293.0
- - - - - chonic (psychosis) 294.8
- - - - - subacute (psychosis) 293.1
- - - - unspecified physical condition 294.9
- - infective 293.9
- - - acute 293.0
- - - subacute 293.1
- - post-traumatic 293.9
- - - acute 293.0
- - - subacute 293.1
- - specified NEC 294.8
- - transient 293.9
- - - specified NEC 293.8
- paranoiac 297.1
- paranoid 297.9
- - alcoholic 291.5
- - climacteric 297.2
- - involutional 297.2
- - menopausal 297.2
- - protracted reactive 298.4
- - psychogenic 298.4
- - - acute 298.3
- - schizophrenic 295.3
- - senile 290.2
- paroxysmal 298.9
- polyneuritic, alcoholic 291.1
- postpartum - see Psychosis, puerperal
- presbyophrenic (type) 290.8
- presenile 290.1
- psychogenic 298.8
- - depressive 298.0
- - paranoid 298.4
- - - acute 298.3
- puerperal
- - specified type - see categories 295-298
- - unspecified type 293.8
- - - acute 293.0
- - - chronic 293.8
- - - subacute 293.1
- reactive (from emotional stress,
  psychological trauma) 298.8
- - confusion 298.2
- - depressive 298.0
- - excitation 298.1
- schizoaffective 295.7
- schizophrenia, schizophrenic (see also
  Schizophrenia) 295.9
- schizophreniform 295.9
- - affective type 295.7
- - confusional type 295.4
- senile NEC 290.2

Puerperal - *continued*
- disorder - *continued*
- - lactation 676.9
- - - specified NEC 676.8
- - nonobstetric NEC (see also Pregnancy, complicated by, conditions in) 648.9
- disruption
- - cesarean wound 674.1
- - episiotomy wound 674.2
- - perineal laceration wound 674.2
- eclampsia 642.6
- - with pre-existing hypertension 642.7
- embolism (pulmonary) 673.2
- - air 673.0
- - amniotic fluid 673.1
- - blood clot 673.2
- - brain or cerebral 674.0
- - cardiac 674.8
- - fat 673.8
- - pyemic 673.3
- - septic 673.3
- endophlebitis - see Puerperal phlebitis
- endotrachelitis 670
- failure
- - lactation 676.4
- - renal, acute 669.3
- fever (meaning sepsis) 670
- - meaning pyrexia (of unknown origin) 672
- fissure, nipple 676.1
- fistula
- - breast 675.1
- - mammary gland 675.1
- - nipple 675.0
- galactophoritis 675.2
- galactorrhea 676.6
- gangrene
- - gas 670
- - uterus 670
- hematoma, subdural 674.0
- hematosalpinx, infectional 670
- hemiplegia, cerebral 674.0
- hemorrhage 666.2
- - brain 674.0
- - bulbar 674.0
- - cerebellar 674.0
- - cerebral 674.0
- - cortical 674.0
- - delayed (uterine) 666.2
- - extradural 674.0
- - internal capsule 674.0
- - intracranial 674.0
- - intrapontine 674.0
- - meningeal 674.0
- - pontine 674.0
- - subarachnoid 674.0
- - subcortical 674.0

Puerperal - *continued*
- hemorrhage - *continued*
- - subdural 674.0
- - uterine, delayed 666.2
- - ventricular 674.0
- hepatorenal syndrome 674.8
- hypertrophy
- - breast 676.3
- - mammary gland 676.3
- induration breast (fibrous) 676.3
- infarction
- - lung - see Puerperal, embolism
- - pulmonary - see Puerperal, embolism
- infection
- - breast 675.1
- - cervix 670
- - fallopian tube 670
- - generalized 670
- - genital tract (major) 670
- - - minor or localized 646.6
- - kidney (bacillus coli) 646.6
- - mammary gland 675.1
- - nipple 675.0
- - ovary 670
- - pelvic 670
- - peritoneum 670
- - renal 646.6
- - tubo-ovarian 670
- - urinary (tract) NEC 646.6
- - - asymptomatic 646.5
- - uterus, uterine 670
- - vagina 646.6
- inflammation - see also Puerperal, infection
- - vein - see Puerperal phlebitis
- ischemia, cerebral 674.0
- lymphangitis 670
- - breast 675.2
- mammillitis 675.2
- mammitis 675.2
- mania 296.0
- mastitis 675.2
- melancholia 296.1
- metritis (septic) (suppurative) 670
- metroperitonitis 670
- metrorrhagia 666.2
- metrosalpingitis 670
- metrovaginitis 670
- milk leg 671.4
- necrosis
- - kidney, tubular 669.3
- - liver (acute) (subacute) (conditions in category 570.-) 674.8
- nephritis or nephrosis (conditions in 580-589) 648.9
- - with hypertension 642.1
- occlusion, pre-cerebral artery 674.0

Puncture - *continued*
- accidental, complicating surgery 998.2
- bladder, nontraumatic 596.6
- by
- - device, implant or graft - see
  Complications, mechanical
- - foreign body left accidentally in
  operation wound 998.4
- - instrument (any) during a procedure,
  accidental 998.2
- internal organs, abdomen, chest, or pelvis
  - see Injury, internal
- kidney, nontraumatic 593.8
Pupillary membrane (persistent) 743.4
Pupillotonia 379.4
Purpura 287.2
- abdominal 287.0
- allergic 287.0
- anaphylactoid 287.0
- annularis telangiectodes 709.1
- arthritic 287.0
- bacterial 287.0
- capillary fragility, idiopathic 287.8
- cryoglobulinemic 273.2
- fibrinolytic (see also Fibrinolysis) 286.6
- fulminans, fulminous 286.6
- gangrenous 287.0
- hemorrhagic, hemorrhagica (see also
  Purpura, thrombocytopenic) 287.3
- - nodular 272.7
- - not due to thrombocytopenia 287.0
- Henoch(-Schonlein) 287.0
- hypergammaglobulinemic
  (Waldenstrom's) 273.0
- idiopathhic 287.3
- - nonthrombocytopenic 287.0
- infectious 287.0
- malignant 287.0
- nervosa 287.0
- newborn NEC 772.6
- nonthrombocytopenic 287.2
- - hemorrhagic 287.0
- - idiopathic 287.0
- nonthrombopenic 287.2
- rheumatica 287.0
- Schonlein(-Henoch) 287.0
- scorbutic 267
- senile 287.2
- simplex 287.2
- symptomatica 287.0
- thrombocytopenic (congenital)
  (essential) (hereditary) (idiopathic)
  (primary) (see also Thrombocytopenia)
  287.3
- - neonatal, transitory 776.1
- - puerperal, postpartum 666.3
- - thrombotic 446.6

Purpura - *continued*
- thrombohemolytic (see also Fibrinolysis)
  286.6
- thrombopenic (congenital) (essential)
  (see also Thrombocytopenia) 287.3
- thrombotic 446.6
- - thrombocytopenic 446.6
- toxic 287.0
- variolosa 050.0
- vascular 287.0
- visceral symptoms 287.0
Purulent - see condition
Pus
- absorption, general - see Septicemia
- in
- - stool 792.1
- - urine 599.0
Pustular rash 782.1
Pustule 686.9
- malignant 022.0
- nonmalignant 686.9
Putnam's disease - see Degeneration,
  combined
Putnam-Dana syndrome - see
  Degeneration, combined
Putrefaction, intestinal 569.8
Putrescent pulp (dental) 522.1
Pyarthritis - see Pyarthrosis
Pyarthrosis 711.0
- tuberculous - see Tuberculosis, joint
Pyelectasis 593.8
Pyelitis (congenital) (uremic) 590.8
- with
- - abortion - see categories 634-639,
    fourth digit .8
- - calculus or stones 592.9
- - contracted kidney 590.0
- - ectopic gestation 639.8
- acute 590.1
- chronic 590.0
- - with calculus 592.9
- complicating pregnancy or puerperium
  646.6
- - fetus or newborn 760.1
- cystica 590.3
- gonococcal 098.1 † 590.8*
- - chronic or duration of 2 months or over
    098.3 † 590.8*
- tuberculous 016.0 † 590.8*
Pyelocystitis (see also Pyelitis) 590.8
Pyelohydronephrosis 591
Pyelonephritis (see also Pyelitis) 590.8
- acute 590.1
- calculous 592.9
- chronic 590.0
- syphilitic 095 † 590.8*
- tuberculous 016.0 † 590.8*

Pyelonephrosis (see also Pyelitis) 590.8
- chronic 590.0
Pyelophlebitis - see Phlebitis
Pyelo-ureteritis cystica 590.3
Pyemia, pyemic (purulent) (see also
  Septicemia) 038.9
- joint 711.0
- liver 572.1
- portal 572.1
- postvaccinal 999.3
- tuberculous - see Tuberculosis, miliary
Pygopagus 759.4
Pykno-epilepsy, pyknolepsy (idiopathic)
  345.0
Pyle's disease 756.8
Pylephlebitis 572.1
Pylethrombophlebitis 572.1
Pyloritis 535.5
Pylorospasm (reflex) 537.8
- congenital or infantile 750.5
- neurotic 306.4
- psychogenic 306.4
Pylorus, pyloric - see condition
Pyoarthrosis - see Pyarthrosis
Pyocele
- mastoid 383.0
- sinus (accessory) (see also Sinusitis)
  473.9
- turbinate (bone) 473.9
- urethra (see also Urethritis) 597.0
Pyocolpos (see also Vaginitis) 616.1
Pyocystitis (see also Cystitis) 595.9
Pyoderma, pyodermia NEC 686.0
- gangrenosum 686.0
- vegetans 686.8
Pyodermatitis 686.0
- vegetans 686.8
Pyogenic - see condition
Pyohemia - see Septicemia
Pyohydronephrosis (see also Pyelitis) 590.8
Pyometra (see also Endometritis) 615.9
Pyometritis (see also Endometritis) 615.9
Pyometrium (see also Endometritis) 615.9

Pyomyositis 728.0
- ossificans 728.1
- tropical 040.8 † 728.0*
Pyonephritis (see also Pyelitis) 590.8
- chronic 590.0
Pyonephrosis (congenital) (see also Pyelitis)
  590.8
- acute 590.1
Pyo-oophoritis (see also Salpingo-
  oophoritis) 614.2
Pyo-ovarium (see also Salpingo-oophoritis)
  614.2
Pyopericarditis 420.9
Pyopericardium 420.9
Pyophlebitis - see Phlebitis
Pyopneumopericardium 420.9
Pyopneumothorax (infectional) 510.9
- with fistula 510.0
- subphrenic (see also Peritonitis) 567.2
- tuberculous 012.0
Pyorrhea (alveolar) (alveolaris) 523.4
- degenerative 523.5
Pyosalpingitis (see also Salpingo-oophoritis)
  614.2
Pyosalpinx (see also Salpingo-oophoritis)
  614.2
Pyosepticemia - see Septicemia
Pyosis Corlett's or Manson's 684
Pyothorax 510.9
- with fistula 510.0
- tuberculous 012.0
Pyoureter 593.8
- tuberculous 016.1 † 593.8*
Pyrexia (of unknown origin) 780.6
- atmospheric 992.0
- during labor 659.2
- heat 992.0
- newborn, environmentally induced 778.4
- puerperal 672
Pyroglobulinemia 273.8
Pyromania 312.2
Pyrosis 787.1
Pyuria (bacterial) 599.0

Q

Q-fever 083.0
- with pneumonia 083.0 † 484.8*
Quadricuspid aortic valve 746.8
Quadriplegia 344.0
- with fracture, spine or vertebra (process) 806.0
- - open 806.1
- brain (current episode) 437.8
- cerebral 437.8
- congenital or infantile (cerebral) (spastic) (spinal) 343.2
- cortical 437.8
- embolic (current episode) (see also Embolism, brain) 434.1
- newborn NEC 767.0
- thrombotic (current episode) (see also Thrombosis, brain) 434.0
- traumatic - see Injury, spinal, cervical

Quadruplet 761.5
- pregnancy (complicating delivery) 651.2
Quarrelsomeness 301.3
Queensland fever 083.0
- seven day 100.8
Quervain's disease 727.0
Queyrat's erythroplasia (M8080/2)
- specified site - see Neoplasm, skin, in situ
- unspecified site 233.5
Quincke's disease or edema - see Edema, angioneurotic
Quinquaud's disease 704.0
Quinsy 475
- gangrenous 475
Quintuplet 761.5
- pregnancy (complicating delivery) 651.8

R

R.D.S. 769
Rabbia 071
Rabia 071
Rabies 071
– inoculation reaction - see Complications, vaccination
Rachischisis 741.9
– with hydrocephalus 741.0
Rachitic - see also condition
– deformities of spine 268.1
– pelvis 268.1
– – with disproportion 653.2
– – – causing obstructed labor 660.1
– – – – fetus or newborn 763.1
Rachitis, rachitism - see also Rickets
– acuta 268.0
– fetalis 756.4
– tarda 268.0
Radial nerve - see condition
Radiation effects or sickness NEC 990
Radiculitis (pressure) (vertebrogenic) 729.2
– accessory nerve 723.4
– anterior crural 724.4
– brachial 723.4
– cervical NEC 723.4
– due to displacement of intervertebral disc - see Neuritis, due to displacement, intervertebral disc
– lumbar NEC 724.4
– lumbosacral 724.4
– rheumatic 729.2
– syphilitic 094.8
– thoracic (with visceral pain) 724.4
Radiculomyelitis (see also Encephalitis) 323.9
– toxic, due to
– – Clostridium tetani 037
– – Corynebacterium diphtheriae 032.8
Radiculopathy (see also Radiculitis) 729.2
Radioactive substances, adverse effect NEC 990
Radiodermal burns (acute, chronic, or occupational) - see Burn
Radiodermatitis 692.8
Radionecrosis NEC 990
Radiotherapy session V58.0
Radium, adverse effect NEC 990
Rage, meaning rabies 071
Raillietiniasis 123.8
Railroad neurosis 300.1

Railway spine 300.1
Raised - see Elevation
Raiva 071
Rales 786.7
Ramifying renal pelvis 753.3
Ramsey-Hunt syndrome 053.1 † 351.1*
– meaning dyssynergia cerebellaris myoclonica 334.2
Ranke's primary infiltration 010.0
Ranula 527.6
– congenital 750.2
Rape (see also Nature and site of injury) 959.9
Rapid
– feeble pulse, due to shock, following injury 958.4
– heart 785.0
– – psychogenic 306.2
– second stage (delivery) 661.3
– – fetus or newborn 763.6
Rarefaction, bone 733.9
Rash 782.1
– canker 034.1
– diaper 691.0
– drug (internal use) 693.0
– – contact 692.3
– ECHO 9 viral 078.8
– enema 692.8
– food (see also Allergy, food) 693.1
– heat 705.1
– napkin 691.0
– nettle 708.8
– pustular 782.1
– rose 782.1
– – epidemic 056.9
– scarlet 034.1
– serum (prophylactic) (therapeutic) 999.5
– wandering, tongue 529.1
Rasmussen's aneurysm 011.2
Rathke's pouch tumor (M9350/1) 237.0
Raymond(-Cestan) syndrome 433.8
Raynaud's
– disease or syndrome 443.0
– gangrene 443.0 † 785.4*
– phenomenon (secondary) 443.0
Reaction
– acute situational maladjustment (see also Reaction, adjustment) 309.9
– adaption (see also Reaction, adjustment) 309.9

Reaction - *continued*
- adjustment 309.9
- - with
- - - conduct disturbance 309.3
- - - - combined with disturbance of
emotions 309.4
- - - mutism, elective 309.8
- - - predominant disturbance (of)
- - - - conduct 309.3
- - - - emotions other than depression
309.2
- - - - mixed, emotions and conduct
309.4
- - - - specified NEC 309.8
- - depressive
- - - with conduct disturbance 309.4
- - - brief 309.0
- - - prolonged 309.1
- affective (see also Psychosis, affective)
296.9
- aggressive 301.3
- allergic (see also Allergy) NEC 995.3
- - drug, medicament and biological - see
Allergy, drug
- - serum 999.5
- anaphylactic - see Shock, anaphylactic
- anesthesia - see Anesthesia, complication
- anger 312.0
- antisocial 301.7
- antitoxin (prophylactic) (therapeutic) -
see Complications, vaccination
- anxiety 300.0
- asthenic 300.5
- compulsive 300.3
- conversion (anesthetic) (autonomic)
(hyperkinetic) (mixed paralytic)
(paresthetic) 300.1
- depressive 300.4
- - affective 296.1
- - manic (see also Psychosis,
manic-depressive) 296.6
- - neurotic 300.4
- - psychoneurotic 300.4
- - psychotic 298.0
- dissociative 300.1
- drug NEC 995.2
- - allergic - see Allergy, drug
- - correct substance properly
administered 995.2
- - overdose or poisoning 977.9
- - - specified drug - see Table of drugs
and chemicals
- - specific to newborn 779.4
- - transmitted via placenta or breast milk
- see Absorption, drug, through
placenta
- - withdrawal 292.0

Reaction - *continued*
- drug NEC - *continued*
- - withdrawal - *continued*
- - - infant of dependent mother 779.5
- - wrong substance given or taken in
error 977.9
- - - specified drug - see Table of drugs
and chemicals
- dyssocial 301.7
- erysipeloid 027.1
- fear 300.2
- - child 313.0
- fluid loss, cerebrospinal 349.0
- foreign
- - body NEC 728.8
- - substance accidentally left during a
procedure (chemical) (powder) (talc)
998.7
- grief 309.0
- group delinquent 312.1
- Herxheimer's 995.0
- hyperkinetic - see Hyperkinesia
- hypochondriacal 300.7
- hypoglycemic, due to insulin 251.0
- - therapeutic misadventure 962.3
- hypomanic 296.0
- hysterical 300.1
- immunization - see Complications,
vaccination
- incompatibility
- - blood group (ABO) (infusion)
(transfusion) 999.6
- - Rh (factor) (infusion) (transfusion)
999.7
- inflammatory - see Infection
- infusion - see Complications, infusion
- inoculation (immune serum) - see
Complications, vaccination
- insulin 995.2
- leukemoid (lymphocytic) (monocytic)
(myelocytic) 288.8
- LSD 305.3
- lumbar puncture 349.0
- manic-depressive (see also Psychosis,
manic-depressive) 296.6
- - depressed 296.1
- neurasthenic 300.5
- neurogenic (see also Neurosis) 300.9
- neurotic NEC 300.9
- neurotic-depressive 300.4
- nitritoid - see Crisis, nitritoid
- obsessive(-compulsive) 300.3
- overanxious, child or adolescent 313.0
- paranoid (chronic) 297.9
- - acute 298.3
- - climacteric 297.2
- - involutional 297.2

Reaction - *continued*
- paranoid - *continued*
-   - menopausal 297.2
-   - senile 290.2
-   - simple 297.0
- personality (see also Disorder, personality) 301.9
- phobic 300.2
- postradiation NEC 990
- psychogenic NEC 300.9
- psychoneurotic (see also Neurosis) 300.9
-   - compulsive 300.3
-   - obsessive 300.3
- psychophysiologic (see also Disorder, psychogenic) 306.9
- psychotic (see also Psychosis) 298.2
-   - due to or associated with physical condition - see Psychosis, organic
- radiation NEC 990
- runaway
-   - socialized 312.1
-   - unsocialized 312.0
- scarlet fever toxin - see Complications, vaccination
- schizophrenic (see also Schizophrenia) 295.9
-   - latent 295.5
- serological for syphillis - see Serology for syphilis
- serum (prophylactic) (therapeutic) 999.5
-   - immediate 999.4
- situational (see also Reaction, adjustment) 309.9
-   - acute 308.3
- somatization (see also Disorder, psychogenic) 306.9
- spinal puncture 349.0
- spite, child 312.0
- stress, acute 308.9
-   - with predominant disturbance (of)
-    - consciousness 308.1
-    - emotions 308.0
-    - mixed 308.4
-    - psychomotor 308.2
-    - specified NEC 308.3
-    - unspecified 308.9
- surgical procedure - see Complications, surgical procedure
- tetanus antitoxin - see Complications, vaccination
- toxin-antitoxin - see Complications, vaccination
- transfusion (blood) (bone marrow) (lymphocytes) (allergic) - see Complications, transfusion
- tuberculin skin test, nonspecific 795.5
- ultraviolet NEC 990

Reaction - *continued*
- unsocialized aggressive 312.0
- vaccination (any) - see Complications, vaccination
- withdrawing, child or adolescent 313.2
- X-ray NEC 990
Reactive depression (see also Reaction, depressive) 300.4
- neurotic 300.4
- psychoneurotic 300.4
- psychotic 298.0
Recanalization, thrombus - see Thrombosis
Receding chin 524.0
Recession
- chamber angle (eye) 364.7
- gingival (generalized) (localized) (postinfective) (postoperative) 523.2
Recklinghausen's disease (M9540/1) 237.7
- bones 252.0
Reclus' disease (cystic) 610.1
Recruitment, auditory 388.4
Rectalgia 569.4
Rectitis 569.4
Rectocele
- female 618.0
- in pregnancy or childbirth 654.4
-   - causing obstructed labor 660.2
-    - fetus or newborn 763.1
- male 569.4
- vagina, vaginal (outlet) 618.0
Rectosigmoid junction - see condition
Rectosigmoiditis 569.8
- ulcerative (chronic) 556
Rectourethral - see condition
Rectovaginal - see condition
Rectovesical - see condition
Rectum, rectal - see condition
Recurrent - see condition
Red-cedar asthma 495.8
Reduced ventilatory or vital capacity 794.2
Reduction function
- kidney (see also Disease, renal) 593.9
- liver 573.8
Redundant, redundancy
- anus 751.5
- cardia 537.8
- clitoris 624.2
- colon 751.5
- foreskin (congenital) 605
- intestine 751.5
- labia 624.3
- organ or site, congenital NEC - see Accessory
- panniculus (abdominal) 278.1
- prepuce (congenital) 605
- pylorus 537.8
- rectum 751.5

Redundant - *continued*
- scrotum 608.8
- sigmoid 751.5
- skin (of face) 701.9
- - eyelids 374.3
- stomach 537.8
- uvula 528.9
- vagina 623.8

Reduplication - see Duplication

Reflex - see also condition
- hyperactive gag 478.2
- vasovagal 780.2

Reflux
- esophageal 530.1
- gastro-esophageal 530.1
- mitral - see Insufficiency, mitral
- ureteral 593.7
- vesico-ureteral 593.7

Reforming, artificial openings - see
  Attention to artificial opening

Refractive error NEC 367.9

Refsum's disease or syndrome 356.3

Refusal of
- food, hysterical 300.1
- treatment because of, due to V62.6
- - patient's decision NEC V64.2
- - reasons of conscience or religion V62.6

Regaud
- tumor (M8082/3) - see Neoplasm,
  nasopharynx, malignant
- type carcinoma (M8082/3) - see
  Neoplasm, nasopharynx, malignant

Regional - see condition

Regulation feeding (infant) (elderly) 783.3
- newborn 779.3

Regurgitation
- aortic (valve) (see also Insufficiency,
  aortic) 424.1
- - syphilitic 093.2 † 424.1*
- food (see also Vomiting) 787.0
- - with reswallowing - see Rumination
- - newborn 779.3
- gastric contents (see also Vomiting) 787.0
- heart - see Endocarditis
- mitral (valve) - see Insufficiency, mitral
- myocardial - see Endocarditis
- pulmonary (valve) (heart) (see also
  Endocarditis, pulmonary) 424.3
- tricuspid - see Endocarditis, tricuspid
- valve, valvular - see Endocarditis
- vesico-ureteral 593.7

Rehabilitation V57.9
- specified NEC V57.8
- vocational V57.2

Reichmann's disease 536.8

Reinsertion, contraceptive device V25.4

Reiter's disease, syndrome, or urethritis
  099.3

Rejection
- food, hysterical 300.1
- transplant 996.8
- - organ (immune or nonimmune cause)
  996.8
- - skin 996.5

Relaxation
- anus (sphincter) 569.4
- - due to hysteria 300.1
- arch (foot) 734
- - congenital 755.6
- back ligaments 728.4
- bladder (sphincter) 596.5
- cardio-esophageal 530.8
- cervix (see also Incompetence, cervix)
  622.5
- diaphragm 519.4
- inguinal rings 550.9
- joint (capsule) (paralytic) 718.9
- - congenital 755.8
- lumbosacral (joint) 724.6
- pelvic floor 618.8
- perineum 618.8
- posture 729.9
- rectum (sphincter) 569.4
- sacroiliac (joint) 724.6
- scrotum 608.8
- urethra (sphincter) 599.8
- uterus (outlet) 618.8
- vagina (outlet) 618.8
- vesical 596.5

Remains
- canal of Cloquet 743.5
- capsule (opaque) 743.5

Remnant
- fingernail 703.8
- - congenital 757.5
- meniscus, knee 717.5
- thyroglossal duct 759.2
- tonsil 474.8
- - infected 474.0
- urachus 753.7

Removal (of)
- catheter (urinary) (indwelling) V53.6
- - from artificial opening - see Attention
    to artificial opening
- device
- - contraceptive V25.4
- - fixation
- - - external V54.8
- - - internal V54.0
- - traction V54.8
- dressing V58.3
- Kirschner wire V54.8
- pin V54.0

Removal - *continued*
- plaster cast V54.8
- plate (fracture) V54.0
- rod V54.0
- screw V54.0
- splint, external V54.8
- suture V58.3
- traction device, external V54.8
Ren
- arcuatus 753.3
- mobile, mobilis (see also Disease, renal)
  593.0
- - congenital 753.3
- unguliformis 753.3
Renal - see condition
Rendu-Osler-Weber disease or syndrome
  448.0
Reninoma (M8361/1) 236.9
Renon-Delille syndrome 253.8
Repair
- pelvic floor, previous, in pregnancy or
  childbirth 654.4
- - fetus or newborn 763.8
- scarred tissue V51
Replacement by artificial or mechanical
  device or prosthesis of
- bladder V43.5
- blood vessel V43.4
- eye globe V43.0
- heart V43.2
- - valve V43.3
- intestine V43.8
- joint V43.6
- - finger V43.6
- - hip (partial) (total) V43.6
- larynx V43.8
- lens V43.1
- limb(s) V43.7
- organ NEC V43.8
- tissue NEC V43.8
Request for expert evidence V68.2
Reserve, decreased or low
- cardiac - see Disease, heart
- kidney (see also Disease, renal) 593.9
Residual - see also condition
- bladder 596.8
- state, schizophrenic 295.6
- urine 788.6
Resorption
- biliary 576.8
- - purulent or putrid (see also
  Cholecystitis) 576.8
- dental (roots) 521.4
- - alveoli 525.8
- septic - see Septicemia
- teeth (external) (internal) (pathological)
  (roots) 521.4

Respiration
- Cheyne-Stokes 786.0
- decreased due to shock, following injury
  958.4
- disorder of, psychogenic 306.1
- failure, insufficient, or poor 786.0
- - newborn NEC 770.8
- sighing, psychogenic 306.1
Respiratory - see condition
Restless legs (syndrome) 333.9
Restriction of housing space V60.1
Rests, ovarian, in fallopian tube 752.1
Restzustand, schizophrenic 295.6
Retained - see Retention
Retardation
- development, developmental, specific
  (see also Disorder, development, specific)
  315.9
- - learning, specific 315.2
- - - arithmetical 315.1
- - - language (skills) 315.3
- - - reading 315.0
- - motor 315.4
- endochondral bone growth 733.9
- growth (see also Retardation, physical)
  783.4
- - fetus 764.9
- - - affecting management of pregnancy
  656.5
- intrauterine growth 764.9
- - affecting management of pregnancy
  656.5
- mental 319
- - mild, I.Q. 50-70 317
- - moderate, I.Q. 35-49 318.0
- - profound, I.Q. under 20 318.2
- - severe, I.Q. 20-34 318.1
- motor, specific 315.4
- physical 783.4
- - child 783.4
- - due to malnutrition 263.2
- - fetus 764.9
- - - affecting management of pregnancy
  656.5
- reading 315.0
Retching (see also Vomiting) 787.0
Retention, retained
- bladder 788.2
- - psychogenic 306.5
- cyst - see Cyst
- dead
- - fetus (at or near term) 656.4
- - - early fetal death 632
- - ovum 631
- decidua (fragments) (following delivery)
  (with hemorrhage) 666.2
- - with abortion - see Abortion, by type

Retention - *continued*
- decidua - *continued*
- - without hemorrhage 667.1
- deciduous tooth 520.6
- dental root 525.3
- fecal (see also Constipation) 564.0
- fluid 276.6
- foreign body - see also Foreign body, retained
- - current trauma - code as Foreign body, by site or type
- membranes (complicating delivery) (with hemorrhage) 666.2
- - with abortion - see Abortion, by type
- - without hemorrhage 667.1
- menses 626.8
- milk (puerperal, postpartum) 676.2
- nitrogen, extrarenal 788.9
- placenta (total) (with hemorrhage) 666.0
- - with abortion - see Abortion, by type
- - portions or fragments (with hemorrhage) 666.2
- - - without hemorrhage 667.1
- - without hemorrhage 667.0
- products of conception
- - early pregnancy (dead ovum) 632
- - following
- - - abortion - see Abortion, by type
- - - delivery 666.2
- - - - with hemorrhage 666.2
- - - - without hemorrhage 667.1
- secundines (following delivery) (with hemorrhage) 666.2
- - with abortion - see Abortion, by type
- - complicating puerperium (delayed hemorrhage) 666.2
- - without hemorrhage 667.1
- smegma, clitoris 624.8
- urine 788.2
- - psychogenic 306.5
- water (in tissues) (see also Edema) 782.3
Reticulation, dust 504
Reticuloendotheliosis
- acute infantile (M9722/3) 202.5
- leukemic (M9940/3) 202.4
- malignant (M9720/3) 202.3
- nonlipid (M9722/3) 202.5
Reticulohistiocytoma 277.8
- giant-cell 277.8
Reticulolymphosarcoma (diffuse) (M9613/3) 200.8
- follicular (M9691/3) 202.0
- nodular (M9691/3) 202.0
Reticulosarcoma (M9640/3) 200.0
- nodular (M9642/3) 200.0
- pleomorphic cell type (M9641/3) 200.0
Reticulosis (skin)

Reticulosis - *continued*
- acute of infancy (M9722/3) 202.5
- histiocytic medullary (M9721/3) 202.3
- lipomelanotic 695.8
- malignant (M9720/3) 202.3
- Sezary (M9701/3) 202.2
Retina, retinal - see condition
Retinitis (see also Chorioretinitis) 363.2
- albuminurica 585 † 363.1*
- arteriosclerotic 440.8
- diabetic 250.4 † 362.0*
- disciformis 362.5
- gravidarum 646.8
- juxtapapillaris 363.0
- luetic - see Retinitis, syphilitic
- pigmentosa 362.7
- punctata albescens 362.7
- renal 585 † 363.1*
- syphilitic (secondary) 091.5 † 363.1*
- - congenital 090.0 † 363.1*
- - early 091.5 † 363.1*
- - late 095 † 363.1*
- syphilitica, central, recurrent 095 † 363.1*
- tuberculous 017.3 † 362.1*
Retinoblastoma (M9510/3) 190.5
- differentiated type (M9511/3) 190.5
- undifferentiated type (M9512/3) 190.5
Retinochoroiditis (see also Chorioretinitis) 363.2
- disseminated 363.1
- - syphilitic 094.8 † 363.1*
- juxtapapillaris 363.0
Retinopathy (background) (Coat's) (exudative) (hypertensive) 362.1
- arteriosclerotic 440.8 † 362.1*
- atherosclerotic 440.8 † 362.1*
- central serous 362.4
- circinate 362.1
- diabetic 250.4 † 362.0*
- of prematurity 362.2
- pigmentary, congenital 362.7
- proliferative 362.2
- - sickle-cell 282.6 † 362.2*
- solar 363.3
Retinoschisis 361.1
- congenital 743.5
Retraction
- cervix (see also Retroversion, uterus) 621.6
- drum (membrane) 384.8
- finger 736.2
- lid 374.4
- lung 518.8
- mediastinum 519.3
- nipple 611.7
- - congenital 757.6
- - puerperal, postpartum 676.0

Retraction - *continued*
- palmar fascia 728.6
- pleura (see also Pleurisy) 511.0
- ring, uterus (Bandl's) (pathological) 661.4
- - fetus or newborn 763.7
- sternum (congenital) 756.3
- - acquired 738.3
- syndrome 378.7
- uterus (see also Retroversion, uterus) 621.6
- valve (heart) - see Endocarditis
Retrobulbar - see condition
Retrocecal - see also condition
- appendix (congenital) 751.5
Retrocession - see Retroversion

Retrodisplacement - see Retroversion
Retroflection, retroflexion - see Retroversion
Retrognathia, retrognathism (mandibular) (maxillary) 524.1
Retrograde menstruation 626.8
Retroperineal - see condition
Retroperitoneal - see condition
Retroperitonitis (see also Peritonitis) 567.9

Retropharyngeal - see condition
Retroplacental - see condition
Retroposition - see Retroversion
Retrosternal thyroid 759.2
Retroversion, retroverted
- cervix (see also Retroversion, uterus) 621.6
- female NEC (see also Retroversion, uterus) 621.6
- iris 364.7
- testis (congenital) 752.5
- uterus, uterine (acute) (acquired) (adherent) (any degree) (asymptomatic) (cervix) (postinfectional) (postpartal, old) 621.6
- - congenital 752.3
- - in pregnancy or childbirth 654.3
- - - causing obstructed labor 660.2
- - - - fetus or newborn 763.1
- - - fetus or newborn 763.8
Reverse peristalsis 787.4
Reye's syndrome 331.8
Rh (factor)
- hemolytic disease 773.0
- incompatibility, immunization or sensitization
- - affecting management of pregnancy 656.1
- - fetus 773.0
- - newborn 773.0
- - transfusion reaction 999.7

Rh - *continued*
- negative mother affecting fetus or newborn 773.0
- transfusion reaction 999.7
Rhabdomyolysis (idiopathic) 728.8
Rhabdomyoma (M8900/0) - see also Neoplasm, connective tissue, benign
- adult (M8904/0) - see Neoplasm, connective tissue, benign
- fetal (M8903/0) - see Neoplasm, connective tissue, benign
- glycogenic (M8904/0) - see Neoplasm, connective tissue, benign
Rhabdomyosarcoma (M8900/3) - see also Neoplasm, connective tissue, malignant
- alveolar (M8920/3) - see Neoplasm, connective tissue, malignant
- embryonal (M8910/3) - see Neoplasm, connective tissue, malignant
- mixed type (M8902/3) - see Neoplasm, connective tissue, malignant
- pleomorphic (M8901/3) - see Neoplasm, connective tissue, malignant
Rhabdosarcoma (M8900/3) - see Rhabdomyosarcoma
Rhesus (factor) incompatibility - see Rh, incompatibility
Rheumaticosis - see Rheumatism
Rheumatism, rheumatic (acute NEC) 729.0
- articular (chronic) NEC 716.9
- - acute or subacute - see Fever, rheumatic
- blennorrhagic 098.5 † 729.0*
- cerebral - see Fever, rheumatic
- chronic NEC 729.0
- desert 114
- febrile - see Fever, rheumatic
- gonococcal 098.5 † 729.0*
- heart (see also Disease, heart, rheumatic) 398.9
- inflammatory (acute) (chronic) (subacute) - see Fever, rheumatic
- intercostal 729.0
- - meaning Tietze's disease 733.6
- joint (chronic) NEC 716.9
- - acute - see Fever, rheumatic
- muscular 729.0
- neuralgic 729.0
- neuromuscular 729.0
- nodose - see Arthritis, nodosa
- nonarticular 729.0
- palindromic (any site) 719.3
- pneumonia 390 † 517.1*
- polyarticular NEC 716.9
- psychogenic 306.0
- sciatic 724.3
- septic - see Fever, rheumatic

Rheumatism - *continued*
- spine 724.9
- subacute NEC 729.0
- tuberculous NEC 015.9
Rheumatoid - see also condition
- lung 714.8 † 517.0*
Rhinitis (atrophic) (catarrhal) (chronic)
  (croupous) (fibrinous) (hyperplastic)
  (hypertrophic) (membranous) (purulent)
  (suppurative) (ulcerative) 472.0
- with sore throat - see Nasopharyngitis
- acute 460
- allergic (nonseasonal) (seasonal) (see also
  Fever, hay) 477.9
- - with asthma 493.0
- granulomatous 472.0
- infective 460
- obstructive 472.0
- pneumococcal 460
- syphilitic 095
- - congenital 090.0
- tuberculous 012.8
- vasomotor (see also Fever, hay) 477.9
Rhino-antritis (chronic) (see also Sinusitis,
  maxillary) 473.0
Rhinodacryolith 375.5
Rhinolith 478.1
- nasal sinus (see also Sinusitis) 473.9
Rhinomegaly 478.1
Rhinopharyngitis (acute) (subacute) (see
  also Nasopharyngitis) 460
- chronic 472.2
- destructive ulcerating 102.5
- mutilans 102.5
Rhinophyma 695.3
Rhinorrhea 478.1
- cerebrospinal (fluid) 349.8
- paroxysmal (see also Fever, hay) 477.9
- spasmodic (see also Fever, hay) 477.9
Rhinosalpingitis 381.5
Rhinoscleroma 040.1
Rhinosporidiosis 117.0
Rhinovirus infection 079.3
Rhizomelique, pseudopolyarthric 446.5
Rhythm
- atrioventricular nodal 427.8
- disorder 427.9
- - coronary sinus 427.8
- - ectopic 427.8
- - nodal 427.8
- escape 427.8
- heart, abnormal 427.9
- idioventricular 426.0
- nodal 427.8
- sleep, inversion 780.5
Rhytidosis facialis 701.8
Rib - see also condition

Rib - *continued*
- cervical 756.2
Riboflavin deficiency 266.0
Rice bodies 718.1
- knee 717.6
Richter's hernia - see Hernia, intestine
Ricinism 988.2
Rickets (active) (acute) (adolescent) (adult)
  (chest wall) (congenital) (current)
  (infantile) (intestinal) 268.0
- celiac 579.0
- fetal 756.4
- hemorrhagic 267
- hypophosphatemic with
  nephrotic-glycosuric dwarfism 270.0
- kidney 588.0
- late effects, any 268.1
- renal 588.0
- scurvy 267
- vitamin D-resistant 275.3
Rickettsial disease NEC 083.9
- specified type NEC 083.8
Rickettsialpox 083.2
Rickettsiosis NEC 083.9
- specified type NEC 083.8
- tick-borne NEC 082.9
- vesicular 083.2
Ricord's chancre 091.0
Riders' bone 733.9
Ridge, alveolus - see also condition
- flabby 525.2
Ridged ear 744.2
Riedel's
- lobe, liver 751.6
- struma 245.3
- thyroiditis or disease 245.3
Rieger's anomaly or syndrome 743.4
Riehl's melanosis 709.0
Rietti-Greppi-Micheli anemia 282.4
Rieux's hernia - see Hernia, abdominal
Riga-Fede disease 529.0
Riggs' disease 523.4
Rigid, rigidity - see also condition
- abdominal 789.4
- articular, multiple, congenital 754.8
- cervix (uteri)
- - in pregnancy or childbirth 654.6
- - - causing obstructed labor 660.2
- - - - fetus or newborn 763.1
- - - fetus or newborn 763.8
- hymen (acquired) (congenital) 623.3
- pelvic floor
- - in pregnancy or childbirth 654.4
- - - causing obstructed labor 660.2
- - - - fetus or newborn 763.1
- - - fetus or newborn 763.8
- perineum or vulva

Rigid - *continued*
- perineum or vulva - *continued*
- − in pregnancy or childbirth 654.8
- − − causing obstructed labor 660.2
- − − − fetus or newborn 763.1
- − − fetus or newborn 763.8
- spine 724.8
- vagina
- − in pregnancy or childbirth 654.7
- − − causing obstructed labor 660.2
- − − − fetus or newborn 763.1
- − − fetus or newborn 763.8
Rigors 780.9
Riley-Day syndrome 742.8
Ring(s)
- aorta 747.2
- Bandl's 661.4
- − fetus or newborn 763.7
- contraction, complicating delivery 661.4
- − fetus or newborn 763.7
- Fleischer's 275.1
- hymenal, tight 623.3
- Kayser-Fleischer (cornea) 371.1
- retraction, uterus, pathological 661.4
- − fetus or newborn 763.7
- Schatzki (esophagus) (lower) (congenital) 750.3
- − acquired 530.3
- Soemering's 366.5
- tracheal, abnormal 748.3
- vascular (congenital) 747.2
- Vossius' 921.3
Ringed hair (congenital) 757.4
Ringworm 110.9
- beard 110.0
- body 110.5
- Burmese 110.9
- corporeal 110.5
- foot 110.4
- groin 110.3
- hand 110.2
- honeycomb 110.0
- nails 110.1
- perianal (area) 110.3
- scalp 110.0
- specified site NEC 110.8
- Tokelau 110.5
Rise, venous pressure 459.8
Risk, suicidal 300.9
Ritter's disease 695.8
Rivalry, sibling 313.3
River blindness 125.3 † 360.1*
Robert's pelvis 755.6
- with disproportion 653.0
- − causing obstructed labor 660.1
- − fetus or newborn 763.1
Robin's syndrome 756.0

Robinson's (hidrotic) ectodermal dysplasia 757.3
Roble's disease 125.3 † 360.1*
Rocky Mountain fever (spotted) 082.0
Roentgen ray, adverse effect NEC 990
Roetheln 056.9
Roger's disease 745.4
Rokitansky's
- disease (see also Necrosis, liver) 570
- tumor 620.2
Rokitansky-Aschoff sinuses (see also Disease, gallbladder) 575.8
Rollet's chancre (syphilitic) 091.0
Romanus lesion 720.1
Romberg's disease 349.8
Roof, mouth - see condition
Rosacea 695.3
- acne 695.3
- keratitis 695.3 † 370.4*
Rosenbach's erysipelatoid or erysipeloid 027.1
Rosenthal's disease 286.2
Roseola 056.9
- infantum 057.8
Rossbach's disease 536.8
- psychogenic 306.4
Rostan's asthma (see also Failure, ventricular, left) 428.1
Rot
- Barcoo (see also Ulcer, skin) 707.9
- knife-grinders' 011.4
Rotation
- anomalous, incomplete or insufficient - see Malrotation
- manual, affecting fetus or newborn 763.8
- spine, incomplete or insufficient 737.8
- tooth, teeth 524.3
- vertebra, incomplete or insufficient 737.8
Roteln 056.9
Roth's meralgia 355.1
Roth-Bernhardt disease or syndrome 355.1
Rothmund's syndrome 757.3
Rothmund-Thomson syndrome 757.3
Rotor's disease or syndrome 277.4
Rotundum ulcus - see Ulcer, stomach
Round
- back (with wedging of vertebrae) 737.1
- − late effect of rickets 268.1
- ulcer (stomach) - see Ulcer, stomach
- worms (large) (infestation) NEC 127.0
Roussy-Levy syndrome 334.3
Rubella 056.9
- complicating pregnancy, childbirth or puerperium 647.5
- complication 056.8
- − neurological 056.0
- − specified NEC 056.7

Rubella - *continued*
- congenital 771.0
- maternal
- - affecting fetus or newborn 760.2
- - - manifest rubella in infant 771.0
- - suspected damage to fetus affecting
  management of pregnancy 655.3
- specified complications NEC 056.7
Rubeola (meaning measles) (see also
  Measles) 055.9
- meaning rubella (see also Rubella) 056.9
- scarlatinosa 057.8
Rubeosis, iris 364.4
Rubinstein-Taybi's syndrome 759.8
Rudimentary (congenital) - see also
  Agenesis
- arm 755.2
- bone 756.9
- cervix uteri 752.4
- eye 743.1
- lobule of ear 744.2
- patella 755.6
- tracheal bronchus 748.3
- uterus 752.3
- - in male 752.7
- - solid or with cavity 752.3
- vagina 752.4
Ruled out condition - see Observation,
  suspected
Rumination 787.0
- neurotic 300.3
- obsessional 300.3
- psychogenic 300.3
Rupia 091.3
- congenital 090.0
- tertiary 095
Rupture, ruptured 553.9
- abdominal viscera NEC 789.9
- - obstetrical trauma 665.5
- abscess (spontaneous) - code by site
  under Abscess
- aneurysm - see Aneurysm
- anus (sphincter) - see Laceration, anus
- aorta, aortic 441.5
- - abdominal 441.3
- - arch 441.1
- - ascending 441.1
- - descending 441.5
- - - abdominal 441.3
- - - thoracic 441.1
- - syphilitic 093.0 † 441.7*
- - thorax, thoracic 441.1
- - transverse 441.1
- - traumatic (thoracic) 901.0
- - - abdominal 902.0
- - valve or cusp (see also Endocarditis,
  aortic) 424.1

Rupture - *continued*
- appendix (with peritonitis) 540.0
- arteriovenous fistula, brain (congenital)
  430
- artery 447.2
- - brain (see also Hemorrhage, brain)
  431
- - coronary (see also Infarct,
  myocardium) 410
- - heart (see also Infarct, myocardium)
  410
- - pulmonary 417.8
- - traumatic (complication) (see also
  Injury, blood vessel) 904.9

- bile duct (see also Disease, biliary) 576.3
- bladder (sphincter) 596.6
- - with abortion - see categories 634-639,
  fourth digit .2
- - nontraumatic 596.6
- - obstetrical trauma 665.5
- - spontaneous 596.6
- - traumatic - see Injury, internal,
  bladder
- blood vessel (see also Hemorrhage) 459.0
- - brain (see also Hemorrhage, brain)
  431
- - heart (see also Infarct, myocardium)
  410
- - traumatic (complication) (see also
  Injury, blood vessel) 904.9
- bone - see Fracture
- bowel 569.8
- brain
- - aneurysm (congenital) (see also
  Hemorrhage, subarachnoid) 430
- - - syphilitic 094.8 † 430*
- - hemorrhagic (see also Hemorrhage,
  brain) 431
- - syphilitic 094.8
- capillaries 448.9
- cardiac (see also Infarct, myocardium)
  410
- cartilage (articular) (current) - see also
  Sprain
- - knee - see Tear, meniscus
- - semilunar - see Tear, meniscus
- cecum (with peritonitis) 540.0

- cerebral aneurysm (congenital) (see also
  Hemorrhage, subarachnoid) 430
- cervix (uteri)
- - with abortion - see categories 634-639,
  fourth digit .2
- - obstetrical trauma - see Laceration,
  cervix, obstetrical trauma
- - traumatic - see Injury, internal, cervix
- chordae tendineae 429.5

Rupture - *continued*
- choroid (direct) (indirect) (traumatic) 363.6
- circle of Willis (see also Hemorrhage, subarachnoid) 430
- colon 569.8
- cornea (traumatic) - see Rupture, eye
- coronary (artery) (thrombotic) (see also Infarct, myocardium) 410
- corpus luteum (infected) (ovary) 620.1
- cyst - see Cyst
- cystic duct (see also Disease, gallbladder) 575.4
- Descemet's membrane 371.3
- - traumatic - see Rupture, eye
- diaphragm - see also Hernia, diaphragm
- - traumatic - see Injury, internal, diaphragm
- diverticulum (intestine) (see also Diverticula) 562.1
- duodenal stump 537.8
- duodenum (ulcer) - see Ulcer, duodenum, with perforation
- ear drum 384.2
- - with otitis media - see Otitis media
- - traumatic - see Wound, open, ear
- esophagus 530.4
- eye (without prolapse of intraocular tissue) 871.0
- - with
- - - exposure of intraocular tissue 871.1
- - - partial loss of intraocular tissue 871.2
- - - prolapse of intraocular tissue 871.1
- fallopian tube 620.8
- - due to pregnancy - see Pregnancy, tubal
- fontanel 767.3
- gallbladder or duct (see also Disease, gallbladder) 575.4
- gastric - see also Rupture, stomach
- - vessel 459.0
- globe (eye) (traumatic) - see Rupture, eye
- graafian follicle (hematoma) 620.0
- heart (auricle) (ventricle) (see also Infarct, myocardium) 410
- hymen 623.8
- internal organ, traumatic - see Injury, internal, by site
- intervertebral disc - see Displacement, intervertebral disc
- - traumatic (current) - see Dislocation, vertebrae
- intestine 569.8
- - traumatic - see Injury, internal, intestine

Rupture - *continued*
- iris 364.7
- - traumatic - see Rupture, eye
- joint capsule - see Sprain
- kidney 866.-
- - birth injury 767.8
- - nontraumatic 593.8
- lacrimal passages 870.2
- - traumatic 870.2
- lens (traumatic) 366.2
- ligament - see also Sprain
- - with open wound - see Wound, open
- liver 864.-
- - birth injury 767.8
- lymphatic vessel 457.8
- marginal sinus (placental) (with hemorrhage) 641.2
- - fetus or newborn 762.1
- meaning hernia - see Hernia
- membrana tympani 384.2
- - with otitis media - see Otitis media
- - traumatic - see Wound, open, ear
- membranes (spontaneous)
- - artificial
- - - delayed delivery following 658.3
- - - - fetus or newborn 761.1
- - - delayed delivery following 658.2
- - - fetus or newborn 761.1
- - premature 658.1
- - - delayed delivery following 658.2
- - - fetus or newborn 761.1
- meningeal artery (see also Hemorrhage, subarachnoid) 430
- meniscus (knee) - see also Tear, meniscus
- - old (see also Derangement, meniscus) 717.5
- - - elbow 718.0
- - - shoulder 718.0
- - site other than knee - code as Sprain
- mesentery 568.8
- mitral - see Insufficiency, mitral
- muscle (traumatic) NEC - see also Sprain
- - with open wound - see Wound, open
- - nontraumatic 728.8
- mycotic aneurysm causing cerebral hemorrhage (see also Hemorrhage, subarachnoid) 430
- myocardium, myocardial (see also Infarct, myocardium) 410
- - traumatic - see Injury, internal, heart
- nontraumatic (meaning hernia) (see also Hernia) 553.9
- obstructed (see also Hernia, by site, with obstruction) 552.9
- - gangrenous (see also Hernia, by site, gangrenous) 551.9
- oesophagus 530.4

Rupture - *continued*
- operation wound 998.3
- ovary, ovarian 620.8
- − corpus luteum 620.1
- − follicle (graafian) 620.0
- oviduct 620.8
- − due to pregnancy - see Pregnancy, tubal
- pancreas 577.8
- − traumatic - see Injury, internal, pancreas
- papillary muscle 429.6
- pelvic
- − floor, complicating delivery 664.1
- − organ NEC - see Injury, pelvic, organs
- penis (traumatic) - see Wound, open, penis
- perineum 624.8
- − during delivery - see Laceration, perineum, complicating delivery
- postoperative 998.3
- prostate (traumatic) - see Injury, internal, prostate
- pulmonary
- − artery 417.8
- − valve (heart) (see also Endocarditis, pulmonary) 424.3
- − vessel 417.8
- pyosalpinx (see also Salpingo-oophoritis) 614.2
- rectum 569.4
- − traumatic - see Injury, internal, rectum
- retina, retinal (traumatic) (without detachment) 361.3
- − with detachment 361.0
- sclera 871.0
- semilunar cartilage, knee 836.2
- − old (see also Derangement, meniscus) 717.5
- sigmoid 569.8
- − traumatic - see Injury, internal, intestine
- sinus Valsalva 747.2
- spinal cord - see also Injury, spinal, by region
- − fetus or newborn 767.4
- spleen 289.5
- − birth injury 767.8
- − congenital 767.8
- − malarial 084.9
- − nontraumatic 289.5
- − spontaneous 289.5
- − traumatic - see Injury, internal, spleen
- splenic vein 459.0
- stomach 537.8
- − traumatic - see Injury, internal, stomach

Rupture - *continued*
- stomach - *continued*
- − ulcer - see Ulcer, stomach, with perforation
- synovium 727.5
- tendon (traumatic) - see also Sprain
- − with open wound - see Wound, open
- − nontraumatic 727.6
- testis (traumatic) 878.2
- − complicated 878.3
- − due to syphilis 095
- thoracic duct 457.8
- tonsil 474.8
- traumatic
- − external site - see Wound, open, by site
- − eye 871.2
- − internal organ (abdomen, chest, or pelvis) - see Injury, internal, by site
- − ligament, muscle, or tendon - see also Sprain
- − − with open wound - see Wound, open
- − meaning hernia - see Hernia
- tricuspid (heart) (valve) - see Endocarditis, tricuspid
- tube, tubal 620.8
- − abscess (see also Salpingo-oophoritis) 614.2
- − due to pregnancy - see Pregnancy, tubal
- tympanum, tympanic (membrane) 384.2
- − with otitis media - see Otitis media
- − traumatic - see Wound, open, ear
- umbilical cord 663.8
- − fetus or newborn 772.0
- ureter (traumatic) - see also Injury, internal, ureter
- − nontraumatic 593.8
- urethra 599.8
- − with abortion - see categories 634-639, fourth digit .2
- − obstetrical trauma 665.5
- − traumatic - see Injury, internal, urethra
- uterosacral ligament 620.8
- uterus (traumatic) - see also Injury, internal, uterus
- − affecting fetus or newborn 763.8
- − after labor 665.1
- − nonpuerperal, nontraumatic 621.8
- − pregnant (during labor) 665.1
- − − before labor 665.0
- vagina 878.6
- − complicated 878.7
- − complicating delivery - see Laceration, vagina, complicating delivery
- valve, valvular (heart) - see Endocarditis
- varicose vein - see Varicose vein
- varix - see Varix

Rupture - *continued*
– vena cava 459.0
– vessel 459.0
– – pulmonary 417.8
– viscus 789.9
– vulva 878.4
– – complicated 878.5

Rupture - *continued*
– vulva - *continued*
– – complicating delivery 664.0
Russell's dysentery 004.8
Russell-Silver syndrome 759.8
Rust's disease 015.0 † 720.8*

S

Saber, sabre
- shin 090.5
- tibia 090.5

Sac lacrimal - see condition

Saccharopinuria 270.7

Saccular - see condition

Sacculation
- aorta (nonsyphilitic) (see also Aneurysm, aorta) 441.6
- - ruptured 441.5
- - syphilitic 093.0 † 441.7*
- bladder 596.3
- colon 569.8
- intralaryngeal (congenital) (ventricular) 748.3
- larynx (congenital) (ventricular) 748.3
- organ or site, congenital - see Distortion
- pregnant uterus 654.4
- - fetus or newborn 763.8
- rectosigmoid 569.8
- sigmoid 569.8
- ureter 593.8
- urethra 599.2

Sachs'
- amaurotic familial idiocy 330.1
- disease 330.1

Sachs-Tay disease 330.1

Sachs-Libman disease 710.0 † 424.9*

Sacralgia 724.6

Sacralization
- fifth lumbar vertebra 756.1
- incomplete (vertebra) 756.1

Sacrodynia 724.6

Sacroiliac joint - see condition

Sacroiliitis NEC 720.2

Sacrum - see condition

Saddle
- back 737.8
- embolus, aorta 444.0
- nose 738.0
- - due to syphilis 090.5

Sadism (sexual) 302.8

Saemisch's ulcer (cornea) 370.0

Sailors' skin 692.7

Saint
- Anthony's fire (see also Erysipelas) 035
- Palogren's disease 723.1
- triad (see also Hernia, diaphragm) 553.3
- Vitus' dance - see Chorea

Salaam tic 781.0

Salicylism
- correct substance properly administered 535.4
- overdose or wrong substance given or taken 965.1

Salivary duct or gland - see condition

Salivation (excessive) (see also Ptyalism) 527.7

Salmonella - see Infection, Salmonella

Salmonellosis 003.0
- pneumonia 003.2 † 484.8*

Salpingitis (catarrhal) (fallopian tube) (follicular) (interstitial) (isthmica nodosa) (nodular) (pseudofollicular) (purulent) (septic) (see also Salpingo-oophoritis) 614.2
- acute 614.0
- chronic 614.1
- ear 381.5
- eustachian (tube) 381.5
- gonococcal (chronic) 098.3 † 614.-*
- - acute 098.1 † 614.0*
- specific (chronic) 098.3 † 614.-*
- - acute 098.1 † 614.0*
- tuberculous 016.4 † 614.2*
- - acute 016.4 † 614.0*
- - chronic 016.4 † 614.1*
- venereal (chronic) 098.3 † 614.-*
- - acute 098.1 † 614.0*

Salpingocele 620.4

Salpingo-oophoritis (purulent) (ruptured) (septic) (suppurative) 614.2
- acute 614.0
- - complication of
- - - abortion - see categories 634-639, fourth digit .0
- - - ectopic gestation 639.0
- - gonococcal 098.1 † 614.0*
- - puerperal, postpartum, childbirth 670
- - tuberculous 016.4 † 614.0*
- chronic 614.1
- - tuberculous 016.4 † 614.1*
- complicating pregnancy 646.6
- - fetus or newborn 760.8
- complication of
- - abortion - see categories 634-639, fourth digit .0
- - ectopic gestation 639.0
- gonococcal (chronic) 098.3 † 614.-*
- - acute 098.1 † 614.0*

Salpingo-oophoritis - *continued*
- old - see Salpingo-oophoritis, chronic
- puerperal 670
- specific - see Salpingo-oophoritis, gonococcal
- tuberculous 016.4 † 614.2*
- - acute 016.4 † 614.0*
- - chronic 016.4 † 614.1*
- venereal - see Salpingo-oophoritis, gonococcal
Salpingo-ovaritis (see also Salpingo-oophoritis) 614.2
Salpingoperitonitis (see also Salpingo-oophoritis) 614.2
Salt-losing
- nephritis (see also Disease, renal) 593.9
- syndrome (see also Disease, renal) 593.9
Salt-rheum - see Eczema
Salzmann's nodular dystrophy 371.4
Sampson's cyst or tumor 617.1
San Joaquin (Valley) fever 114
Sandblasters'
- asthma 502
- lung 502
Sander's disease 297.1
Sandhoff's disease 272.7
Sanfilippo syndrome 277.5
Sanger-Brown ataxia 334.2
Sao Paulo fever or typhus 082.0
Saponification, mesenteric 567.8
Sapremia - see Septicemia
Sarcocele (benign)
- syphilitic 095
- - congenital 090.5
Sarcoepiplocele (see also Hernia) 553.9
Sarcoepiplomphalocele - see Hernia, umbilicus
Sarcoid (any site) 135
- Boeck's 135
- Darier-Roussy 135
- Spiegler-Fendt 686.8
Sarcoidosis 135
Sarcoma (M8800/3) - see also Neoplasm, connective tissue, malignant
- alveolar soft part (M9581/3) - see Neoplasm, connective tissue, malignant
- ameloblastic (M9330/3) 170.1
- - upper jaw (bone) 170.0
- botryoid (M8910/3) - see Neoplasm, connective tissue, malignant
- botryoides (M8910/3) - see Neoplasm, connective tissue, malignant
- cerebellar (M9480/3) 191.6
- - circumscribed (arachnoidal) (M9471/3) 191.6
- circumscribed (arachnoidal) cerebellar (M9471/3) 191.6

Sarcoma - *continued*
- clear cell, of tendons and aponeuroses (M9044/3) - see Neoplasm, connective tissue, malignant
- embryonal (M8991/3) - see Neoplasm, connective tissue, malignant
- endometrial (stromal) (M8930/3) 182.0
- - isthmus 182.1
- endothelial (M9130/3) - see also Neoplasm, connective tissue, malignant
- - bone (M9260/3) - see Neoplasm, bone, malignant
- epithelioid cell (M8804/3) - see Neoplasm, connective tissue, malignant
- Ewing's (M9260/3) - see Neoplasm, bone, malignant
- germinoblastic (diffuse) (M9632/3) 202.8
- - follicular (M9697/3) 202.0
- giant cell (M8802/3) - see also Neoplasm, connective tissue, malignant
- - bone (M9250/3) - see Neoplasm, bone, malignant
- glomoid (M8710/3) - see Neoplasm, connective tissue, malignant
- granulocytic (M9930/3) 205.3
- hemangioendothelial (M9130/3) - see Neoplasm, connective tissue, malignant
- hemorrhagic, multiple (M9140/3) - see Neoplasm, skin, malignant
- Hodgkin's (M9662/3) 201.2
- immunoblastic (M9612/3) 200.8
- Kaposi's (M9140/3) - see Neoplasm, skin, malignant
- Kupffer cell (M9124/3) 155.0
- leptomeningeal (M9530/3) - see Neoplasm, meninges, malignant
- lymphangioendothelial (M9170/3) - see Neoplasm, connective tissue, malignant
- lymphoblastic (M9630/3) 200.1
- lymphocytic (M9620/3) 200.1
- mast cell (M9740/3) 202.6
- melanotic (M8720/3) - see Melanoma
- meningeal (M9530/3) - see Neoplasm, meninges, malignant
- meningothelial (M9530/3) - see Neoplasm, meninges, malignant
- mesenchymal (M8800/3) - see also Neoplasm, connective tissue, malignant
- - mixed (M8990/3) - see Neoplasm, connective tissue, malignant
- mesothelial (M9050/3) - see Neoplasm, malignant
- monstrocellular (M9481/3)
- - specified site - see Neoplasm, malignant
- - unspecified site 191.9

Sarcoma - *continued*
- myeloid (M9930/3) 205.3
- neurogenic (M9540/3) - see Neoplasm, connective tissue, malignant
- odontogenic (M9270/3) 170.1
- - upper jaw (bone) 170.0
- osteoblastic (M9180/3) - see Neoplasm, bone, malignant
- osteogenic (M9180/3) - see also Neoplasm, bone, malignant
- - juxtacortical (M9190/3) - see Neoplasm, bone, malignant
- - periosteal (M9190/3) - see Neoplasm, bone, malignant
- periosteal (M8812/3) - see also Neoplasm, bone, malignant
- - osteogenic (M9190/3) - see Neoplasm, bone, malignant
- plasma cell (M9731/3) 203.8
- pleomorphic cell (M8802/3) - see Neoplasm, connective tissue, malignant
- reticuloendothelial (M9720/3) 202.3
- reticulum cell (M9640/3) 200.0
- - nodular (M9642/3) 200.0
- - pleomorphic cell type (M9641/3) 200.0
- round cell (M8803/3) - see Neoplasm, connective tissue, malignant
- small cell (M8803/3) - see Neoplasm, connective tissue, malignant
- spindle cell (M8801/3) - see Neoplasm, connective tissue, malignant
- stromal (endometrial) (M8930/3) 182.0
- - isthmus 182.1
- synovial (M9040/3) - see also Neoplasm, connective tissue, malignant
- - biphasic type (M9043/3) - see Neoplasm, connective tissue, malignant
- - epitheloid cell type (M9042/3) - see Neoplasm, connective tissue, malignant
- - spindle cell type (M9041/3) - see Neoplasm, connective tissue, malignant
Sarcomatosis
- meningeal (M9539/3) - see Neoplasm, meninges, malignant
- specified site NEC (M8800/3) - see Neoplasm, connective tissue, malignant
- unspecified site (M8800/6) 171.9
Sarcosinemia 270.8
Sarcosporidiosis 136.5
Saturnine - see condition
Saturnism 984.-
- specified type of lead - see Table of drugs and chemicals

Satyriasis 302.8
Sauriasis - see Ichthyosis
Savill's disease 695.8
Scabies (any site) 133.0
Scald - see Burn
Scalp - see condition
Scaphocephaly 756.0
Scapulalgia 733.9
Scar, scarring (see also Cicatrix) 709.2
- adherent 709.2
- atrophic 709.2
- cervix
- - in pregnancy or childbirth 654.6
- - - causing obstructed labor 660.2
- - - - fetus or newborn 763.1
- - - fetus or newborn 763.8
- chorioretinal 363.3
- choroid 363.3
- congenital 757.3
- conjunctiva 372.6
- cornea 371.0
- - xerophthalmic 371.0
- - - vitamin A deficiency 264.6 † 371.0*
- due to
- - previous cesarean section, complicating pregnancy or childbirth 654.2
- - - fetus or newborn 763.8
- duodenum (cap) 537.3
- hypertrophic 701.4
- keloid 701.4
- labia 624.4
- lung (base) 518.8
- macula 363.3
- muscle 728.8
- myocardium, myocardial 412
- painful 709.2
- posterior pole 363.3
- postnecrotic 571.9
- psychic 300.9
- retina 363.3
- trachea 478.9
- uterus 621.8
- - in pregnancy or childbirth 654.2
- - - fetus or newborn 763.8
- vulva 624.4
Scarabiasis 134.1
Scarlatina (see also Fibrosis, lung) 034.1
- anginosa 034.1
- maligna 034.1
- myocarditis (acute) 034.1 † 422.0*
- - old (see also Myocarditis) 429.0
- ulcerosa 034.1
Scarlatinella 057.8
Schamberg's
- dermatitis 709.0
- dermatosis, pigmentary 709.0

Schwannoma (M9560/0) - see also
   Neoplasm, connective tissue, benign
 - malignant (M9560/3) - see Neoplasm,
   connective tissue, malignant
Schwartz syndrome 756.8
Sciatic - see condition
Sciatica (infectional) 724.3
 - due to displacement of intervertebral disc
   722.1
Sclera - see condition
Sclerectasia 379.1
Scleredema
 - adultorum 710.1
 - Buschke's 710.1
 - newborn 778.1
Sclerema
 - adiposum (newborn) 778.1
 - adultorum 710.1
 - edematosum (newborn) 778.1
 - newborn 778.1
Scleriasis - see Scleroderma
Scleritis (annular) (anterior)
   (granulomatous) (posterior) (suppurative)
   379.0
 - syphilitic 095 † 379.0*
 - tuberculous (nodular) 017.3 † 379.0*
Sclerochoroiditis 379.0
Scleroconjunctivitis 379.0
Sclerodactylia 701.0
Scleroderma, sclerodermia (acrosclerotic)
   (diffuse) (generalized) (progressive)
   (pulmonary) 710.1
 - circumscribed 701.0
 - localized 701.0
 - newborn 778.1
Sclerokeratitis 379.0
 - tuberculous 017.3 † 379.0*
Scleroma, trachea 040.1
Scleromalacia perforans 379.0
Scleromyxedema 701.8
Sclerose en plaques 340
Sclerosis, sclerotic
 - adrenal (gland) 255.8
 - Alzheimer's 331.0
 - - dementia in 290.1
 - amyotrophic (lateral) 335.2
 - aorta, aortic 440.0
 - - valve (see also Endocarditis, aortic)
   424.1
 - artery, arterial, arteriolar, arteriovascular
   - see Arteriosclerosis
 - ascending
 - - multiple 340
 - brain 341.9
 - - artery, arterial 437.0
 - - atrophic lobar 331.0
 - - - dementia in 290.1

Sclerosis - *continued*
 - brain - *continued*
 - - diffuse 341.1
 - - - familial (chronic) (infantile) 330.0
 - - - infantile (chronic) (familial) 330.0
 - - - Pelizaeus-Merzbacher type 330.0
 - - disseminated 340
 - - infantile (diffuse) (degenerative) 330.0
 - - insular 340
 - - Krabbe's 330.0
 - - miliary 340
 - - multiple 340
 - - Pelizaeus-Merzbacher 330.0
 - - presenile (Alzheimer's) 331.0
 - - - dementia in 290.1
 - - progressive familial 330.0
 - - senile 437.0
 - - tuberous 759.5
 - bulbar, progressive 340
 - bundle of His 426.5
 - cardiac 414.0
 - cardiorenal 404.9
 - cardiovascular (see also Disease,
   cardiovascular) 429.2
 - - renal 404.9
 - centrolobar, familial 330.0
 - cerebellar - see Sclerosis, brain
 - cerebral - see Sclerosis, brain
 - cerebrospinal 340
 - - disseminated 340
 - - multiple 340
 - cerebrovascular 437.0
 - choroid 363.4
 - combined (spinal cord) - see also
   Degeneration, combined
 - - multiple 340
 - concentric, Balo's 341.1
 - cornea 371.4
 - coronary (artery) 414.0
 - corpus cavernosum
 - - female 624.8
 - - male 607.8
 - diffuse NEC 341.1
 - disease, heart 414.0
 - disseminated 340
 - dorsal 340
 - dorsolateral (spinal cord) - see
   Degeneration, combined
 - extrapyramidal 333.9
 - eye, senile nuclear 366.1
 - Friedreich's (spinal cord) 334.0
 - funicular (spermatic cord) 608.8
 - general (vascular) - see Arteriosclerosis
 - gland (lymphatic) 457.8
 - hepatic 571.9
 - hereditary
 - - cerebellar 334.2

Sclerosis - *continued*
- hereditary - *continued*
- - spinal 334.0
- insular 340
- - pancreas 251.8
- islands of Langerhans 251.8
- kidney - see Sclerosis, renal
- larynx 478.7
- lateral 335.2
- - amyotrophic 335.2
- - descending 335.2
- - primary 335.2
- - spinal 335.2
- liver 571.9
- lobar, atrophic (of brain) 331.0
- - dementia in 290.1
- lung (see also Fibrosis, lung) 515
- mastoid 383.1
- mitral - see Endocarditis, mitral
- Monckeberg's 440.2
- multiple (brain stem) (cerebral) (generalized) (spinal cord) 340
- myocardium, myocardial 414.0
- ovary 620.8
- pancreas 577.8
- penis 607.8
- peripheral arteries 440.2
- plaques 340
- pluriglandular 258.8
- polyglandular 258.8
- posterior (spinal cord) (syphilitic) 094.0

- posterolateral (spinal cord) - see Degeneration, combined
- prepuce 607.8
- presenile (Alzheimer's) 331.0
- - dementia in 290.1
- primary, lateral 335.2
- progressive, systemic 710.1

- pulmonary (see also Fibrosis, lung) 515
- - artery 416.0
- - valve (heart) (see also Endocarditis, pulmonary) 424.3
- renal 587
- - with
- - - cystine storage disease 270.0
- - - hypertension (see also Hypertension, kidney) 403.9
- - - hypertensive heart disease (conditions in 402) 404.9
- - - arteriolar (hyaline) (see also Hypertension, kidney) 403.9
- - - hyperplastic (see also Hypertension, kidney) 403.9
- retina (senile) (vascular) 362.1
- senile - see Arteriosclerosis
- spinal (cord) (progressive) 336.8

Sclerosis - *continued*
- spinal - *continued*
- - combined - see also Degeneration, combined
- - - multiple 340
- - - syphilitic 094.8
- - disseminated 340
- - dorsolateral - see Degeneration, combined
- - hereditary (mixed form) 334.0
- - lateral (amyotrophic) 335.2
- - multiple 340
- - posterior (syphilitic) 094.0
- stomach 537.8
- subendocardial, congenital 425.3
- systemic (progressive) 710.1
- - with lung involvement 710.1 † 517.2*
- tricuspid (heart) (valve) - see Endocarditis, tricuspid
- tuberous (brain) 759.5
- tympanic membrane 384.8
- valve, valvular (heart) - see Endocarditis
- vascular - see Arteriosclerosis
- vein 459.8
Sclerotenonitis 379.0
Scoliosis (acquired) (postural) 737.3
- congenital 754.2
- idiopathic 737.3
- paralytic 737.3
- rachitic 268.1
- tuberculous 015.0 † 737.4*
Scoliotic pelvis 738.6
- with disproportion 653.0
- - causing obstructed labor 660.1
- - fetus or newborn 763.1
Scorbutus, scorbutic (see also Scurvy) 267
- anemia 281.8
Scotoma (arcuated) (Bjerrum) (central) (ring) 368.4
- scintillating 368.1
Scratch - see Injury, superficial
Screening (for) V82.9
- alcoholism V79.1
- anemia, deficiency NEC V78.1
- - iron V78.0
- anomaly, congenital V82.8
- antenatal - see Antenatal, screening
- arterial hypertension V81.1
- arthropod-borne viral disease NEC V73.5
- bacterial conjunctivitis V74.4
- bacteriuria, asymptomatic V81.5
- bronchitis, chronic V81.3
- brucellosis V74.8
- cardiovascular condition NEC V81.2
- cataract V80.2
- cholera V74.0

Screening - *continued*
- chromosomal anomalies
- - athletes V70.3
- - by amniocentesis, antenatal V28.0
- - postnatal V82.4
- condition
- - cardiovascular NEC V81.2
- - eye NEC V80.2
- - genitourinary NEC V81.6
- - neurological V80.0
- - respiratory NEC V81.4
- - skin V82.0
- - specified NEC V82.8
- congenital
- - anomaly NEC V82.8
- - - eye problems V80.2
- - dislocation of hip V82.3
- contamination NEC (see also Poisoning) V82.5
- cystic fibrosis V77.6
- dengue fever V73.5
- depression V79.0
- developmental handicap V79.8
- - in early childhood V79.3
- diabetes mellitus V77.1
- diphtheria V74.3
- disease or disorder V82.9
- - bacterial V74.9
- - - specified NEC V74.8
- - blood V78.9
- - - specified NEC V78.8
- - blood-forming organ V78.9
- - - specified NEC V78.8
- - cardiovascular NEC V81.2
- - - hypertensive V81.1
- - - ischemic V81.0
- - Chagas' V75.3
- - ear NEC V80.3
- - endocrine NEC V77.9
- - eye NEC V80.2
- - genitourinary NEC V81.6
- - heart NEC V81.2
- - - hypertensive V81.1
- - - ischemic V81.0
- - immunity NEC V77.9
- - infectious NEC V75.9
- - mental V79.9
- - - specified NEC V79.8
- - metabolic NEC V77.9
- - - inborn NEC V77.7
- - neurological V80.0
- - nutritional NEC V77.9
- - rheumatic NEC V82.2
- - rickettsial V75.0
- - sickle cell (trait) V78.2
- - specified NEC V82.8
- - thyroid V77.0

Screening - *continued*
- disease or disorder - *continued*
- - vascular NEC V81.2
- - - ischemic V81.0
- - venereal V74.5
- - viral V73.9
- - - arthropod-borne NEC V73.5
- - - specified NEC V73.8
- dislocation of hip, congenital V82.3
- drugs in athletes V70.3
- emphysema V81.3
- encephalitis, viral (mosquito- or tick-borne) V73.5
- fever
- - dengue V73.5
- - hemorrhagic V73.5
- - yellow V73.4
- filariasis V75.6
- galactosemia V77.4
- genitourinary condition NEC V81.6
- glaucoma V80.1
- gout V77.5
- helminthiasis, intestinal V75.7
- hematopoietic malignancy V76.8
- hemoglobinopathies NEC V78.3
- hemorrhagic fever V73.5
- Hodgkin's disease V76.8
- hormones in athletes V70.3
- hypertension V81.1
- infection
- - mycotic V75.4
- - parasitic NEC V75.8
- ingestion of radioactive substance V82.5
- intestinal helminthiasis V75.7
- leishmaniasis V75.2
- leprosy V74.2
- leptospirosis V74.8
- leukemia V76.8
- lymphoma V76.8
- malaria V75.1
- malignant neoplasm (of) V76.9
- - bladder V76.3
- - blood V76.8
- - breast V76.1
- - cervix V76.2
- - hematopoietic system V76.8
- - lymph (glands) V76.8
- - respiratory organs V76.0
- - specified sites NEC V76.4
- malnutrition V77.2
- measles V73.2
- mental
- - disorder V79.9
- - - specified NEC V79.8
- - retardation V79.2
- metabolic errors, inborn V77.7
- multiphasic V82.6

Secondary neoplasm - *continued*
- urinary organs NEC 198.1
- vesical (orifice) 198.1
Secretion
- catecholamine, by pheochromocytoma 255.6
- hormone
- - antidiuretic, inappropriate (syndrome) 253.6
- - by
- - - carcinoid tumor 259.2
- - - pheochromocytoma 255.6
- - ectopic NEC 259.3
- urinary
- - excessive 788.4
- - suppression 788.5
Section
- cesarean
- - affecting fetus or newborn 763.4
- - post mortem, affecting fetus or newborn 761.6
- - previous, in pregnancy or childbirth 654.2
- - - fetus or newborn 763.8
- nerve, traumatic - see Injury, nerve, by site
Segmentation, incomplete (congenital) - see also Fusion
- bone NEC 756.9
- lumbosacral (joint) 756.1
- vertebra 756.1
- - lumbosacral 756.1
Seizure 780.3
- akinetic 345.0
- apoplexy, apoplectic (see also Disease, cerebrovascular, acute) 436
- atonic 345.0
- autonomic 300.1
- brain or cerebral (see also Disease, cerebrovascular, acute) 436
- convulsive (see also Convulsions) 780.3
- cortical (focal) (motor) 345.5
- epileptic (see also Epilepsy) 345.9
- epileptiform, epileptoid 780.3
- - focal 345.5
- febrile 780.3
- heart - see Disease, heart
- hysterical 300.1
- jacksonian (focal) 345.5
- - motor type 345.5
- - sensory type 345.5
- newborn 779.0
- paralysis (see also Disease, cerebrovascular, acute) 436
- uncinate 345.4
Self-mutilation 300.9
Semicoma 780.0

Seminoma (M9061/3)
- anaplastic type (M9062/3)
- - specified site - see Neoplasm, malignant
- - unspecified site 186.9
- specified site - see Neoplasm, malignant
- spermatocytic (M9063/3)
- - specified site - see Neoplasm, malignant
- - unspecified site 186.9
- unspecified site 186.9
Senear-Usher disease 694.4
Senectus 797
Senescence 797
Senile (see also Condition) 797
- cervix (atrophic) 622.8
- degenerative atrophy, skin 701.3
- endometrium (atrophic) 621.8
- fallopian tube (atrophic) 620.8
- heart (failure) 797
- ovary (atrophic) 620.3
- wart (see also Keratosis, seborrheic) 702
Senility 797
- with
- - acute confusional state 290.3
- - mental changes NEC 290.9
- - psychosis NEC (see also Psychosis, senile) 290.2
- premature 259.8
Sensation
- burning (see also Disturbance, sensation) 782.0
- - tongue 529.6
- loss of (see also Disturbance, sensation) 782.0
- prickling (see also Disturbance, sensation) 782.0
- tingling (see also Disturbance, sensation) 782.0
Sense loss (touch) (see also Disturbance, sensation) 782.0
- smell 781.1
- taste 781.1
Sensibility disturbance (cortical) (deep) (vibratory) (see also Disturbance, sensation) 782.0
Sensitiver beziehungswahn 297.8
Sensitivity - see also Allergy
- carotid sinus 337.0
- cold, autoimmune 283.0
- methemoglobin 289.7
Sensitization, auto-erythrocytic 287.2
Separation
- anxiety, abnormal 309.2
- apophysis, traumatic - code as Fracture, closed
- choroid 363.7

Separation - *continued*
- costochondral - see Dislocation, costochondral
- epiphysis, epiphyseal, traumatic - code as Fracture, by site, closed
- fracture - see Fracture
- infundibulum cardiac from right ventricle by a partition 746.8
- joint (traumatic) (current) - code by site under Dislocation
- placenta (normally implanted) - see Placenta, separation
- pubic bone, obstetrical trauma 665.6
- retina, retinal - see Detachment, retina
- sternoclavicular (traumatic) - see Dislocation, sternoclavicular
- symphysis pubis, obstetrical trauma 665.6
- tracheal ring, incomplete (congenital) 748.3
Sepsis (generalized) (see also Septicemia) 038.9
- with
- - abortion - see categories 634-639, fourth digit .0
- - ectopic gestation 639.0
- buccal 528.3
- dental 522.4
- following infusion, injection, transfusion, or vaccination 999.3
- Friedlander's 038.4
- intraocular 360.0
- localized
- - in operation wound 998.5
- - skin (see also Abscess) 682.9
- malleus 024
- newborn NEC 771.8
- of tracheostomy stoma 519.0
- oral 528.3
- pelvic, puerperal, postpartum, childbirth 670
- puerperal, postpartum, childbirth (pelvic) 670
- skin, localized (see also Abscess) 682.9
- umbilical (newborn) (organism unspecified) 771.4
- - tetanus 771.3
- urinary 599.0
Septate - see Septum
Septic - see also condition
- arm (with lymphangitis) 682.3
- embolus - see Embolism
- finger (with lymphangitis) 681.0
- foot (with lymphangitis) 682.7
- gallbladder (see also Cholecystitis) 575.8
- hand (with lymphangitis) 682.4
- joint 711.0
- kidney (see also Infection, kidney) 590.9

Septic - *continued*
- leg (with lymphangitis) 682.6
- mouth 528.3
- nail 681.9
- - finger 681.0
- - toe 681.1
- sore (see also Abscess) 682.9
- - throat 034.0
- - - milk borne 034.0
- - - streptococcal 034.0
- spleen (acute) 289.5
- teeth 522.4
- throat 034.0
- thrombus - see Thrombosis
- toe (with lymphangitis) 681.1
- tonsils 474.0
- umbilical cord 771.8
- uterus (see also Endometritis) 615.9
Septicemia, septicemic (generalized) (suppurative) 038.9
- with
- - abortion - see categories 634-639, fourth digit .0
- - ectopic gestation 639.0
- anaerobic 038.3
- anthrax 022.3
- Bacillus coli 038.4
- complicating labor 659.3
- cryptogenetic 038.9
- Erysipelothrix (insidiosa) (rhusiopathiae) 027.1
- Escherichia coli 038.4
- following infusion, injection, transfusion, or vaccination 999.3
- Friedlander's (bacillus) 038.4
- gangrenous 038.9
- gonococcal 098.8
- gram-negative (organism) 038.4
- - anaerobic 038.3
- herpes (simplex) 054.5
- herpetic 054.5
- Listeria monocytogenes 027.0
- meningeal - see Meningitis
- meningococcal (fulminating) (chronic) 036.2
- newborn NEC 771.8
- pneumococcal 038.2
- - with pneumonia 481
- postoperative 998.5
- puerperal, postpartum 670
- Salmonella (aertrycke) (callinarum) (choleraesuis) (enteritidis) (suipestifer) (typhimurium) 003.1
- Shigella (see also Dysentery, bacillary) 004.9
- specified organism NEC 038.8
- staphylococcal 038.1

Septicemia - *continued*
- streptococcal (anaerobic) 038.0
- viral 079.8
Septum, septate (congenital) - see also
  Anomaly, specified type NEC
- anal 751.2
- aqueduct of Sylvius 742.3
- - with spina bifida 741.0
- uterus (see also Double uterus) 752.2
- vagina 752.4
- - in pregnancy or childbirth 654.7
- - - causing obstructed labor 660.2
- - - - fetus or newborn 763.1
- - - fetus or newborn 763.8
Sequestration
- lung (congenital) 748.5
- orbit 376.1
- pulmonary artery (congenital) 747.3
Sequestrum
- bone 730.1
- dental 525.8
- jaw bone 526.4
- sinus (accessory) (nasal) (see also
  Sinusitis) 473.9
Sequoiosis asthma 495.8
Serology for syphilis
- doubtful
- - with signs or symptoms - code by site
  and stage under Syphilis
- - follow-up of latent syphilis - see
  Syphilis, latent
- false positive 795.6
- negative, with signs or symptoms - code
  by site and stage under Syphilis
- positive 097.1
- - with signs or symptoms - code by site
  and stage under Syphilis
- - false 795.6
- - follow-up of latent syphilis - see
  Syphilis, latent
- - only finding - see Syphilis, latent
- reactivated 097.1
Seroma - see Hematoma
Seropurulent - see condition
Serositis, multiple 569.8
- peritoneal 568.8
- pleural - see Pleurisy
Serous - see condition
Sertoli cell
- adenoma (M8640/0)
- - specified site - see Neoplasm, benign
- - unspecified site
- - - female 220
- - - male 222.0
- carcinoma (M8640/3)
- - specified site - see Neoplasm,
  malignant

Sertoli cell - *continued*
- carcinoma - *continued*
- - unspecified site 186.9
- tumor (M8640/0)
- - with lipid storage (M8641/0)
- - - specified site - see Neoplasm, benign
- - - unspecified site
- - - - female 220
- - - - male 222.0
- - specified site - see Neoplasm, benign
- - unspecified site
- - - female 220
- - - male 222.0
Sertoli-Leydig cell tumor (M8631/0)
- specified site - see Neoplasm, benign
- unspecified site
- - female 220
- - male 222.0
Serum
- allergy, allergic reaction 999.5
- - shock 999.4
- arthritis 999.5
- complication or reaction NEC 999.5
- disease NEC 999.5
- hepatitis 070.3 † 573.1*
- - with hepatic coma 070.2 † 573.1*
- intoxication 999.5
- jaundice (homologous) 070.3 † 573.1*
- - with hepatic coma 070.2 † 573.1*
- neuritis 999.5
- poisoning NEC 999.5
- rash NEC 999.5
- sickness NEC 999.5
Sesamoiditis 733.9
Sever's disease or osteochondrosis 732.5
Sex chromosome mosaics 758.8
Sextuplet 761.5
- pregnancy (complicating delivery) 651.8
Sexuality, pathologic (see also Deviation,
  sexual) 302.9
Sezary, disease, reticulosis or syndrome
  (M9701/3) 202.2
Shadow, lung 793.1
Shaking palsy or paralysis (see also
  Parkinsonism) 332.0
Shallowness, acetabulum 736.3
Shaver's disease 503
Sheath (tendon) - see condition
Shedding
- nail 703.8
- premature, primary (deciduous) teeth
  520.6
Sheehan's disease or syndrome 253.2
Shelf, rectal 569.4
Shell teeth 520.5
Shellshock (current) (see also Reaction,
  stress, acute) 308.9

Shellshock - *continued*
- lasting state 300.1
Shield kidney 753.3
Shift, mediastinal 793.2
Shiga's
- bacillus 004.0
- dysentery 004.0
Shigella (dysentery) (see also Dysentery, bacillary) 004.9
Shigellosis (see also Dysentery, bacillary) 004.9
Shin splints 844.9
Shingles (see also Herpes zoster) 053.9
Shipyard eye or disease 077.1 † 370.4*
Shirodkar suture, in pregnancy 654.5
Shock 785.5
- allergic - see Shock, anaphylactic
- anaphylactic 995.0
- - chemical - see Table of drugs and chemicals
- - correct medicinal substance properly administered 995.0
- - drug or medicinal substance
- - - correct substance properly administered 995.0
- - - overdose or wrong substance given or taken 977.9
- - - - specified drug - see Table of drugs and chemicals
- - following sting(s) 989.5
- - immunization 999.4
- - serum 999.4
- anaphylactoid - see Shock, anaphylactic
- anesthetic
- - correct substance properly administered 995.4
- - overdose or wrong substance given 968.-
- - - specified anesthetic - see Table of drugs and chemicals
- birth, fetus or newborn NEC 779.8
- cardiogenic 785.5
- chemical substance - see Table of drugs and chemicals
- complicating
- - abortion - see categories 634-639, fourth digit .5
- - ectopic or molar pregnancy 639.5
- - labor and delivery 669.1
- culture 309.2
- drug 995.0
- - correct substance properly administered 995.0
- - overdose or wrong drug given or taken 977.9
- - - specified drug - see Table of drugs and chemicals

Shock - *continued*
- electric 994.8
- endotoxic 785.5
- - due to surgical procedure 998.0
- following injury (immediate) (delayed) 958.4
- hematologic 785.5
- hypovolemic 785.5
- - surgical 998.0
- - traumatic 958.4
- insulin 251.0
- lightning 994.0
- lung 518.5
- obstetric 669.1
- - complicating abortion - see categories 634-639, fourth digit .5
- paralytic (see also Disease, cerebrovascular, acute) 436
- pleural (surgical) 998.0
- - due to trauma 958.4
- postoperative 998.0
- psychic (see also Reaction, stress, acute) 308.9
- septic 785.5
- - due to
- - - surgical procedure 998.0
- - - transfusion 999.8
- spinal - see also Injury, spinal, by region
- - with spinal bone injury - see Fracture, vertebra, by region, with spinal cord lesion
- surgical 998.0
- therapeutic misadventure NEC (see also Complications) 998.8
- transfusion - see Complications, transfusion
- traumatic (immediate) (delayed) 958.4
Shoemakers' chest 738.3
Short, shortening, shortness
- arm 736.8
- - congenital 755.2
- breath 786.0
- common bile duct, congenital 751.6
- cord (umbilical) 663.4
- - affecting fetus or newborn 762.6
- cystic duct, congenital 751.6
- esophagus (congenital) 750.4
- femur (acquired) 736.8
- - congenital 755.3
- frenulum linguae 750.0
- frenum linguae 750.0
- hamstrings 727.8
- hip (acquired) 736.3
- - congenital 755.6
- leg (acquired) 736.8
- - congenital 755.3
- metatarsus (congenital) 754.7

Short - *continued*
- metatarsus - *continued*
- - acquired 736.7
- organ or site, congenital NEC - see Distortion
- palate (congenital) 750.2
- radius (acquired) 736.0
- - congenital 755.2
- round ligament 629.8
- stature, constitutional (hereditary) 783.4
- tendon 727.8
- - Achilles (acquired) 727.8
- - - congenital 754.7
- - congenital 756.8
- thigh (acquired) 736.8
- - congenital 755.3
- tibialis anticus 727.8
- umbilical cord 663.4
- - affecting fetus or newborn 762.6
- urethra 599.8
- uvula (congenital) 750.2
- vagina 623.8
Shortsightedness 367.1
Shoulder - see condition
Shovel shaped incisors 520.2
Shower, thromboembolic - see Embolism
Shunt
- arterial-venous (dialysis) V45.1
- arteriovenous, pulmonary (acquired) NEC 417.0
- - congenital 747.3
- - traumatic (complication) 901.4
- cerebral ventricle (communicating) in situ V45.2
- surgical, prosthetic, with complications - see Complications, shunt
Shutdown, renal 586
- complicating
- - abortion - see categories 634-639, fourth digit .3
- - ectopic or molar pregnancy 639.3
- following labor and delivery 669.3
Shy-Drager syndrome 333.0
Sialadenitis (any gland) (chronic) (suppurative) 527.2
Sialadenosis (periodic) 527.2
Sialectasia 527.8
Sialitis 527.2
Sialoadenitis 527.2
Sialoangitis 527.2
Sialodochitis (fibrinosa) 527.2
Sialodocholithiasis 527.5
Sialolithiasis 527.5
Sialorrhea (see also Ptyalism) 527.7
Sialosis 527.8
Siamese twin 759.4
Sicca syndrome 710.2

Sick 799.9
- or handicapped person in family V61.4
Sickle cell anemia (see also Disease, sickle cell) 282.6
Sicklemia (see also Disease, sickle cell) 282.6
Sickness
- air (travel) 994.6
- airplane 994.6
- alpine 993.2
- altitude 993.2
- aviators' 993.2
- balloon 993.2
- car 994.6
- compressed air 993.3
- decompression 993.3
- milk 988.8
- morning 643.0
- motion 994.6
- mountain 993.2
- protein (see also COmplications, vaccination) 999.5
- radiation NEC 990
- roundabout (motion) 994.6
- sea 994.6
- serum NEC 999.5
- sleeping (African) 086.5
- - by Trypanosoma 086.5
- - - gambiense 086.3
- - - rhodesiense 086.4
- - Gambian 086.3
- - Rhodesian 086.4
- sweating 078.2
- swing (motion) 994.6
- train (railway) (travel) 994.6
- travel (any vehicle) 994.6
Siderosis (lung) 503
- eye (globe) 360.2
Siemens' syndrome 757.3
Sigmoid
- flexure - see condition
- kidney 753.3
Sigmoiditis - see Enteritis
Silicosis, silicotic (simple) (complicated) 502
- non-nodular 503
- pulmonum 502
Silicotuberculosis 011.4
Silo-filler's disease 506.9
Silver syndrome 759.8
Simmonds' cachexia or disease 253.2
Simon's disease 272.6
Simple, simplex - see condition
Sinding-Larsen disease or osteochondrosis 732.4
Singers' node or nodule 478.5
Single
- atrium 745.6

Sloughing - *continued*
- appendix 543
- bladder 596.8
- fascia 728.9
- phagedena (see also Gangrene) 785.4
- rectum 569.4
- scrotum 608.8
- tendon 727.9
- ulcer (see also Ulcer, skin) 707.9
Slow
- feeding newborn 779.3
- fetal growth NEC 764.9
- - affecting management of pregnancy 656.5
Slowing, urinary stream 788.6
Sluder's neuralgia 337.0
Slurred, slurring speech 784.5
Small(ness)
- introitus, vagina 623.3
- kidney, unknown cause 589.9
- - bilateral 589.1
- - unilateral 589.0
- ovary 620.8
- pelvis
- - with disproportion 653.1
- - - causing obstructed labor 660.1
- - - fetus or newborn 763.1
- placenta - see Placenta, insufficiency
- uterus 621.8
Small-for-dates - see also Light-for-dates
- affecting management of pregnancy 656.5
Smallpox (see also Variola) 050.9
- hemorrhagic (pustular) 050.0
- malignant 050.0
- modified 050.2
- vaccination complications - see Complications, vaccination
Smith's fracture (separation) - see Fracture, radius, lower end
Smith-Lemli-Opitz syndrome 759.8
Smoker's
- cough 491.0
- throat 472.1
Smothering spells 786.0
Snapping
- finger 727.0
- hip 719.6
- jaw 524.6
- knee 717.9
Sneddon-Wilkinson disease or syndrome 694.1
Sneezing 784.9
- intractable 478.1
Sniffing
- cocaine 304.2
- glue (airplane) 304.6

Snoring 786.0
Snow blindness 370.2
Snuffles (non-syphilitic) 460
- syphilitic (infant) 090.0
Social migrant V60.0
Sodoku 026.0
Soemering's ring 366.5
Soft - see also condition
- nails 703.8
Softening
- bone 268.2
- brain (necrotic) (progressive) 434.9
- - arteriosclerotic 437.0
- - congenital 742.4
- - embolic NEC (see also Embolism, brain) 434.1
- - hemorrhagic (see also Hemorrhage, brain) 431
- - occlusive 434.9
- - thrombotic NEC (see also Thrombosis, brain) 434.0
- cartilage 733.9
- cerebellar - see Softening, brain
- cerebral - see Softening, brain
- cerebrospinal - see Softening, brain
- myocardial, heart (see also Degeneration, myocardial) 429.1
- spinal cord 336.8
- stomach 537.8
Soldier's heart 306.2
Solitary kidney (congenital) 753.0
Somatization reaction, somatic reation - see Disorder, psychogenic
Somnambulism 307.4
- hysterical 300.1
Somnolence 780.5
- nonorganic origin 307.4
- periodic 349.8
Sonne dysentery 004.3
Soor 112.0
Sore
- Delhi 085.1
- desert (see also Ulcer, skin) 707.9
- eye 379.9
- Lahore 085.1
- mouth 528.9
- - canker 528.2
- - denture 528.9
- muscle 729.1
- Naga (see also Ulcer, skin) 707.9
- oriental 085.1
- pressure 707.0
- skin NEC 709.9
- soft 099.0
- throat 462
- - with influenza, flu, or grippe 487.1
- - acute 462

Sore - *continued*
− throat - *continued*
− − chronic 472.1
− − Coxsackie (virus) 074.0
− − diphtheritic 032.0
− − epidemic 034.0
− − gangrenous 462
− − herpetic 054.7
− − influenzal 487.1
− − malignant 462
− − purulent 462
− − putrid 462
− − septic 034.0
− − streptococcal (ulcerative) 034.0
− − ulcerated 462
− − viral NEC 462
− − − Coxsackie 074.0
− tropical (see also Ulcer, skin) 707.9
− veldt (see also Ulcer, skin) 707.9
Soto's syndrome 756.8
Spacing, abnormal, tooth, teeth 524.3
Spade-like hand (congenital) 754.8
Spading nail 703.8
− congenital 757.5
Spanemia 285.9
Spanish collar 605
Sparganosis 123.5
Spasm(s), spastic, spasticity (see also Condition) 781.0
− accommodation 367.5
− ampulla of Vater (see also Disease, gallbladder) 576.8
− anus, ani (sphincter) (reflex) 564.6
− − psychogenic 306.4
− artery NEC 443.9
− − cerebral 435
− Bell's 351.0
− bladder (sphincter, external or internal) 596.8
− bowel 564.1
− − psychogenic 306.4
− bronchus, bronchiole 519.1
− cardia 530.0
− cardiac - see Angina
− carpopedal (see also Tetany) 781.7
− cecum 564.1
− cerebral (arteries) (vascular) 435
− cervix, complicating delivery 661.4
− − fetus or newborn 763.7
− ciliary body (of accommodation) 367.5
− colon 564.1
− − psychogenic 306.4
− common duct (see also Disease, biliary) 576.8
− compulsive 307.2
− conjugate 378.8
− coronary (artery) - see Angina

Spasm(s) - *continued*
− diaphragm (reflex) 786.8
− − psychogenic 306.1
− duodenum 564.8
− esophagus (diffuse) 530.5
− − psychogenic 306.4
− facial 351.8
− fallopian tube 620.8
− gastrointestinal (tract) 536.8
− − psychogenic 306.4
− glottis 478.7
− − hysterical 300.1
− − psychogenic 306.1
− − − specified as conversion reaction 300.1
− − reflex through recurrent laryngeal nerve 478.7
− habit 307.2
− heart - see Angina
− hourglass - see Contraction, hourglass
− hysterical 300.1
− infantile 345.6
− internal oblique, eye 378.5
− intestinal 564.1
− − psychogenic 306.4
− larynx, laryngeal 478.7
− − hysterical 300.1
− − psychogenic 306.1
− − − specified as conversion reaction 300.1
− levator palpebrae superioris 374.4
− lightning 345.6
− muscle 728.8
− nervous 306.0
− nodding 307.3
− occupation 300.8
− oculogyric 378.8
− oesophagus (diffuse) 530.5
− − psychogenic 306.4
− ophthalmic artery 362.3
− orbicularis 781.0
− perineal 625.8
− peroneo-extensor (see also Flat, foot) 734
− pharynx (reflex) 478.2
− − hysterical 300.1
− − psychogenic 306.1
− − − specified as conversion reaction 300.1
− psychogenic 306.0
− pylorus 537.8
− − adult hypertrophic 537.0
− − congenital or infantile 750.5
− − psychogenic 306.4
− rectum (sphincter) 564.6
− − psychogenic 306.4
− retinal (artery) 362.3

Spasm(s) - *continued*
- sacroiliac 724.6
- sigmoid 564.1
- - psychogenic 306.4
- sphincter of Oddi (see also Disease, gallbladder) 576.5
- stomach 536.8
- - neurotic 306.4
- throat 478.2
- - hysterical 300.1
- - psychogenic 306.1
- - - specified as conversion reaction 300.1
- tic 307.2
- tongue 529.8
- torsion 333.6
- trigeminal nerve (see also Neuralgia, trigeminal) 350.1
- ureter 593.8
- urethra (sphincter) 599.8
- uterus 625.8
- - complicating labor 661.4
- - - fetus or newborn 763.7
- vagina 625.1
- - psychogenic 306.5
- vascular NEC 443.9
- vasomotor NEC 443.9
- vein NEC 459.8
- viscera 789.0
Spasmodic - see condition
Spasmus nutans 307.3
Spastic - see also Spasm
- child 343.9
Spasticity - see also Spasm
- cerebral, child 343.9
Speaker's throat 784.4
Specific, specified - see condition
Speech defect, disorder, disturbance, impediment NEC 784.5
- psychogenic 307.9
Sperm counts V26.2
Spermatic cord - see condition
Spermatocele 608.1
- congenital 752.8
Spermatocystitis 608.4
Spermatocytoma (M9063/3)
- specified site - see Neoplasm, malignant
- unspecified site 186.9
Spermatorrhea 608.8
Sphacelus (see also Gangrene) 785.4
Sphenoidal - see condition
Sphenoiditis (chronic) (see also Sinusitis, sphenoidal) 473.3
Sphenopalatine ganglion neuralgia 337.0
Sphericity, increased lens (congenital) 743.3
Spherocytosis (congenital) (familial) (hereditary) 282.0

Spherocytosis - *continued*
- hemoglobin disease 282.7
- sickle cell (disease) 282.6
Spherophakia 743.3
Sphincter - see condition
Sphincteritis, sphincter of Oddi (see also Cholecystitis) 576.8
Sphingolipidosis 272.7
Sphingomyelinosis 272.7
Spicule tooth 520.2
Spider
- finger 755.5
- nevus 448.1
- vascular 448.1
Spiegler-Fendt sarcoid 686.8
Spielmeyer-Stock disease 330.1
Spielmeyer-Vogt disease 330.1
Spina bifida (aperta) 741.9
- with hydrocephalus 741.0
- fetus (suspected), affecting management of pregnancy 655.0
- occulta 756.1
Spindle, Krukenberg's 371.1
Spine, spinal - see condition
Spiradenoma (eccrine) (M8403/0) - see Neoplasm, skin, benign
Spirillosis NEC (see also Fever, relapsing) 087.9
Spirillum minus 026.0
Spirochetal - see condition
Spirochetosis 104.9
- bronchopulmonary 104.8
- icterohemorrhagic 100.0
- lung 104.8
Spitting blood (see also Hemoptysis) 786.3
Splanchnomegaly 569.8
Splanchnoptosis 569.8
Spleen, splenic - see condition
Splenic flexure syndrome 569.8
Splenitis 289.5
- interstitial 289.5
- malarial (see also Malaria) 084.6
- malignant 289.5
- nonspecific 289.5
- tuberculous 017.7
Splenocele 289.5
Splenomegalia - see Splenomegaly
Splenomegalic - see condition
Splenomegaly 789.2
- congenital 759.0
- congestive, chronic 289.5
- Egyptian 120.1
- Gaucher's 272.7
- idiopathic 789.2
- malarial (see also Malaria) 084.6
- neutropenic 288.0
- Niemann-Pick 272.7

Splenomegaly - *continued*
- syphilitic 095
- - congenital 090.0
Splenopathy 289.5
Splenopneumonia - see Pneumonia
Splenoptosis 289.5
Splinter - code by site under Injury,
  superficial
Split, splitting
- heart sounds 427.8
- lip, congenital 749.1
- - with cleft palate 749.2
- nails 703.8
- urinary stream 788.6
Spoiled child reaction 312.0
Spondylarthrosis 721.9
Spondylitis 720.9
- ankylopoietica 720.0
- ankylosing (chronic) 720.0
- atrophic 720.9
- chronic (traumatic) 721.9
- deformans (chronic) 721.9
- gonococcal 098.5 † 720.8*
- gouty 274.0 † 712.0*
- hypertrophic 721.9
- infectious NEC 720.9
- Kummell's 721.7
- Marie-Strumpell 720.0
- muscularis 720.9
- ossificans ligamentosa 721.6
- osteoarthritica 721.9
- rheumatoid 720.0
- rhizomelica 720.0
- sacroiliac NEC 720.2
- senescent 721.9
- senile 721.9
- static 721.9
- traumatic (chronic) 721.9
- tuberculous 015.0 † 720.8*
- typhosa 002.0 † 720.8*
Spondyloarthrosis 721.9
Spondylolisthesis (congenital)
  (lumbosacral) 756.1
- with disproportion 653.3
- - causing obstructed labor 660.1
- - fetus or newborn 763.1
- acquired 738.4
- degenerative 738.4
- traumatic 756.1
- - acute (lumbar) - see Fracture,
    vertebra, lumbar
- - - site other than lumbosacral - code by
      region under Fracture, vertebra
Spondylolysis (congenital) 756.1
- acquired 738.5
- cervical 756.1
- lumbosacral region 756.1

Spondylolysis - *continued*
- lumbosacral region - *continued*
- - with disproportion 653.3
- - - causing obstructed labor 660.1
- - - fetus or newborn 763.1
Spondylopathy
- inflammatory 720.9
- traumatic 721.7
Spondylose rhizomelique 720.0
Spondylosis 721.9
- with
- - disproportion 653.3
- - - causing obstructed labor 660.1
- - - fetus or newborn 763.1
- - myelopathy NEC 721.9 † 336.3*
- cervical 721.0
- - with myelopathy 721.1 † 336.3*
- inflammatory 720.9
- lumbar, lumbosacral 721.3
- - with myelopathy 721.4 † 336.3*
- sacral 721.3
- - with myelopathy 721.4 † 336.3*
- thoracic 721.2
- - with myelopathy 721.4 † 336.3*
- traumatic 721.7
Sponge
- inadvertently left in operation wound
  998.4
- kidney (medullary) 753.1
Sponge-divers' disease 989.5
Spongioblastoma (M9422/3)
- multiforme (M9440/3)
- - specified site - see Neoplasm,
    malignant
- - unspecified site 191.9
- polare (M9423/3)
- - specified site - see Neoplasm,
    malignant
- - unspecified site 191.9
- primitive polar (M9443/3)
- - specified site - see Neoplasm,
    malignant
- - unspecified site 191.9
- specified site - see Neoplasm, malignant
- unspecified site 191.9
Spongiocytoma (M9400/3)
- specified site - see Neoplasm, malignant
- unspecified site 191.9
Spongioneuroblastoma (M9504/3) - see
  Neoplasm, malignant
Spontaneous - see also condition
- fracture (cause unknown) 733.1
Spoon nail 703.8
- congenital 757.5
Sporadic - see condition
Sporotrichosis (cutaneous) (disseminated)
  (lymphatic) (pulmonary) (skeletal) 117.1

Sporotrichum schenckii infection 117.1
Spots
- atrophic (skin) 701.3
- Bitot's (in the young child) 264.1 † 372.5*
- cafe au lait 709.0
- Cayenne pepper 448.1
- cotton wool, retina 362.8
- de Morgan's 448.1
- Fuchs' black (myopic) 360.2
- interpalpebral 372.5
- liver 709.0
- Mongolian (pigmented) 757.3
Spotted fever - see Fever, spotted
Spotting, intermenstrual NEC 626.4
- irregular 626.6
- regular 626.5
Sprain, strain (joint) (ligament) (muscle)
  (tendon) 848.9
- Achilles tendon 845.0
- acromioclavicular 840.0
- ankle 845.0
- - and foot 845.0
- anterior longitudinal, cervical 847.0
- arm 840.9
- - upper 840.9
- - - and shoulder 840.9
- astragalus 845.0
- atlanto-axial 847.0
- atlanto-occipital 847.0
- atlas 847.0
- axis 847.0
- back 847.9
- breast bone 848.4
- broad ligament - see Injury, internal,
  broad ligament
- calcaneofibular 845.0
- carpal 842.0
- carpometacarpal 842.1
- cartilage
- - costal, without mention of injury to
    sternum 848.3
- - - involving sternum 848.4
- - knee 844.9
- - - with current tear (see also Tear,
    meniscus) 836.2
- - semilunar (knee) 844.8
- - - with current tear (see also Tear,
    meniscus) 836.2
- - septal, nose 848.0
- - thyroid region 848.2
- - xiphoid 848.4
- cervical, cervicodorsal, cervicothoracic
  847.0
- chondrocostal, without mention of injury
  to sternum 848.3
- - involving sternum 848.4
- chondrosternal 848.4

Sprain - *continued*
- clavicle 840.9
- coccyx 847.4
- collar bone 840.9
- coraco-acromial 840.8
- coracoclavicular 840.1
- coracohumeral 840.2
- coronary, knee 844.8
- costal cartilage 848.3
- crico-arytenoid articulation 848.2
- cricothyroid articulation 848.2
- cruciate knee 844.2
- deltoid
- - ankle 845.0
- - shoulder 840.8
- dorsal 847.1
- elbow 841.9
- - and forearm 841.9
- femur (proximal end) 843.9
- - distal end 844.9
- fibula (proximal end) 844.9
- - distal end 845.0
- fibulocalcaneal 845.0
- finger(s) 842.1
- foot 845.1
- forearm 841.9
- - and elbow 841.9
- glenoid 840.8
- hand 842.1
- hip 843.9
- - and thigh 843.9
- humerus (proximal end) 840.9
- - distal end 841.9
- iliofemoral 843.0
- infraspinatus 840.3
- innominate
- - acetabulum 843.8
- - pubic junction 848.5
- - sacral junction 846.1
- internal
- - collateral, ankle 845.0
- - semilunar cartilage 844.8
- - - with current tear (see also Tear,
    meniscus) 836.2
- interphalangeal
- - finger 842.1
- - toe 845.1
- ischiocapsular 843.1
- jaw (cartilage) (meniscus) 848.1
- knee 844.9
- - and leg 844.9
- lateral collateral, knee 844.0
- leg 844.9
- - and knee 844.9
- ligamentum teres femoris 843.8
- lumbar (spine) 847.2
- lumbosacral 846.0

Sprue - *continued*
- tropical 579.1
Spur
- bone 726.9
- calcaneal 726.7
- iliac crest 726.5
- nose (septum) 478.1
- - bone 726.9
- septal 478.1
Sputum, excessive (cause unknown) 786.4
Squamous - see also condition
- epithelium in
- - cervical canal (congenital) 752.4
- - uterine mucosa (congenital) 752.3
Squashed nose 738.0
- congenital 754.0
Squint (see also Strabismus) 378.9
- accommodative 378.0
Stab - see also Wound, open
- internal organs - see Injury, internal, by
  site, with open wound
Staehli's pigment line 371.1
Staggering gait 781.2
- hysterical 300.1
Staghorn calculus 592.0
Stain, port wine 757.3
Staining
- tooth, teeth (hard tissues) 521.7
- - due to
- - - accretions 523.6
- - - deposits (betel) (black) (green)
      (materia alba) (orange) (tobacco)
      (soft) 523.6
- - - metals (copper, silver) 521.7
- - - pulpal bleeding 521.7
Stammering 307.0
Standstill
- auricular 426.6
- cardiac (see also Arrest, cardiac) 427.5
- sinoatrial 426.6
- ventricular (see also Arrest, cardiac)
  427.5
Stannosis 503
Stanton's disease 025
Staphylitis (acute) (catarrhal) (chronic)
  (gangrenous) (membranous) (suppurative)
  (ulcerative) 528.3
Staphylococcemia 038.1
Staphylococcus, staphylococcal - see
  condition
Staphyloma 379.1
- anterior 379.1
- ciliary 379.1
- cornea 371.7
- equatorial 379.1
- posterior 379.1
- sclera 379.1

Stargardt's disease 362.7
Starvation (inanition) (due to lack of food)
  994.2
- edema 262
- voluntary NEC 307.1
Stasis
- bile (see also Disease, biliary) 576.8
- bronchus (see also Bronchitis) 490
- cardiac (see also Failure, heart,
  congestive) 428.0
- cecum 564.8
- colon 564.8
- dermatitis - see Varix, with stasis
  dermatitis
- duodenal 536.8
- eczema - see Varicose vein
- foot 991.4
- gastric 536.8
- ileocecal coil 564.8
- ileum 564.8
- intestinal 564.8
- jejunum 564.8
- liver 571.9
- - cirrhotic - see Cirrhosis, liver
- lymphatic 457.8
- portal 571.9
- pulmonary 514
- stomach 536.8
- ulcer 454.0
- urine 788.2
- venous 459.9
State
- affective and paranoid, mixed, organic
  psychotic 294.8
- agitated 307.9
- - acute reaction to stress 308.2
- anxiety (neurotic) 300.0
- apprehension 300.0
- climacteric, female 627.2
- clouded
- - epileptic 345.9
- - paroxysmal (idiopathic) 345.9
- compulsive (with obsession) (mixed)
  300.3
- confusional 298.2
- - acute 293.0
- - - with senility 290.3
- - epileptic 293.0
- - reactive (from emotional stress,
    psychological trauma) 298.2
- - subacute 293.1
- constitutional psychopathic 301.9
- convulsive (see also Convulsions) 780.3
- depressive NEC 311
- - neurotic 300.4
- dissociative 300.1
- hallucinatory, induced by drug 292.1

Stenosis - *continued*
- aortic - *continued*
- − rheumatic 395.0
- − − with
- − − − insufficiency, incompetency or regurgitation 395.2
- − − − − with mitral (valve) disease 396
- − − − − mitral (valve) disease 396
- − − specified cause NEC 424.1
- − − syphilitic 093.2 † 424.1*
- aqueduct of Sylvius 742.3
- − − with spina bifida 741.0
- − − acquired 331.4
- bile duct or biliary passage (see also Obstruction, biliary) 576.2
- bladder neck (acquired) 596.0
- − congenital 753.6
- brain 348.8
- bronchus 519.1
- − syphilitic 095
- cardia (stomach) 537.8
- − congenital 750.7
- cardiovascular (see also Disease, cardiovascular) 429.2
- cervix, cervical (canal) 622.4
- − congenital 752.4
- − in pregnancy or childbirth 654.6
- − − causing obstructed labor 660.2
- − − − fetus or newborn 763.1
- − − fetus or newborn 763.8
- colon (see also Obstruction, intestine) 560.9
- − congenital 751.2
- colostomy 569.6
- common (bile) duct (see also Obstruction, biliary) 576.2
- coronary (artery) 414.0
- cystic duct (see also Obstruction, gallbladder) 575.2
- due to (presence of) any device, implant or graft classifiable to 996.0-996.5 996.7
- duodenum 537.3
- − congenital 751.1
- ejaculatory duct NEC 608.8
- endocervical os - see Stenosis, cervix
- enterostomy 569.6
- esophagus 530.3
- − congenital 750.3
- − syphilitic 095
- − − congenital 090.5
- external ear canal 380.5
- gallbladder (see also Obstruction, gallbladder) 575.2
- glottis 478.7
- heart valve - see also Endocarditis
- − congenital NEC 746.8
- hymen 623.3

Stenosis - *continued*
- infundibulum cardiac 746.8
- intestine (see also Obstruction, intestine) 560.9
- − congenital (small) 751.1
- − − large 751.2
- lacrimal duct, punctum or sac 375.5
- − congenital 743.6
- lacrimonasal duct 375.5
- − congenital 743.6
- larynx 478.7
- − congenital 748.3
- − syphilitic 095
- − − congenital 090.5
- mitral (chronic) (inactive) (valve) (see also Endocarditis, mitral) 394.0
- − with
- − − aortic valve disease 396
- − − incompetency, insufficiency or regurgitation 394.2
- − − − with aortic valve disease 396
- − active or acute 391.1
- − − with rheumatic or Sydenham's chorea 392.0
- − congenital 746.5
- − specified cause, except rheumatic 424.0
- − syphilitic 093.2 † 424.0*
- myocardium, myocardial (see also Degeneration, myocardial) 429.1
- nares (anterior) (posterior) 478.1
- − congenital 748.0
- nasal duct 375.5
- − congenital 743.6
- nasolacrimal duct 375.5
- − congenital 743.6
- oesophagus - see Stenosis, esophagus
- − congenital 750.3
- organ or site, congenital NEC - see Atresia
- pulmonary (artery) (congenital) 747.3
- − acquired 417.8
- − in tetralogy of Fallot 745.2
- − infundibular 746.8
- − valve (see also Endocarditis, pulmonary) 424.3
- − − congenital 746.0
- − vessel NEC 417.8
- pulmonic (congenital) 746.0
- pylorus (hypertrophic) 537.0
- − adult 537.0
- − congenital 750.5
- − infantile 750.5
- rectum (sphincter) (see also Stricture, rectum) 569.2
- renal artery 440.1
- salivary duct (any) 527.8

Stenosis - *continued*
- spinal 724.0
- - cervical 723.0
- stomach, hourglass 537.6
- subaortic 746.8
- - hypertrophic 425.1
- supra-aortic 747.2
- trachea 519.1
- - congenital 748.3
- - syphilitic 095
- - tuberculous 012.8
- tricuspid (valve) (see also Endocarditis, tricuspid) 397.0
- - congenital 746.1
- tubal 628.2
- ureter (see also Stricture, ureter) 593.3
- urethra (see also Stricture, urethra) 598.9
- vagina 623.2
- - congenital 752.4
- - in pregnancy or childbirth 654.7
- - - causing obstructed labor 660.2
- - - - fetus or newborn 763.1
- - - fetus or newborn 763.8
- valve (cardiac) (heart) (see also Endocarditis) 424.9
- - congenital NEC 746.8
- - - urethra 753.6
- vena cava (inferior) (superior) 459.2
- - congenital 747.4
- vulva 624.8
Stercolith (see also Fecalith) 560.3
- appendix 543
Stercoraceous, stercoral ulcer 569.8
- anus or rectum 569.4
Stereotypies NEC 307.3
Sterility
- female - see Infertility, female
- male 606
Sterilization, admission for V25.2
Sternalgia (see also Angina) 413
Sternopagus 759.4
Sternum bifidum 756.3
Steroid
- effects (adverse) (iatrogenic)
- - cushingoid
- - - correct substance properly administered 255.0
- - - overdose or wrong substance given or taken 962.0
- - diabetes
- - - correct substance properly administered 251.8
- - - overdose or wrong substance given or taken 962.0
- - due to
- - - correct substance properly administered 255.8

Steroid - *continued*
- effects - *continued*
- - due to - *continued*
- - - overdose or wrong substance given or taken 962.0
- - fever
- - - correct substance properly administered 780.6
- - - overdose or wrong substance given or taken 962.0
- - withdrawal
- - - correct substance properly administered 255.4
- - - overdose or wrong substance given or taken 962.0
- responder 365.0
Stevens-Johnson disease 695.1
Stewart-Morel syndrome 733.3
Sticker's disease 057.0
Sticky eye 372.0
Stiff neck (see also Torticollis) 723.5
Stiffness, joint 719.5
- ankle 719.5
- elbow 719.5
- finger 719.5
- hip 719.5
- knee 719.5
- multiple sites 719.5
- sacroiliac 724.6
- shoulder 719.5
- specified NEC 719.5
- spine 724.8
- surgical fusion except spine V45.4
- - spine V45.4
- wrist 719.5
Stigmata congenital syphilis 090.5
Still's disease or syndrome 714.3
Stillbirth NEC 779.9
Stilling's syndrome 378.7
Sting (animal) (bee) (fish) (insect) (jellyfish) (Portuguese man-o-war) (wasp) (venomous) 989.5
- anaphylactic shock or reaction 989.5
- plant 692.6
Stippled epiphyses 756.5
Stitch
- abscess 998.5
- burst (in operation wound) 998.3
- in back 724.5
Stokes' disease 242.0
Stokes-Adams syndrome 426.9
Stokvis(-Talma) disease 289.7
Stomach - see condition
Stomatitis 528.0
- angular 528.5
- - due to dietary or vitamin deficiency 266.0

Stomatitis - *continued*
- aphthous 528.2
- candidal 112.0
- denture 528.9
- diphtheritic 032.0
- due to thrush 112.0
- epidemic 078.4
- epizootic 078.4
- follicular 528.0
- gangrenous 528.1
- herpetic 054.2
- herpetiformis 528.2
- malignant 528.0
- membranous acute 528.0
- monilial 112.0
- mycotic 112.0
- necrotic 528.1
- necrotizing ulcerative 101
- parasitic 112.0
- septic 528.0
- spirochetal 101
- suppurative (acute) 528.0
- ulcerative 528.0
- ulceromembranous 101
- vesicular 528.0
- - with exanthem 074.3
- Vincent's 101
Stomatocytosis 282.8
Stomatomycosis 112.0
Stomatorrhagia 528.9
Stone(s) - see also Calculus
- bladder 594.1
- - diverticulum 594.0
- cystine 270.0
- kidney 592.0
- prostate 602.0
- pulp (dental) 522.2
- renal 592.0
- salivary duct or gland (any) 527.5
- ureter 592.1
- urethra (impacted) 594.2
- urinary (duct) (impacted) (passage) 592.9
- - bladder 594.1
- - - diverticulum 594.0
- - lower tract NEC 594.9
- xanthin 277.2
Stonecutters' lung 502
Stonemasons'
- asthma, disease, or lung 502
- phthisis 011.4
Stoppage
- bowel or intestine (see also Obstruction, intestine) 560.9
- heart (see also Arrest, cardiac) 427.5
- urine 788.2
Strabismus (alternating) (congenital) (nonparalytic) 378.9

Strabismus - *continued*
- concomitant NEC 378.3
- - convergent 378.0
- - divergent 378.1
- convergent 378.0
- divergent 378.1
- due to adhesions, scars 378.6
- intermittent 378.2
- latent 378.4
- mechanical 378.6
- paralytic 378.5
- vertical 378.3
Strain - see also Sprain
- eye NEC 368.1
- heart - see Disease, heart
- meaning gonorrhea - see Gonorrhea
- physical NEC V62.8
- postural 729.9
- psychological NEC V62.8
Strangulation, strangulated 994.7
- appendix 543
- asphyxiation or suffocation by 994.7
- bladder neck 596.0
- bowel - see Strangulation, intestine
- colon - see Strangulation, intestine
- cord (umbilical) - see Compression, umbilical cord
- food or foreign body (see also Asphyxia, food) 933.1
- hernia - see also Hernia, by site, with obstruction
- - gangrenous - see Hernia, by site, gangrenous
- intestine 560.2
- - with hernia - see also Hernia, by site, with obstruction
- - - gangrenous - see Hernia, by site, gangrenous
- - congenital (small) 751.1
- - - large 751.2
- mesentery 560.2
- mucus (see also Asphyxia, mucus) 933.1
- omentum 560.2
- organ or site, congenital NEC - see Atresia
- ovary 620.8
- penis 607.8
- - foreign body 939.3
- rupture 552.9
- - gangrenous 551.9
- stomach due to hernia (see also Hernia, by site, with obstruction) 552.9
- - gangrenous (see also Hernia, by site, gangrenous) 551.9
- umbilical cord - see Compression, umbilical cord
- vesico-urethral orifice 596.0

Strangury 788.1
Strawberry gallbladder (see also Disease,
  gallbladder) 575.6
Streak, ovarian 752.0
Strephosymbolia 315.0
− secondary to organic lesion 784.6
Streptobacillus moniliformis 026.1
Streptococcemia 038.0
Streptococcicosis 041.0
Streptococcus, streptococcal - see condition
Streptomycosis - see Actinomycosis
Streptothrix - see Actinomycosis
Streptotrichosis - see Actinomycosis
Stress reaction (acute) - see Reaction, stress,
  acute
Stretching, nerve - see Injury, nerve, by site
Striae
− albicantes 701.3
− atrophicae 701.3
− distensae (cutis) 701.3
Stricture 799.8
− anus (sphincter) 569.2
− − congenital 751.2
− − infantile 751.2
− aorta (ascending) (see also Stenosis,
  aorta) 747.2
− aortic (valve) (see also Stenosis, aortic)
  424.1
− − congenital 746.3
− aqueduct of Sylvius 742.3
− − with spina bifida 741.0
− − acquired 331.4
− artery 447.1
− − basilar - see Narrowing, artery, basilar
− − carotid - see Narrowing, artery, carotid
− − congenital (peripheral) 747.6
− − − cerebral 747.8
− − − coronary 746.8
− − − retinal 743.5
− − − umbilical 747.5
− − coronary 414.0
− − precerebral NEC - see Narrowing,
  artery, precerebral NEC
− − pulmonary 747.3
− − − acquired 417.8
− − vertebral - see Narrowing, artery,
  vertebral
− auditory canal (external) (congenital)
  744.0
− − acquired 380.5
− bile duct or passage (postoperative) (see
  also Obstruction, biliary) 576.2
− bladder 596.8
− − neck 596.0
− bowel (see also Obstruction, intestine)
  560.9
− bronchus 519.1

Stricture - continued
− bronchus - continued
− − syphilitic 095
− cardia (stomach) 537.8
− − congenital 750.7
− cardiac - see also Disease, heart
− − orifice (stomach) 537.8
− cecum (see also Obstruction, intestine)
  560.9
− cervix, cervical (canal) 622.4
− − congenital 752.4
− − in pregnancy or childbirth 654.6
− − − causing obstructed labor 660.2
− − − − fetus or newborn 763.1
− − − fetus or newborn 763.8
− colon (see also Obstruction, intestine)
  560.9
− − congenital 751.2
− common duct (see also Obstruction,
  biliary) 576.2
− coronary (artery) 414.0
− − congenital 746.8
− cystic duct (see also Obstruction,
  gallbladder) 575.2
− duodenum 537.3
− − congenital 751.1
− ear canal (external) (congenital) 744.0
− − acquired 380.5
− ejaculatory duct 608.8
− esophagus 530.3
− − congenital 750.3
− − syphilitic 095
− − − congenital 090.5
− eustachian tube 381.6
− − congenital 744.2
− fallopian tube 628.2
− − gonococcal 098.3 † 614.-*
− − tuberculous 016.4
− gallbladder or duct (see also Obstruction,
  gallbladder) 575.2
− glottis 478.7
− heart - see also Disease, heart
− − valve - see also Endocarditis
− − − congenital NEC 746.8
− hepatic duct (see also Obstruction,
  biliary) 576.2
− hourglass, of stomach 537.6
− hymen 623.3
− hypopharynx 478.2
− intestine (see also Obstruction, intestine)
  560.9
− − congenital (small) 751.1
− − − large 751.2
− − ischemic 557.1
− lacrimal apparatus 375.5
− − congenital 743.6
− larynx 478.7

Stricture - *continued*
- larynx - *continued*
- - congenital 748.3
- - syphilitic 095
- - - congenital 090.5
- lung 518.8
- meatus
- - ear (congenital) 744.0
- - - acquired 380.5
- - osseous (ear) (congenital) 744.0
- - - acquired 380.5
- - urinarius (see also Stricture, urethra) 598.9
- - - congenital 753.6
- mitral (valve) (see also Stenosis, mitral) 394.0
- - congenital 746.5
- nares (anterior) (posterior) 478.1
- - congenital 748.0
- nasal duct 375.5
- - congenital 743.6
- nasolacrimal duct 375.5
- - congenital 743.6
- nasopharynx 478.2
- - syphilitic 095
- nose 478.1
- nostril (anterior) (posterior) 478.1
- - congenital 748.0
- oesophagus 530.3
- - congenital 750.3
- - syphilitic 095
- - - congenital 090.5
- organ or site, congenital NEC - see Atresia
- os uteri (see also Stricture, cervix) 622.4
- osseous meatus (ear) (congenital) 744.0
- - acquired 380.5
- oviduct - see Stricture, fallopian tube
- pelviureteric junction 593.3
- pharynx (dilatation) 478.2
- prostate 602.8
- pulmonary
- - artery 747.3
- - - acquired 417.8
- - - noncongenital 417.8
- - valve (see also Endocarditis, pulmonary) 424.3
- - - congenital 746.0
- - vessel NEC 417.8
- punctum lacrimale 375.5
- - congenital 743.6
- pylorus (hypertrophic) 537.0
- - adult 537.0
- - congenital 750.5
- - infantile 750.5
- rectosigmoid 569.8
- rectum (sphincter) 569.2

Stricture - *continued*
- rectum - *continued*
- - congenital 751.2
- - due to
- - - chemical burn 947.3
- - - irradiation 569.2
- - - lymphogranuloma venereum 099.1
- - gonococcal 098.7
- - inflammatory 099.1
- - syphilitic 095
- - tuberculous 014
- renal artery 440.1
- salivary duct or gland (any) 527.8
- sigmoid (flexure) (see also Obstruction, intestine) 560.9
- spermatic cord 608.8
- stoma, following
- - colostomy 569.6
- - enterostomy 569.6
- - gastrostomy 997.4
- - tracheostomy 519.0
- stomach 537.8
- - congenital 750.7
- - hourglass 537.6
- subglottic 478.7
- syphilitic NEC 095
- tendon (sheath) 727.9
- trachea 519.1
- - congenital 748.3
- - syphilitic 095
- - tuberculous 012.8
- tricuspid (valve) (see also Endocarditis, tricuspid) 397.0
- - congenital 746.1
- tunica vaginalis 608.8
- ureter (postoperative) 593.3
- - congenital 753.2
- - tuberculous 016.1
- ureteropelvic junction 593.3
- - congenital 753.2
- ureterovesical orifice 593.3
- - congenital 753.2
- urethra (anterior) (meatal) (organic) (posterior) (spasmodic) 598.9
- - associated with schistosomiasis 120.- † 598.0*
- - congenital (valvular) 753.6
- - gonococcal 098.2 † 598.0*
- - gonorrheal 098.2 † 598.0*
- - infective 598.0
- - late effect of injury 598.1
- - postcatheterization 598.2
- - postobstetric 598.1
- - postoperative 598.2
- - specified cause NEC 598.8
- - syphilitic 095
- - traumatic 598.1

Stricture - *continued*
- urethra - *continued*
- - valvular, congenital 753.6
- urinary meatus 598.9
- - congenital 753.6
- uterus, uterine 621.5
- - os (external) (internal) - see Stricture, cervix
- vagina (outlet) 623.2
- - congenital 752.4
- valve (cardiac) (heart) (see also Endocarditis) 424.9
- - congenital (cardiac) (heart) NEC 746.8
- - - urethra 753.6
- vas deferens 608.8
- - congenital 752.8
- vein 459.2
- vena cava (inferior) (superior) NEC 459.2
- - congenital 747.4
- vesico-urethral orifice 596.0
- - congenital 753.6
- vulva (acquired) 624.8
Stridor 786.1
- congenital (larynx) 748.3
Stridulous - see condition
Stroke (see also Disease, cerebrovascular, acute) 436
- apoplectic (see also Disease, cerebrovascular, acute) 436
- brain (see also Disease, cerebrovascular, acute) 436
- epileptic - see Epilepsy
- heart - see Disease, heart
- heat 992.0
- lightning 994.0
- paralytic (see also Disease, cerebrovascular, acute) 436
Stromatosis, endometrial (M8931/1) 236.0
Strongyloides stercoralis infestation 127.2
Strongyloidiasis 127.2
Strongyloidosis 127.2
Strongylus (gibsoni) infestation 127.7
Strophulus 779.8
- pruriginosus 698.2
Struck by lightning 994.0
Struma (see also Goiter) 240.9
- Hashimoto 245.2
- lymphomatosa 245.2
- nodosa (simplex) 241.9
- - endemic 241.9
- - sporadic 241.9
- - toxicosa 242.3
- ovarii (M9090/0) 220
- - and carcinoid (M9091/1) 236.2
- - malignant (M9090/3) 183.0

Struma - *continued*
- Riedel's 245.3
- scrofulous 017.2
- tuberculous 017.2
- - abscess 017.2
- - adenitis 017.2
- - lymphangitis 017.2
- - ulcer 017.2
Strumipriva cachexia (see also Hypothyroidism) 244.9
Strumpell-Marie spine 720.0
Strumpell-Westphal pseudosclerosis 275.1
Stuart deficiency disease 286.3
Stuart-Prower factor deficiency (see also Defect, coagulation) 286.3
Student's elbow 727.2
Stupor 780.0
- catatonic 295.2
- circular - see Psychosis, manic-depressive, circular
- manic 296.6
- manic-depressive (see also Psychosis, manic-depressive) 296.6
- mental (anergic) (delusional) 298.9
- psychogenic 298.8
- reaction to exceptional stress (transient) 308.2
- traumatic NEC - see also Injury, intracranial
- - with spinal (cord)
- - - lesion - see Injury, spinal, by region
- - - shock - see Injury, spinal, by region
Sturge(-Weber)(-Dimitri) disease or syndrome 759.6
Sturge-Kalischer-Weber syndrome 759.6
Stuttering 307.0
Sty, stye 373.1
- external 373.1
- internal 373.1
- meibomian 373.1
Subacidity, gastric 536.8
- psychogenic 306.4
Subacute - see condition
Subarachnoid - see condition
Subcortical - see condition
Subcutaneous, subcuticular - see condition
Subdural - see condition
Subendocardium - see condition
Subependymoma (M9383/1) 237.5
Suberosis 495.3
Subglossitis - see Glossitis
Subinvolution (uterus) 621.1
- breast (postlactational) (postpartum) 611.8
- chronic 621.1
- puerperal 674.8
Sublingual - see condition

Sublinguitis 527.2
Subluxation - see also Dislocation
- congenital NEC - see also Malposition, congenital
- - hip 754.3
- - joint
- - - lower limb 755.6
- - - shoulder 755.5
- - - upper limb 755.5
- lens 379.3
- rotary, cervical region of spine - see Fracture, vertebra, cervical
Submaxillary - see condition
Submersion (fatal) (nonfatal) 994.1
Submucous - see condition
Subnormal accommodation 367.4

Subnormality, mental (see also Retardation, mental) 319
- mild 317
- moderate 318.0
- profound 318.2
- severe 318.1
Subphrenic - see condition
Subscapular nerve - see condition
Subseptus uterus 752.3

Substernal thyroid (see also Goiter) 240.9
- congenital 759.2
Substitution disorder 300.1
Subtentorial - see condition
Subthyroidism (acquired) (see also Hypothyroidism) 244.9
- congenital 243

Succenturiata placenta - see Placenta, abnormal
Sucking thumb, child 307.9
Sudamen, sudamina 705.1
Sudanese kala-azar 085.0
Sudden
- death, cause unknown 798.1
- - during childbirth 669.9
- - infant 798.0
- - puerperal, postpartum 674.9
- heart failure (see also Failure, heart) 428.9
- infant death syndrome 798.0

Sudeck's atrophy, disease, or syndrome 733.7
Suffocation - see also Asphyxia
- by
- - bed clothes 994.7
- - bunny bag 994.7
- - cave-in 994.7
- - constriction 994.7
- - drowning 994.1
- - inhalation

Suffocation - *continued*
- by - *continued*
- - inhalation - *continued*
- - - food or foreign body (see also Asphyxia, food or foreign body) 933.1
- - - gases, fumes, or vapors NEC 987.9
- - - - specified agent - see Table of drugs and chemicals
- - - oil or gasoline (see also Asphyxia, food or foreign body) 933.1
- - overlying 994.7
- - plastic bag 994.7
- - pressure 994.7
- - strangulation 994.7
- during birth 768.1
- mechanical 994.7
Sugar
- blood
- - high 790.2
- - low 251.2
- in urine 791.5
Suicide, suicidal (attempted)
- by poisoning - see Table of drugs and chemicals
- risk 300.9
- tendencies 300.9
- trauma NEC (see also Nature and site of injury) 959.9
Sulfatidosis 330.0
Sulfhemoglobinemia, sulphemoglobinemia (acquired) (congenital) 289.7
Summer - see condition
Sunburn 692.7
Sunken acetabulum 718.8
Sunstroke 992.0
Superfecundation 651.9
Superfetation 651.9
Superinvolution uterus 621.8
Supernumerary (congenital)
- aortic cusps 746.8
- auditory ossicles 744.0
- bone 756.9
- breast 757.6
- carpal bones 755.5
- cusps, heart valve NEC 746.8
- - pulmonary 746.0
- digit(s) 755.0
- ear 744.1
- fallopian tube 752.1
- finger 755.0
- hymen 752.4
- kidney 753.3
- lacrimonasal duct 743.6
- lobule (ear) 744.1
- muscle 756.8
- nipple(s) 757.6

Supernumerary - *continued*
- organ or site not listed - see Accessory
- ovary 752.0
- oviduct 752.1
- pulmonic cusps 746.0
- rib 756.3
- - cervical or first 756.2
- - - syndrome 756.2
- roots (of teeth) 520.2
- tarsal bones 755.6
- teeth 520.1
- - causing crowding 524.3
- testis 752.8
- thumb 755.0
- toe 755.0
- uterus 752.2
- vagina 752.4
- vertebra 756.1
Supervision (of)
- contraceptive method previously
  prescribed V25.4
- dietary (for) V65.3
- - allergy V65.3
- - colitis V65.3
- - diabetes mellitus V65.3
- - gastritis V65.3
- - hypercholesterolemia V65.3
- - hypoglycemia V65.3
- - intolerance V65.3
- - obesity V65.3
- lactation V24.1
- pregnancy - see Pregnancy, supervision of

Supplemental teeth 520.1
- causing crowding 524.3
Suppression
- lactation 676.5
- menstruation 626.8
- ovarian secretion 256.3
- renal 586
- urine, urinary secretion 788.5

Suppuration, suppurative - see also
  condition
- accessory sinus (chronic) (see also
  Sinusitis) 473.9
- adrenal (gland) 255.8
- antrum (chronic) (see also Sinusitis,
  maxillary) 473.0
- bladder (see also Cystitis) 595.8
- bowel 569.8
- brain 324.0
- breast 611.0
- - puerperal, postpartum 675.1
- dental periosteum 526.5
- ear (middle) NEC 382.4
- - external 380.1
- - internal 386.3

Suppuration - *continued*
- ethmoidal (chronic) (sinus) (see also
  Sinusitis, ethmoidal) 473.2
- fallopian tube (see also
  Salpingo-oophoritis) 614.2
- frontal (chronic) (sinus) (see also
  Sinusitis, frontal) 473.1
- gallbladder (see also Cholecystitis) 575.0
- gum 523.3
- hernial sac - see Hernia, by site
- intestine 569.8
- joint 711.0
- labyrinthine 386.3
- lung 513.0
- mammary gland 611.0
- - puerperal, postpartum 675.1
- maxilla, maxillary 526.4
- - sinus (chronic) (see also Sinusitis,
  maxillary) 473.0
- muscle 728.0
- nasal sinus (chronic) (see also Sinusitis)
  473.9
- pancreas 577.0
- parotid gland 527.2
- pelvis, pelvic
- - female (see also Disease, pelvis,
  inflammatory) 614.4
- - male (see also Peritonitis) 567.2
- pericranial (see also Osteomyelitis) 730.2
- salivary duct or gland (any) 527.2
- sinus (see also Sinusitis) 473.9
- sphenoidal (chronic) (sinus) (see also
  Sinusitis, sphenoidal) 473.3
- thymus (gland) 254.1
- thyroid (gland) 245.0
- tonsil 474.0
- uterus (see also Endometritis) 615.9
- wound - code as Wound, open,
  complicated
- - dislocation - code as Dislocation,
  compound
- - fracture - code as Fracture, open
- - scratch or other superficial injury -
  code as Injury, superficial, infected
Suprarenal (gland) - see condition
Suprascapular nerve - see condition
Suprasellar - see condition
Surfer knots 919.8
- infected 919.9
Surgery
- elective V50.9
- - specified type NEC V50.8
- not done - see Procedure, surgical, not
  done
- plastic
- - corrective, restorative V51
- - cosmetic V50.1

Surgery - *continued*
- plastic - *continued*
- - following healed injury or operation V51
- previous, in pregnancy or childbirth
- - cervix 654.6
- - - causing obstructed labor 660.2
- - - - fetus or newborn 763.1
- - pelvic soft tissues NEC 654.9
- - - causing obstructed labor 660.2
- - - - fetus or newborn 763.1
- - - fetus or newborn 763.8
- - perineum or vulva 654.8
- - uterus 654.2
- - - causing obstructed labor 660.2
- - - - fetus or newborn 763.1
- - vagina 654.7
Surgical
- abortion - see Abortion, therapeutic
- emphysema 998.8
- operation NEC 799.9
- procedures, complication or misadventure - see Complications, surgical procedures
- shock 998.0
Suspected condition, ruled out (see also Observation, suspected) V71.9
Suspended uterus
- in pregnancy or childbirth 654.4
- - causing obstructed labor 660.2
- - - fetus or newborn 763.1
- - fetus or newborn 763.8
Sutton and Gull's disease - see Hypertension, kidney
Sutton's disease 709.0
Suture
- burst (in operation wound) 998.3
- inadvertently left in operation wound 998.4
Swab inadvertently left in operation wound 998.4
Swallowed foreign body (see also Foreign body) 938
Swallowing difficulty (see also Dysphagia) 787.2
Swan neck hand (intrinsic) 736.0
Sweat, sweats
- fetid 705.8
- gland disease NEC 705.9
- night 780.8
Sweating
- disease or sickness 078.2
- excessive 780.8
- miliary 078.2
Swelling
- abdomen, abdominal (not referable to any particular organ) 789.3

Swelling - *continued*
- ankle 719.0
- arm 729.8
- Calabar 125.2
- cervical gland 785.6
- chest 786.6
- extremity (lower) (upper) 729.8
- finger 729.8
- foot 729.8
- glands 785.6
- hand 729.8
- head 784.2
- inflammatory - see Inflammation
- joint 719.0
- - tuberculous - see Tuberculosis, joint
- leg 729.8
- limb 729.8
- neck 784.2
- pelvic 789.3
- scrotum 608.8
- superficial, localized (skin) 782.2
- testis 608.8
- toe 729.8
- tubular (see also Disease, renal) 593.9
- wandering, due to Gnathostoma (spinigerum) 128.1
- white - see Tuberculosis, arthritis
Swift(-Feer) disease 985.0
Swimmers'
- ear 380.1
- itch 120.3
Swollen - see Swelling
Sycosis 704.8
- barbae (not parasitic) 704.8
- contagiosa 110.0
- lupoides 704.8
- mycotic 110.0
- parasitic 110.0
- vulgaris 704.8
Sydenham's chorea - see Chorea, Sydenham's
Symblepharon 372.6
- congenital 743.6
Sympathetic - see condition
Sympatheticotonia 337.9
Sympathicoblastoma (M9500/3)
- specified site - see Neoplasm, malignant
- unspecified site 194.0
Sympathicogonioma (M9500/3) - see Sympathicoblastoma
Sympathoblastoma (M9500/3) - see Sympathicoblastoma
Sympathogonioma (M9500/3) - see Sympathicoblastoma
Symphalangy 755.1
Symptoms specified NEC 780.9
- involving

Symptoms specified NEC - *continued*
- involving - *continued*
- - abdomen NEC 789.9
- - cardiovascular system NEC 785.9
- - chest NEC 786.9
- - digestive system NEC 787.9
- - head and neck NEC 784.9
- - musculoskeletal system NEC 781.9
- - nervous system NEC 781.9
- - nutrition, metabolism and delopment
   NEC 783.9
- - pelvis NEC 789.9
- - respiratory system NEC 786.9
- - skin and integument NEC 782.9
- - urinary system NEC 788.9
- neurotic 300.9
Sympus 759.8
Synarthrosis 719.8
Syncephalus 759.4
Synchondrosis, abnormal 756.9
Synchysis (vitreous humor) 379.2
- scintillans 379.2
- senile 379.2
Syncope 780.2
- bradycardia 427.8
- cardiac 780.2
- carotid sinus 337.0
- complicating delivery 669.2
- due to lumbar puncture 997.0
- fatal 798.1
- heart 780.2
- heat 992.1
- tussive 786.2
- vasoconstriction 780.2
Syndactylism, syndactyly (finger or toe)
   755.1
Syndrome - see also Disease
- abdominal
- - acute 789.0
- - migraine 346.2
- - muscle deficiency 756.8
- Achard-Thiers 255.2
- acute abdominal 789.0
- Adair-Dighton 756.5
- Adams-Stokes(-Morgagni) 426.9
- Adie(-Holmes) 379.4
- adiposogenital 253.8
- adrenal
- - hemorrhage 036.3 † 255.5*
- - meningococcic 036.3 † 255.5*
- adrenocortical 255.3
- adrenogenital (acquired) 255.2
- - congenital 255.2
- afferent loop NEC 537.8
- air blast concussion - see Injury, internal
- Albright(-McCune)(-Sternberg) 756.5
- alcohol withdrawal 291.8

Syndrome - *continued*
- Alder's 288.2
- Aldrich(-Wiskott) 279.1
- Alport's 759.8
- Alvarez 435
- alveolocapillary block 516.3
- amnestic (confabulatory) 291.1
- amyostatic 275.1
- angina (see also Angina) 413
- anterior
- - chest wall 786.5
- - spinal artery 435
- - - compression 721.1 † 336.3*
- - tibial (compartment) 958.8
- antibody deficiency 279.0
- - agammaglobulinemic 279.0
- - congenital 279.0
- - hypogammaglobulinemic 279.0
- anti-mongolism 758.3
- aortic
- - arch 446.7
- - bifurcation 444.0
- Apert's 755.5
- argentaffin 259.2
- Argyll Robertson's (syphilitic) 094.8 †
   379.4*
- - nonsyphilitic 379.4
- arm-shoulder (see also Neuropathy,
   peripheral, autonomic) 337.9
- Arnold-Chiari 741.0
- Arrillaga-Ayerza 416.0
- arteriomesenteric duodenum occlusion
   537.8
- aspiration, of newborn, massive or
   meconium 770.1
- ataxia-telangiectasia 334.8
- auriculotemporal 350.8
- autosomal - see also Abnormal,
   autosomes NEC
- - deletion 758.3
- Avellis' 344.8
- Ayerza's 416.0
- Baastrup's 721.5
- Babinski's 093.8
- Babinski-Nageotte 344.8
- Bagratuni's 446.5
- Banti's - see Cirrhosis, liver
- Baron Munchhausen 301.5
- Barre-Guillain 357.0
- Barre-Lieou 723.2
- basilar artery 435
- Bassen-Kornzweig 272.5
- battered baby or child 995.5
- Baumgarten-Cruveilhier 571.5
- Beckwith(-Wiedemann) 759.8
- Behcet's 136.1
- Benedikt's 344.8

Syndrome - *continued*
- Bernard-Horner 337.9
- Bernhardt-Roth 355.1
- Bernheim's (see also Failure, heart, congestive) 428.0
- Bertolotti's 756.1
- Bianchi's 784.6
- Biedl-Bardet 759.8
- Biemond's 759.8
- bilateral polycystic ovarian 256.4
- Bing-Horton's 346.2
- black widow spider bite 989.5
- Blackfan-Diamond 284.0
- blast (concussion) - see Blast, injury
- blind loop 579.2
- Bloch-Sulzberger 757.3
- Bloom(-MacHacek)(-Torre) 757.8
- blue diaper 270.0
- Bonnevie-Ullrich 758.6
- Bonnier's 386.1
- Bouillaud's 391.9
- Bouveret's 427.2
- brachial plexus 353.0
- brain (acute) (chronic) (organic) (nonpsychotic) (with neurotic reaction) (with behavioral reaction) 310.9
- - with presenile brain disease 290.1
- - chronic alcoholic 291.2
- - congenital - see Retardation, mental
- - post-traumatic
- - - nonpsychotic 310.2
- - - psychotic (see also Psychosis, organic) 294.9
- Brenneman's 289.2
- Briquet's 300.8
- broad ligament laceration 620.6
- Brock's 518.0
- Brown's sheath 378.6
- Brown-Sequard 344.8
- Brugsch's 757.3
- bubbly lung 770.7
- Budd-Chiari 453.0
- bulbar 335.2
- Burnett's 999.9
- burning feet 266.2
- Bywater's 958.5
- Caffey's 756.5
- Caplan 714.8 † 517.0*
- carcinoid 259.2
- cardiopulmonary-obesity 278.8
- cardiorenal 404.-
- cardiorespiratory distress (idiopathic), newborn 769
- cardiovascular renal 404.-
- carotid
- - artery (internal) 435
- - sinus 337.0

Syndrome - *continued*
- carpal tunnel 354.0
- Carpenter's 759.8
- cat-cry 758.3
- cauda equina 344.6
- causalgia 354.4
- cerebellomedullary malformation 741.0
- cervical (root) (spine) NEC 723.8
- - disc 722.7 † 336.3*
- - posterior, sympathicus 723.2
- - rib 756.2
- - sympathetic paralysis NEC 337.9
- - traumatic (acute) NEC 847.0
- cervicobrachial (diffuse) 723.3
- cervicocranial 723.2
- cervicodorsal outlet 353.2
- Cestan's 344.8
- Charcot's 443.9
- Charcot-Marie-Tooth 356.1
- Chediak-Higashi(-Steinbrink) 288.2
- Chiari's 453.0
- Chiari-Frommel 676.6
- child maltreatment (emotional) (nutritional) 995.5
- chromosome 4 short arm deletion 758.3
- Claude Bernard-Horner 337.9
- Claude's 352.6
- climacteric 627.2
- clumsiness 315.4
- Cockayne's 759.8
- coeliac artery compression 447.4
- Cogan's 370.5
- cold injury 778.2
- Collet(-Sicard) 352.6
- compartmental (anterior) (deep) (posterior) (tibial) 958.8
- compression 958.5
- - cauda equina 344.6
- concussion 310.2
- congenital
- - affecting more than one system NEC 759.8
- - facial diplegia 352.6
- - muscular hypertrophy-cerebral 759.8
- congestion-fibrosis (pelvic) 625.5
- Conn's 255.1
- conus medullaris 336.8
- coronary, insufficiency or intermediate (see also Insufficiency, coronary) 411
- Costen's 524.6
- costochondral junction 733.6
- costoclavicular 353.0
- craniovertebral 723.2
- Creutzfeldt-Jakob 046.1 † 331.5*
- - with dementia 290.1
- cri-du-chat 758.3
- Crigler-Najjar 277.4

Syndrome - *continued*
- crush 958.5
- Cruveilhier-Baumgarten 571.5
- Cushing's (iatrogenic) (idiopathic) (pituitary-dependent) 255.0
- da Costa's 306.2
- Dana-Putnam - see Degeneration, combined
- Dandy-Walker 742.3
- − − with spina bifida 741.0
- Danlos' 756.8
- de Lange's 759.8
- de Toni-Fanconi(-Debre) 270.0
- defibrination (see also Fibrinolysis) 286.6
- − − with
- − − − abortion - see categories 634-639 - fourth digit .1
- − − − ectopic gestation 639.1
- Dejerine-Roussy 348.8
- Dejerine-Thomas 333.0
- demyelinating NEC 341.9
- depersonalization 300.6
- Di George's 279.1
- diabetes-dwarfism-obesity 258.1
- diencephalohypophyseal NEC 253.8
- discogenic - see Displacement, intervertebral disc
- Donohue's 259.8
- dorsolateral medullary (see also Disease, cerebrovascular, acute) 436
- Down's 758.0
- Dressler's (see also Insufficiency, coronary) 411
- drug withdrawal, infant of dependent mother 779.5
- dry eye 375.1
- Duane's 378.7
- Dubin-Johnson 277.4
- Duchenne's 335.2
- due to abnormality
- − − autosomal NEC (see also Abnormal, autosomes NEC) 758.5
- − − − D1 758.1
- − − − E3 758.2
- − − − G 758.0
- − − − 13 758.1
- − − − 18 758.2
- − − − 21 or 22 758.0
- − − chromosomal 758.9
- − − − sex 758.8
- dumping (postgastrectomy) 564.2
- dyspraxia 315.4
- dystrophia dystocia 654.9
- ectopic ACTH 255.0
- Eddowes' 756.5
- Edward's 758.2
- efferent loop 537.8

Syndrome - *continued*
- effort (aviators') (psychogenic) 306.2
- Ehlers-Danlos 756.8
- Eisenmenger's 745.4
- Ekbom 333.9
- Ellison-Zollinger 251.5
- Ellis-van Creveld 756.5
- entrapment - see Neuropathy, entrapment
- epidemic vomiting 078.8
- Epstein's - see Nephrosis
- erythrocyte fragmentation 283.1
- exhaustion 300.5
- extrapyramidal 333.9
- eye retraction 378.7
- eyelid-malar-mandible 756.0
- Faber's 280
- facet 724.8
- falx (see also Hemorrhage, brain) 431
- familial eczema-thrombocytopenia 279.1
- Fanconi(-de Toni)(-Debre) 270.0
- fatigue 300.5
- Feil-Klippel 756.1
- Felty's 714.1
- first arch 756.0
- Fitzhugh-Curtis 098.8
- Forbes-Albright 253.1
- Foville's (peduncular) 344.8
- Franceschetti 756.0
- Fraser's 759.8
- Freeman Sheldon 759.8
- Frey's 350.8
- Friderichsen-Waterhouse 036.3 † 255.5*
- Frolich's 253.8
- Froin's 336.8
- Frommel-Chiari 676.6
- frontal lobe 310.0
- functional
- − − bowel 564.9
- − − prepuberal castrate 752.8
- ganglion (basal ganglion brain) 333.9
- Ganser's, hysterical 300.1
- Gardner-Diamond 287.2
- gastro-esophageal laceration-hemorrhage 530.7
- gastrojejunal loop obstruction 537.8
- Gelineau's 347
- genito-anorectal 099.1
- Gerhardt's 478.3
- Gilles de la Tourette 307.2
- glucuronyl transferase 277.4
- Goldberg-Maxwell 257.8
- Goldenhaar's 756.0
- Goldflam-Erb 358.0
- Goodpasture's 446.2
- Gopalan's 266.2
- Gorlin-Chaudry-Moss 759.8

Syndrome - *continued*
- Gougerot-Carteaud 701.8
- Gradenigo's 382.0
- gray or grey (newborn) 779.4
- Guerin-Stern 754.8
- Guillain-Barre(-Strohl) 357.0
- Gunn's 742.8
- gustatory sweating 350.8
- Hallerman-Streiff 756.0
- Hamman-Rich 516.3
- Hand-Schuller-Christian 277.8
- Hanot-Chauffard(-Troisier) 275.0
- Harada's 363.2
- harlequin color-change 757.3
- Hayem-Widal 283.9
- Hegglin's 288.2
- Heller's 299.1
- hemolytic-uremic 283.1
- Henoch(-Schonlein) 287.0
- hepatic flexure 569.8
- hepatorenal 572.4
- - following delivery 674.8
- - specified due to a procedure 997.4
- Herter-Gee 579.0
- Heyd's 572.4
- Hoffman's 244.9 † 359.5*
- Hoffmann-Bouveret 427.2
- Horner's 337.9
- - traumatic 954.0
- Hunt's 053.1 † 351.1*
- - dyssynergia cerebellaris myoclonica 334.2
- - herpetic geniculate ganglionitis 053.1 † 351.1*
- Hunter-Hurler 277.5
- Hurler's (in bones) 277.5
- Hutchinson-Boeck 135
- Hutchinson-Gilford 259.8
- hydralazine
- - correct substance properly administered 695.4
- - overdose or wrong substance given or taken 972.6
- hydraulic concussion (abdominal) (see also Injury, internal, abdomen) 868.0
- hyperabduction 447.8
- hyperkalemic 276.7
- hyperkinetic - see also Hyperkinesia
- - heart 429.8
- hypermobility 728.5
- hypersomnia-bulimia 349.8
- hypersympathetic 337.9
- hyperventilation 306.1
- hypokalemic 276.8
- hypopituitarism 253.2
- hypoplastic left-heart 746.7
- hypopotassemia 276.8

Syndrome - *continued*
- hypotension, maternal 669.2
- idiopathic cardiorespiratory distress, newborn 769
- Imerslund(-Grasbeck) 281.1
- immobility (paraplegic) 728.3
- immunity deficiency, combined 279.2
- inappropriate secretion of antidiuretic hormone 253.6
- infant of diabetic mother 775.0
- infantilism 253.3
- inferior vena cava 459.2
- influenza-like 487.1
- intermediate coronary (see also Insufficiency, coronary) 411
- interspinous ligament 724.8
- irritable
- - bowel 564.1
- - heart 306.2
- - weakness 300.5
- Jaccoud's 714.4
- Jackson's 344.8
- Jaffe-Lichtenstein 252.0
- Jakob-Creutzfeldt 046.1 † 331.5*
- - with dementia 290.1
- Jaybi's 759.8
- jugular foramen 352.6
- Kanner's 299.0
- Kartagener's 759.3
- Kast's 756.4
- Kimmelstiel-Wilson 250.3 † 581.8*
- Kleine-Levin 349.8
- Klein-Wardenburg 270.2
- Klinefelter's 758.7
- Klippel-Feil 756.1
- Klippel-Trenaunay 759.8
- Klumpke(-Dejerine) 767.6
- Korsakoff's (nonalcoholic) 294.0
- - alcoholic 291.1
- labyrinthine 386.5
- Langdon Down 758.0
- Larsen's 755.8
- lateral
- - cutaneous nerve of thigh 355.1
- - medullary (see also Disease, cerebrovascular, acute) 436
- Launois' 253.0
- Laurence-Moon(-Biedl) 759.8
- Legg-Calve-Perthes 732.1
- lenticular 275.1
- Leriche's 444.0
- Leri-Weill 756.5
- Lermoyez's 386.0
- Lesch-Nyhan 277.2
- Lichtheim's - see Degeneration, combined

Syndrome - *continued*
- otolith 386.1
- oto-palatal-digital 759.8
- pain - see Pain
- papillary muscle (see also Infarct, myocardium) 410
- Papillon-Leage and Psaume 759.8
- paralysis agitans 332.0
- paralytic 344.9
- − specified NEC 344.8
- Parinaud's 378.8
- − oculoglandular 372.0
- Parkinson's (see also Parkinsonism) 332.0
- parkinsonian (see also Parkinsonism) 332.0
- Parry-Romberg 349.8
- Parsonage-Aldren-Turner 353.5
- Patau's 758.1
- Paterson(-Brown)(-Kelly) 280
- Pelger-Huet 288.2
- pellagroid 265.2
- Pellegrini-Stieda 726.6
- Pellizzi's 259.8
- pelvic congestion-fibrosis 625.5
- Pendred's 243
- penta X 758.8
- peptic ulcer - see Ulcer, peptic
- periodic 277.3
- Petges-Clejat or Petges-Clegat 710.3
- Peutz-Jeghers 759.6
- phantom limb 353.6
- Pick's
- − heart 423.2
- − liver 423.2
- Pickwickian 278.8
- Pierre Robin 756.0
- pineal 259.8
- placental
- − dysfunction 762.2
- − insufficiency 762.2
- − transfusion 762.3
- Plummer-Vinson 280
- pluricarential of infancy 260
- plurideficiency 260
- pluriglandular (compensatory) 258.8
- polycarential of infancy 260
- polyglandular 258.8
- pontine 348.8
- popliteal web 756.8
- post-artificial-menopause 627.4
- postcardiotomy 429.4
- postcholecystectomy 576.0
- postcommissurotomy 429.4
- postconcussional 310.2
- postcontusional 310.2
- postencephalitic 310.8

Syndrome - *continued*
- posterior cervical sympathicus 723.2
- postgastrectomy (dumping) 564.2
- postgastric surgery 564.2
- postinfarction (see also Insufficiency, coronary) 411
- postlaminectomy 722.8
- postleukotomy 310.0
- postmastectomy lymphedema 457.0
- postmyocardial infarct (see also Insufficiency, coronary) 411
- postoperative NEC 998.9
- postpartum panhypopituitary 253.2
- postphlebitic 459.1
- postvagotomy 564.2
- postvalvulotomy 429.4
- postviral NEC 780.7
- potassium intoxication 276.7
- Potter's 753.0
- pre-infarction (see also Insufficiency, coronary) 411
- premature senility 259.8
- premenstrual tension 625.4
- Profichet's 729.9
- progressive pallidal degeneration 333.0
- prune belly 756.7
- pseudoturner's 759.8
- psycho-organic 293.9
- − acute 293.0
- − nonpsychotic severity 310.1
- − − specified focal (partial) NEC 310.8
- − subacute 293.1
- pulmonary
- − arteriosclerosis 416.0
- − renal (hemorrhagic) 446.2
- pulseless 446.7
- pyloroduodenal 537.8
- pyramidopallidonigral 332.0
- radicular NEC 729.2
- − lower limbs 724.4
- − upper limbs 723.4
- − − newborn 767.4
- Ramsey Hunt's - see Syndrome, Hunt's
- Raymond(-Cestan) 433.8
- Raynaud 443.0
- Refsum's 356.3
- Reiter's 099.3
- Rendu-Osler-Weber 448.0
- Renon-Delille 253.8
- respiratory distress (idiopathic) (newborn) 769
- − adult 518.5
- restless legs 333.9
- retraction 378.7
- Reye's 331.8
- Rieger's 743.4

Syndrome - *continued*
- trisomy NEC - *continued*
- - G 758.0
- - 13 or D(1) 758.1
- - 18 or E(3) 758.2
- - 20 758.5
- - 21 758.0
- - 22 758.0
- tropical wet feet 991.4
- Turck's 378.7
- Turner(-Varny) 758.6
- twin (to twin) transfusion 762.3
- Ullrich(-Bonnevie)(-Turner) 758.6
- Ullrich-Feichtiger 759.8
- underwater blast injury (abdominal) (see also Injury, internal, abdomen) 868.0
- Unverricht(-Lundborg) 333.2
- Unverricht-Wagner 710.3
- upward gaze 378.8
- uremia, chronic 585
- urethral 597.8
- urethro-oculo-articular 099.3
- urohepatic 572.4
- vago-hypoglossal 352.6
- van der Hoeve's 756.5
- vasomotor 443.9
- vasovagal 780.2
- VATER 759.8
- vena cava (inferior) (superior) (obstruction) 459.2
- Vernet's 352.6
- vertebral
- - artery 435
- - - compression 721.1 † 336.3*
- - lumbar 724.4
- - steal 435
- vertebrogenic (pain) 724.5
- vertiginous NEC 386.9
- Villaret's 352.6
- Vinson-Plummer 280
- virus 079.9
- visceral larva migrans 128.0
- visual disorientation 368.8
- vitamin B6 deficiency 266.1
- vitreous touch 997.9
- Vogt's 333.7
- Vogt-Koyanagi 364.2
- von Bechterew-Strumpell 720.0
- von Hippel(-Lindau) 759.6
- Wagner-Unverricht 710.3
- Waldenstrom's (macroglobulinemia) 273.3
- Wallenberg's (see also Disease, cerebrovascular, acute) 436
- Wardenburg-Klein 270.2
- Waterhouse(-Friderichsen) 036.3 † 255.5*

Syndrome - *continued*
- Weber's 344.8
- Weber-Christian 729.3
- Weber-Cockayne 757.3
- Weber-Gubler 344.8
- Weber-Leyden 344.8
- Weber-Osler 448.0
- Wegener's 446.4
- Weingarten's 518.3
- Weiss-Baker 337.0
- Werdnig-Hoffmann 335.0
- Wermer's 258.0
- Werner 259.8
- Wernicke's 265.1
- Westphal-Strumpell 275.1
- whiplash 847.0
- whistling face 759.8
- Wilkinson-Sneddon 694.1
- Wilson's 275.1
- Wilson-Mikity 770.7
- Wiskott-Aldrich 279.1
- withdrawal
- - alcohol 291.8
- - drug 292.0
- - - infant of dependent mother 779.5
- Woakes 471.1
- Wolff-Parkinson-White 426.7
- Wright 447.8
- xiphoidalgia 733.9
- XO 758.6
- XXXXY 758.8
- XXY 758.7
- yellow vernix - see Distress, fetal
- Zieve's 571.1
- Zollinger-Ellison 251.5
Synechia (anterior) (posterior) (pupil) 364.7
- intra-uterine 621.5
Synesthesia (see also Disturbance, sensation) 782.0
Synodontia 520.2
Synophthalmus 759.8
Synorchidism 752.8
Synorchism 752.8
Synostosis (congenital) 756.5
- astragalo-scaphoid 755.6
- radio-ulnar 755.5
Synovial - see condition
Synovioma (malignant) (M9040/3) - see also Neoplasm, connective tissue, malignant
- benign (M9040/0) - see Neoplasm, connective tissue, benign
Synoviosarcoma (M9040/3) - see Neoplasm, connective tissue, malignant
Synovitis 727.0
- chronic crepitant, wrist 727.2

Synovitis - *continued*
- due to
- - crystals - see Arthritis, due to crystals
- gonococcal 098.5 † 727.0*
- gouty 274.0 † 712.0*
- syphilitic 095
- - congenital 090.0
- traumatic, current - see Sprain
- tuberculous - see Tuberculosis, synovitis
- villonodular 719.2
Syphilide 091.3
- congenital 090.0
- newborn 090.0
- tubercular 095
- - congenital 090.0
Syphilis, syphilitic (acquired) 097.9
- abdomen (late) 095
- acoustic nerve 094.8
- adenopathy (secondary) 091.4
- adrenal (gland) 095
- - with cortical hypofunction 095
- age under 2 years NEC (see also Syphilis, congenital) 090.9
- - acquired 097.9
- alopecia (secondary) 091.8
- anemia 095
- aneurysm (artery) (ruptured) 093.8
- - aorta 093.0 † 441.7*
- - central nervous system 094.8
- - congenital 090.5
- anus 095
- - primary 091.1
- - secondary 091.3
- aorta (arch) (abdominal) (pulmonary) (thoracic) 093.8
- - aneurysm 093.0 † 441.7*
- aortic (insufficiency) (regurgitation) (stenosis) 093.8
- - aneurysm 093.0 † 441.7*
- arachnoid (adhesive) 094.2 † 320.7*
- artery 093.8
- - cerebral 094.8
- - spinal 094.8
- asymptomatic - see Syphilis, latent
- ataxia (locomotor) 094.0
- atrophoderma maculatum 091.3
- auricular fibrillation 093.8
- Bell's palsy 094.8
- bladder 095
- bone 095 † 730.8*
- - secondary 091.6
- brain 094.8
- breast 095
- bronchus 095
- bubo 091.0
- bulbar palsy 094.8
- bursa (late) 095

Syphilis - *continued*
- cardiac decompensation 093.8
- cardiovascular (early) (late) (primary) (secondary) (tertiary) 093.9
- - specified type and site NEC 093.8
- causing death under 2 years of age (see also Syphilis, congenital) 090.9
- - stated to be acquired NEC 097.9
- central nervous system (early) (late) (latent) (primary) (recurrent) (relapse) (secondary) (tertiary) 094.9
- - with
- - - ataxia 094.0
- - - paralysis general 094.1
- - - - juvenile 090.4
- - - paresis (general) 094.1
- - - - juvenile 090.4
- - - tabes (dorsalis) 094.0
- - - - juvenile 090.4
- - - taboparesis 094.1
- - - - juvenile 090.4
- - aneurysm 094.8
- - congenital 090.4
- - juvenile 090.4
- - remission in (sustained) 094.9
- - serology doubtful, negative, or positive 094.9
- - specified nature or site NEC 094.8
- - vascular 094.8
- cerebral 094.8
- - meningovascular 094.2 † 320.7*
- - nerves 094.8
- - sclerosis 094.8
- - thrombosis 094.8
- cerebrospinal 094.8
- - tabetic type 094.0
- cerebrovascular 094.8
- cervix 095
- chancre (multiple) 091.0
- - extragenital 091.2
- - Rollet's 091.0
- Charcot's joint 094.0 † 713.5*
- choked disc 094.8 † 377.0*
- chorioretinitis 091.5 † 363.1*
- - late 095 † 363.1*
- choroiditis - see Syphilitic chorioretinitis
- choroidoretinitis - see Syphilitic chorioretinitis
- ciliary body (secondary) 091.5 † 364.1*
- - late 095 † 364.1*
- colon (late) 095
- combined sclerosis 094.8
- complicating pregnancy, childbirth or puerperium 647.0
- - fetus or newborn 760.2
- condyloma (latum) 091.3
- congenital 090.9

Syphilis - *continued*
- congenital - *continued*
- − with
- − − − paresis (general) 090.4
- − − − tabes (dorsalis) 090.4
- − − − taboparesis 090.4
- − − chorioretinitis, choroiditis 090.0 †
  363.1*
- − − early, or less than 2 years after birth
  NEC 090.2
- − − − with manifestations 090.0
- − − − latent (without manifestations)
  090.1
- − − − − negative spinal fluid test 090.1
- − − − − serology, positive 090.1
- − − − symptomatic 090.0
- − − interstitial keratitis 090.3 † 370.5*
- − − juvenile neurosyphilis 090.4
- − − late, or 2 years or more after birth
  NEC 090.7
- − − − chorioretinitis, choroiditis 090.5 †
  363.1*
- − − − interstitial keratitis 090.3 † 370.5*
- − − − juvenile neurosyphilis 090.4
- − − − latent (without manifestations)
  090.6
- − − − − negative spinal fluid test 090.6
- − − − − serology, positive 090.6
- − − − symptomatic or with manifestations
  NEC 090.5
- conjugal 097.9
- − tabes 094.0
- conjunctiva 095 † 372.1*
- cord bladder 094.0
- cornea, late 095 † 370.5*
- coronary (artery) 093.8
- − sclerosis 093.8
- cranial nerve 094.8
- cutaneous - see Syphilis, skin
- d'emblee 095
- dacryocystitis 095 † 375.4*
- degeneration, spinal cord 094.8
- dementia
- − paralytica 094.1
- − − juvenilis 090.4
- destruction of bone 095 † 730.8*
- dilatation, aorta 093.0 † 441.7*
- due to blood transfusion 097.9
- dura mater 094.8
- ear 095
- − inner 095
- − − nerve (eighth) 094.8
- − − neurorecurrence 094.8
- early NEC 091.0
- − cardiovascular 093.9
- − central nervous system 094.9
- − − paresis 094.1

Syphilis - *continued*
- early NEC - *continued*
- − − central nervous system - *continued*
- − − − tabes 094.0
- − − latent (without manifestations) (less
  than 2 years after infection) 092.9
- − − − negative spinal fluid test 092.9
- − − − serological relapse after treatment
  092.0
- − − − serology positive 092.9
- − − paresis 094.1
- − − relapse (treated, untreated) 091.7
- − − skin 091.3
- − − symptomatic NEC 091.8
- − − − extragenital chancre 091.2
- − − − primary, except extragenital chancre
  091.0
- − − − secondary (see also Syphilis,
  secondary) 091.3
- − − − − relapse (treated, untreated) 091.7
- − − tabes 094.0
- − − ulcer 091.3
- eighth nerve 094.8
- endocarditis 093.2 † 424.9*
- − aortic 093.2 † 424.1*
- − pulmonary 093.2 † 424.3*
- epididymis (late) 095
- epiglottis 095
- epiphysitis (congenital) 090.0
- esophagus 095
- eustachian tube 095
- eye 095 † 363.1*
- eyelid 095 † 373.5*
- − with gumma 095 † 373.5*
- − ptosis 094.8 † 374.3*
- fallopian tube 095
- fracture 095 † 730.8*
- gallbladder (late) 095
- gastric 095
- − crisis 094.0
- − polyposis 095
- general 097.9
- − paralysis 094.1
- − − juvenile 090.4
- genital (primary) 091.0
- gumma NEC 095
- − cardiovascular system 093.9
- − central nervous system 094.9
- − congenital 090.5
- heart 093.8
- − block 093.8
- − decompensation 093.8
- − disease 093.8
- − failure 093.8
- − valve NEC 093.2 † 424.9*
- hemianesthesia 094.8
- hemianopsia 095 † 368.4*

Syphilis - *continued*
– hemiparesis 094.8
– hemiplegia 094.8ˑ
– hepatic artery 093.8
– hepatis 095 † 573.2*
– hereditaria tarda (see also Syphilis, congenital, late) 090.7
– hereditary (see also Syphilis, congenital) 090.9
– – interstitial keratitis 090.3 † 370.5*
– hyalitis 095 † 379.2*
– inactive - see Syphilis, latent
– infantum NEC 090.9

– inherited - see Syphilis, congenital
– internal ear 095
– intestine (late) 095
– iris, iritis (secondary) 091.5 † 364.1*
– – late 095 † 364.1*
– joint (late) 095
– keratitis (congenital) (interstitial) (early) (late) 090.3 † 370.5*
– kidney 095 † 583.8*
– lacrimal passages 095 † 375.4*

– laryngeal paralysis 095
– larynx 095
– late 097.0
– – cardiovascular 093.9
– – central nervous system 094.9
– – latent or 2 years or more after infection (without manifestations) 096
– – – negative spinal fluid test 096
– – – serology positive 096
– – paresis 094.1
– – specified site NEC 095
– – symptomatic or with symptoms 095
– – tabes 094.0
– latent 097.1
– – central nervous system 094.9
– – date of infection unspecified 097.1
– – early, or less than 2 years after infection 092.9
– – late, or 2 years or more after infection 096
– – serology
– – – doubtful
– – – – with signs or symptoms - code by site and stage under Syphilis
– – – – follow-up of latent syphilis 097.1
– – – – – central nervous system 094.9
– – – – – date of infection unspecified 097.1
– – – – – early, or less than 2 years after infection 092.9
– – – – – late, or 2 years or more after infection 096
– – – positive, only finding 097.1

Syphilis - *continued*
– latent - *continued*
– – serology - *continued*
– – – positive - *continued*
– – – – date of infection unspecified 097.1
– – – – early, or less than 2 years after infection 097.1
– – – – late, or 2 years or more after infection 097.1
– lens 095
– leukoderma 091.3
– – late 095
– lienis 095
– lip 091.3
– – chancre 091.2
– – late 095
– – primary 091.2
– Lissauer's paralysis 094.1
– liver 095 † 573.2*
– – secondary 091.6 † 573.2*
– locomotor ataxia 094.0
– lung 095 † 517.8*
– lymph gland (early) (secondary) 091.4
– – late 095
– lymphadenitis (secondary) 091.4
– macular atrophy of skin 091.3
– – striated 095
– maternal, affecting fetus or newborn 760.2
– – manifest syphilis in infant - see category 090
– mediastinum (late) 095
– meninges (adhesive) (brain) (spinal cord) 094.2 † 320.7*
– meningitis 094.2 † 320.7*
– – acute 091.8 † 320.7*
– – congenital 090.4 † 320.7*
– meningo-encephalitis 094.2 † 320.7*
– meningovascular 094.2 † 320.7*
– – congenital 090.4 † 320.7*
– mesarteritis 093.8
– – brain 094.8
– – spine 094.8
– middle ear 095
– mitral stenosis 093.2 † 424.0*
– monoplegia 094.8
– mouth (secondary) 091.3
– – late 095
– mucocutaneous 091.3
– – late 095
– mucous
– – membrane 091.3
– – – late 095
– – patches 091.3
– – – congenital 090.0
– muscle 095 † 728.0*

Syphilis - *continued*
- myocardium 093.8 † 422.0*
- nasal sinus 095
- neonatorum NEC 090.9
- nerve palsy (any cranial nerve) 094.8
- nervous system, central 094.9
- neuritis 095
- neurorecidive of retina 094.8 † 363.1*
- neuroretinitis 094.8 † 363.1*
- nodular superficial 095
- nonvenereal endemic 104.0
- nose 095
- − saddle back deformity 090.5
- − septum 095
- − − perforated 095
- occlusive arterial disease 093.8
- oesophagus 095
- ophthalmic 095 † 363.1*
- ophthalmoplegia 094.8 † 378.5*
- optic nerve (atrophy) (neuritis) (papilla) 094.8 † 377.1*
- orbit (late) 095 † 376.1*
- organic 097.9
- osseous (late) 095 † 730.8*
- osteochondritis (congenital) 090.0
- osteoporosis 095 † 730.8*
- ovary 095
- oviduct 095
- palate 095
- pancreas (late) 095
- pancreatitis 095
- paralysis 094.8
- − general 094.1
- − juvenile 090.4
- paresis (general) 094.1
- − juvenile 090.4
- paresthesia 094.8
- Parkinson's disease or syndrome 094.8 † 332.1*
- paroxysmal tachycardia 093.8
- pemphigus (congenital) 090.0
- penis 091.0
- − chancre 091.0
- − late 095
- pericardium 093.8 † 420.0*
- perichondritis, larynx 095
- periosteum 095 † 730.8*
- − congenital 090.0 † 730.8*
- − early 091.6 † 730.3*
- − secondary 091.6 † 730.3*
- peripheral nerve 095
- petrous bone (late) 095 † 730.8*
- pharynx 095
- − secondary 091.3
- pituitary (gland) 095
- placenta 095
- pleura (late) 095

Syphilis - *continued*
- pontine lesion 094.8
- portal vein 093.8
- primary NEC 091.2
- − anal 091.1
- − and secondary (see also Syphilis, secondary) 091.9
- − cardiovascular 093.9
- − central nervous system 094.9
- − extragenital chancre NEC 091.2
- − fingers 091.2
- − genital 091.0
- − lip 091.2
- − specified site NEC 091.2
- − tonsils 091.2
- prostate 095
- ptosis (eyelid) 094.8 † 374.3*
- pulmonary (late) 095 † 517.8*
- − artery 093.8
- pulmonum 095 † 517.8*
- pyelonephritis 095 † 590.8*
- recently acquired, symptomatic NEC 091.8
- rectum 095
- respiratory tract 095
- retina
- − late 095 † 363.1*
- − neurorecidive 094.8 † 363.1*
- retrobulbar neuritis 094.8 † 377.3*
- salpingitis 095
- sclera (late) 095 † 379.0*
- sclerosis
- − cerebral 094.8
- − coronary 093.8
- − multiple 094.8
- − subacute 094.8
- scotoma (central) 095 † 368.4*
- scrotum 095
- secondary (and primary) 091.9
- − adenopathy 091.4
- − anus 091.3
- − bone 091.6
- − cardiovascular 093.9
- − central nervous system 094.9
- − chorioretiniis, choroiditis 091.5 † 363.1*
- − hepatitis 091.6 † 573.2*
- − liver 091.6 † 573.2*
- − lymphadenitis 091.4
- − meningitis, acute 091.8 † 320.7*
- − mouth 091.3
- − mucous membranes 091.3
- − periosteum 091.6 † 730.3*
- − periostitis 091.6 † 730.3*
- − pharynx 091.3
- − relapse (treated, untreated) 091.7
- − skin 091.3

Syringoma - *continued*
- chondroid (M8940/0) - see Neoplasm, benign
Syringomyelia 336.0
Syringomyelitis (see also Encephalitis) 323.9
Syringomyelocele 741.9
- with hydrocephalus 741.0

Syringopontia 336.0
System, systemic - see also condition
- disease, combined - see Degeneration, combined
- lupus erythematosis 710.0
- - inhibitor 286.6

T

Tab - see Tag
Tabacism 989.8
Tabacosis 989.8
Tabardillo 080
 - flea-borne 081.0
 - louse-borne 080
Tabes, tabetic
 - with
 - - central nervous system syphilis 094.0
 - - Charcot's joint 094.0 † 713.5*
 - - cord bladder 094.0
 - - crisis, viscera (any) 094.0
 - - paralysis, general 094.1
 - - paresis (general) 094.1
 - - perforating ulcer 094.0
 - arthropathy 094.0 † 713.5*
 - bladder 094.0
 - bone 094.0
 - cerebrospinal 094.0
 - congenital 090.4
 - conjugal 094.0
 - dorsalis 094.0
 - - neurosyphilis 094.0
 - early 094.0
 - juvenile 090.4
 - latent 094.0
 - mesenterica 014
 - paralysis insane, general 094.1
 - spasmodic 094.0
 - - not dorsal or dorsalis 343.9
 - syphilis (cerebrospinal) 094.0
Taboparalysis 094.1
Taboparesis (remission) 094.1
 - with
 - - Charcot's joint 094.1 † 713.5*
 - - cord bladder 094.1
 - - perforating ulcer 094.1
 - juvenile 090.4
Tachycardia 785.0
 - atrial 427.8
 - auricular 427.8
 - nodal 427.8
 - paroxysmal 427.2
 - - atrial 427.0
 - - atrioventricular (AV) 427.0
 - - junctional 427.0
 - - nodal 427.0
 - - supraventricular 427.0
 - - ventricular 427.1
 - psychogenic 306.2

Tachycardia - *continued*
 - sick sinus 427.8
 - sinoauricular 427.8
 - sinus 427.8
 - supraventricular 427.8
 - ventricular 427.1
Tachypnea 786.0
 - hysterical 300.1
 - psychogenic 306.1
 - transitory, of newborn 770.6
Taenia (infection) (infestation) (see also Infestation, taenia) 123.3
 - diminuta 123.6
 - nana 123.6
 - saginata 123.2
 - solium (intestinal form) 123.0
 - - larval form 123.1
Taeniasis (intestine) (see also Infestation, taenia) 123.3
Taenzer's disease 757.4
Tag (hypertrophied skin) (infected) 701.9
 - adenoid 474.8
 - anus 455.9
 - hemorrhoidal 455.9
 - hymen 623.8
 - perineal 624.8
 - rectum 455.9
 - skin 701.9
 - - accessory 757.3
 - - congenital 757.3
 - tonsil 474.8
 - urethra, urethral 599.8
 - vulva 624.8
Tahyna fever 062.5 † 323.3*
Takayasu's disease or syndrome 446.7
Talipes (congenital) 754.7
 - acquired (any type except planus) 736.7
 - asymmetric 754.7
 - calcaneovalgus 754.6
 - calcaneovarus 754.5
 - calcaneus 754.7
 - cavus 754.7
 - equinovalgus 754.6
 - equinovarus 754.5
 - equinus 754.7
 - percavus 754.7
 - planovalgus 754.6
 - planus (acquired) (any degree) 734
 - - congenital 754.6
 - - due to rickets 268.1

Talipes - *continued*
- valgus 754.6
- varus 754.5
Talma's disease 728.8
Tamponade heart (see also Pericarditis)
  423.9
Tanapox 078.8
Tangier disease 272.5
Tantrum (childhood) 312.0

Tapeworm (infection) (infestation) (see also
  Infestation, tapeworm) 123.9
Tapia's syndrome 352.6
Tarsalgia 729.2
Tarsitis (eyelid) 373.8
- syphilitic 095 † 373.8*
- tuberculous 017.0 † 373.4*
Tartar (teeth) 523.6
Tattoo (mark) 709.0
Taurodontism 520.2
Taussig-Bing heart or syndrome 745.1

Taybi's syndrome 759.8
Taylor's disease 701.8
Tay-Sachs
- amaurotic familial idiocy 330.1
- disease 330.1
Tear, torn (traumatic) - see also Wound,
  open
- anus, anal (sphincter) 863.8
- - with open wound into cavity 863.9
- - complicating delivery 664.2
- - - with mucosa 664.3
- - nontraumatic, nonpuerperal 565.0
- articular cartilage, old 718.0
- bladder
- - complicating abortion - see categories
    634-639, fourth digit .2
- - obstetrical trauma 665.5
- bowel
- - complicating abortion - see categories
    634-639, fourth digit .2
- - obstetrical trauma 665.5
- broad ligament
- - complicating abortion - see categories
    634-639, fourth digit .2
- - obstetrical trauma 665.6
- bucket handle (knee) (meniscus) - see
  Tear, meniscus
- capsule, joint - see Sprain
- cartilage - see also Sprain
- - articular, old 718.0
- - knee - see Tear, meniscus
- cervix
- - complicating abortion - see categories
    634-639, fourth digit .2
- - obstetrical trauma (current) 665.3
- - old 622.3

Tear - *continued*
- internal organ (abdomen, chest, or pelvis)
  - see Injury, internal, by site
- ligament - see also Sprain
- - with open wound - see Wound, open
- meniscus (knee) (current injury) 836.2
- - bucket handle 836.0
- - - old 717.0
- - lateral 836.1
- - - old 717.4
- - medial 836.0
- - - anterior horn 836.0
- - - - old 717.1
- - - bucket handle 836.0
- - - - old 717.0
- - - old 717.3
- - - posterior horn 836.0
- - - - old 717.2
- - old NEC 717.5
- - site other than knee - code as Sprain
- muscle - see also Sprain
- - with open wound - see Wound, open
- pelvic
- - floor, complicating delivery 664.1
- - organ NEC
- - - complicating abortion - see
      categories 634-639, fourth digit .2
- - - obstetrical trauma 665.5
- perineum - see Laceration, perineum
- periurethral tissue
- - with abortion - see categories 634-639,
    fourth digit .2
- - obstetrical trauma 665.5
- rectovaginal septum - see Laceration,
  rectovaginal septum
- retina, retinal (giant) (with detachment)
  361.0
- - horseshoe (without detachment) 361.3
- - without detachment 361.3
- semilunar cartilage, knee (see also Tear,
  meniscus) 717.5
- tendon - see also Sprain
- - with open wound - see Wound, open
- tentorial, at birth 767.0
- umbilical cord
- - affecting fetus or newborn 772.0
- - complicating delivery 663.8
- urethra
- - with abortion - see categories 634-639,
    fourth digit .2
- - obstetrical trauma 665.5
- uterus - see Injury, internal, uterus
- vagina - see Laceration, vagina
- vulva, complicating delivery 664.0
Tear-stone 375.5
Teeth - see also condition
- grinding 306.8

Teething syndrome 520.7

Telangiectasia, telangiectasis (verrucus) 448.9
- ataxic (cerebellar) 334.8
- hemorrhagic, hereditary (congenital) (senile) 448.0
- spider 448.1

Telescoped bowel or intestine (see also Intussusception) 560.0

Teletherapy, adverse effect NEC 990

Temperature
- body, high (of unknown origin) (see also Pyrexia) 780.6
- cold, trauma from 991.9
- - newborn 778.2
- - specified effect NEC 991.8

Temple - see condition

Temporal - see condition

Temporosphenoidal - see condition

Tendency
- bleeding (see also Defect, coagulation) 286.9
- homosexual 302.0
- paranoid 301.0
- suicide 300.9

Tenderness, abdominal 789.0

Tendinitis, tendonitis (see also Tenosynovitis) 726.9
- achilles 726.7
- adhesive 726.9
- - shoulder 726.0
- calcific 727.8
- gluteal 726.5
- patellar 726.6
- psoas 726.5
- tibialis (anterior) (posterior) 726.7
- trochanteric 726.5

Tendon - see condition

Tendosynovitis - see Tenosynovitis

Tendovaginitis - see Tenosynovitis

Tenesmus 787.9
- rectal 787.9
- vesical 788.9

Tennis elbow 726.3

Tenonitis - see also Tenosynovitis
- eye (capsule) 376.0

Tenontosynovitis - see Tenosynovitis

Tenontothecitis - see Tenosynovitis

Tenophyte 727.9

Tenosynovitis 727.0
- adhesive 726.9
- - shoulder 726.0
- ankle 727.0
- bicipital 726.1
- buttock 727.0
- due to crystals - see Arthritis due to crystals

Tenosynovitis - *continued*
- elbow 727.0
- finger 727.0
- foot 727.0
- gonococcal 098.5 † 727.0*
- hand 727.0
- hip 727.0
- knee 727.0
- shoulder 726.2
- - adhesive 726.0
- spine 727.0
- supraspinatous 726.1
- toe 727.0
- tuberculous - see Tuberculosis, tenosynovitis
- wrist 727.0

Tenovaginitis - see Tenosynovitis

Tension
- arterial, high (see also Hypertension) 401.9
- headache 307.8
- nervous 799.2
- premenstrual 625.4
- state 300.9

Tentorium - see condition

Teratencephalus 759.8

Teratism 759.7

Teratoblastoma (malignant) (M9080/3) - see Neoplasm, malignant

Teratocarcinoma (M9081/3) - see also Neoplasm, malignant
- liver 155.0

Teratoma (solid) (M9080/1) - see also Neoplasm, uncertain behavior
- adult (cystic) (M9080/0) - see Neoplasm benign
- and embryonal carcinoma, mixed (M9081/3) - see Neoplasm, malignant
- benign (M9080/0) - see Neoplasm, benign
- combined with choriocarcinoma (M9101/3) - see Neoplasm, malignant
- cystic (adult) (M9080/0) - see Neoplasm, benign
- differentiated type (M9080/0) - see Neoplasm, benign
- embryonal (M9080/3) - see also Neoplasm, malignant
- - liver 155.0
- immature (M9080/3) - see Neoplasm, malignant
- liver (M9080/3) 155.0
- - adult, benign, cystic, differentiated type or mature (M9080/0) 211.5
- malignant (M9080/3) - see also Neoplasm, malignant

Teratoma - *continued*
- malignant - *continued*
- - anaplastic type (M9082/3) - see
  Neoplasm, malignant
- - intermediate type (M9083/3) - see
  Neoplasm, malignant
- - trophoblastic (M9102/3)
- - - specified site - see Neoplasm,
    malignant
- - - unspecified site 186.9
- - undifferentiated type (M9082/3) - see
  Neoplasm, malignant
- mature (M9080/0) - see Neoplasm,
  benign
- ovary (M9080/0) 220
- - embryonal, immature or malignant
  (M9080/3) 183.0
- suprasellar (M9080/3) - see Neoplasm,
  malignant
- testis (M9080/3) 186.9
- - adult, benign, cystic, differentiated
  type or mature (M9080/0) 222.0
- - undescended 186.0
Termination
- anomalous - see also Malposition,
  congenital
- - portal vein 747.4
- - right pulmonary vein 747.4
- pregnancy (legal) (therapeutic) 635.-
- - fetus NEC 779.6
- - illegal 636.-
Ternidens diminutus infestation 127.7

Terrors, night (child) 307.4
Tertiary - see condition
Test(s)
- blood-alcohol V70.4
- blood-drug V70.4
- developmental, infant or child V20.2
- fertility V26.2
- skin, diagnostic
- - allergy V72.7
- - bacterial disease - see Screening, by
  name of disease
- - hypersensitivity V72.7
- - Wassermann V74.5
- - positive (see also Serology for syphilis,
  positive) 097.1
- - - false 795.6
Testicle, testicular, testis - see condition

Tetanus, tetanic (cephalic) (convulsions)
037
- with
- - abortion - see categories 634-639,
  fourth digit .0
- - ectopic gestation 639.0
- inoculation V03.7

Tetanus - *continued*
- inoculation - *continued*
- - reaction (due to serum) - see
  Complications, vaccination
- neonatorum 771.3
- puerperal, postpartum, childbirth 670
Tetany 781.7
- alkalosis 276.3
- associated with rickets 268.0
- convulsions 781.7
- - hysterical 300.1
- functional (hysterical) 300.1
- hyperkinetic 781.7
- - hysterical 300.1
- hyperpnea 786.0
- - hysterical 300.1
- - psychogenic 306.1
- hyperventilation 786.0
- - hysterical 300.1
- - psychogenic 306.1
- hysterical 300.1
- neonatal 775.4
- parathyroid (gland) 252.1
- parathyroprival 252.1
- postoperative 252.1
- post-thyroidectomy 252.1
- psychogenic 306.1
- - specified as conversion reaction 300.1
Tetralogy of Fallot 745.2
Tetraplegia - see Quadriplegia
Thalassanemia 282.4
Thalassemia (alpha) (beta) (disease) (Hb C)
(Hb D) (Hb E) (Hb H) (Hb I) (Hb S) (high
fetal gene) (high fetal hemoglobin)
(intermedia) (major) (minor) (mixed)
(sickle cell) (trait) (with
hemoglobinopathy) 282.4
- with other abnormal hemoglobin NEC
  282.4
Thalassemic variants 282.4
Thecoma (M8600/0) 220
- malignant (M8600/3) 183.0
Thelitis 611.0
- puerperal, postpartum 675.0
Therapeutic - see condition
Therapy V57.9
- breathing V57.0
- occupational V57.2
- physical NEC V57.1
- speech V57.3
- vocational V57.2
Thermic - see condition
Thermoplegia 992.0
Thesaurismosis, glycogen (see also Disease,
glycogen storage) 271.0
Thiaminic deficiency 265.1
Thibierge-Weissenbach syndrome 710.1

Thickening
- bone 733.9
- breast 611.7
- hymen 623.3
- larynx 478.7
- nail 703.8
- - congenital 757.5
- periosteal 733.9
- pleura (see also Pleurisy) 511.0
- skin 782.8
- subepiglottic 478.7
- tongue 529.8
- valve, heart - see Endocarditis
Thiele syndrome 724.6
Thigh - see condition
Thinning vertebra 733.0
Thirst 783.5
- due to deprivation of water 994.3
Thomsen's disease 359.2
Thomson's disease 757.3
Thoracic - see also condition
- kidney 753.3
Thoracogastroschisis (congenital) 759.8
Thoracopagus 759.4
Thorax - see condition
Thorn syndrome (see also Disease, renal) 593.9
Thornwaldt's
- cyst 478.2
- disease 478.2
Thorson-Biorck syndrome 259.2

Threadworm (infection) (infestation) 127.4
Threatened
- abortion 640.0
- - with subsequent abortion 634.-
- - fetus 762.1
- labor 644.0
- - fetus or newborn 761.8
- - premature 644.1
- miscarriage 640.0
- - fetus 762.1
- premature delivery 644.1
- - fetus or newborn 761.8
Thresher lung 495.0
Thrix annulata (congenital) 757.4

Throat - see condition
Thrombo-angiitis 443.1
- obliterans (general) 443.1
- - cerebral 437.1
- - vessels
- - - brain 437.1
- - - spinal cord 437.1
Thromboarteritis - see Arteritis
Thromboasthenia (hereditary) (hemorrhagic) (Glanzmann) 287.1
Thrombocytasthenia (Glanzmann) 287.1

Thrombocythemia (essential) (hemorragic) (idiopathic) (primary) (M9962/1) 238.7
Thrombocytopathy 287.1
- dystrophic 287.1
- granulopenic 287.1
Thrombocytopenia, thrombocytopenic 287.5
- congenital 287.3
- dilutional 287.4
- due to
- - drugs 287.4
- - extracorporeal circulation of blood 287.4
- - massive blood transfusion 287.4
- - platelet alloimmunization 287.4
- essential 287.3
- hereditary 287.3
- neonatal, transitory 776.1
- - due to
- - - exchange transfusion 776.1
- - - idiopathic maternal thrombocytopenia 776.1
- - - isoimmunization 776.1
- primary 287.3
- puerperal, postpartum 666.3
- secondary 287.4
Thrombocytosis, essential 289.9
Thromboembolism - see Embolism
Thrombopathy (Bernard-Soulier) 287.1
- constitutional 286.4
- Willebrand-Jurgens' 286.4
Thrombopenia (see also Thrombocytopenia) 287.5
Thrombophlebitis 451.9
- antepartum (superficial) 671.2
- - deep 671.3
- - fetus or newborn 760.3
- cavernous (venous) sinus - see Thrombophlebitis, intracranial venous sinus
- cerebral (sinus) (vein) 325
- - nonpyogenic 437.8
- due to implanted device 996.7
- during or resulting from a procedure NEC 997.2
- femoral 451.1
- following infusion, perfusion or transfusion 999.2
- hepatic (vein) 451.8
- idiopathic, recurrent 453.1
- ilio-femoral 451.1
- intracranial venous sinus (any) 325
- - nonpyogenic 437.6
- lateral (venous) sinus - see Thrombophlebitis, intracranial venous sinus
- leg 451.2

Thrombophlebitis - *continued*
- leg - *continued*
- - deep (vessels) 451.1
- - superficial (vessels) 451.0
- longitudinal (venous) sinus - see
  Thrombophlebitis, intracranial venous
  sinus
- lower extremity 451.2
- - deep (vessels) 451.1
- - superficial (vessels) 451.0
- migrans, migrating 453.1
- pelvic
- - with
- - - abortion - see categories 634-639,
    fourth digit .0
- - - ectopic gestation 639.0
- - - puerperal 671.4
- portal (vein) 572.1
- postoperative 997.2
- pregnancy (superficial) 671.2
- - deep 671.3
- - fetus or newborn 760.3
- puerperal, postpartum, chilbirth
  (superficial) 671.2
- - deep 671.4
- - pelvic 671.4
- - specified site NEC 671.5
- sinus (intracranial) - see
  Thrombophlebitis, intracranial venous
  sinus
- specified site NEC 451.8
Thrombosis, thrombotic (marantic)
  (multiple) (progressive) (septic) (vein)
  (vessel) 453.9
- with childbirth or during the puerperium -
  see Thrombosis, puerperal, postpartum,
  childbirth
- antepartum - see Thrombosis, pregnancy
- aorta, aortic 444.1
- - abdominal 444.0
- - bifurcation 444.0
- - saddle 444.0
- - thoracic 444.1
- - valve - see Endocarditis, aortic
- apoplexy (see also Thrombosis, brain)
  434.0
- appendix, septic 540.9
- - with peritonitis, perforation, or rupture
  540.0
- artery, arteries (postinfectional) 444.9
- - auditory, internal 433.8
- - basilar (see also Occlusion, artery,
  basilar) 433.0
- - carotid (common) (internal) (see also
  Occlusion, artery, carotid) 433.1
- - cerebellar (anterior inferior) (posterior
  inferior) (superior) 433.8

Thrombosis - *continued*
- artery - *continued*
- - cerebral (see also Thrombosis, brain)
  434.0
- - choroidal (anterior) 433.8
- - communicating posterior 433.8
- - coronary (see also Infarct,
  myocardium) 410
- - - due to syphilis 093.8
- - extremity (lower) (upper) 444.2
- - hepatic 444.8
- - hypophyseal 433.8
- - meningeal, anterior or posterior 433.8
- - mesenteric (with gangrene) 557.0
- - of extremities 444.2
- - ophthalmic 362.3
- - pontine 433.8
- - precerebral NEC - see Occlusion,
  artery, precerebral NEC
- - pulmonary 415.1
- - retinal 362.3
- - spinal, anterior or posterior 433.8
- - traumatic (complication) (early) (see
  also Injury, blood vessel) 904.9
- - vertebral (see also Occlusion, artery,
  vertebral) 433.2
- auricular (see also Infarct, myocardium)
  410
- basilar (artery) (see also Occlusion,
  artery, basilar) 433.0
- bland NEC 453.9
- brain (artery) (stem) 434.0
- - due to syphilis 094.8
- - puerperal, postpartum, childbirth
  674.0
- - sinus (see also Thrombosis, intracranial
  venous sinus) 325
- capillary 448.9
- cardiac (see also Infarct, myocardium)
  410
- - due to syphilis 093.8
- - valve - see Endocarditis
- carotid (artery) (common) (internal) (see
  also Occlusion, artery, carotid) 433.1
- cavernous (venous) sinus - see
  Thrombosis, intracranial venous sinus
- cerebral (see also Thrombosis, brain)
  434.0
- coronary (artery) (see also Infarct,
  myocardium) 410
- - due to syphilis 093.8
- corpus cavernosum 607.8
- cortical (see also Thrombosis, brain)
  434.0
- due to (presence of) any device, implant
  or graft classifiable to 996.0-996.5 996.7
- endocardial - see Infarct, myocardium

Thrombosis - *continued*
- eye 362.3
- femoral 453.8
- - artery 444.2
- heart (chamber) (see also Infarct, myocardium) 410
- hepatic 453.0
- - artery 444.8
- iliac 453.8
- - artery 444.8
- intestine (with gangrene) 557.0
- intracranial (see also Thrombosis, brain) 434.0
- - venous sinus (any) 325
- - - nonpyogenic origin 437.6
- intramural - see Infarct, myocardium
- jugular (bulb) 453.8
- kidney (see also Lesion, kidney) 593.8
- - artery 593.8
- lateral (venous) sinus - see Thrombosis, intracranial venous sinus
- leg 451.2
- - deep (vessels) 451.1
- - superficial (vessels) 451.0
- liver 453.0
- - artery 444.8
- longitudinal (venous) sinus - see Thrombosis, intracranial venous sinus
- lower extremity - see Thrombosis, leg
- lung 415.1
- meninges (brain) (see also Thrombosis, brain) 434.0
- mesenteric (artery) (with gangrene) 557.0
- mitral - see Insufficiency, mitral
- mural (see also Infarct, myocardium) 410
- - due to syphilis 093.8
- omentum (with gangrene) 557.0
- ophthalmic (artery) 362.3
- parietal (see also Infarct, myocardium) 410
- penis, penile 607.8
- peripheral arteries 444.2
- portal 452
- - due to syphilis 093.8
- precerebral artery - see also Occlusion, artery, precerebral NEC
- pregnancy 671.9
- - deep-vein 671.3
- - superficial 671.2
- puerperal, postpartum, childbirth 671.9
- - brain (artery) 674.0
- - - venous 671.5
- - cardiac 674.8
- - cerebral (artery) 674.0
- - - venous 671.5
- - deep-vein 671.4

Thrombosis - *continued*
- puerperal - *continued*
- - pelvic 671.4
- - pulmonary (artery) 673.2
- - specified site NEC 671.5
- - superficial 671.2
- pulmonary (artery) (vein) 415.1
- renal (see also Lesion, kidney) 593.8
- - artery 593.8
- - vein 453.3
- resulting from presence of shunt or other internal prosthetic device 996.7
- retina, retinal (artery) 362.3
- scrotum 608.8
- seminal vesicle 608.8
- sigmoid (venous) sinus - see Thrombosis, intracranial venous sinus
- silent NEC 453.9
- sinus, intracranial (any) (see also Thrombosis, intracranial venous sinus) 325
- specified site NEC 453.8
- spermatic cord 608.8
- spinal cord 336.1
- - due to syphilis 094.8
- - pyogenic origin 324.1
- spleen, splenic 289.5
- - artery 444.8
- testis 608.8
- traumatic (complication) (early) (see also Injury, blood vessel) 904.9
- tricuspid - see Endocarditis, tricuspid
- tunica vaginalis 608.8
- umbilical cord (vessels) 663.6
- - affecting fetus or newborn 762.6
- vas deferens 608.8
- vena cava (inferior) (superior) 453.2
Thrombus - see Thrombosis
Thrush 112.0
Thumb - see also condition
- sucking (child problem) 307.9
Thymergasia (see also Psychosis, manic-depressive) 296.6
Thymitis 254.8
Thymoma (benign) (M8580/0) 212.6
- malignant (M8580/3) 164.0
Thymus, thymic (gland) - see condition
Thyrocele (see also Goiter) 240.9
Thyroglossal - see also condition
- cyst 759.2
- duct, persistent 759.2
Thyroid (gland) (body) - see condition
Thyroiditis 245.9
- acute 245.0
- - nonsuppurative 245.0
- autoimmune 245.2
- chronic 245.8

Thyroiditis - *continued*
- chronic - *continued*
- - lymphadenoid 245.2
- - lymphocytic 245.2
- de Quervain 245.1
- fibrous (chronic) 245.3
- giant
- - cell 245.1
- - follicular 245.1
- granulomatous (subacute) (de Quervain) 245.1
- iatrogenic 245.4
- invasive 245.3
- ligneous 245.3
- lymphocytic (chronic) 245.2
- lymphoid 245.2
- lymphomatous 245.2
- pseudotuberculous 245.1
- pyogenic 245.0
- Riedel's 245.3
- subacute 245.1
- suppurative 245.0
- tuberculous 017.5
- woody 245.3
Thyrolingual duct, persistent 759.2
Thyrotoxic
- heart failure (see also Thyrotoxicosis) 242.9 † 425.7*
- storm (see also Thyrotoxicosis) 242.9
Thyrotoxicosis (recurrent) 242.9
- with
- - goiter (diffuse) - see Goiter, toxic
- due to
- - ectopic thyroid nodule 242.4
- - ingestion of (excessive) thyroid material 242.8
- - specified cause NEC 242.8
- factitia 242.8
- heart 242.- † 425.7*
- neonatal 775.3
Tibia vara 736.4
Tic 307.2
- breathing 307.2
- child problem 307.2
- convulsive 307.2
- degenerative (generalized) (localized) 333.3
- - facial 351.8
- douloureux (see also Neuralgia, trigeminal) 350.1
- - atypical 350.2
- habit 307.2
- lid 307.2
- occupational 300.8
- orbicularis 307.2
- organic origin 333.3
- postchoreic - see Chorea

Tic - *continued*
- salaam 781.0
- spasm 307.2
Tick-borne - see condition
Tietze's disease or syndrome 733.6
Tight fascia (lata) 728.9
Tightness
- anus 564.8
- foreskin (congenital) 605
- hymen 623.3
- introitus 623.3
- rectal sphincter 564.8
- tendon 727.8
- - achilles (heel) 727.8
- urethral sphincter 598.9
Tilting vertebra 737.9
Tin miners' lung 503
Tinea (intersecta) (tarsi) 110.9
- amiantacea 110.0
- asbestina 110.0
- barbae 110.0
- beard 110.0
- black dot 110.0
- blanca 111.2
- capitis 110.0
- decalvans (see also Alopecia) 704.0
- flava 111.0
- foot 110.4
- furfuracea 111.0
- imbricata (tokelau) 110.5
- lepothrix 039.0
- manuum 110.2
- microsporic (see also Dermatophytosis) 110.9
- nigra 111.1
- nodosa 111.3
- pedis 110.4
- scalp 110.0
- specified site NEC 110.8
- sycosis 110.0
- tonsurans 110.0
- trichophytic (see also Dermatophytosis) 110.9
- unguium 110.1
- versicolor 111.0
Tingling sensation (see also Disturbance, sensation) 782.0
Tinnitus (audible) (aurium) (subjective) 388.3
Tipping pelvis 738.6
- with disproportion 653.0
- - causing obstructed labor 660.1
- - - fetus or newborn 763.1
Tiredness 780.7
Tissue - see condition
Tobacco heart 989.8
Tocopherol deficiency 269.1

Todd's
- cirrhosis - see Cirrhosis, biliary
- paralysis 344.8
Toe - see condition
Toilet, artificial opening - see Attention to artificial opening
Tokelau ringworm 110.5
Tollwut 071
Tommaselli's disease
- correct substance properly administered 599.7
- overdose or wrong substance given or taken 961.4
Tongue - see also condition
- worms 134.1
Tonguetie 750.0
Tonic pupil 379.4
Toni-Fanconi syndrome 270.0

Tonsil - see condition
Tonsillitis (acute) (catarrhal) (croupous) (follicular) (gangrenous) (infective) (lacunar) (lingual) (malignant) (membranous) (phlegmonous) (pneumococcal) (pseudomembranous) (purulent) (septic) (staphylococcal) (subacute) (suppurative) (toxic) (ulcerative) (vesicular) (viral) 463
- with influenza, flu, or grippe 487.1
- chronic 474.0
- diphtheritic 032.0
- hypertrophic 474.0
- influenzal 487.1
- parenchymatous 475
- streptococcal 034.0
- tuberculous 012.8
- Vincent's 101
Tonsillopharyngitis 465.8

Tooth, teeth - see condition
Toothache 525.9
Topagnosis 782.0
Tophi (gouty) NEC 274.0 † 712.0*
- ear 274.8 † 380.8*
- heart 274.8 † 425.7*
Torn - see Tear, torn
Torsion
- accessory tube 620.5
- adnexa (female) 620.5
- aorta (congenital) 747.2
- bile duct (see also Disease, biliary) 576.8
- - congenital 751.6
- bowel, colon or intestine 560.2
- cervix (see also Malposition, uterus) 621.6
- dystonia - see Dystonia, torsion
- epididymis 608.2
- fallopian tube 620.5

Torsion - *continued*
- gallbladder (see also Disease, gallbladder) 575.8
- - congenital 751.6
- hydatid of morgagni 620.5
- kidney (pedicle) 593.8
- Meckel's diverticulum (congenital) 751.0
- mesentery 560.2
- omentum 560.2
- organ or site, congenital NEC - see Anomaly, specified type NEC
- ovary (pedicle) 620.5
- - congenital 752.0
- oviduct 620.5
- penis 607.8
- - congenital 752.8
- spasm - see Dystonia, torsion
- spermatic cord 608.2
- spleen 289.5
- testis 608.2
- tibia 736.8
- umbilical cord - see Compression, umbilical cord
- uterus (see also Malposition, uterus) 621.6
Torticollis (intermittent) (spastic) 723.5
- congenital 756.8
- - sternomastoid 754.1
- due to birth injury 767.8
- hysterical 300.1
- psychogenic 306.0
- - specified as conversion reaction 300.1
- rheumatic 723.5
- rheumatoid 714.0
- spasmodic 333.8
- traumatic, current NEC 847.0
Tortuous
- artery 447.1
- organ or site, congenital NEC - see Distortion
- retina vessel (congenital) 743.5
- ureter 593.4
- urethra 599.8
- vein - see Varicose vein
Torula, torular (infection) 117.5
- histolytica 117.5
- lung 117.5
Torulosis 117.5
Torus (mandibularis) (palatinus) 526.8
Tower skull 756.0
- with exophthalmos 756.0
Toxemia 799.8
- bacterial - see Septicemia
- biliary (see also Disease, biliary) 576.8
- burn - see Burn
- congenital NEC 779.8
- eclamptic 642.6

Toxemia - *continued*
- eclamptic - *continued*
- - with pre-existing hypertension 642.7
- erysipelatous (see also Erysipelas) 035
- fatigue 799.8
- fetus or newborn NEC 779.8
- food (see also Poisoning, food) 005.9
- gastric 537.8
- gastrointestinal 558
- intestinal 558
- kidney (see also Disease, renal) 593.9
- lung 518.8
- malarial NEC (see also Malaria) 084.6
- maternal (of pregnancy), affecting fetus or newborn 760.0
- myocardial - see Myocarditis, toxic
- of pregnancy (pre-eclamptic) (mild) 642.4
- - with
- - - convulsions 642.6
- - - pre-existing hypertension 642.7
- - fetus or newborn 760.0
- - severe 642.5
- pre-eclamptic - see Toxemia, of pregnancy
- puerperal, postpartum - see Toxemia, of pregnancy
- pulmonary 518.8
- septic (see also Septicemia) 038.9
- staphylococcal 038.1
- - due to food 005.0
- stasis 799.8
- stomach 537.8
- uremic (see also Uremia) 586
- urinary 586
Toxic (poisoning) - see also condition
- from drug or poison - see Table of drugs and chemicals
- thyroid (gland) (see also Thyrotoxicosis) 242.9
Toxicemia - see Toxemia
Toxicity
- fava bean 282.2
- from drug or poison - see Table of drugs and chemicals
Toxicosis (see also Toxemia) 799.8
- capillary, hemorrhagic 287.0
Toxocariasis 128.0
Toxoplasmosis (acquired) 130
- with pneumonia 130 † 484.8*
- congenital, active 771.2
- maternal, affecting fetus or newborn 760.2
- - manifest toxoplasmosis in infant or fetus 771.2
- suspected damage to fetus affecting management of pregnancy 655.4

Trabeculation, bladder 596.8
Trachea - see condition
Tracheitis (acute) (catarrhal) (infantile) (membranous) (plastic) (pneumococcal) (viral) 464.1
- with
- - bronchitis 490
- - - acute or subacute 466.0
- - - chronic 491.8
- - - tuberculous - see Tuberculosis, pulmonary
- - laryngitis (acute) 464.2
- - - chronic 476.1
- - - tuberculous 012.3
- chronic 491.8
- - with
- - - bronchitis (chronic) 491.8
- - - laryngitis (chronic) 476.1
- - due to external agent - see condition, respiratory, chronic, due to
- diphtheritic 032.3
- due to external agent - see Inflammation, respiratory, upper, due to
- streptococcal 034.0
- syphilitic 095
- tuberculous 012.8
Trachelitis (nonvenereal) (see also Cervicitis) 616.0
- trichomonal 131.0 † 616.0*
Tracheobronchial - see condition
Tracheobronchitis (see also Bronchitis) 490
- acute or subacute 466.0
- chronic 491.8
- influenzal 487.1
- senile 491.8
Tracheobronchopneumonitis - see Pneumonia, broncho
Tracheocele (external) (internal) 519.1
- congenital 748.3
Tracheomalacia 519.1
- congenital 748.3
Tracheopharyngitis (acute) 465.8
- chronic 478.9
- - due to external agent - see condition, respiratory, chronic, due to
- due to external agent - see Inflammation, respiratory, upper, due to
Tracheostenosis 519.1
Tracheostomy (status) V44.0
- attention to V55.0
- malfunctioning 519.0
Trachoma, trachomatous 076.9 † 372.0*
- active (stage) 076.1 † 372.0*
- contraction of conjunctiva 076.1 † 372.0*
- dubium 076.0
- initial (stage) 076.0
- Turck's 476.0

Train sickness 994.6
Training, orthoptic V57.4
Trait
− hemoglobin
− − abnormal NEC 282.7
− − − with thalassemia 282.4
− − C (see also Disease, hemoglobin C)
    282.7
− − − with elliptocytosis 282.7
− − S (Hb-S) 282.5
− Lepore 282.4
− − with other abnormal hemoglobin NEC
    282.4
− sickle cell 282.5
− − with
− − − elliptocytosis 282.5
− − − spherocytosis 282.5
Traits, paranoid 301.0
Tramp V60.0
Trance 780.0
− hysterical 300.1
Transfusion
− blood
− − reaction or complication - see
    Complications, transfusion
− − without reported diagnosis V58.2
− reaction (adverse) - see Complications,
    transfusion
Transient (homeless) (see also Condition)
    V60.0
Transitional, lumbosacral joint or vertebra
    756.1
Translocation
− autosomes NEC 758.5
− − balanced in normal individual 758.4
− − D1 758.1
− − E3 758.2
− − G 758.0
− − 13 758.1
− − 18 758.2
− − 21 or 22 758.0
− balanced autosomal in normal individual
    758.4
− chromosomes NEC 758.9
− Down's syndrome 758.0
Translucency, iris 364.5
Transmission of chemical substances
    through the placenta - see Absorption,
    chemical, through placenta
Transplant
− bone V42.4
− − marrow V42.8
− complication NEC (see also
    Complications, graft) 996.7
− − organ (failure) (immune or
    nonimmune cause) (infection)
    (rejection) 996.8

Transplant - *continued*
− complication NEC - *continued*
− − skin NEC 996.7
− − − infection 996.6
− − − rejection 996.5
− cornea V42.5
− hair V50.0
− heart V42.1
− − valve V42.2
− intestine V42.8
− kidney V42.0
− liver V42.7
− lung V42.6
− organ V42.9
− − specified NEC V42.8
− pancreas V42.8
− skin V42.3
− tissue V42.9
− − specified NEC V42.8
Transplants, ovarian, endometrial 617.1
Transposed - see Transposition

Transposition (congenital) - see also
    Malposition, congenital
− abdominal viscera 759.3
− aorta (dextra) 745.1
− appendix 751.5
− arterial trunk 745.1
− colon 751.5
− great vessels (complete) (partial) 745.1
− − both originating from right ventricle
    745.1
− heart 746.8
− − with complete transposition of viscera
    759.3
− intestine (large) (small) 751.5
− stomach 750.7
− − with general transposition of viscera
    759.3
− tooth, teeth 524.3
− vessels (complete) (partial) 745.1
− viscera (abdominal) (thoracic) 759.3
Trans-sexualism 302.5
Transverse - see also condition
− arrest (deep), in labor 660.3
− − fetus or newborn 763.1
− lie 652.3
− − before labor, affecting fetus or
    newborn 761.7
− − causing obstructed labor 660.0
− − − fetus or newborn 763.1
Transvestism, transvestitism 302.3

Trapped placenta (with hemorrhage) 666.0
− without hemorrhage 667.0
Trauma, traumatism (see also Injury) 959.9
− birth - see Birth injury NEC
− complicating

Trauma - *continued*
- complicating - *continued*
- - abortion - see categories 634-639, fourth digit .2
- - ectopic or molar pregnancy 639.2
- during delivery NEC 665.9
- maternal, during pregnancy, affecting fetus or newborn 760.5
- previous major, affecting management of pregnancy, childbirth, puerperium V23.8
Traumatic - see condition
Treacher-Collins syndrome 756.0
Treitz's hernia - see Hernia, abdominal
Trematode infestation NEC 121.9
Trematodiasis NEC 121.9
Trembles 988.8
Tremor 781.0
- essential (benign) 333.1
- familial 333.1
- hereditary 333.1
- hysterical 300.1
- intention 333.1
- mercurial 985.0
- muscle 728.8
- Parkinson's (see also Parkinsonism) 332.0
- psychogenic 306.0
- - specified as conversion reaction 300.1
- senilis 797
- specified type NEC 333.1
Trench
- foot 991.4
- mouth 101
Treponema pallidum infection (see also Syphilis) 097.9
Treponematosis 102.9
- due to
- - T. pallidum - see Syphilis
- - T. pertenue (yaws) (see also Yaws) 102.9
Triad
- Kartagener 759.3
- Saint's (see also Hernia, diaphragm 553.3
Trichiasis 704.2
- cicatricial 704.2
- eyelid 374.0
Trichinella spiralis (infection) (infestation) 124
Trichinelliasis 124
Trichinellosis 124
Trichiniasis 124
Trichinosis 124
Trichobezoar 938
- intestine 936
- stomach 935.2
Trichocephaliasis 127.3
Trichocephalosis 127.3

Trichocephalus infestation 127.3
Trichoclasis 704.2
Trichoepithelioma (M8100/0) - see also Neoplasm, skin, benign
- malignant (M8100/3) - see Neoplasm, skin, malignant
Trichofolliculoma (M8101/0) - see Neoplasm, skin, benign
Tricholemmoma (M8102/0) - see Neoplasm, skin, benign
Trichomoniasis 131.9
- bladder 131.0 † 595.4*
- intestinal 007.3
- prostate 131.0 † 601.4*
- seminal vessels 131.0
- specified site NEC 131.8
- urethra 131.0 † 597.8*
- urogenitalis 131.0
- vagina 131.0 † 616.1*
Trichomycosis 039.0
- axillaris 039.0
- nodosa 111.2
- nodularis 111.2
- rubra 039.0
Trichonocardiosis (axillaris) (palmellina) 039.0
Trichonodosis 704.2
Trichophytid, trichophyton infection (see also Dermatophytosis) 110.9
Trichophytobezoar 938
- intestine 936
- stomach 935.2
Trichophytosis - see Dermatophytosis
Trichoptilosis 704.2
Trichorrhexis (nodosa) 704.2
Trichosporosis nodosa 111.2
Trichostasis spinulosa (congenital) 757.4
Trichostrongyliasis (small intestine) 127.6
Trichostrongylosis 127.6
Trichostrongylus (instabilis) infection 127.6
Trichotillomania 300.3
Trichromat, anomalous (congenital) 368.5
Trichromatopsia, anomalous (congenital) 368.5
Trichuriasis 127.3
Trichuris trichiura (infection) (infestation) (any site) 127.3
Tricuspid (valve) - see condition
Trifid - see also Accessory
- kidney (pelvis) 753.3
- tongue 750.1
Trigger finger (acquired) 727.0
- congenital 756.8
Trigonitis (bladder) (pseudomembranous) 595.3
Trigonocephaly 756.0
Trilocular heart 746.8

Tripartita placenta - see Placenta, abnormal
Triple - see also Accessory
− kidneys 753.3
− uteri 752.2
− X female 758.8
Triplegia 344.8
− congenital or infantile 343.8
Triplet 761.5
− pregnancy (complicating delivery) 651.1
Triplication - see Accessory
Trismus 781.0
− neonatorum 771.3
− newborn 771.3
Trisomy (syndrome) NEC 758.5
− autosomes NEC 758.5
− D(1) 758.1
− E(3) 758.2
− G (group) 758.0
− 13 (partial) 758.1
− 18 (partial) 758.2
− 21 (partial) 758.0
− 22 758.0
Tritanomaly 368.5
Tritanopia 368.5
Trombidiosis 133.8
Trophedema (hereditary) 757.0
Trophoblastic disease (see also
  Hydatidiform mole) 630
− previous, affecting management of
  pregnancy V21.1
Trophoneurosis NEC 356.9
− disseminated 710.1
Tropical - see also condition
− maceration feet (syndrome) 991.4
− wet foot (syndrome) 991.4
Trouble - see also Disease
− bowel 569.9
− heart - see Disease, heart
− intestine 569.9
− kidney (see also Disease, renal) 593.9
− nervous 799.2
− sinus (see also Sinusitis) 473.9
Truancy, childhood
− socialized 312.1
− unsocialized 312.0
Truncus
− arteriosus (persistent) 745.0
− communis 745.0
Trunk - see condition
Trypanosoma infestation - see
  Trypanosomiasis
Trypanosomiasis 086.9
− with meningoencephalitis 086.- † 323.4*
− African 086.5
− − by Trypanosoma 086.5
− − − gambiense 086.3
− − − rhodesiense 086.4

Trypanosomiasis - *continued*
− American 086.2
− − with
− − − heart involvement 086.0 † 425.6*
− − − other organ involvement 086.1
− − without mention of organ involvement
    086.2
− Brazilian - see Trypanosomiasis,
  American
− by Trypanosoma
− − cruzi - see Trypanosomiasis, American
− − gambiense 086.3
− − rhodesiense 086.4
− gambiensis, Gambian 086.3
− rhodesiensis, Rhodesian 086.4
− South American - see Trypanosomiasis,
  American
T-shaped incisors 520.2
Tsutsugamushi 081.2
Tube, tubal, tubular - see condition
− ligation, admission for V25.2
Tubercle - see also Tuberculosis
− brain, solitary 013.8 † 348.8*
− Darwin's 744.2
− Ghon, primary infection 010.0
Tuberculid, tuberculide (indurating,
  subcutaneous) (lichenoid) (miliary)
  (papulonecrotic) (primary) (skin) 017.0
Tuberculoma - see also Tuberculosis
− brain (any part) (calcified) 013.8 † 348.8*
− meninges (cerebral) (spinal) 013.1 †
    349.2*
− spinal cord 013.8 † 336.3*
Tuberculosis, tubercular, tuberculous
  (calcification) (calcified) (caseous)
  (chromogenic acid fast bacilli) (congenital)
  (degeneration) (disease) (fibrocaseous)
  (fistula) (gangrene) (interstitial) (isolated
  circumscribed lesions) (necrosis)
  (parenchymatous) (ulcerative) 011.9
− abdomen 014
− − lymph gland 014
− abscess 011.9
− − arm 017.8
− − bone 015.9 † 730.6*
− − − hip 015.1 † 730.5*
− − − knee 015.2 † 730.5*
− − − sacrum 015.0 † 730.4*
− − − specified site NEC 015.7 † 730.6*
− − − spinal 015.0 † 730.4*
− − − vertebra 015.0 † 730.4*
− − brain 013.8 † 324.0*
− − breast 017.8
− − Cowper's gland 016.3
− − dura (mater) 013.8 † 324.9*
− − − cerebral 013.8 † 324.0*
− − − spinal 013.8 † 324.1*

Tuberculosis - *continued*
- abscess - *continued*
- - epidural 013.8 † 324.9*
- - - cerebral 013.8 † 324.0*
- - - spinal 013.8 † 324.1*
- - frontal sinus - see Tuberculosis, sinus
- - genital organs NEC 016.9
- - - female 016.4
- - - male 016.3
- - genitourinary 016.9
- - gland (lymphatic) - see Tuberculosis, lymph gland
- - hip 015.1
- - iliopsoas 015.0 † 730.4*
- - intestine 014
- - ischiorectal 014
- - joint NEC 015.9
- - - hip 015.1
- - - knee 015.2
- - - specified NEC 015.8
- - - vertebral 015.0 † 730.4*
- - kidney 016.0
- - knee 015.2
- - lumbar 015.0 † 730.4*
- - lung 011.2
- - - primary, progressive 010.8
- - meninges (cerebral) (spinal) 013.0 † 320.4*
- - pelvic 016.9
- - perianal 014
- - - fistula 014
- - perinephritic 016.0
- - perineum 017.8
- - perirectal 014
- - psoas 015.0 † 730.4*
- - rectum 014
- - retropharyngeal 012.8
- - sacrum 015.0 † 730.4*
- - scrofulous 017.2
- - scrotum 016.3
- - skin 017.0
- - - primary 017.0
- - spinal cord 013.8 † 324.1*
- - spine or vertebra (column) 015.0 † 730.4*
- - strumous 017.2
- - subdiaphragmatic 014
- - testis 016.3
- - thigh 017.8
- - urinary 016.1
- - - kidney 016.0
- - uterus 016.4
- accessory sinus - see Tuberculosis, sinus
- Addison's disease 017.6 † 255.4*
- adenitis (see also Tuberculosis, lymph gland) 017.2
- adenoids 012.8

Tuberculosis - *continued*
- adenopathy (see also Tuberculosis, lymph gland) 017.2
- - tracheobronchial 012.1
- - - primary progressive 010.8
- adherent pericardium 017.8
- adnexa (uteri) 016.4
- adrenal (capsule) (gland) 017.6 † 255.4*
- air passage NEC 012.8
- alimentary canal 014
- anemia 017.8
- ankle (joint) 015.8
- - bone 015.7 † 730.5*
- anus 014
- apex (see also Tuberculosis, pulmonary) 011.9
- apical (see also Tuberculosis, pulmonary) 011.9
- appendicitis 014
- appendix 014
- arachnoid 013.0 † 320.4*
- artery 017.8
- arthritis (chronic) (synovial) 015.9 † 711.4*
- - hip 015.1 † 711.4*
- - knee 015.2 † 711.4*
- - specified site NEC (ankle) (wrist) 015.8 † 711.4*
- - spine or vertebra (column) 015.0 † 711.4*
- articular - see Tuberculosis, joint
- ascites 014
- asthma (see also Tuberculosis, pulmonary) 011.9
- axilla, axillary 017.2
- - gland 017.2
- bilateral (see also Tuberculosis, pulmonary) 011.9
- bladder 016.1 † 595.4*
- bone 015.9 † 730.6*
- - hip 015.1 † 730.5*
- - knee 015.2 † 730.5*
- - limb NEC 015.7 † 730.5*
- - sacrum 015.0 † 730.4*
- - specified NEC 015.7 † 730.6*
- - spine or vertebral column 015.0 † 730.4*
- bowel 014
- - miliary 014
- brain 013.8 † 348.8*
- breast 017.8
- broad ligament 016.4
- bronchi, bronchial, bronchus 011.3
- - ectasia, ectasis 011.5
- - fistula 011.3
- - - primary, progressive 010.8
- - gland 012.1

Tuberculosis - *continued*
- bronchi - *continued*
- - gland - *continued*
- - - primary, progressive 010.8
- - isolated 012.2
- - lymph gland or node 012.1
- - - primary, progressive 010.8
- bronchiectasis 011.5
- bronchitis 011.3
- bronchopleural 012.0
- bronchopneumonia, bronchopneumonic 011.6
- bronchorrhagia 011.3
- bronchotracheal 011.3
- - isolated 012.2
- bronze disease 017.6 † 255.4*
- buccal cavity 017.8
- bulbourethral gland 016.3
- bursa (see also Tuberculosis, joint) 015.9

- cachexia NEC (see also Tuberculosis, pulmonary) 011.9
- cardiomyopathy 017.8 † 425.8*
- caries (see also Tuberculosis, bone) 015.9 † 730.6*
- cartilage (see also Tuberculosis, bone) 015.9 † 730.6*
- - intervertebral 015.0 † 730.4*
- catarrhal (see also Tuberculosis, pulmonary) 011.9
- cecum 014
- cellular tissue (primary) 017.0
- cellulitis (primary) 017.0
- central nervous system 013.9
- cerebellum 013.8 † 348.8*
- cerebral 013.8 † 348.8*
- - meninges 013.0 † 320.4*
- cerebrospinal 013.8 † 348.8*
- - meninges 013.0 † 320.4*
- cerebrum 013.8 † 348.8*
- cervical 017.2
- - gland 017.2
- - lymph nodes 017.2
- cervicis uteri 016.4
- cervicitis (uteri) 016.4
- cervix 016.4
- chest (see also Tuberculosis, pulmonary) 011.9
- childhood type or first infection 010.0

- choroid 017.3 † 363.1*
- choroiditis 017.3 † 363.1*
- ciliary body 017.3 † 364.1*
- colitis 014
- colliers' 011.4
- colliquativa (primary) 017.0
- colon 014
- complex, primary 010.0

Tuberculosis - *continued*
- complicating pregnancy, childbirth or puerperium 647.3
- - fetus or newborn 760.2
- congenital 771.2
- conjunctiva 017.3 † 370.3*
- connective tissue 017.8
- - bone - see Tuberculosis, bone
- cornea (ulcer) 017.3 † 370.3*
- Cowper's gland 016.3
- coxae 015.1
- coxalgia 015.1
- cul-de-sac of Douglas 014
- curvature, spine 015.0 † 737.4*
- cutis (colliquativa) (primary) 017.0
- cyst, ovary 016.4
- cystitis 016.1 † 595.4*
- dactylitis 015.7 † 730.5*
- diarrhea 014
- diffuse (see also Tuberculosis, miliary) 018.9
- digestive tract 014
- disseminated (see also Tuberculosis, miliary) 018.9
- duodenum 014
- dura (mater) 013.0 † 320.4*
- - abscess 013.8 † 324.9*
- - - cerebral 013.8 † 324.0*
- - - spinal 013.8 † 324.1*
- dysentery 014
- ear (inner) (middle) 017.4 † 382.3*
- - bone 015.7 † 730.6*
- - external (primary) 017.0
- - skin (primary) 017.0
- elbow 015.8
- empyema 012.0
- encephalitis 013.8 † 323.4*
- endarteritis 017.8
- endocarditis 017.8 † 424.9*
- - aortic 017.8 † 424.1*
- - mitral 017.8 † 424.0*
- - pulmonary 017.8 † 424.3*
- - tricuspid 017.8 † 424.2*
- endocardium (see also Tuberculosis, endocarditis) 017.8 † 424.9*
- endocrine glands NEC 017.8
- endometrium 016.4
- enteric, enterica 014
- enteritis 014
- enterocolitis 014
- epididymis 016.2 † 604.9*
- epididymitis 016.2 † 604.9*
- epidural abscess 013.8 † 324.9*
- - cerebral 013.8 † 324.0*
- - spinal 013.8 † 324.1*
- epiglottis 012.3
- episcleritis 017.3 † 379.0*

Tuberculosis - *continued*
- erythema (induratum) (nodosum)
  (primary) 017.1
- esophagus 017.8 † 530.1*
- eustachian tube 017.4 † 382.3*
- exudative 012.0
- - primary, progressive 010.1
- eye 017.3
- - glaucoma 017.3 † 365.6*
- eyelid (primary) 017.0
- - lupus 017.0 † 373.4*
- fallopian tube 016.4 † 614.2*
- - acute 016.4 † 614.0*
- - chronic 016.4 † 614.1*
- fascia 017.8
- fauces 012.8
- finger 017.8
- first infection 010.0
- florida 011.6
- foot 017.8
- gallbladder 017.8
- galloping (see also Tuberculosis,
  pulmonary) 011.9
- ganglionic 015.9
- gastritis 017.8
- gastrocolic fistula 014.- † 014*
- gastroenteritis 014
- gastrointestinal tract 014
- general, generalized 018.9
- - acute 018.0
- - chronic 018.8
- genital organs NEC 016.9
- - female 016.4
- - male 016.3
- genitourinary NEC 016.9
- genu 015.2
- glandulae suprarenalis 017.6 † 255.4*
- glandular, general 017.2
- glottis 012.3
- grinders' 011.4
- groin 017.2
- gum 017.8
- hand 017.8
- heart 017.8 † 425.8*
- hematogenous - see Tuberculosis, miliary
- hemoptysis - code by type under
  Tuberculosis, pulmonary 011.9
- hemorrhage NEC - code by type under
  Tuberculosis, pulmonary 011.9
- hemothorax 012.0
- hepatitis 017.8
- hilar lymph nodes 012.1
- - primary, progressive 010.8
- hip (joint) (disease) 015.1
- - bone 015.1 † 730.5*
- hydrocephalus 013.0 † 320.4*
- hydropneumothorax 012.0

Tuberculosis - *continued*
- hydrothorax 012.0
- hypoadrenalism 017.6 † 255.4*
- hypopharynx 012.8
- ileocecal (hyperplastic) 014
- ileocolitis 014
- ileum 014
- iliac spine (superior) 015.0 † 730.4*
- immunological findings only 010.0
- incipient NEC (see also Tuberculosis,
  pulmonary) 011.9
- indurativa (primary) 017.1
- infantile 010.0
- infection 011.9
- - without clinical manifestation 010.0
- infraclavicular gland 017.2
- inguinal gland 017.2
- inguinalis 017.2
- intestine (any part) 014
- iris 017.3 † 364.1*
- iritis 017.3 † 364.1*
- ischiorectal 014
- jaw 015.7 † 730.6*
- jejunum 014
- joint 015.9
- - hip 015.1
- - knee 015.2
- - specified NEC 015.8
- - vertebral 015.0 † 730.4*
- keratitis 017.3 † 370.3*
- - interstitial 017.3 † 370.5*
- keratoconjunctivitis 017.3 † 370.3*
- kidney 016.0
- knee (joint) 015.2
- kyphoscoliosis 015.0 † 737.4*
- kyphosis 015.0 † 737.4*
- laryngitis 012.3
- larynx 012.3
- leptomeninges, leptomeningitis (cerebral)
  (spinal) 013.0 † 320.4*
- lichenoides (primary) 017.0
- linguae 017.8
- lip 017.8
- liver 017.8
- lordosis 015.0 † 737.4*
- lung - see Tuberculosis, pulmonary
- luposa 017.0
- - eyelid 017.0 † 373.4*
- lymph gland or node (peripheral) 017.2
- - abdomen 014
- - bronchial 012.1
- - - primary, progressive 010.8
- - cervical 017.2
- - hilar 012.1
- - - primary, progressive 010.8
- - intrathoracic 012.1
- - - primary, progressive 010.8

Tuberculosis - *continued*
- pharyngitis 012.8
- pharynx 012.8
- phlyctenulosis (conjunctiva) 017.3 †
  370.3*
- phthisis NEC (see also Tuberculosis,
  pulmonary) 011.9
- pituitary gland 017.8
- placenta 016.4
- pleura, pleural, pleurisy, pleuritis
  (fibrinous) (obliterative) (purulent)
  (simple plastic) (with effusion) 012.0
- – primary, progressive 010.1
- pneumonia, pneumonic 011.6
- pneumothorax (spontaneous) (tense
  valvular) 011.7
- polyserositis 018.9
- – acute 018.0
- – chronic 018.8
- potters' 011.4
- prepuce 016.3
- primary 010.9
- – complex 010.0
- – complicated 010.8
- – – with pleurisy or effusion 010.1
- – progressive NEC 010.8
- – – with pleurisy or effusion 010.1
- – skin 017.0
- proctitis 014
- prostate 016.3 † 601.4*
- prostatitis 016.3 † 601.4*
- pulmonaris (see also Tuberculosis,
  pulmonary) 011.9
- pulmonary (artery) (incipient)
  (malignant) (multiple round foci)
  (pernicious) (reinfection stage) 011.9
- – cavitated or with cavitation 011.2
- – – primary, progressive 010.8
- – childhood type or first infection 010.0
- – fibrosis or fibrotic 011.4
- – infiltrative 011.0
- – – primary, progressive 010.8
- – nodular 011.1
- – specified NEC 011.8
- – status following surgical collapse of
  lung NEC 011.9
- pyelitis 016.0 † 590.8*
- pyelonephritis 016.0 † 590.8*
- pyemia - see Tuberculosis, miliary
- pyonephrosis 016.0 † 590.8*
- pyopneumothorax 012.0
- pyothorax 012.0
- rectum (with abscess) 014
- – fistula 014
- reinfection stage (see also Tuberculosis,
  pulmonary) 011.9
- renal 016.0 † 583.8*

Tuberculosis - *continued*
- renis 016.0 † 583.8*
- respiratory NEC (see also Tuberculosis,
  pulmonary) 011.9
- – specified site NEC 012.8
- retina 017.3 † 362.1*
- retroperitoneal 014
- – gland 014
- – lymph gland or node 014
- rheumatism NEC 015.9
- rhinitis 012.8
- sacro-iliac (joint) 015.8
- sacrum 015.0 † 730.4*
- salivary gland 017.8
- salpingitis 016.4 † 614.2*
- – acute 016.4 † 614.0*
- – chronic 016.4 † 614.1*
- sandblasters' 011.4
- sclera 017.3 † 379.0*
- scoliosis 015.0 † 737.4*
- scrofulous 017.2
- scrotum 016.3
- seminal tract or vesicle 016.3 † 608.8*
- senile NEC (see also Tuberculosis,
  pulmonary) 011.9
- septic NEC (see also Tuberculosis,
  miliary) 018.9
- shoulder (joint) 015.8
- – blade 015.7 † 730.6*
- sigmoid 014
- sinus (any nasal) 012.8
- – bone 015.7 † 730.6*
- – epididymis 016.2 † 604.9*
- skeletal NEC 015.9 † 730.6*
- skin (any site) (primary) 017.0
- spermatic cord 016.3
- spinal
- – column 015.0 † 730.4*
- – cord 013.8 † 323.4*
- – disease 015.0 † 730.4*
- – medulla 013.8 † 323.4*
- – membrane 013.0 † 320.4*
- – meninges 013.0 † 320.4*
- spine 015.0 † 730.4*
- spleen 017.7
- splenitis 017.7
- spondylitis 015.0 † 720.8*
- sternoclavicular joint 015.8
- stomach 017.8
- stonemasons' 011.4
- struma 017.2
- subcutaneous tissue (cellular) (primary)
  017.0
- subcutis (primary) 017.0
- subdeltoid bursa 017.8
- submaxillary 017.8
- – region 017.8

Tuberculosis - *continued*
- supraclavicular gland 017.2
- suprarenal (capsule) (gland) 017.6 †
  255.4*
- swelling, joint (see also Tuberculosis,
  joint) 015.9
- symphysis pubis 015.8
- synovitis 015.9 † 727.0*
- - hip 015.1 † 727.0*
- - knee 015.2 † 727.0*
- - specified site NEC 015.8 † 727.0*
- - spine or vertebra 015.0 † 727.0*
- systemic - see Tuberculosis, miliary
- tarsitis 017.0 † 373.4*
- tendon (sheath) - see Tuberculosis,
  tenosynovitis
- tenosynovitis 015.9 † 727.0*
- - hip 015.1 † 727.0*
- - knee 015.2 † 727.0*
- - specified site NEC 015.8 † 727.0*
- - spine or vertebra 015.0 † 727.0*
- testis 016.3 † 608.8*
- throat 012.8
- thymus gland 017.8
- thyroid gland 017.5
- toe 017.8
- tongue 017.8
- tonsil (lingual) 012.8
- tonsillitis 012.8
- trachea, tracheal 012.8
- - gland 012.1
- - - primary, progressive 010.8
- - isolated 012.2
- tracheobronchial 011.3
- - glandular 012.1
- - - primary, progressive 010.8
- - isolated 012.2
- - lymph gland or node 012.1
- - - primary, progressive 010.8
- tubal 016.4 † 614.2*
- - acute 016.4 † 614.0*
- - chronic 016.4 † 614.1*
- tunica vaginalis 016.3
- typhlitis 014
- ulcer (skin) (primary) 017.0
- - bowel or intestine 014
- - specified site NEC - code by site under
  Tuberculosis 011.9
- unspecified site - see Tuberculosis,
  pulmonary
- ureter 016.1 † 593.8*
- urethra, urethral (gland) 016.1
- urinary organ or tract 016.1
- uterus 016.4
- uveal tract 017.3 † 363.1*
- uvula 017.8
- vagina 016.4

Tuberculosis - *continued*
- vas deferens 016.3
- vein 017.8
- verruca (primary) 017.0
- verrucosa (cutis) (primary) 017.0
- vertebra (column) 015.0 † 730.4*
- vesiculitis 016.3 † 608.8*
- viscera NEC 014
- vulva 016.4
- wrist (joint) 015.8
- - bone 015.7 † 730.5*
Tuberculum
- occlusal 520.2
- paramolare 520.2
Tuberous sclerosis (brain) 759.5
Tubo-ovarian - see condition
Tuboplasty, after previous sterilization
  V26.0
Tubotympanitis 381.1
Tularemia 021
- conjunctivitis 021 † 372.0*
- ophthalmic 021
- pneumonia (any) 021 † 484.4*
Tumefaction - see also Swelling
- liver (see also Hypertrophy, liver) 789.1
Tumor (M8000/1) - see also Neoplasm,
  unspecified nature
- Abrikossoff's (M9580/0) - see also
  Neoplasm, connective tissue, benign
- - malignant (M9580/3) - see Neoplasm,
  connective tissue, malignant
- acinar cell (M8550/1) - see Neoplasm,
  uncertain behavior
- acinic cell (M8550/1) - see Neoplasm,
  uncertain behavior
- adenomatoid (M9054/0) - see also
  Neoplasm, benign
- - odontogenic (M9300/0) 213.1
- - - upper jaw (bone) 213.0
- adnexal (skin) (M8390/0) - see
  Neoplasm, skin, benign
- adrenal
- - cortical (benign) (M8370/0) 227.0
- - - malignant (M8370/3) 194.0
- - rest (M8671/0) - see Neoplasm, benign
- alpha-cell (M8152/0)
- - malignant (M8152/3)
- - - pancreas 157.4
- - - specified site NEC - see Neoplasm,
  malignant
- - - unspecified site 157.4
- - pancreas 211.7
- - specified site NEC - see Neoplasm,
  benign
- - unspecified site 211.7
- aneurysmal (see also Aneurysm) 442.9
- aortic body (M8691/1) 237.3

Tumor - *continued*
- aortic body - *continued*
- - malignant (M8691/3) 194.6
- argentaffin (M8241/1) - see Neoplasm, uncertain behavior
- basal cell (M8090/1) - see also Neoplasm, skin, uncertain behavior
- benign (M8000/0) - see Neoplasm, benign
- beta-cell (M8151/0)
- - malignant (M8151/3)
- - - pancreas 157.4
- - - specified site NEC - see Neoplasm, malignant
- - - unspecified site 157.4
- - - pancreas 211.7
- - specified site NEC - see Neoplasm, benign
- - unspecified site 211.7
- blood - see Hematoma
- Brenner (M9000/0) 220
- - borderline malignancy (M9000/1) 236.2
- - malignant (M9000/3) 183.0
- - proliferating (M9000/1) 236.2
- Brooke's (M8100/0) - see Neoplasm, skin, benign
- brown fat (M8880/0) 214
- Burkitt's (M9750/3) 200.2
- calcifying epithelial odontogenic (M9340/0) 213.1
- - upper jaw (bone) 213.0
- carcinoid (M8240/1) - see Carcinoid
- carotid body (M8692/1) 237.3
- - malignant (M8692/3) 194.5
- cells (M8001/1) - see also Neoplasm, unspecified nature
- - benign (M8001/0) - see Neoplasm, benign
- - malignant (M8001/3) - see Neoplasm, malignant
- - uncertain whether benign or malignant (M8001/1) - see Neoplasm, unspecified nature
- cervix in pregnancy or childbirth 654.6
- - causing obstructed labor 660.2
- - - fetus or newborn 763.1
- - fetus or newborn 763.8
- chondromatous giant cell (M9230/0) - see Neoplasm, bone, benign
- chromaffin (M8700/0) - see also Neoplasm, benign
- - malignant (M8700/3) - see Neoplasm, malignant
- Cock's peculiar 706.2
- Codman's (M9230/0) - see Neoplasm, bone, benign

Tumor - *continued*
- dentigerous, mixed (M9282/0) 213.1
- - upper jaw (bone) 213.0
- dermoid (M9084/0) - see Neoplasm, benign
- - with malignant transformation (M9084/3) 183.0
- desmoid (extra-abdominal) (M8821/1) - see also Neoplasm, connective tissue, uncertain behavior
- - abdominal (M8822/1) - see Neoplasm, connective tissue, uncertain behavior
- embryonal (mixed) (M9080/1) - see also Neoplasm, uncertain behavior
- - liver (M9080/3) 155.0
- endodermal sinus (M9071/3)
- - specified site - see Neoplasm, malignant
- - unspecified site
- - - female 183.0
- - - male 186.9
- epithelial
- - benign (M8010/0) - see Neoplasm, benign
- - malignant (M8010/3) - see Neoplasm, malignant
- Ewing's (M9260/3) - see Neoplasm, bone, malignant
- fatty - see Lipoma
- fibroid (M8890/0) - see Leiomyoma
- G cell (M8153/1)
- - malignant (M8153/3)
- - - pancreas 157.4
- - - specified site NEC - see Neoplasm, malignant
- - - unspecified site 157.4
- - specified site - see Neoplasm, uncertain behavior
- - unspecified site 235.5
- giant cell (type) (M8003/1) - see also Neoplasm, unspecified nature
- - bone (M9250/1) 238.0
- - - malignant (M9250/3) - see Neoplasm, bone, malignant
- - chondromatous (M9230/0) - see Neoplasm, bone, benign
- - malignant (M8003/3) - see Neoplasm, malignant
- - soft parts (M9251/1) - see Neoplasm, connective tissue, uncertain behavior
- - - malignant (M9251/3) - see Neoplasm, connective tissue, malignant
- glomus (M8711/0) 228.0
- - jugulare (M8690/1) 237.3
- - - malignant (M8690/3) 194.6

Tumor - *continued*
- odontogenic - *continued*
- − adenomatoid (M9300/0) 213.1
- − − upper jaw (bone) 213.0
- − benign (M9270/0) 213.1
- − − upper jaw (bone) 213.0
- − calcifying epithelial (M9340/0) 213.1
- − − upper jaw (bone) 213.0
- − malignant (M9270/3) 170.1
- − − upper jaw (bone) 170.0
- − squamous (M9312/0) 213.1
- − − upper jaw (bone) 213.0
- ovarian stromal (M8590/1) 236.2
- ovary
- − in pregnancy or childbirth 654.4
- − − causing obstructed labor 660.2
- − − − fetus or newborn 763.1
- − − fetus or newborn 763.8
- pacinian (M9507/0) - see Neoplasm, skin, benign
- Pancoast's (M8010/3) 162.3
- papillary - see Papilloma
- pelvic, in pregnancy or childbirth 654.9
- − causing obstructed labor 660.2
- − − fetus or newborn 763.1
- − fetus or newborn 763.8
- phantom 300.1
- plasma cell (M9731/1) 238.6
- − benign (M9731/0) - see Neoplasm, benign
- − malignant (M9731/3) 203.8
- polyvesicular vitelline (M9071/3)
- − specified site - see Neoplasm, malignant
- − unspecified site
- − − female 183.0
- − − male 186.9
- Pott's puffy (see also Osteomyelitis) 730.2
- Rathke's pouch (M9350/1) 237.0
- Regaud's (M8082/3) - see Neoplasm, nasopharynx, malignant
- rete cell (M8140/0) 222.0
- retinal anlage (M9363/0) - see Neoplasm, benign
- salivary gland type, mixed (M8940/0) - see also Neoplasm, benign
- − malignant (M8940/3) - see Neoplasm, malignant
- Sampson's 617.1
- Schloffer's (see also Peritonitis) 567.2
- Schminke's (M8082/3) - see Neoplasm, nasopharynx, malignant
- sebaceous (see also Cyst, sebaceous) 706.2
- secondary (M8000/6) - see Secondary neoplasm

Tumor - *continued*
- Sertoli cell (M8640/0)
- − with lipid storage (M8641/0)
- − − specified site - see Neoplasm, benign
- − − unspecified site
- − − − female 220
- − − − male 222.0
- − specified site - see Neoplasm, benign
- − unspecified site
- − − female 220
- − − male 222.0
- Sertoli-Leydig cell (M8631/0)
- − specified site - see Neoplasm, benign
- − unspecified site
- − − female 220
- − − male 222.0
- sex cord(-stromal) (M8590/1) - see Neoplasm, uncertain behavior
- skin appendage (M8390/0) - see Neoplasm, skin, benign
- soft tissue
- − benign (M8800/0) - see Neoplasm, connective tissue, benign
- − malignant (M8800/3) - see Neoplasm, connective tissue, malignant
- sternomastoid 754.1
- sweat gland (M8400/1) - see also Neoplasm, skin, uncertain behavior
- − benign (M8400/0) - see Neoplasm, skin, benign
- − malignant (M8400/3) - see Neoplasm, skin, malignant
- syphilitic, brain 094.8
- − congenital 090.4
- testicular stromal (M8590/1) 236.4
- theca cell (M8600/0) 220
- theca cell-granulosa cell (M8621/1) 236.2
- theca-lutein (M8610/0) 220
- turban (M8200/0) 216.4
- uterus in pregnancy or childbirth 654.1
- − causing obstructed labor 660.2
- − − fetus or newborn 763.1
- − fetus or newborn 763.8
- vagina in pregnancy or childbirth 654.7
- − causing obstructed labor 660.2
- − − fetus or newborn 763.1
- − fetus or newborn 763.8
- varicose (see also Varicose vein) 454.9
- von Recklinghausen's (M9540/1) 237.7
- vulva in pregnancy or childbirth 654.8
- − causing obstructed labor 660.2
- − − fetus or newborn 763.8
- Warthin's (M8561/0) 210.2
- white (see also Tuberculosis, arthritis) 015.9 † 711.4*
- White-Darier 757.3

Tumor - *continued*
- Wilms' (M8960/3) 189.0
- yolk sac (M9071/3)
- - specified site - see Neoplasm, malignant
- - unspecified site
- - - female 183.0
- - - male 186.9
Tumorlet (M8040/1) - see Neoplasm, uncertain behavior
Tungiasis 134.1
Tunica vasculosa lentis 743.5
Turban tumor (M8200/0) 216.4
Turck's
- syndrome 378.7
- trachoma 476.0
Turner's
- hypoplasia, hypoplasis (tooth) 520.4
- syndrome 758.6
- tooth 520.4
Turner-Varny syndrome 758.6
Turricephaly 756.0
Tussis convulsiva (see also Whooping cough) 033.9
Twin 761.5
- conjoined 759.4
- pregnancy (complicating delivery) 651.0
Twist, twisted
- bowel, colon or intestine 560.2
- hair (congenital) 757.4
- mesentery or omentum 560.2
- - gangrenous - see Hernia, by site, gangrenous
- organ or site, congenital NEC - see Anomaly, specified type NEC
- ovarian pedicle 620.5
- - congenital 752.0
- umbilical cord - see Compression, umbilical cord
Tylosis 700
- linguae 528.6
- palmaris et plantaris 757.3
Tympanites (abdominal) (intestine) 787.3
Tympanitis 384.8
- with otitis media - see Otitis media
- acute 384.0
- chronic 384.1
Tympanosclerosis 385.0
Tympanum - see condition
Tympany
- abdomen 787.3
- chest 786.7
Typhlitis (see also Appendicitis) 541
Typhoenteritis 002.0
Typhoid (abortive) (ambulant) (any site) (fever) (hemorrhagic) (infection) (intermittent) (malignant) (rheumatic) 002.0

Typhoid - *continued*
- abdominal 002.0
- clinical (Widal and blood test negative) 002.0
- inoculation reaction - see Complications, vaccination
- mesenteric lymph nodes 002.0
- pneumonia 002.0 † 484.8*
- spine 002.0 † 720.8*
- Widal negative 002.0
Typhomalaria (fever) (see also Malaria) 084.6
Typhomania 002.0
Typhoperitonitis 002.0
Typhus (fever) 081.9
- abdominal, abdominalis 002.0
- African tick 082.1
- brain 081.9
- cerebral 081.9
- classical 080
- endemic (flea-borne) 081.0
- epidemic (louse-borne) 080
- exanthematic NEC 080
- exanthematicus NEC 080
- - brillii NEC 081.1
- - mexicanus NEC 081.0
- - pediculo vestimenti causa 080
- - typus murinus 081.0
- flea-borne 081.0
- India tick 082.1
- Kenya tick 082.1
- louse-borne 080
- Mexican 081.0
- - flea-borne 081.0
- - louse-borne 080
- - tabardillo 080
- mite-borne 081.2
- murine 081.0
- North Asian tick-borne 082.2
- petechial 081.9
- Queensland tick 082.3
- rat 081.0
- recrudescent 081.1
- recurrent (see also Fever, relapsing) 087.9
- Sao Paulo 082.0
- scrub (China) (India) (Malay) (New Guinea) 081.2
- shop (of Malaya) 081.0
- Siberian tick 082.2
- tick-borne NEC 082.9
- tropical 081.2
Tyrosinosis 270.2
Tyrosinuria 270.2

U

Uhl's disease 746.8
Ulcer, ulcerated, ulcerating, ulceration,
ulcerative 707.9
- abdomen (wall) (see also Ulcer, skin)
707.8
- ala, nose 478.1
- alveolar process 526.5
- amebic (intestine) (see also Amebiasis)
006.9
- - skin 006.6
- anastomotic - see Ulcer, gastrojejunal
- anorectal 569.4
- antral - see Ulcer, stomach
- anus (sphincter) (solitary) 569.4
- - varicose - see Varicose, ulcer, anus
- aphthous (oral) (recurrent) 528.2
- - genital organ(s)
- - - female 616.8
- - - male 608.8
- arm (see also Ulcer, skin) 707.8
- artery 447.2
- atrophic NEC - see Ulcer, skin
- bile duct (see also Disease, biliary) 576.8
- bladder (solitary) (sphincter) 596.8
- - bilharzial 120.- † 595.4*
- - submucosal (see also Cystitis) 595.1
- - tuberculous 016.1 † 595.4*
- bleeding NEC 533.4
- bone 730.9
- bowel (see also Ulcer, intestine) 569.8
- breast 611.0
- bronchus 519.1
- buccal (cavity) (traumatic) 528.9
- burn - see Ulcer, duodenum
- Buruli 031.1
- buttock (see also Ulcer, skin) 707.8
- - decubitus 707.0
- cancerous (M8000/3) - see Neoplasm,
malignant
- cardia - see Ulcer, stomach
- cardio-esophageal (peptic) 530.2
- cecum (see also Ulcer, intestine) 569.8
- cervix (uteri) (trophic) 622.0
- - with mention of cervicitis 616.0
- chancroidal 099.0
- chest (wall) (see also Ulcer, skin) 707.8
- chiclero 085.4
- chin (see also Ulcer, skin) 707.8
- chronic (cause unknown) - see Ulcer, skin
- Cochin-China 085.1

Ulcer - continued
- colon (see also Ulcer, intestine) 569.8
- conjunctiva (acute) (postinfectional)
372.0
- cornea (annular) (catarrhal) (central)
(infectional) (marginal) (ring) (serpent)
(serpiginous) (with perforation) 370.0
- - dendritic 054.4 † 370.1*
- - phlyctenular, tuberculous 017.3 †
370.3*
- - tuberculous 017.3 † 370.3*
- corpus cavernosum (chronic) 607.8
- crural - see Ulcer, lower extremity
- Curling's - see Ulcer, duodenum
- Cushing's - see Ulcer, peptic
- decubitus (any site) 707.0
- dendritic 054.4 † 370.1*
- diabetes, diabetic (mellitus) 250.-
- Dieulafoy's - see Ulcer, stomach
- due to
- - infection NEC - see Ulcer, skin
- - radiation - see Ulcer, by site
- - trophic disturbance (any region) - see
Ulcer, skin
- - X-ray - see Ulcer, by site
- duodenum, duodenal (eroded) (peptic)
532.9
- - with
- - - hemorrhage 532.4
- - - - and perforation 532.6
- - - perforation 532.5
- - acute 532.3
- - - with
- - - - hemorrhage 532.0
- - - - - and perforation 532.2
- - - - perforation 532.1
- - chronic 532.7
- - - with
- - - - hemorrhage 532.4
- - - - - and perforation 532.6
- - - - perforation 532.5
- dysenteric NEC 009.0
- elusive 595.1
- epiglottis 478.7
- esophagus (peptic) 530.2
- - due to ingestion of aspirin, chemical or
medicament 530.2
- - fungal 530.2
- - infectional 530.2
- - varicose 456.1

Ulcer - *continued*
- esophagus - *continued*
- - varicose - *continued*
- - - bleeding 456.0
- eye NEC 360.0
- - dendritic 054.4 † 370.1*
- eyelid (region) 373.0
- face (see also Ulcer, skin) 707.8
- fauces 478.2
- fistulous NEC - see Ulcer, skin
- foot (indolent) (see also Ulcer, lower extremity) 707.1
- - perforating 707.1
- - - leprous 030.1
- - - syphilitic 094.0
- - varicose 454.0
- - - inflamed of infected 454.2
- frambesian, initial 102.0
- gallbladder or duct (see also Disease, gallbladder) 575.8
- gangrenous (see also Gangrene) 785.4
- gastric - see Ulcer, stomach
- gastrocolic - see Ulcer, gastrojejunal
- gastroduodenal - see Ulcer, peptic
- gastroesophageal - see Ulcer, stomach
- gastrohepatic - see Ulcer, stomach
- gastrointestinal - see Ulcer, gastrojejunal
- gastrojejunal (peptic) 534.9
- - with
- - - hemorrhage 534.4
- - - - and perforation 534.6
- - - perforation 534.5
- - acute 534.3
- - - with
- - - - hemorrhage 534.0
- - - - - and perforation 534.2
- - - - perforation 534.1
- - chronic 534.7
- - - with
- - - - hemorrhage 534.4
- - - - - and perforation 534.6
- - - - perforation 534.5
- gastrojejunocolic - see Ulcer, gastrojejunal
- gingiva 523.8
- gingivitis 523.1
- glottis 478.7
- groin (see also Ulcer, skin) 707.8
- gum 523.8
- hand (see also Ulcer, skin) 707.8
- heel 707.1
- - decubitus 707.0
- hip (see also Ulcer, skin) 707.8
- - decubitus 707.0
- Hunner's 595.1
- hypopharynx 478.2
- hypopyon (chronic) (subacute) 370.0

Ulcer - *continued*
- hypostaticum - see Ulcer, varicose
- ileum (see also Ulcer, intestine) 569.8
- intestine, intestinal 569.8
- - amebic (see also Amebiasis) 006.9
- - duodenal - see Ulcer, duodenum
- - marginal 569.8
- - perforating 569.8
- - small, primary 569.8
- - stercoraceous 569.8
- - stercoral 569.8
- - tuberculous 014
- - typhoid (fever) 002.0
- - varicose 456.8
- jejunum, jejunal - see Ulcer, gastrojejunal
- keratitis 370.0
- knee - see Ulcer, lower extremity
- labium (majus) (minus) 616.5
- laryngitis (see also Laryngitis) 464.0
- larynx (aphthous) (contact) 478.7
- - diphtheritic 032.3
- leg - see Ulcer, lower extremity
- lip 528.5
- lower extremity (atrophic) (chronic) (neurogenic) (perforating) (pyogenic) (trophic) (tropical) 707.1
- - decubitus 707.0
- - varicose 454.0
- - - inflamed or infected 454.2
- luetic - see Ulcer, syphilitic
- lung 518.8
- - tuberculous 011.2
- malignant (M8000/3) - see Neoplasm, malignant
- marginal NEC - see Ulcer, gastrojejunal
- meatus (urinarius) 597.8
- Meckel's diverticulum 751.0
- Meleney's (chronic undermining) 686.0
- Mooren's (cornea) 370.0
- mouth (traumatic) 528.9
- nasopharynx 478.2
- neck (see also Ulcer, skin) 707.8
- neurogenic NEC - see Ulcer, skin
- nose, nasal (passage) (infectional) 478.1
- - septum 478.1
- - - varicose 456.8
- - skin - see Ulcer, skin
- - spirochetal NEC 104.8
- oesophagus (peptic) 530.2
- - due to ingestion of aspirin, chemical or medicament 530.2
- - fungal 530.2
- - infectional 530.2
- - varicose 456.1
- - - bleeding 456.0
- oral mucosa (traumatic) 528.9

Ulcer - *continued*
- palate 528.9
- - soft 528.9
- penetrating NEC 533.5
- penis (chronic) 607.8
- peptic (site unspecified) 533.9
- - with
- - - hemorrhage 533.4
- - - - and perforation 533.6
- - - perforation 533.5
- - acute 533.3
- - - with
- - - - hemorrhage 533.0
- - - - - and perforation 533.2
- - - - perforation 533.1
- - chronic 533.7
- - - with
- - - - hemorrhage 533.4
- - - - - and perforation 533.6
- - - - perforation 533.5
- perforating NEC 533.5
- - skin 707.9
- perineum (see also Ulcer, skin) 707.8
- peritonsillar 474.8
- phagedenic (tropical) NEC - see Ulcer, skin
- pharynx 478.2
- phlebitis - see Phlebitis
- plaster 707.0
- popliteal space - see Ulcer, lower extremity
- postpyloric - see Ulcer, duodenum
- prepuce 607.8
- prepyloric - see Ulcer, stomach
- pressure 707.0
- pseudopeptic - see Ulcer, peptic
- pyloric - see Ulcer, stomach
- rectosigmoid 569.8
- rectum (sphincter) (solitary) 569.4
- - stercoraceous 569.4
- - varicose - see Varicose, ulcer, anus
- retina (see also Chorioretinitis) 363.2
- rodent (M8090/3) - see also Neoplasm, skin, malignant
- round - see Ulcer, stomach
- sacrum (region) (see also Ulcer, skin) 707.8
- scalp (see also Ulcer, skin) 707.8
- sclera 379.0
- scrofulous 017.2
- scrotum 608.8
- - tuberculous 016.3
- - varicose 456.4
- seminal vesicle 608.8
- sigmoid 569.8
- skin (atrophic) (chronic) (neurogenic) (perforating) (pyogenic) (trophic) 707.9

Ulcer - *continued*
- skin - *continued*
- - with gangrene (see also Gangrene) 785.4
- - amebic 006.6
- - decubitus 707.0
- - lower extremity 707.1
- - tuberculous (primary) 017.0
- - varicose - see Ulcer, varicose
- sloughing NEC - see Ulcer, skin
- solitary, anus or rectum (sphincter) 569.4
- sore throat 462
- - streptococcal 034.0
- spermatic cord 608.8
- spine (tuberculous) 015.0 † 730.4*
- stasis (venous) 454.0
- - inflamed or infected 454.2
- stercoraceous 569.8
- stercoral 569.8
- - anus or rectum 569.4
- stoma, stomal - see Ulcer, gastrojejunal
- stomach (eroded) (peptic) (round) 531.9
- - with
- - - hemorrhage 531.4
- - - - and perforation 531.6
- - - perforation 531.5
- - acute 531.3
- - - with
- - - - hemorrhage 531.0
- - - - - and perforation 531.2
- - - - perforation 531.1
- - chronic 531.7
- - - with
- - - - hemorrhage 531.4
- - - - - and perforation 531.6
- - - - perforation 531.5
- stomatitis 528.0
- stress - see Ulcer, peptic
- strumous (tuberculous) 017.2
- submental (see also Ulcer, skin) 707.8
- syphilitic (any site) (early) (secondary) 091.3
- - late 095
- - perforating 095
- - - foot 094.0
- testis 608.8
- thigh - see Ulcer, lower extremity
- throat 478.2
- - diphtheritic 032.0
- toe - see Ulcer, lower extremity
- tongue (traumatic) 529.0
- tonsil 474.8
- - diphtheritic 032.0
- trachea 519.1
- trophic - see Ulcer, skin
- tropical NEC 707.9
- tuberculous - see Tuberculosis, ulcer

Ulcer - *continued*
- tunica vaginalis 608.8
- turbinate 730.9
- typhoid (fever) 002.0
- - perforating 002.0
- umbilical (newborn) 771.4
- unspecified site NEC - see Ulcer, skin
- urethra (meatus) (see also Urethritis) 597.8
- uterus 621.8
- - cervix 622.0
- - - with mention of cervicitis 616.0
- - neck 622.0
- - - with mention of cervicitis 616.0
- vagina 616.8
- valve, heart 421.0
- varicose (lower extremity, any part) 454.0
- - anus - see Varicose, ulcer, anus
- - esophagus 456.1
- - - bleeding 456.0
- - inflamed or infected 454.2
- - nasal septum 456.8
- - rectum - see Varicose, ulcer, anus
- - scrotum 456.4
- - specified site NEC 456.8
- vas deferens 608.8
- vulva (acute) (infectional) 616.5
- - Behcet's syndrome 136.1 † 616.5*
- - herpetic 054.1 † 616.5*
- vulvobuccal, recurring 616.5
- X-ray - see Ulcer, by site
- yaws 102.4

Ulcus - see also Ulcer
- cutis tuberculosum 017.0
- duodeni - see Ulcer, duodenum
- durum 091.0
- - extragenital 091.2
- gastrojejunale - see Ulcer, gastrojejunal
- hypostaticum - see Ulcer, varicose
- molle (cutis) (skin) 099.0
- serpens corneae (pneumococcal) 370.0
- ventriculi - see Ulcer, stomach
Ulegyria 742.4
Ulerythema
- acneiforme 701.8
- ophryogenes 757.4

Ullrich(-Bonnevie)(-Turner) syndrome 758.6
Ullrich-Feichtiger syndrome 759.8
Ulnar - see condition
Ulorrhagia 523.8
Ulorrhea 523.8
Unavailability of medical facilities (at) V63.9
- due to

Unavailability of medical facilities - *cont.*
- due to - *continued*
- - investigation by social service agency V63.8
- - lack of services at home V63.1
- - remoteness from facility V63.0
- - waiting list V63.2
- home V63.1
- outpatient clinic V63.0
Uncinariasis (see also Ancylostomiasis) 126.9
Unconscious(ness) 780.0
Under observation - see Observation
Underdevelopment - see also Undeveloped
- sexual 259.0
Undernourishment 269.9
Undernutrition 269.9
Underweight 783.4
- for gestational age - see Light-for-dates
Underwood's disease 778.1
Undescended - see also Malposition, congenital
- cecum 751.4
- colon 751.4
- testicle 752.5
Undetermined cause 799.9
Undeveloped, undevelopment - see also Hypoplasia
- brain (congenital) 742.1
- cerebral (congenital) 742.1
- fetus or newborn 764.9
- heart 746.8
- lung 748.5
- testis 257.2
- uterus 259.0
Undiagnosed (disease) 799.9
Unemployment, anxiety concerning V62.0
Unequal leg (length) (acquired) 736.8
- congenital 755.3
Unerupted tooth, teeth 520.6
Unextracted dental root 525.3
Unguis incarnatus 703.0
Unicollis uterus 752.3
Unicornis uterus 752.3
Unicorporeus uterus 752.3
Uniformis uterus 752.3
Unilateral - see also condition
- development, breast 611.8
- organ or site, congenital NEC - see Agenesis
- vagina 752.4
Unilateralis uterus 752.3
Unilocular heart 746.8
Union, abnormal - see also Fusion
- larynx and trachea 748.3
Universal mesentery 751.4
Unknown 799.9

Unknown - *continued*
- cause 799.9
- diagnosis 799.9
Unsoundness of mind (see also Psychosis) 298.9
Unspecified cause 799.9
Unstable
- back NEC 724.9
- joint 718.9
- lie 652.0
- - fetus or newborn 761.7
- lumbosacral joint (congenital) 756.1
- - acquired 724.6
- sacroiliac 724.6
- spine NEC 724.9
Untruthfulness, child problem 312.0
Unverricht(-Lundborg) disease or epilepsy 333.2
Unverricht-Wagner syndrome 710.3
Upper respiratory - see condition
Upset
- gastrointestinal 536.8
- - psychogenic 306.4
- - virus (see also Enteritis, viral) 008.8
- intestinal (large) (small) 564.9
- - psychogenic 306.4
- menstruation 626.9
- mental 300.9
- stomach 536.8
- - psychogenic 306.4
Urachus - see also condition
- patent 753.7
- persistent 753.7
Uratic arthritis 274.0 † 712.0*
Urbach's lipoid proteinosis 272.8
Urbach-Oppenheim disease 250.7 † 709.8*
Urbach-Wiethe disease 272.8
Urea, blood, high - see Uremia
Uremia, uremic (absorption) (amaurosis) (amblyopia) (aphasia) (apoplexy) (coma) (delirium) (dementia) (dropsy) (dyspnea) (fever) (intoxication) (mania) (paralysis) (poisoning) (toxemia) (vomiting) 586
- chronic 585
- complicating
- - abortion - see categories 634-639, fourth digit .3
- - ectopic or molar pregnancy 639.3
- - hypertension (see also Hypertension, kidney) 403.9
- - labor and delivery 639.3
- congenital 779.8
- extrarenal 788.9
- hypertensive (see also Hypertension, kidney) 403.9
- maternal nec, affecting fetus or newborn 760.1

Uremia - *continued*
- prerenal 788.9
Ureter, ureteral - see condition
Ureteralgia 788.0
Ureterectasis 593.8
Ureteritis 593.8
- cystica 590.3
- due to calculus 592.1
- gonococcal (acute) 098.1
- - chronic or duration of 2 months or over 098.3
- nonspecific 593.8
Ureterocele 593.8
- congenital 753.2
Ureterolith 592.1
Ureterolithiasis 592.1
Urethra, urethral - see condition
Urethralgia 788.9
Urethritis (abacterial) (acute) (allergic) (anterior) (chronic) (nonvenereal) (posterior) (recurrent) (simple) (subacute) (ulcerative) (undifferentiated) 597.8
- diplococcal 098.0
- - chronic or duration of 2 months or over 098.2
- gonococcal 098.0
- - chronic or duration of 2 months or over 098.2
- nongonococcal (sexually transmitted) 099.4
- - Reiter's 099.3
- nonspecific (sexually transmitted) 099.4
- not sexually transmitted 597.8
- Reiter's 099.3
- trichomonal or due to Trichomonas (vaginalis) 131.0 † 597.8*
- venereal NEC 099.4
Urethrocele
- female 618.0
- male 599.5
Urethrorectal - see condition
Urethrorrhagia 599.8
Urethrotrigonitis 595.3
Urethrovaginal - see condition
Urhidrosis, uridrosis 705.8
Uric acid
- diathesis 274.9
- in blood 790.6
Uricacidemia 790.6
Uricemia 790.6
Uricosuria 791.9
Urinary - see condition
Urine
- blood in (see also Hematuria) 599.7
- discharge excessive 788.4
- extravasation 788.8
- incontinence 788.3

V

Vaccination
- complication or reaction - see
Complications, vaccination
- not done (contraindicated) V64.0
- - because of patient's decision V64.2
- prophylactic (against) V05.9
- - arthropod-borne viral
- - - disease NEC V05.1
- - - encephalitis V05.0
- - cholera (alone) V03.0
- - - with typhoid-paratyphoid (cholera
+ TAB) V06.0
- - common cold V04.7
- - diphtheria-tetanus-pertussis combined
(DTP) V06.1
- - - with
- - - - poliomyelitis (DTP + polio)
V06.3
- - - - typhoid-paratyphoid (DTP +
TAB) V06.2
- - diphtheria alone V03.5
- - disease (single) NEC V05.9
- - - bacterial NEC V03.9
- - - - specified NEC V03.8
- - - combinations NEC V06.9
- - - - specified NEC V06.8
- - - specified NEC V05.8
- - encephalitis, viral, arthropod-borne
V05.0
- - influenza V04.8
- - leishmaniasis V05.2
- - measles alone V04.2
- - measles-mumps-rubella (MMR) V06.4
- - mumps alone V04.6
- - pertussis alone V03.6
- - plague V03.3
- - poliomyelitis V04.0
- - rabies V04.5
- - rubella alone V04.3
- - smallpox V04.1
- - tetanus toxoid alone V03.7
- - tuberculosis (BCG) V03.2
- - tularemia V03.4
- - typhoid-paratyphoid alone (TAB)
V03.1
- - yellow fever V04.4
Vaccinia (generalized) 999.0
- congenital 771.2
- eyelid 999.0 † 373.5*
- localized 999.3

Vaccinia - *continued*
- not from vaccination 051.0
- - eyelid 051.0 † 373.5*
Vacuum in sinus (accessory) (nasal) (see
also Sinusitis) 473.9
Vagabond V60.0
Vagabonds' disease 132.1
Vagina, vaginal - see condition
Vaginalitis (tunica) 608.4
Vaginismus (reflex) 625.1
- hysterical 300.1
- psychogenic 306.5
Vaginitis (acute) (atrophic) (chronic)
(circumscribed) (diffuse)
(emphysematous) (hemophilus vaginalis)
(nonspecific) (nonvenereal) (senile)
(ulcerative) 616.1
- with
- - abortion - see categories 634-639,
fourth digit .0
- - ectopic gestation 639.0
- adhesive, congenital 752.4
- atrophic, postmenopausal 627.3
- blennorrhagic 098.0
- - chronic or duration of 2 months or over
098.2
- complicating pregnancy or puerperium
646.6
- - fetus or newborn 760.8
- due to Trichomonas (vaginalis) 131.0 †
616.1*
- gonococcal 098.0
- - chronic or duration of 2 months or over
098.2
- granuloma 099.2
- monilia 112.1 † 616.1*
- mycotic 112.1 † 616.1*
- postmenopausal atrophic 627.3
- senile 627.3
- syphilitic (early) 091.0
- - late 095
- trichomonal 131.0 † 616.1*
- tuberculous 016.4
- venereal NEC 099.8
Vagotonia 352.3
Vallecula - see condition
Valley fever 114
Valsuani's disease 648.2
Valve, valvular (formation) - see also
condition

Varix - *continued*
- inflamed or infected - *continued*
- - ulcerated 454.2
- labia (majora) 456.6
- orbit 456.8
- - congenital 747.6
- ovary 456.5
- papillary 448.1
- pelvis 456.5
- pharynx 456.8
- placenta - see Placenta, abnormal
- rectum - see Hemorrhoids
- renal papilla 456.8
- retina 362.1
- scrotum (ulcerated) 456.4
- sigmoid colon 456.8
- specified site NEC 456.8
- spinal (cord) (vessels) 456.8
- spleen, splenic (vein) (with phlebolith) 456.8
- sublingual 456.3
- ulcerated 454.0
- - inflamed or infected 454.2
- umbilical cord, affecting fetus or newborn 762.6
- uterine ligament 456.5
- vocal cord 456.8
- vulva 456.6
- - in pregnancy, childbirth or puerperium 671.1
Vas deferens - see condition
Vas deferentitis 608.4
Vasa previa 663.5
- hemorrhage from, affecting fetus or newborn 772.0
Vascular - see also condition
- loop on papilla (optic) 743.5
- sheathing, retina 362.1
- spider 448.1
Vascularity, pulmonary, congenital 747.3
Vasculitis 447.6
- allergic 287.0
- cryoglobulinemic 273.2
- disseminated 447.6
- kidney 447.8
- nodular 695.2
- retina 362.1
- rheumatic - see Fever, rheumatic
Vasitis 608.4
- nodosa 608.4
- tuberculous 016.3
Vasodilation 443.9
Vasomotor - see condition
Vasoplasty, after previous sterilization V26.0
Vasospasm 443.9
- cerebral (artery) 435

Vasospasm - *continued*
- peripheral NEC 443.9
- retina (artery) 362.3
Vasospastic - see condition
Vasovagal attack (paroxysmal) 780.2
- psychogenic 306.2
VATER syndrome 759.8
Vater's ampulla - see condition
Vegetation, vegetative
- adenoid (nasal fossa) 474.2
- endocarditis (acute) (any valve) (chronic) (subacute) 421.0
- heart (mycotic) (valve) 421.0
Veil, Jackson's 751.4
Vein, venous - see condition
Veldt sore (see also Ulcer, skin) 707.9
Velpeau's hernia - see Hernia, femoral
Venofibrosis 459.8
Venom, venomous
- bite or sting (animal or insect) 989.5
- poisoning 989.5
Venous - see condition
Ventouse delivery NEC 669.5
- fetus or newborn 763.3
Ventral - see condition
Ventricle, ventricular - see also condition
- escape 427.6
Ventriculitis, cerebral (see also Meningitis) 322.9
Vernet's syndrome 352.6
Verneuil's disease 095
Verruca (filiformis) (plana) (plana juvenilis) (plantaris) (vulgaris) 078.1
- acuminata (any site) 078.1
- necrogenica (primary) 017.0
- seborrheica 702
- senile 702
- tuberculosa (primary) 017.0
- venereal 078.1
- viral 078.1
Verrucosities (see also Verruca) 078.1
Verruga
- peruana 088.0
- peruviana 088.0
Verse's disease 275.4 † 722.9*
Version
- before labor, affecting fetus or newborn 761.7
- cephalic (correcting previous malposition) 652.1
- - affecting fetus or newborn 761.7
- cervix (see also Malposition, uterus) 621.6
- uterus (postinfectional) (postpartal, old) (see also Malposition, uterus) 621.6
- - forward - see Anteversion, uterus
- - lateral - see Lateroversion, uterus

Vertebra, vertebral - see condition
Vertigo 780.4
– auditory 386.1
– aural 386.1
– benign paroxysmal 386.1
– central 386.2
– cerebral 386.2
– epidemic 078.8 † 386.1*
– epileptic - see Epilepsy
– hysterical 300.1
– labyrinthine 386.1
– Meniere's 386.0
– menopausal 627.2
– otogenic 386.1
– peripheral 386.1
Vesania (see also Psychosis) 298.9
Vesical - see condition
Vesicle
– cutaneous 709.8
– seminal - see condition
– skin 709.8
Vesicocolic - see condition
Vesicoperineal - see condition
Vesicorectal - see condition
Vesico-urethrorectal - see condition
Vesicovaginal - see condition
Vesicular - see condition
Vesiculitis (seminal) 608.0
– amebic 006.8
– gonorrheal (acute) 098.1 † 608.0*
– – chronic or duration of 2 months or over
      098.3
– trichomonal 131.0
– tuberculous 016.3 † 608.8*
Vestibulitis 386.3
– ear 386.3
– nose (external) 478.1
Vestige, vestigial - see also Persistence
– branchial 744.4
– structures in vitreous 743.5
Vidal's disease 698.3
Villaret's syndrome 352.6
Villous - see condition
Vincent's
– angina 101
– bronchitis 101
– disease 101
– gingivitis 101
– infection (any site) 101
– laryngitis 101
– stomatitis 101
– tonsillitis 101
Vinson-Plummer syndrome 280
Viosterol deficiency (see also Deficiency,
   calciferol) 268.9
Virchow's disease 733.9
Viremia 790.8

Virilism (adrenal) 255.2
– with
– – adrenal
– – – hyperplasia 255.2
– – – insufficiency (congenital) 255.2
– – cortical hyperfunction 255.2
– – 11 hydroxylase defect 255.2
– – 21 hydroxylase defect 255.2
– – 3B hydroxysteroid dehydrogenase
        defect 255.2
Virilization (female) (see also Virilism)
   255.2
Virus, viral - see also condition
– infection (see also Infection, virus) 079.9
– septicemia 079.9
Viscera, visceral - see condition
Visceroptosis 569.8
Visible peristalsis 787.4
Vision, visual
– binocular, suppression 368.3
– blurred, blurring 368.8
– – hysterical 300.1
– defect, defective NEC 369.9
– disorientation (syndrome) 368.8
– disturbance NEC 368.9
– – hysterical 300.1
– field, limitation 368.4
– hallucinations 368.1
– halos 368.1
– loss 369.9
– – both eyes 369.3
– – complete - see Blindness
– – one eye 369.8
– – sudden 368.1
– low (both eyes) 369.2
– – one eye (other eye normal) 369.7
– – – blindness, other eye 369.1
– perception, simultaneous without fusion
   368.3
Vitality, lack or want of 780.7
– newborn 779.8
Vitamin deficiency NEC (see also
   Deficiency, vitamin) 269.2
Vitelline duct, persistent 751.0
Vitiligo 709.0
– eyelid 374.5
– vulva 624.8
Vitreous - see also condition
– touch syndrome 997.9
Vocal cord - see condition
Vocational rehabilitation V57.2
Vogt's (Cecile) disease or syndrome 333.7
Vogt-Koyanagi syndrome 364.2
Vogt-Spielmeyer
– amaurotic familial idiocy 330.1
– disease 330.1
Voice

Voice - *continued*
- change (see also Dysphonia) 784.4
- loss (see also Aphonia) 784.4
Volhynian fever 083.1
Volkmann's ischemic contracture or
paralysis (complicating trauma) 958.6
Voluntary starvation 307.1
Volvulus (bowel) (colon) (intestine) 560.2
- congenital 751.5
- duodenum 537.3
- fallopian tube 620.5
- oviduct 620.5
- stomach (due to absence of gastrocolic
ligament) 537.8
Vomiting 787.0
- allergic 535.4
- bilious (cause unknown) 787.0
- - following gastro-intestinal surgery
564.3
- blood (see also Hematemesis) 578.0
- causing asphyxia, choking, or suffocation
(see also Asphyxia, food) 933.1
- cyclical 536.2
- - psychogenic 306.4
- epidemic 078.8
- fecal matter 569.8
- following gastrointestinal surgery 564.3
- functional 536.8
- - psychogenic 306.4
- habit 536.2
- hysterical 300.1
- nervous 306.4
- neurotic 306.4
- newborn 779.3
- of or complicating pregnancy 643.9
- - due to
- - - organic disease 643.8
- - - specific cause NEC 643.8
- - early - see Hyperemesis, gravidarum
- - late 643.2
- pernicious or persistent 536.2
- - complicating pregnancy - see
Hyperemesis, gravidarum
- - psychogenic 306.4
- psychic 306.4
- psychogenic 307.5
- stercoral 569.8
- uncontrollable 536.2
- - psychogenic 306.4
- uremic - see Uremia
- winter 078.8

Vomito negro (see also Fever, yellow) 060.9
Von Bechterew(-Strumpell) disease or
syndrome 720.0
Von Bezold's abscess 383.0
Von Economo's disease 049.8 † 323.4*
Von Gierke's disease 271.0
Von Gies' joint 095
Von Graefe's disease 378.8
Von Hippel(-Lindau) disease or syndrome
759.6
Von Jaksch's
- anemia 285.8
- disease 285.8
Von Recklinghausen's
- disease (M9540/1) 237.7
- - bones 252.0
- tumor (M9540/1) 237.7
Von Recklinghausen-Applebaum disease
275.0
Von Willebrand(-Jurgens)(-Minot) disease
or syndrome 286.4
Vossius' ring 921.3
Vrolik's disease 756.5
Vulva - see condition
Vulvitis (acute) (allergic) (aphthous)
(atrophic) (chronic) (gangrenous)
(hypertrophic) (intertriginous) (senile)
616.1
- adhesive, congenital 752.4
- blennorrhagic 098.0
- - chronic or duration of 2 months or over
098.2
- complicating pregnancy, childbirth or
puerperium 646.6
- due to Ducrey's bacillus 099.0
- gonococcal 098.0
- - chronic or duration of 2 months or over
098.2
- leukoplakic 624.0
- monilial 112.1 † 616.1*
- syphilitic (early) 091.0
- - late 095
- trichomonal 131.0 † 616.1*
Vulvorectal - see condition
Vulvovaginitis (see also Vulvitis) 616.1
- amebic 006.8
- gonococcal (acute) 098.0
- herpetic 054.1 † 616.1*
- monilial 112.1 † 616.1*
- trichomonal (vaginalis) 131.0 † 616.1*

W

Weber-Osler syndrome 448.0
Wedge-shaped or wedging vertebrae 733.0
Wegener's granulomatosis or syndrome
  446.4
Weight
– gain (abnormal) (excessive) 783.1
– – during pregnancy 646.1
– less than 1000 grams at birth 765.0
– loss (cause unknown) 783.2
Weightlessness 994.9
Weil(l)-Marchesani syndrome 759.8
Weil's disease 100.0
Weingarten's syndrome 518.3
Weiss-Baker syndrome 337.0
Wen (see also Cyst, sebaceous) 706.2

Wenckebach's phenomenon 426.1
Werdnig-Hoffmann
– atrophy, muscle 335.0
– syndrome or disease 335.0
Werlhof's disease (see also Purpura,
  thrombocytopenic) 287.3
Wermer's syndrome or disease 258.0
Werner's disease or syndrome 259.8
Wernicke's
– encephalopathy 265.1
– polioencephalitis, superior 265.1
– syndrome 265.1
Wernicke-Posadas disease 114
West African fever 084.8
Westphal-Strumpell syndrome 275.1

Wet feet, tropical (syndrome) (maceration)
  991.4
Wharton's duct - see condition
Wheal 709.8
Wheezing 786.0
Whiplash injury or syndrome 847.0
Whipple's disease 040.2
Whipworm 127.3
White - see also condition
– leg, puerperal, postpartum, childbirth
  671.4
– mouth 112.0
– spot lesions, teeth 521.0
Whitehead 706.2
Whitlow (with lymphangitis) 681.0
– herpetic 054.6
Whitmore's disease or fever 025
Whooping cough 033.9
– with pneumonia 033.- † 484.3*
– Bordetella
– – bronchoseptica 033.8
– – parapertussis 033.1
– – pertussis 033.0
Widening aorta (see also Aneurysm, aorta)
  441.6
– ruptured 441.5

Wilkinson-Sneddon disease or syndrome
  694.1
Willan's lepra 696.1
Willebrand-Jurgens thrombopathy 286.4
Wilms' tumor (M8960/3) 189.0
Wilson's
– disease or syndrome 275.1
– hepatolenticular degeneration 275.1
– lichen ruber 697.0
Wilson-Mikity syndrome 770.7

Window - see also Imperfect closure
– aorticopulmonary 745.0
Winged scapula 736.8
Winter - see condition
Wiskott-Aldrich syndrome 279.1
Withdrawal symptoms, syndrome
– alcohol 291.8
– drug or narcotic 292.0
– newborn, infant of dependent mother
  779.5
– steroid NEC
– – correct substance properly
    administered 255.4
– – overdose or wrong substance given or
    taken 962.0
Witts' anemia 280
Witzelsucht 301.9
Woakes
– ethmoiditis 471.1
– syndrome 471.1
Wolfe-Parkinson-White syndrome 426.7

Wolhynian fever 083.1
Wolman's disease 272.7
Wood asthma 495.8
Woolly, wooly hair (congenital) (nevus)
  757.4
Word
– blindness (congenital) (developmental)
  315.0
– – secondary to organic lesion 784.6
– deafness (congenital) (developmental)
  315.3
– – secondary to organic lesion 784.6

Worm(s) (colic) (fever) (infection)
  (infestation) (see also Infestation) 128.9
– guinea 125.7
– in intestine NEC 127.9
Worm-eaten soles 102.3

Worn out (see also Exhaustion) 780.7
Worried well V65.5
Wound, open (by cutting or piercing
  instrument) (by firearms) (dissection)
  (incised) (penetrating) (perforating)
  (puncture) (with initial hemorrhage, not
  internal) 879.8

Note – For open wounds penetrating to internal organs of abdomen, chest or pelvis – *see* Injury, internal, by site, with open wound.

The following fourth-digit subdivisions are for use with categories 875–877, 880–886 and 890–895:

.0 *Without mention of complication*
.1 *Complicated*
.2 *With tendon involvement* (for use with categories 880–884 and 890–894 only)

"Complicated" includes open wounds with mention of delayed healing, delayed treatment, foreign body, or major infection.

Wound - *continued*
- face - *continued*
- - specified part NEC - *continued*
- - - complicated 873.5
- finger(s) (nail) (subungual) 883.-
- flank 879.4
- - complicated 879.5
- foot (any part except toe(s) alone) 892.-
- - toe(s) alone 893.-
- forearm 881.-
- forehead 873.4
- - complicated 873.5

- genital organs (external) NEC 878.8
- - complicated 878.9
- globe (eye) (see also Wound, open, eyeball) 871.9
- groin 879.4
- - complicated 879.5
- gum(s) 873.6
- - complicated 873.7
- hand 882.-
- - finger(s) (and thumb(s)) alone 883.-
- head NEC 873.8
- - with intracranial injury 854.1
- - - due to or associated with skull fracture NEC 803.3
- - - - base 801.3
- - - - vault 800.3
- - complicated 873.9
- - scalp - see Wound, open, scalp
- heel 892.-
- hip 890.-
- hymen 878.6
- - complicated 878.7
- hypochondrium 879.4
- - complicated 879.5
- hypogastric region 879.2
- - complicated 879.3
- iliac (region) 879.4
- - complicated 879.5
- incidental to
- - dislocation - code as Dislocation, compound
- - fracture - code as Fracture, open
- - intracranial injury - code as Injury, intracranial, with open wound
- - nerve injury - code as Injury, nerve

- inguinal region 879.4
- - complicated 879.5
- instep 892.-
- intraocular 871.9
- - with
- - - partial loss (of intraocular tissue) 871.2
- - - prolapse or exposure (of intraocular tissue) 871.1

Wound - *continued*
- intraocular - *continued*
- - laceration (see also Laceration, eyeball 871.4
- - penetrating 871.7
- - - with foreign body (nonmagnetic) 871.6
- - - - magnetic 871.5
- - without prolapse (of intraocular tissue) 871.0
- iris - see Wound, open, intraocular
- jaw (fracture not involved) 873.4
- - with fracture - see Fracture, jaw
- - complicated 873.5
- knee 891.-
- labium (majus) (minus) 878.4
- - complicated 878.5
- lacrimal apparatus, gland, or sac 870.2
- - with laceration of eyelid 870.2
- larynx 874.0
- - complicated 874.1
- leg (multiple) 891.-
- - thigh 890.-
- lens (eye) 366.2
- limb
- - lower (multiple) NEC 894.-
- - upper (multiple) NEC 884.-
- lip 873.4
- - complicated 873.5
- loin 876.-
- lumbar region 876.-
- malar region 873.4
- - complicated 873.5
- mastoid region 873.4
- - complicated 873.5
- midthoracic region 875.-
- mouth 873.6
- - complicated 873.7
- multiple, unspecified site 879.8

Note – Multiple open wounds of sites classifiable to the same four-digit category should be classified to that category unless they are in different limbs.

Multiple open wounds of sites classifiable to different four-digit categories, or in different limbs, should be coded separately.

Wound - *continued*
- multiple - *continued*
- - complicated 879.9
- nail
- - finger(s) 883.-
- - thumb 883.-
- - toe(s) 893.-
- nape (neck) 874.8

Wound - *continued*
− trunk - *continued*
− − specified part NEC - *continued*
− − − complicated 879.7
− tunica vaginalis 878.2
− − complicated 878.3
− tympanic membrane 872.6
− − complicated 872.7
− tympanum 872.6
− − complicated 872.7
− umbilical region 879.2
− − complicated 879.3
− uvula 873.6
− − complicated 873.7
− vagina 878.6
− − complicated 878.7
− vitreous (humor) 871.2
− vulva 878.4

Wound - *continued*
− vulva - *continued*
− − complicated 878.5
− wrist 881.-
Wright's syndrome 447.8
Wrist - see condition
Wrong drug (given in error) NEC 977.9
− specified drug or substance - see Table of
  drugs and chemicals
Wry neck - see Torticollis
Wuchereria infestation 125.0
− bancrofti 125.0
− Brugia malayi 125.1
− malayi 125.1
Wuchereriasis 125.0
Wuchereriosis 125.0
Wuchernde struma langhans (M8332/3)
  193

X

Xanthelasma 272.2
− eyelid 272.2 † 374.5*
− palpebrarum 272.2 † 374.5*
Xanthelasmoidea 757.3
Xanthinuria 277.2
Xanthofibroma (M8831/0) - see Neoplasm,
  connective tissue, benign
Xanthoma(s), xanthomatosis 272.2
− bone 272.7
− cutaneotendinous 272.7
− disseminatum 272.7
− eruptive 272.2
− familial 272.7
− hereditary 272.7
− hypercholesterolemic 272.0
− hyperlipidemic 272.4
− infantile 272.7
− joint 272.7
− juvenile 272.7
− multiple 272.7
− tendon (sheath) 272.7
− tuberosum 272.2
− tubo-eruptive 272.2
Xanthosis 709.0
Xenophobia 300.2
Xeroderma (congenital) (see also
  Ichthyosis) 757.3
− acquired 701.1
− − eyelid 373.3

Xeroderma - *continued*
− pigmentosum 757.3
− vitamin A deficiency 264.8 † 701.1*
Xerophthalmia 372.5
− vitamin A deficiency 264.7 † 372.5*
Xerosis
− conjunctiva 372.5
− − with Bitot's spot 372.5
− − − with vitamin A deficiency 264.1 †
      372.5*
− − vitamin A deficiency 264.0 † 372.5*
− cornea 371.4
− − with corneal ulceration 370.0
− − − vitamin A deficiency 264.3 † 370.0*
− − vitamin A deficiency 264.2 † 371.4*
− cutis 706.8
− skin 706.8
Xerostomia 527.7
Xiphopagus 759.4
XO syndrome 758.6
X-ray
− effects, adverse NEC 990
− of chest
− − for suspected tuberculosis V71.2
− − routine V72.5
XXXXY syndrome 758.8
XXY syndrome 758.7
Xylulosuria 271.8

Y

Yawning 786.0
– psychogenic 306.1
Yaws 102.9
– bone or joint lesions 102.6
– butter 102.1
– chancre 102.0
– cutaneous, less than five years after
  infection 102.2
– early (cutaneous) (macular)
  (maculopapular) (micropapular)
  (papular) 102.2
– – frambeside 102.2
– – skin lesions NEC 102.2
– eyelid 102.- † 373.4*
– ganglion 102.6
– gangosis, gangosa 102.5
– gumma, gummata 102.4
– – bone 102.6
– gummatous
– – frambeside 102.4
– – osteitis 102.6
– – periostitis 102.6
– hydrarthrosis 102.6
– hyperkeratosis (early) (late) 102.3
– initial lesions 102.0

Yaws - *continued*
– juxta-articular nodules 102.7
– late nodular (ulcerated) 102.4
– latent (without clinical manifestations)
  (with positive serology) 102.8
– mother 102.0
– mucosal 102.7
– multiple papillomata 102.1
– nodular, late (ulcerated) 102.4
– osteitis 102.6
– papilloma, plantar or palmar 102.1
– periostitis (hypertrophic) 102.6
– ulcers 102.4
– wet crab 102.1
Yellow
– atrophy 570
– – chronic 571.8
– – resulting from administration of blood,
     plasma, serum or other biological
     substance 070.3 † 573.1*
– – – with hepatic coma 070.2 † 573.1*
– fever - see Fever, yellow
– jack (see also Fever, yellow) 060.9
– jaundice - see Jaundice
Yersinia septica 027.8

Z

Zenker's diverticulum (esophagus) 530.6
Ziehen-Oppenheim disease 333.6
Zieve's syndrome 571.1
Zollinger-Ellison syndrome 251.5
Zona (see also Herpes, zoster) 053.9
Zoophobia 300.2

Zoster (herpes) (see also Herpes, zoster)
  053.9
Zuelzer(-Ogden) anemia (megaloblastic)
  281.2
Zygomycosis 117.7
Zymotic - see condition

SECTION II

ALPHABETICAL INDEX TO EXTERNAL CAUSES OF INJURY

(E CODE)

ALPHABETICAL INDEX TO EXTERNAL CAUSES
OF INJURY

(E CODE)

A

Abandonment
– causing exposure to weather conditions - see Exposure
– child, with intent to injure or kill   E968.4
– helpless person, infant, newborn   E904.0
– – with intent to injure or kill   E968.4
Abortion, criminal, injury to child   E968.8

Abuse, child   E967.9
– by
– – parent(s)   E967.0
– – specified person(s), except parent(s)   E967.1
– – unspecified person   E967.9

Accident (to)   E928.9
– aircraft (in transit) (powered)   E841.-
– – at landing, take-off   E840.-
– – due to, caused by cataclysm - see categories   E908, E909
– – late effect of   E929.1
– – unpowered (see also Collision, aircraft, unpowered)   E842.-
– – while alighting, boarding   E843.-
– amphibious vehicle
– – on
– – – land - see Accident, motor vehicle
– – – water - see Accident, watercraft
– animal-drawn vehicle NEC   E827.-
– animal, ridden NEC   E828.-
– balloon (see also Collision, aircraft, unpowered)   E842.-
– caused by, due to

Accident - *continued*
– caused by - *continued*
– – abrasive wheel (metalworking)   E919.3
– – animal NEC   E906.9
– – – being ridden (in sport or transport)   E828.-
– – avalanche NEC   E909
– – band saw   E919.4
– – bench saw   E919.4
– – bore, earth-drilling or mining (land) (seabed)   E919.1
– – bulldozer   E919.7
– – cataclysmic
– – – earth surface movement or eruption   E909
– – – storm   E908
– – chain
– – – hoist   E919.2
– – – – agricultural operations   E919.0
– – – – mining operations   E919.1
– – – – saw   E920.1
– – circular saw   E919.4
– – cold (excessive) (see also Cold, exposure to)   E901.9
– – combine   E919.0
– – conflagration - see Conflagration
– – corrosive liquid, substance NEC   E924.1
– – cotton gin   E919.8
– – crane   E919.2
– – – agricultural operations   E919.0

Accident - *continued*
- caused by - *continued*
- - saw E920.4
- - - band E919.4
- - - bench E919.4
- - - chain E920.1
- - - circular E919.4
- - - hand E920.4
- - - - powered E920.1
- - - powered, except hand E919.4
- - - radial E919.4
- - sawing machine, metal E919.3
- - shaft
- - - hoist E919.1
- - - lift E919.1
- - - transmission E919.6
- - shears E920.4
- - - hand E920.4
- - - - powered E920.1
- - - mechanical E919.3
- - shovel E920.4
- - - steam E919.7
- - spinning machine E919.8
- - steam - see also Burning, steam
- - - engine E919.5
- - - shovel E919.7
- - thresher E919.0
- - thunderbolt NEC E907
- - tractor E919.0
- - - when in transport under its own
      power - see categories E810-E825
- - transmission belt, cable, chain, gear,
      pinion, pulley, shaft E919.6
- - turbine (gas) (water driven) E919.5
- - under-cutter E919.1
- - weaving machine E919.8
- - winch E919.2
- - - agricultural operations E919.0
- - - mining operations E919.1
- diving E883.0
- - with insufficient air supply E913.2
- glider (hang) (see also Collision, aircraft,
    unpowered) E842.-
- hovercraft
- - on
- - - land - see Accident, motor vehicle
- - - water - see Accident, watercraft
- ice yacht (see also Accident, vehicle
    NEC) E848
- in
- - medical, surgical procedure
- - - as, or due to misadventure - see
      Misadventure
- - - causing an abnormal reaction or
      later complication without mention
      of misadventure - see Reaction,
      abnormal

Accident - *continued*
- kite carrying a person (see also Collision,
    aircraft, unpowered) E842.-
- land yacht (see also Accident, vehicle
    NEC) E848
- late effect of - see Late effect
- launching pad E845.-
- machine, machinery (see also Accident,
    caused by, due to, by specific type of
    machine) E919.9
- - agricultural including animal powered
    E919.0
- - earth moving or scraping E919.7
- - earth-drilling E919.1
- - excavating E919.7
- - involving transport under own power
    on highway or transport vehicle - see
    categories E810-E825, E840-E845
- - lifting (appliances) E919.2
- - metalworking E919.3
- - mining E919.1
- - prime movers, except electric motors
    E919.5
- - - electric motors - see Accident,
      machine, by specific type of machine
- - recreational E919.8
- - specified NEC E919.8
- - transmission E919.6
- - watercraft (deck) (engine room)
    (galley) (laundry) (loading) E836.-
- - woodworking or forming E919.4
- motor vehicle (on public highway)
    (traffic) E819.-
- - due to cataclysm - see categories
    E908, E909
- - involving
- - - collision (see also Collision, motor
      vehicle) E812.-
- - nontraffic, not on public highway - see
    categories E820-E825
- - not involving collision - see categories
    E816-E819
- nonmotor vehicle NEC E829.-
- - nonroad - see Accident, vehicle NEC
- - road, except pedal cycle, animal-drawn
    vehicle or animal being ridden E829.-
- nonroad vehicle NEC - see Accident,
    vehicle NEC
- not elsewhere classifiable, involving
- - cable car (not on rails) E847
- - - on rails E829.-
- - coal car in mine E846
- - handtruck - see Accident, vehicle NEC
- - logging car E846
- - sled(ge), meaning snow or ice vehicle
    E848
- - tram, mine or quarry E846

Accident - *continued*
- not elsewhere classifiable - *continued*
- - truck
- - - mine or quarry   E846
- - - self-propelled, industrial   E846
- - - station baggage   E846
- - tub, mine or quarry   E846
- - vehicle NEC   E848
- - - snow and ice   E848
- - - used only on industrial premises
      E846
- - wheelbarrow   E848
- off-road type motor vehicle (not on
  public highway) NEC   E821.-
- - on public highway - see categories
      E810-E819
- pedal cycle   E826.-
- railway   E807.-
- - due to cataclysm - see categories
      E908, E909
- - involving
- - - burning by engine, locomotive, train
      (see also Explosion, railway
      engine)   E803.-
- - - collision (see also Collision,
      railway)   E800.-
- - - derailment (see also Derailment,
      railway)   E802.-
- - - explosion (see also Explosion,
      railway engine)   E803.-
- - - fall (see also Fall from railway
      rolling stock)   E804.-
- - - fire (see also Explosion, railway
      engine)   E803.-
- - - hitting by, being struck by
- - - - object falling in, on, from, rolling
        stock, train, vehicle   E806.-
- - - - rolling stock, train, vehicle
        E805.-
- - - overturning, railway rolling stock,
      train, vehicle (see also Derailment,
      railway)   E802.-
- - - running off rails, railway (see also
      Derailment, railway)   E802.-
- - - specified circumstances NEC
      E806.-
- - - train or vehicle hit by
- - - - avalanche   E909
- - - - falling object (earth, rock, tree)
        E806.-
- - - - - due to cataclysm - see
          categories   E908, E909
- - - - landslide   E909
- ski(ing)   E885
- - jump   E884.9
- - lift or tow (with chair or gondola)
      E847

Accident - *continued*
- snow vehicle, motor driven (not on public
  highway)   E820.-
- - on public highway - see categories
      E810-E819
- spacecraft   E845.-
- specified cause NEC   E928.8
- street car   E829.-
- traffic NEC   E819.-
- vehicle (with pedestrian) NEC   E848
- - battery powered airport passenger
      vehicle   E846
- - battery powered truck (baggage)
      (mail)   E846
- - powered commercial or industrial
      (with other vehicle or object within
      commercial or industrial premises)
      E846
- watercraft   E838.-
- - due to, caused by cataclysm - see
      categories   E908, E909
- - machinery   E836.-
- - with
- - - drowning or submersion resulting
      from
- - - - accident other than to watercraft
        E832.-
- - - - accident to watercraft   E830.-
- - - injury, except drowning or
      submersion, resulting from
- - - - accident other than to watercraft -
        see categories   E833-E838
- - - - accident to watercraft   E831.-
Acid throwing   E961
Acosta syndrome   E902.0
Aero-otitis media - see Effects of air
  pressure
Aeroneurosis   E902.1
Aerosinusitis - see Effects of air pressure
After-effect, late - see Late effect
Air
- blast in war operations   E993
- embolism (traumatic) NEC   E928.9
- - in
- - - infusion or transfusion   E874.1
- - - perfusion   E874.2
- sickness   E903
Alpine sickness   E902.0
Altitude sickness - see Effects of air
  pressure
Anaphylactic shock, anaphylaxis (see also
  Table of drugs and chemicals)   E947.9
- due to bite or sting (venomous) - see
  Bite, venomous NEC
Andes disease   E902.-
Apoplexy
- heat - see Heat

Arachnidism E905.1
Arson E968.0
Arthritis, serum - see Serum arthritis
Asphyxia, asphyxiation
– by
– – chemical in war operations E997.2
– – explosion - see Explosion
– – food (bone) (seed) (regurgitated food) E911
– – foreign object, except food E912
– – fumes in war operations E997.2
– – gas - see also Table of drugs and chemicals
– – – in war operations E997.2
– – – legal
– – – – execution E978
– – – – intervention (tear) E972
– – mechanical means (see also Suffocation) E913.9
– from
– – conflagration - see Conflagration
– – fire - see also Fire
– – – in war operations E990.-
– – ignition - see Ignition
Aspiration
– foreign body - see Foreign body, aspiration
– mucus, not of newborn (with asphyxia, obstruction respiratory passage, suffocation) E912
– phlegm (with asphyxia, obstruction respiratory passage, suffocation) E912
– vomitus (with asphyxia, obstruction respiratory passage, suffocation) E911
Assassination (attempt) (see also Assault) E968.9
Assault (homicidal) (by) (in) E968.9
– acid E961
– – swallowed E962.1
– bite (of human being) E968.8
– bomb ((placed in) car or house) E965.8
– – antipersonnel E965.5
– – letter E965.7
– – petrol E965.6
– brawl (hand) (fists) (foot) E960.0
– burning, burns (by fire) E968.0
– – acid E961
– – – swallowed E962.1
– – caustic, corrosive substance E961
– – – swallowed E962.1
– – chemical from swallowing caustic, corrosive substance E962.1
– – hot liquid E968.3
– – scalding E968.3
– – vitriol E961
– – – swallowed E962.1
– caustic, corrosive substance E961

Assault - *continued*
– caustic - *continued*
– – swallowed E962.1
– cut, any part of body E966
– dagger E966
– drowning E964
– explosive(s) E965.9
– – dynamite E965.8
– – bomb (see also Assault, bomb) E965.8
– fight (hand) (fists) (foot) E960.0
– – with weapon E968.9
– – – blunt or thrown E968.2
– – – cutting or piercing E966
– – – firearm - see Shooting, homicide
– fire E968.0
– firearm(s) - see Shooting, homicide
– garrotting E963
– gunshot (wound) - see Shooting, homicide
– hanging E963
– injury NEC E968.9
– – to child due to criminal abortion E968.8
– knife E966
– late effect of E969
– ligature E963
– poisoning E962.9
– – drugs or medicaments E962.0
– – gas(es) or vapors, except drugs and medicaments E962.2
– – solid or liquid substances, except drugs and medicaments E962.1
– puncture, any part of body E966
– pushing
– – before moving object, train, vehicle E968.8
– – from high place E968.1
– rape E960.1
– scalding E968.3
– shooting - see Shooting, homicide
– stab, any part of body E966
– strangulation E963
– submersion E964
– suffocation E963
– violence NEC E968.9
– vitriol E961
– – swallowed E962.1
– weapon E968.9
– – blunt or thrown E968.2
– – cutting or piercing E966
– firearm - see Shooting, homicide
– wound E968.9
– – cutting E966
– – gunshot - see Shooting, homicide
– – knife E966
– – piercing E966

Assault - *continued*
- wound - *continued*
- - puncture E966
- - stab E966
Attack by animal NEC E906.9
Avalanche E909

Avalanche - *continued*
- falling on or hitting
- - motor vehicle (in motion) (on public
   highway) E909
- - railway train E909
Aviators' disease E902.1

B

Barotitis, barodontalgia, barosinusitis,
  barotrauma (otitic) (sinus) - see Effects of
  air pressure
Battered
- baby or child (syndrome) - see Abuse,
  child
- person other than baby or child - see
  Assault
Bayonet wound (see also Cut by bayonet)
  E920.3
- in
- - legal intervention E974
- - war operations E995
Bean in nose E912
Bed set on fire NEC E898.0
Beheading (by guillotine)
- homicide E966
- legal execution E978
Bending, injury in E927
Bends E902.0
Bite
- animal (nonvenomous) NEC E906.3
- - venomous NEC E905.9
- arthropod (nonvenomous) NEC E906.4
- - venomous - see Sting
- black widow spider E905.1
- cat E906.3
- centipede E905.4
- cobra E905.0
- dog E906.0
- fer de lance E905.0
- gila monster E905.0
- human being E968.8
- insect (nonvenomous) E906.4
- - venomous - see Sting
- krait E905.0
- late effect of - see Late effect
- lizard E906.2
- - venomous E905.0
- marine animal
- - nonvenomous E906.3
- - - snake E906.2
- - venomous E905.6
- - - snake E905.0
- millipede E906.4

Bite - *continued*
- millipede - *continued*
- - venomous E905.4
- moray eel E906.3
- rat E906.1
- rattlesnake E905.0
- rodent, except rat E906.3
- serpent - see Bite, snake
- shark E906.3
- snake (venomous) E905.0
- - nonvenomous E906.2
- - sea E905.0
- spider E905.1
- - nonvenomous E906.4
- tarantula (venomous) E905.1
- venomous NEC E905.9
- - by specific animal - see category E905
- viper E905.0
Blast (air) in war operations E993
- from nuclear explosion E996
- underwater E992
Blizzard E908
Blow E928.9
- by law-enforcing agent, police (on duty)
  E975
- - with blunt object E973
Blowing up (see also Explosion) E923.9
Brawl (hand) (fists) (foot) E960.0
Breakage (accidental)
- cable of cable car not on rails E847
- ladder (causing fall) E881.0
- part (any) of
- - animal-drawn vehicle E827.-
- - ladder (causing fall) E881.0
- - motor vehicle
- - - in motion (on public highway)
     E818.-
- - - - not on public highway E825.-
- - nonmotor road vehicle, except
     animal-drawn vehicle or pedal cycle
     E829
- - off-road type motor vehicle (not on
     public highway) NEC E821.-
- - - on public highway E818.-
- - pedal cycle E826.-

Breakage - *continued*
- part - *continued*
- - scaffolding (causing fall) E881.1
- - snow vehicle, motor-driven (not on public highway) E820.-
- - - on public highway E818.-
- - vehicle NEC - see Accident, vehicle NEC

Broken
- glass, injury by E920.8
- power line (causing electric shock) E925.1

Bumping against, into (accidentally)
- object (moving) (projected) (stationary) E917.9
- - caused by crowd (with fall) E917.1
- - in
- - - running water E917.2
- - - sports E917.0
- - with fall E888
- person(s) E917.9
- - with fall E886.9
- - - in sports E886.0
- - as, or caused by, a crowd (with fall) E917.1
- - in sports E917.0
- - - with fall E886.0

Burning, burns (accidental) (by) (from) (on) E899
- acid (any kind) E924.1
- - swallowed - see Table of drugs and chemicals
- bedclothes (see also Fire, specified NEC) E898.0
- blowlamp (see also Fire, specified NEC) E898.1
- blowtorch (see also Fire, specified NEC) E898.1
- boat, ship, watercraft - see categories E830, E831, E837
- bonfire (controlled) E897
- - uncontrolled E892
- candle (see also Fire, specified NEC) E898.1
- caustic liquid, substance E924.1
- - swallowed - see Table of drugs and chemicals
- chemical E924.1
- - from swallowing caustic, corrosive substance - see Table of drugs and chemicals
- - in war operations E997.2
- cigar(s) or cigarette(s) (see also Fire, specified NEC) E898.1
- clothes, clothing, nightdress - see Ignition, clothes
- - with conflagration - see Conflagration

Burning - *continued*
- conflagration - see Conflagration
- corrosive liquid, substance E924.1
- - swallowed - see Table of drugs and chemicals
- electric current (see also Electric shock) E925.9
- fire, flames (see also Fire) E899
- flare, Verey pistol E922.8
- heat
- - from appliance (electrical) E924.8
- - in local application or packing during medical or surgical procedure E873.5
- homicide (attempt) (see also Assault, burning) E968.0
- hot
- - liquid E924.0
- - - caustic or corrosive E924.1
- - object (not producing fire or flames) E924.8
- - substance E924.9
- - - caustic or corrosive E924.1
- - - liquid (metal) NEC E924.0
- - - specified NEC E924.8
- ignition - see also Ignition
- - clothes, clothing, nightdress - see also Ignition, clothes
- - - with conflagration - see Conflagration
- - highly inflammable material (benzine) (fat) (gasoline) (kerosene) (paraffin) (petrol) E894
- in war operations (from fire-producing device or conventional weapon) E990.9
- - from nuclear explosion E996
- - petrol bomb E990.0
- inflicted by other person
- - stated as
- - - homicidal, intentional (see also Assault, burning) E968.0
- - - undetermined whether accidental or intentional E988.1
- internal, from swallowed caustic, corrosive liquid, substance - see Table of drugs and chemicals
- lamp (see also Fire, specified NEC) E898.1
- late effect of NEC E929.4
- lighter (cigar) (cigarette) (see also Fire, specified NEC) E898.1
- lightning E907
- liquid (boiling) (hot) (molten) E924.0
- - caustic, corrosive (external) E924.1
- - - swallowed - see Table of drugs and chemicals

Burning - *continued*
- local application of externally applied
  substance in medical or surgical care
  E873.5

- machinery - see Accident, machine
- matches (see also Fire, specified NEC)
  E898.1

- medicament, externally applied   E873.5
- metal, molten   E924.0
- object (hot)   E924.8
- - producing fire or flames - see Fire
- pipe (smoking) (see also Fire, specified
  NEC)   E898.1
- radiation - see Radiation
- railway engine, locomotive, train (see also
  Explosion, railway engine)   E803.-
- self-inflicted (unspecified whether
  accidental or intentional)   E988.1
- - caustic or corrosive substance NEC
  E988.7
- - stated as intentional, purposeful
  E958.1
- - - caustic or corrosive substance NEC
  E958.7
- stated as undetermined whether
  accidental or intentional   E988.1

Burning - *continued*
- stated as undetermined whether - *cont.*
- - caustic or corrosive substance NEC
  E988.7
- steam   E924.0
- - pipe   E924.8
- substance (hot)   E924.9
- - boiling or molten   E924.0
- - caustic, corrosive (external)   E924.1
- - - swallowed - see Table of drugs and
  chemicals
- suicidal (attempt) NEC   E958.1
- - caustic substance   E958.7
- - late effect of   E959
- therapeutic misadventure
- - overdose of radiation   E873.2
- torch, welding (see also Fire, specified
  NEC)   E898.1
- trash fire (see also Burning, bonfire)
  E897
- vapor   E924.0
- vitriol   E924.1
- x-rays   E926.3
- - in medical, surgical procedure - see
  Misadventure, failure, in dosage,
  radiation
Butted by animal   E906.8

C

Cachexia, lead or saturnine   E866.0
- from pesticide NEC (see also Table of
  drugs and chemicals)   E863.4
Caisson disease   E902.2
Capital punishment (any means)   E978
Car sickness   E903
Casualty (not due to war) NEC   E928.9
- war (see also War operations)   E995
Cat
- bite   E906.3
- scratch   E906.8
Cataclysmic (any injury)
- earth surface movement or eruption
  E909
- storm or flood resulting from storm
  E908
Catching fire - see Ignition
Caught
- between
- - objects (moving) (stationary and
  moving)   E918

Caught - *continued*
- - - and machinery - see Accident,
  machine
- by cable car, not on rails   E847
- in
- - machinery (moving parts of) - see
  Accident, machine
- - object   E918
Cave-in (causing asphyxia, suffocation (by
  pressure)) (see also Suffocation due to
  cave-in)   E913.3
- struck or crushed by   E916
- - with asphyxia or suffocation (see also
  Suffocation due to cave-in)   E913.3
- with injury other than asphyxia or
  suffocation   E916
Change(s) in air pressure - see also Effects
  of air pressure
- sudden, in aircraft (ascent) (descent)
  (causing aeroneurosis or aviators'
  disease)   E902.1

Chilblains NEC E901.0
– due to manmade conditions E901.1
Choking (on) (any object except food or
vomitus) E912
– apple E911
– bone E911
– food, any type (regurgitated) E911
– mucus or phlegm E912
– seed E911
Civil insurrection - see War operations
Cloudburst (any injury) E908
Cold, exposure to (accidental) (excessive)
(extreme) (place) E901.9
– causing chilblains or immersion foot
E901.0
– due to
– – manmade conditions E901.1
– – specified cause NEC E901.8
– – weather (conditions) E901.0
– late effect of NEC E929.5
– self-inflicted (undetermined whether
accidental or intentional) E988.3
– – suicidal E958.3
– suicide E958.3
Colic, lead, painter's or saturnine - see
category E866
Collapse
– building E916
– – burning E891.8
– – – private E890.8
– due to heat - see Heat
– machinery - see Accident, machine
– postoperative NEC E878.9
– structure, burning NEC E891.8
Collision (accidental)

Note – In the case of collisions between
different types of vehicles, persons and objects, priority in classification is in the following order:
    Aircraft
    Watercraft
    Motor vehicle
    Railway vehicle
    Pedal cycle
    Animal-drawn vehicle
    Animal being ridden
    Street car or other nonmotor road
      vehicle
    Other vehicle
    Pedestrian or person using pedestrian
      conveyance
    Object (except where falling from or
      set in motion by vehicle etc. listed
      above)

In the listing below, the combinations are
listed only under the vehicle etc. having
priority. For definitions, see Volume 1,
p. 547.

Collision - *continued*
– aircraft (with object or vehicle) (fixed)
(movable) (moving) E841.-
– – powered (in transit) (with unpowered
aircraft) E841.-
– – – while landing, taking off E840.-
– – unpowered E842.-
– – while landing, taking off E840.-
– – with
– – – person (while landing, taking off)
(without accident to aircraft)
E844.-
– animal being ridden (in sport or
transport) E828.-
– – and
– – – animal (being ridden) (herded)
(unattended) E828.-
– – – nonmotor road vehicle, except pedal
cycle or animal-drawn vehicle
E828.-
– – – object (fallen) (fixed) (movable)
(moving) not falling from or set in
motion by vehicle of higher priority
E828.-
– – – pedestrian (conveyance or vehicle)
E828.-
– animal-drawn vehicle E827.-
– – and
– – – animal (being ridden) (herded)
(unattended) E827.-
– – – nonmotor road vehicle, except pedal
cycle E827.-
– – – object (fallen) (fixed) (movable)
(moving) not falling from or set in
motion by vehicle of higher priority
E827.-
– – – pedestrian (conveyance or vehicle)
E827.-
– – – streetcar E827.-
– motor vehicle (on public highway) (traffic
accident) E812.-
– – after leaving, running off, public
highway (without antecedent collision)
(without re-entry) E816.-
– – – with antecedent collision on public
highway - see categories
E810-E815
– – – with re-entrance collision with
another motor vehicle E811.-
– – and

Collision - *continued*
- off-road type motor vehicle - *continued*
- - and - *continued*
- - - other object or vehicle nec, fixed or movable, not set in motion by aircraft, motor vehicle on highway or snow vehicle, motor-driven E821.-
- - - pedal cycle E821.-
- - - pedestrian (conveyance) E821.-
- - - railway train E821.-
- - on public highway - see Collision, motor vehicle

- pedal cycle E826.-
- - and
- - - animal (carrying person, property) (herded) (unattended) E826.-
- - - animal-drawn vehicle E826.-
- - - another pedal cycle E826.-
- - - nonmotor road vehicle E826.-
- - - object (fallen) (fixed) (movable) (moving) not falling from, set in motion by, aircraft, motor vehicle, railway train E826.-
- - - pedestrian (conveyance) E826.-
- - - person (using pedestrian conveyance) E826.-
- - - street car E826.-

- pedestrian(s) (conveyance) E917.9
- - and
- - - crowd, human stampede (with fall) E917.1
- - - machinery - see Accident, machine
- - - object (fallen) (moving) (projected) (stationary) not falling from or set in motion by any vehicle listed in categories E800-E848 E917.9
- - - - caused by a crowd E917.1
- - - - in
- - - - - running water E917.2
- - - - - - with drowning or submersion - see Submersion
- - - - - sports E917.0
- - - - with fall E888
- - - vehicle, nonmotor, nonroad E848
- - in
- - - running water E917.2
- - - - with drowning or submersion - see Submersion
- - - sports E917.0
- - - - with fall E886.0
- - with fall E886.9
- - - in sports E886.0
- person(s) (using pedestrian conveyance) (see also Collision, pedestrian) E917.9

Collision - *continued*
- railway (rolling stock) (train) (vehicle) (with (subsequent) derailment, explosion, fall or fire) E800.-
- - with antecedent derailment E802.-
- - and
- - - animal (carrying person) (herded) (unattended) E801.-
- - - another railway train or vehicle E800.-
- - - buffers E801.-
- - - fallen tree on railway E801.-
- - - farm machinery, nonmotor (in transport) (stationary) E801.-
- - - gates E801.-
- - - nonmotor vehicle E801.-
- - - object (fallen) (fixed) (movable) (moving) not falling from, set in motion by, aircraft or motor vehicle NEC E801.
- - - pedal cycle E801.-
- - - pedestrian (conveyance) E805.-
- - - person (using pedestrian conveyance) E805.-
- - - platform E801.-
- - - rock on railway E801.-
- - - street car E801.-
- snow vehicle, motor-driven (not on public highway) E820.-
- - and
- - - animal (being ridden) (-drawn vehicle) E820.-
- - - another off-road motor vehicle E820.-
- - - other motor vehicle, not on public highway E820.-
- - - other object or vehicle nec, fixed or movable, not set in motion by aircraft or motor vehicle on highway E820.-
- - - pedal cycle E820.-
- - - pedestrian (conveyance) E820.-
- - - railway train E820.-
- - on public highway - see Collision, motor vehicle
- street car(s) E829.-
- - and
- - - animal, herded, not being ridden, unattended E829.-
- - - nonmotor road vehicle NEC E829.-
- - - object (fallen) (fixed) (movable) (moving) not falling from or set in motion by aircraft, animal-drawn vehicle, animal being ridden, motor vehicle, pedal cycle or railway train E829.-

Crash - *continued*
- aircraft - *continued*
- − in war operations E994
- − on runway NEC E840.-
- − stated as
- − − homicidal E968.8
- − − suicidal E958.6
- − − undetermined whether accidental or
        intentional E988.6
- − unpowered E842.-
- − glider E842.-
- motor vehicle - see also Accident, motor
  vehicle
- − homicidal E968.8
- − suicidal E958.5
- − undetermined whether accidental or
      intentional E988.5
Crushed (accidentally) E928.9
- between
- − boat(s), ship(s), watercraft (and dock
      or pier) (without accident to
      watercraft) E838.-
- − − after accident to, or collision,
          watercraft E831.-
- − objects (moving) (stationary and
      moving) E918
- by
- − avalanche NEC E909
- − boat, ship, watercraft after accident to,
      collision, watercraft E831.-
- − cave-in E916
- − − with asphyxiation or suffocation (see
          also Suffocation due to cave-in)
          E913.3
- − crowd, human stampede E917.1
- − falling
- − − aircraft (see also Accident, aircraft)
          E841.-
- − − − in war operations E994
- − − earth, material E916
- − − − with asphyxiation or suffocation
            (see also Suffocation due to
            cave-in) E913.3
- − − object E916
- − − − on ship, watercraft E838.-
- − − − while loading, unloading
            watercraft E838.-
- − landslide NEC E909
- − lifeboat after abandoning ship E831.-
- − machinery - see Accident, machine
- − railway rolling stock, train, vehicle
      (part of) E805.-
- − street car E829.-
- − vehicle NEC - see Accident, vehicle
      NEC
- in
- − machinery - see Accident, machine

Crushed - *continued*
- in - *continued*
- − object E918
- − transport accident - see categories
      E800-E848
- late effect of NEC E929.9
Cut, cutting (any part of body) (accidental)
  E920.9
- by
- − arrow E920.8
- − axe E920.4
- − bayonet (see also Bayonet wound)
      E920.3
- − blender E920.2
- − broken glass E920.8
- − can opener E920.4
- − − powered E920.2
- − chisel E920.4
- − circular saw E919.4
- − cutting or piercing instrument - see also
      Category E920
- − − late effect of E929.8
- − dagger E920.3
- − dart E920.8
- − drill - see Accident caused by drill
- − edge of stiff paper E920.8
- − electric
- − − beater E920.2
- − − fan E920.2
- − − knife E920.2
- − − mixer E920.2
- − fork E920.4
- − garden fork E920.4
- − hand saw or tool (not powered)
      E920.4
- − − powered E920.1
- − hedge clipper E920.4
- − − powered E920.1
- − hoe E920.4
- − ice pick E920.4
- − knife E920.3
- − − electric E920.2
- − lathe turnings E920.8
- − lawn mower E920.4
- − − powered E920.0
- − − − riding E919.8
- − machine - see Accident, machine
- − meat
- − − grinder E919.8
- − − slicer E919.8
- − nails E920.8
- − needle E920.4
- − object, edged, pointed, sharp - see
      category E920
- − paper cutter E920.4
- − piercing instrument - see category
      E920

Cut - *continued*
- by - *continued*
- - piercing instrument - *continued*
- - - late effect of E929.8
- - pitchfork E920.4
- - powered
- - - can opener E920.2
- - - garden cultivator E920.1
- - - - riding E919.8
- - - hand saw E920.1
- - - hand tool NEC E920.1
- - - hedge clipper E920.1
- - - household appliance or implement
  E920.2
- - - lawn mower (hand) E920.0
- - - - riding E919.8
- - - rivet gun E920.1
- - - staple gun E920.1
- - rake E920.4
- - saw
- - - circular E919.4
- - - hand E920.4
- - scissors E920.4
- - screwdriver E920.4
- - sewing machine (electric) (powered)
  E920.2
- - - not powered E920.4

Cut - *continued*
- by - *continued*
- - shears E920.4
- - shovel E920.4
- - spade E920.4
- - splinters E920.8
- - sword E920.3
- - tin can lid E920.8
- - wood slivers E920.8
- homicide (attempt) E966
- inflicted by other person
- - stated as
- - - intentional, homicidal E966
- - - undetermined whether accidental or
  intentional E986
- late effect of NEC E929.8
- legal
- - execution E978
- - intervention E974
- self-inflicted (unspecified whether
  accidental or intentional) E986
- - stated as intentional, purposeful E956
- stated as undetermined whether
  accidental or intentional E986
- suicidal (attempt) E956
- war operations E995
Cyclone (any injury) E908

D

Death due to injury occurring one year or
  more previous - see Late effect
Decapitation (accidental circumstances)
  NEC E928.9
- homicidal E966
- legal execution (by guillotine) E978
Deprivation - see also Privation
- homicidal intent E968.4
Derailment (accidental)
- railway (rolling stock) (train) (vehicle)
  (with subsequent collision) E802.-
- - with
- - - collision (antecedent) (see also
  Collision, railway) E800.-
- - - explosion (subsequent) (without
  antecedent collision) E802.-
- - - - antecedent E803.-
- - - fall (without collision (antecedent))
  E802.-
- - - fire (without collision
  (antecedent)) E802.-
- street car E829.-

Descent
- parachute (voluntary) (without accident
  to aircraft) E844.-
- - due to accident to aircraft - see
  categories E840-E842
Desertion
- child, with intent to injure or kill E968.4
- helpless person, infant, newborn E904.0
- - with intent to injure or kill E968.4
Destitution - see Privation
Disability, late effect or sequela of injury -
  see Late effect
Disease
- Andes E902.0
- aviators' E902.1
- caisson E902.2
- range E902.0
Divers' disease, palsy, paralysis, squeeze
  E902.0
Dog bite E906.0
Dragged by
- cable car (not on rails) E847

Dragged by - *continued*
- cable car - *continued*
- - on rails E829.-
- motor vehicle (on highway) E814.-
- - not on highway, nontraffic accident
  E825.-

Dragged by - *continued*
- street car E829.-
Drinking poison (accidental) - see Table of
drugs and chemicals
Drowning - see Submersion
Dust in eye E914

E

Earth falling (on) (with asphyxia or
suffocation (by pressure)) (see also
Suffocation due to cave-in) E913.3

- as, or due to, a cataclysm (involving any
  transport vehicle) - see categories E908,
  E909
- not due to cataclysmic action E913.3
- - motor vehicle (in motion) (on public
  highway) E818.-
- - - not on public highway E825.-
- - nonmotor road vehicle NEC E829.-
- - pedal cycle E826.-
- - railway rolling stock, train, vehicle
  E806.-
- - street car E829.-
- - struck or crushed by E916
- - - with asphyxiation or suffocation
  E913.3
- with injury other than asphyxia,
  suffocation E916

Earthquake (any injury) E909

Effect(s) (adverse) of
- air pressure E902.9
- - at high altitude E902.9
- - - in aircraft E902.1
- - - residence or prolonged visit (causing
  conditions as listed in E902.0)
  E902.0
- - due to
- - - diving E902.2
- - - specified cause NEC E902.8
- - in aircraft E902.1
- cold, excessive (exposure to) (see also
  Cold, exposure to) E901.9
- heat (excessive) (see also Heat) E900.9
- hot
- - place - see Heat
- - weather E900.0
- insolation E900.0
- insulation - see Heat
- late - see Late effect of
- motion E903

Effect(s) - *continued*
- nuclear explosion or weapon in war
  operations (blast) (fireball) (heat)
  (radiation) (direct) (secondary) E996
- radiation - see Radiation
- travel E903
Electric shock, electrocution (accidental)
(from exposed wire, faulty appliance, high
voltage cable, live rail, open socket) (by)
(in) E925.9
- appliance or wiring
- - domestic E925.0
- - factory E925.2
- - farm (building) E925.8
- - - house E925.0
- - home E925.0
- - industrial (conductor) (control
  apparatus) (transformer) E925.2
- - outdoors E925.8
- - public building E925.8
- - residential institution E925.8
- - school E925.8
- - specified place NEC E925.8
- caused by other person
- - stated as
- - - intentional, homicidal E968.8
- - - undetermined whether accidental or
  intentional E988.4
- electric power generating plant,
  distribution station E925.1
- homicidal (attempt) E968.8
- legal execution E978
- lightning E907
- machinery E925.9
- - domestic E925.0
- - factory E925.2
- - farm E925.8
- - home E925.0
- misadventure in medical or surgical
  procedure
- - in electroshock therapy E873.4
- self-inflicted (undetermined whether
  accidental or intentional) E988.4
- - stated as intentional E958.4

Electric shock - *continued*
- stated as undetermined whether
  accidental or intentional   E988.4
- suicidal (attempt)   E958.4
- transmission line   E925.1
Electrocution - see Electric shock
Embolism
- air (traumatic) NEC - see Air embolism
Encephalitis
- lead or saturnine   E866.0
- - from pesticide NEC   E863.4
Entanglement
- in
- - bedclothes, causing suffocation
      E913.0
- - wheel of pedal cycle   E826.-
Entry of foreign body, material, any - see
  Foreign body
Execution, legal (any method)   E978
Exhaustion
- cold - see Cold, exposure to
- due to excessive exertion   E927
- heat - see Heat
Explosion (accidental) (in) (of) (on)
  E923.9
- acetylene   E923.2
- aerosol can   E921.8
- air tank (compressed) (in machinery)
  E921.1
- aircraft (in transit) (powered)   E841.-
- - at landing, take-off   E840.-
- - in war operations   E994
- - unpowered   E842.-
- anesthetic gas in operating theatre
  E923.2
- automobile tire NEC   E921.8
- - causing transport accident - see
      categories   E810-E825
- blasting (cap) (materials)   E923.1
- boiler (machinery), not on transport
  vehicle   E921.0
- - steamship - see Explosion, watercraft
- bomb   E923.8
- - in war operations   E993
- - - after cessation of hostilities   E998
- - - atom, hydrogen or nuclear   E996
- - - injury by fragments from   E991.9
- - - - antipersonnel bomb   E991.3
- butane   E923.2
- caused by
- - other person
- - - stated as
- - - - intentional, homicidal - see
        Assault, explosive
- - - - undetermined whether accidental
        or homicidal   E985.5
- coal gas   E923.2

Explosion - *continued*
- detonator   E923.1
- dynamite   E923.1
- explosive (material) NEC   E923.9
- - gas(es)   E923.2
- - missile   E923.8
- - - in war operations   E993
- - - - injury by fragments from   E991.9
- - - - - antipersonnel bomb   E991.3
- - used in blasting operations   E923.1
- fire-damp   E923.2
- fireworks   E923.0
- gas   E923.2
- - cylinder (in machinery)   E921.1
- - pressure tank (in machinery)   E921.1
- gasoline (fumes) (tank) not in moving
  motor vehicle   E923.2
- grain store   E923.8
- grenade   E923.8
- - in war operations   E993
- - - injury by fragments from   E991.9
- homicide (attempt) - see Assault,
  explosive
- hot water heater, tank (in machinery)
  E921.0
- in mine (of explosive gases) NEC
  E923.2
- late effect of NEC   E929.8
- machinery - see also Accident, machine
- - pressure vessel - see Explosion,
      pressure vessel
- methane   E923.2
- missile   E923.8
- - in war operations   E993
- - - injury by fragments from   E991.9
- motor vehicle (part of)
- - in motion (on public highway)   E818.-
- - - not on public highway   E825.-
- munitions (dump) (factory)   E923.8
- - in war operations   E993
- of mine   E923.8
- - in war operations
- - - after cessation of hostilities   E998
- - - at sea or in harbor   E992
- - - land   E993
- - - - after cessation of hostilities
        E998
- - - - injury by fragments from   E991.9
- - - marine   E992
- own weapons in war operations   E993
- - injury by fragments from   E991.9
- - - antipersonnel bomb   E991.3
- pressure
- - cooker   E921.8
- - gas tank (in machinery)   E921.1
- - vessel (in machinery)   E921.9

Explosion - *continued*
- pressure - *continued*
- − vessel - *continued*
- − − on transport vehicle - see
     categories E800-E848
- − − specified type NEC E921.8
- propane E923.2
- railway engine, locomotive, train (boiler)
  (with subsequent collision, derailment,
  fall) E803.-
- − with
- − − collision (antecedent) (see also
     Collision, railway) E800.-
- − − derailment (antecedent) E802.-
- − − fire (without collision or derailment
     (antecedent)) E803.-
- secondary fire resulting from - see Fire
- self-inflicted (unspecified whether
  accidental or intentional) E985.5
- − stated as intentional, purposeful
     E955.5
- shell (artillery) E923.8
- − in war operations E993
- − − injury by fragments from E991.9
- stated as undetermined whether caused
  accidentally or purposely inflicted
  E985.5
- steam or water lines (in machinery)
  E921.0

Explosion - *continued*
- suicide (attempted) E955.5
- torpedo E923.8
- − in war operations E992
- transport accident - see categories
  E800-E848
- war operations - see War operations,
  explosion
- watercraft (boiler) E837.-
- − causing drowning, submersion (after
     jumping from watercraft) E830.-
Exposure (weather) (conditions) (rain)
  (wind) E904.3
- excessive
- − cold (see also Cold, exposure to)
     E901.9
- − − self-inflicted - see Cold, exposure to,
     self-inflicted
- − heat E900.0
- helpless person, infant, newborn due to
  abandonment or neglect E904.0
- noise E928.1
- prolonged in deepfreeze unit or
  refrigerator E901.1
- radiation - see Radiation
- resulting from transport accident - see
  categories E800-E848
- vibration E928.2
- with homicidal intent E968.4

F

Fall, falling (accidental) E888
- building E916
- − burning E891.8
- − − private E890.8
- down
- − escalator E880.0
- − ladder E881.0
- − − in boat, ship, watercraft E833.-
- − staircase E880.9
- − stairs, steps - see Fall from stairs
- earth (with asphyxia or suffocation (by
  pressure)) (see also Earth, falling)
  E913.3
- from, off
- − aircraft (at landing, take-off) (in
     transit) (while alighting, boarding)
     E843.-
- − − resulting from accident to aircraft -
     see categories E840-E842
- − animal (in sport or transport) E828.-
- − animal-drawn vehicle E827.-

Fall - *continued*
- from - *continued*
- − balcony E882
- − bed E884.2
- − bicycle E826.-
- − boat, ship, watercraft (into water)
     E832.-
- − − after accident to, collision, fire on
     E830.-
- − − − and subsequently struck by (part
        of) boat E831.-
- − − and subsequently struck by (part of)
     boat E838.-
- − − burning, crushed, sinking E830.-
- − − − and subsequently struck by (part
        of) boat E831.-
- − bridge E882
- − building E882
- − − burning E891.8
- − − − private E890.8
- − bunk in boat, ship, watercraft E834.-

Fall - *continued*
- from - *continued*
- − vehicle NEC - *continued*
- − − stationary E884.9
- − viaduct E882
- − wall E882
- − window E882

- in, on
- − aircraft (at landing, take-off) (in transit) E843.-
- − − resulting from accident to aircraft - see categories E840-E842
- − boat, ship, watercraft E835.-
- − − due to accident to watercraft E831.-
- − − on ladder, stairs E833.-
- − − one level to another NEC E834.-
- − cutting or piercing instrument or machine - see Cut
- − deck (of boat, ship, watercraft) E835.-
- − − due to accident to watercraft E831.-
- − escalator E880.0
- − gangplank E835.-
- − glass, broken E920.8
- − knife - see Cut, knife
- − ladder E881.0
- − − in boat, ship, watercraft E833.-
- − − − due to accident to watercraft E831.-
- − object, edged, pointed or sharp - see Cut
- − pitchfork E920.4
- − railway rolling stock, train, vehicle (while alighting, boarding) E804.-
- − − with
- − − − collision (see also Collision, railway) E800.-
- − − − derailment (see also Derailment, railway) E802.-
- − − − explosion (see also Explosion, railway engine) E803.-
- − scaffolding E881.1
- − scissors E920.4
- − staircase, stairs, steps (see also Fall from stairs) E880.9
- − street car E829.-
- − water transport (see also Fall in boat) E835.-

- into
- − cavity E883.9
- − dock E883.9
- − − from boat, ship, watercraft (see also Fall from boat) E832.-
- − hold (of ship) E834.-

Fall - *continued*
- into - *continued*
- − hold - *continued*
- − − due to accident to watercraft E831.-
- − hole E883.9
- − manhole E883.2
- − moving part of machinery - see Accident, machine
- − opening in surface NEC E883.9
- − pit E883.9
- − quarry E883.9
- − shaft E883.9
- − storm drain E883.2
- − tank E883.9
- − water (with drowning or submersion) NEC E910.9
- − well E883.1

- late effect of NEC E929.3

- object (see also Hit by object falling) E916

- over
- − animal E885
- − cliff E884.1
- − embankment E884.9
- − small object E885

- overboard (see also Fall from boat) E832.-
- rock E916
- same level NEC E888
- − aircraft (any kind) E843.-
- − − resulting from accident to aircraft - -see categories E840-E842
- − boat, ship, watercraft E835.-
- − − due to accident to, collision, watercraft E831.-
- − from
- − − collision, pushing, shoving, by or with other person(s) E886.9
- − − − as, or caused by, a crowd E917.1
- − − − in sports E886.0
- − − slipping, stumbling, tripping E885
- snowslide E916
- − as avalanche E909
- stone E916
- through
- − hatch (on ship) E834.-
- − − due to accident to watercraft E831.-
- − roof E882
- − window E882
- timber E916
- while alighting from, boarding, entering, leaving
- − aircraft (any kind) E843.-

Fire - *continued*
- specified NEC - *continued*
- - with - *continued*
- - - ignition - *continued*
- - - - highly inflammable material (benzine) (fat) (gasoline) (kerosene) (paraffin) (petrol) E894
- started by other person
- - stated as
- - - undetermined whether or not with intent to injure or kill E988.1
- - - with intent to injure or kill E968.0
- suicide (attempted) E958.1
- - late effect of E959
- tunnel (uncontrolled) E892

Fireball effects from nuclear explosion in war operations E996

Fireworks (explosion) E923.0

Flash burns from explosion (see also Explosion) E923.9

Flood (any injury) (resulting from storm) E908
- caused by collapse of dam or manmade structure E909
Forced landing (aircraft) E840.-
Foreign body, object or material (entrance into (accidental))
- air passage (causing injury) E915
- - nose (with asphyxia, obstruction, suffocation) E912
- - - causing injury without asphyxia, obstruction, suffocation E915
- - with asphyxia, obstruction, suffocation E912
- - - food or vomitus E911
- alimentary canal (causing injury) (with obstruction) E915
- - mouth E915
- - - with asphyxia, obstruction, suffocation E912
- - - - food E911
- - pharynx E915
- - - with asphyxia, obstruction, suffocation E912
- - - - food E911
- - with asphyxia, obstruction respiratory passage, suffocation E912
- - - food E911
- aspiration (with asphyxia, obstruction respiratory passage, suffocation) E912
- - causing injury without asphyxia, obstruction respiratory passage, suffocation E915
- - food (regurgitated) (vomited) E911

Foreign body - *continued*
- aspiration - *continued*
- - food - *continued*
- - - causing injury without asphyxia, obstruction respiratory passage, suffocation E915
- - mucus (not of newborn) E912
- - phlegm E912
- bladder (causing injury or obstruction) E915
- bronchus, bronchi - see Foreign body, air passage
- conjunctival sac E914
- digestive system - see Foreign body, alimentary canal
- ear (causing injury or obstruction) E915
- esophagus (causing injury or obstruction) E915
- eye (any part) E914
- eyelid E914
- hairball (stomach) (with obstruction) E915
- ingestion - see Foreign body, alimentary canal
- inhalation - see Foreign body, aspiration
- intestine (causing injury or obstruction) E915
- iris E914
- lacrimal apparatus E914
- larynx - see Foreign body, air passage
- late effect of NEC E929.8
- lung - see Foreign body, air passage
- mouth - see Foreign body, alimentary canal, mouth
- nasal passage - see Foreign body, air passage, nose
- nose - see Foreign body, air passage, nose
- ocular muscle E914
- oesophagus (causing injury or obstruction) E915
- operation wound (left in) - see Misadventure, foreign object
- orbit E914
- pharynx - see Foreign body, alimentary canal, pharynx
- rectum (causing injury or obstruction) E915
- stomach (hairball) (causing injury or obstruction) E915
- tear ducts or glands E914
- trachea - see Foreign body, air passage
- urethra (causing injury or obstruction) E915
- vagina (causing injury or obstruction) E915
Found dead, injured
- from exposure (to) - see Exposure

Found dead - *continued*
- on
- - public highway   E819.-
- - railway right of way   E807.-
Fracture (circumstances unknown or unspecified)   E887
- due to specified external means - see Manner of accident

Fracture - *continued*
- late effect of NEC   E929.3
- occurring in water transport NEC   E835.-
Freezing - see Cold, exposure to
Frostbite   E901.0
- due to manmade conditions   E901.1
Frozen - see Cold, exposure to

G

Garrotting, homicidal (attempted)   E963
Gored   E906.8

Gunshot wound (see also Shooting)   E922.9

H

Hailstones, injured by   E904.3
Hairball (stomach) (with obstruction)   E915
Hang gliding   E842.-
Hanged himself (see also Hanging, self-inflicted)   E983.0
Hanging (accidental)   E913.8
- caused by other person
- - in accidental circumstances   E913.8
- - stated as
- - - intentional, homicidal   E963
- - - undetermined whether accidental or intentional   E983.0
- homicide (attempt)   E963
- in bed or cradle   E913.0
- legal execution   E978
- self-inflicted (unspecified whether accidental or intentional)   E983.0
- - in accidental circumstances   E913.8
- - stated as intentional, purposeful   E953.0
- stated as undetermined whether accidental or intentional   E983.0
- suicidal (attempt)   E953.0
Heat (apoplexy) (collapse) (cramps) (effects of) (excessive) (exhaustion) (fever)   E900.9
- due to
- - manmade conditions (as listed in E900.1, except boat, ship, watercraft)   E900.1
- - weather (conditions)   E900.0
- from

Heat - *continued*
- from - *continued*
- - electric heating apparatus causing burning   E924.8
- - nuclear explosion in war operations   E996
- generated in, boiler, engine, evaporator, fire room of boat, ship, watercraft   E838.-
- inappropriate in local application or packing in medical or surgical procedure   E873.5
- late effect of NEC   E929.5
Hemorrhage
- delayed following medical or surgical treatment without mention of misadventure - see Reaction, abnormal
- during medical or surgical treatment as misadventure - see Misadventure, cut
High
- altitude, effects   E902.9
- level of radioactivity, effects - see Radiation
- pressure effects - see also Effects of air pressure
- - from rapid descent in water (causing caisson or divers' disease, palsy or paralysis)   E902.2
- temperature, effects - see Heat
Hit, hitting (accidental) by
- aircraft (propeller) (without accident to aircraft)   E844.-
- - unpowered   E842.-

Hot
- liquid, object, substance, accident caused by - see also Accident, caused by, hot, by type of substance
- - late effect of E929.8
- place, effects - see Heat
- weather, effects E900.0
Humidity, causing problem E904.3
Hunger E904.1

Hunger - *continued*
- resulting from
- - abandonment or neglect E904.0
- - transport accident - see categories E800-E848
Hurricane (any injury) E908
Hypobarism, hypobaropathy - see Effects of air pressure
Hypothermia - see Cold, exposure to

I

Ictus
- caloris - see Heat
- solaris E900.0
Ignition (accidental)
- anesthetic gas in operating theatre E923.2
- bedclothes E898.0
- - with
- - - conflagration - see Conflagration
- - - ignition (of)
- - - - clothing - see Ignition, clothes
- - - - highly inflammable material (benzine) (fat) (gasoline) (kerosene) (paraffin) (petrol) E894
- benzine E894
- clothes, clothing (from controlled fire) (in building) E893.9
- - from
- - - bonfire E893.2
- - - highly inflammable material E894
- - - sources or material as listed in E893.8 E893.8
- - - trash fire E893.2
- - - uncontrolled fire - see Conflagration
- - in
- - - private dwelling E893.0
- - - specified building or structure, except private dwelling E893.1
- - not in building or structure E893.2
- - with conflagration - see Conflagration
- explosive material - see Explosion
- fat E894
- gasoline E894
- kerosene E894
- material
- - explosive - see Explosion
- - highly inflammable E894
- - - with
- - - - conflagration - see Conflagration
- - - - explosion E923.2

Ignition - *continued*
- nightdress - see Ignition, clothes
- paraffin E894
- petrol E894

Immersion - see Submersion

Implantation of quills of porcupine E906.8
Inanition (from) E904.9
- hunger - see Lack of food
- resulting from homicidal intent E968.4
- thirst - see Lack of water
Inattention after, at birth E904.0
- homicidal, infanticidal intent E968.4
Infanticide (see also Assault) E968.9
Ingestion
- foreign body (causing injury) (with obstruction) - see Foreign body, alimentary canal
- poisonous substance NEC - see Table of drugs and chemicals
Inhalation
- excessively cold substance, manmade E901.1
- foreign body - see Foreign body, aspiration
- liquid air, hydrogen, nitrogen E901.1
- mucus, not of newborn (with asphyxia, obstruction respiratory passage, suffocation) E912
- phlegm (with asphyxia, obstruction respiratory passage, suffocation) E912
- poisonous gas - see Table of drugs and chemicals
- vomitus (with asphyxia, obstruction respiratory passage, suffocation) E911
Injury, injured (accidental(ly)) NEC E928.9
- by, caused by, from
- - air rifle (B-B gun) E917.9
- - animal (not being ridden) NEC E906.9

Injury - *continued*
- by - *continued*
- - animal - *continued*
- - - being ridden (in sport or transport) E828.-
- - assault (see also Assault) E968.9
- - avalanche E909
- - bayonet (see also Bayonet wound) E920.3
- - being thrown against some part of, or object in
- - - motor vehicle (in motion) (on public highway) E818.-
- - - - not on public highway E825.-
- - - nonmotor road vehicle NEC E829.-
- - - off-road motor vehicle NEC E821.-
- - - railway train E806.-
- - - snow vehicle, motor-driven E820.-
- - - street car E829.-
- - bending E927
- - broken glass E920.8
- - bullet - see Shooting
- - cave-in (see also Suffocation due to cave-in) E913.3
- - - earth surface movement or eruption E909
- - - storm E908
- - - without asphyxiation or suffocation E916
- - cloudburst E908
- - cutting or piercing instrument (see also Cut) E920.9
- - cyclone E908
- - earthquake E909
- - electric current (see also Electric shock) E925.9
- - explosion (see also Explosion) E923.9
- - fire - see Fire
- - flare, Verey pistol E922.8
- - flood E908
- - foreign body - see Foreign body
- - hailstones E904.3
- - hurricane E908
- - landslide E909
- - law-enforcing agent, police, in course of legal intervention - see Legal intervention
- - lightning E907
- - live rail or live wire - see Electric shock
- - machinery - see also Accident, machine
- - - aircraft, without accident to aircraft E844.-

Injury - *continued*
- by - *continued*
- - machinery - *continued*
- - - boat, ship, watercraft (deck) (engine room) (galley) (laundry) (loading) E836.-
- - missile
- - - explosive E923.8
- - - firearm - see Shooting
- - - in war operations - see War operations, missile
- - moving part of motor vehicle (in motion) (on public highway) E818.-
- - - not on public highway, nontraffic accident E825.-
- - - while alighting, boarding, entering, leaving - see Fall from motor vehicle, while alighting, boarding
- - nail E920.8
- - noise E928.1
- - object
- - - fallen on
- - - - motor vehicle (in motion) (on public highway) E818.-
- - - - - not on public highway E825.-
- - - falling - see Hit by object falling
- - radiation - see Radiation
- - railway rolling stock, train, vehicle (part of) E805.-
- - - door or window E806.-
- - rotating propeller, aircraft E844.-
- - rough landing of off-road type motor vehicle (after leaving ground or rough terrain) E821.-
- - - snow vehicle E820.-
- - saber (see also Wound, saber) E920.3
- - shot - see Shooting
- - sound waves E928.1
- - splinter or sliver, wood E920.8
- - straining E927
- - street car (door) E829.-
- - suicide (attempt) E958.9
- - sword E920.3
- - third rail - see Electric shock
- - thunderbolt E907
- - tidal wave E909
- - - caused by storm E908
- - tornado E908
- - torrential rain E908
- - twisting E927
- - vehicle NEC - see Accident, vehicle NEC
- - vibration E928.2
- - volcanic eruption E909
- - weapon burst, in war operations E993
- - weightlessness (in spacecraft, real or simulated) E928.0

Injury - *continued*
- by - *continued*
- - wood splinter or sliver   E920.8
- due to
- - civil insurrection - see War operations
- - - occurring after cessation of
      hostilities   E998
- - war operations - see War operations
- - - occurring after cessation of
      hostilities   E998
- homicidal (see also Assault)   E968.9
- in, on
- - civil insurrection - see War operations
- - fight   E960.0
- - parachute descent (voluntary) (without
    accident to aircraft)   E844.-
- - - with accident to aircraft - see
      categories E840-E842
- - public highway   E819.-
- - railway right of way   E807.-
- - war operations - see War operations
- inflicted (by)
- - in course of arrest (attempted),
    suppression of disturbance,
    maintenance of order, by
    law-enforcing agents - see Legal
    intervention
- - law-enforcing agent (on duty) - see
    Legal intervention
- - other person
- - - stated as
- - - - accidental   E928.9
- - - - homicidal, intentional - see
        Assault
- - - - undetermined whether accidental
        or intentional - see Injury stated
        as undetermined
- - police (on duty) - see Legal
    intervention
- late effect of   E929.9
- purposely (inflicted) by other person(s) -
  see Assault
- self-inflicted (unspecified whether
  accidental or intentional)   E988.9
- - stated as
- - - accidental   E928.9
- - - intentionally, purposely   E958.9

Injury - *continued*
- specified cause NEC   E928.8
- stated as
- - undetermined whether accidentally or
    purposely inflicted (by)   E988.9
- - - cut (any part of body)   E986
- - - cutting or piercing instrument
      (classifiable to   E920) E986
- - - drowning   E984
- - - explosive(s) (missile)   E985.5
- - - falling from high place   E987.9
- - - - manmade structure, except
        residential   E987.1
- - - - natural site   E987.2
- - - - residential premises   E987.0
- - - hanging   E983.0
- - - knife   E986
- - - late effect of   E989
- - - puncture (any part of body)   E986
- - - shooting - see Shooting stated as
      undetermined whether accidental or
      intentional
- - - specified means NEC   E988.8
- - - stab (any part of body)   E986
- - - strangulation - see Suffocation
      stated as undetermined whether
      accidental or intentional
- - - submersion   E984
- - - suffocation - see Suffocation stated
      as undetermined whether accidental
      or intentional
- to child due to criminal abortion   E968.8
Insufficient nourishment - see also Lack of
food
- homicidal intent   E968.4
Insulation, effects - see Heat
Interruption of respiration by
- food lodged in esophagus   E911
- foreign body, except food, in esophagus
  E912
Intervention, legal - see Legal intervention
Intoxication, drug or poison - see Table of
drugs and chemicals
Irradiation - see Radiation

J

Jammed (accidentally)
- between objects (moving) (stationary and
  moving)   E918

Jammed - *continued*
- in object   E918

Jumped or fell from high place, so stated - see Jumping from high place
Jumping
− before train, vehicle or other moving object (unspecified whether accidental or intentional) E988.0
− − stated as
− − − intentional, purposeful E958.0
− − − suicidal (attempt) E958.0
− from
− − aircraft
− − − by parachute (voluntarily) (without accident to aircraft) E844.-
− − − due to accident to aircraft - see categories E840-E842
− − boat, ship, watercraft (into water)
− − − after accident to, fire on, watercraft E830.-
− − − − and subsequently struck by (part of) boat E831.-
− − − burning, crushed, sinking E830.-
− − − − and subsequently struck by (part of) boat E831.-
− − − voluntarily, without accident (to boat) with injury other than drowning or submersion E883.0
− − − − with drowning or submersion - see Submersion
− − building
− − − burning E891.8
− − − − private E890.8
− − cable car (not on rails) E847
− − − on rails E829.-
− − high place

Note − The following fourth-digit subdivisions are for use with categories E957 and E987:
.0 residential premises
.1 Other manmade structures
.2 Natural sites
.9 Unspecified.

Jumping - *continued*
− from - *continued*
− − high place - *continued*
− − − in accidental circumstances or in sport - see categories E880-E884
− − − stated as
− − − − in undetermined circumstances E987.-
− − − − suicidal (attempt) E957.-
− − − − with intent to injure self E957.-
− − motor vehicle (in motion) (on public highway) - see Fall from motor vehicle
− − nonmotor road vehicle NEC E829.-
− − street car E829.-
− − structure, burning NEC E891.8
− into water
− − from, off watercraft - see Jumping from boat
− − with injury other than drowning or submersion E883.0
− − − drowning or submersion - see Submersion
Justifiable homicide - see Assault

K

Kicked by
− animal E906.8
− person(s) (accidentally) E917.9
− − as, or caused by, a crowd (with fall) E917.1
− − in fight E960.0
− − in sports (with fall) E917.0
− − with intent to injure or kill E960.0
Kicking against
− object (moving) (projected) (stationary) E917.9
− − in sports E917.0
− person - see Striking against person
Killed, killing (accidentally) NEC (see also Injury) E928.9

Killed - *continued*
− in
− − action - see War operations
− − brawl, fight (hand) (fists) (foot) E960.0
− − − by weapon - see also Assault
− − − − cutting, piercing E966
− − − − firearm - see Shooting, homicide
− self
− − stated as
− − − accident E928.9
− − − suicide - see Suicide
− − unspecified whether accidental or suicidal E988.9

Knocked down (accidentally) (by) NEC
E928.9
- animal (not being ridden) E906.8
- - being ridden (in sport or transport)
  E828.-
- blast from explosion (see also
  Explosion) E923.9
- crowd, human stampede E917.1

Knocked down - *continued*
- late effect of - see Late effect
- person (accidentally) E917.9
- - in brawl, fight E960.0
- - in sports E917.0
- transport vehicle - see Vehicle involved
  under hit, by
- while boxing E917.0

L

Laceration NEC E928.9
Lack of
- air (refrigerator or closed place),
  suffocation by E913.2
- care (helpless person) (infant)
  (newborn) E904.0
- - homicidal intent E968.4
- food except as result of transport
  accident E904.1
- - helpless person, infant, newborn due to
  abandonment or neglect E904.0
- water except as result of transport
  accident E904.2
- - helpless person, infant, newborn due to
  abandonment or neglect E904.0
Landslide E909
- falling on, hitting
- - motor vehicle (any) (in motion) (on or
  off public highway) E909
- - railway rolling stock, train, vehicle
  E909
Late effect of
- accident NEC (accident classifiable to
  E928.9) E929.9
- - specified NEC (accident classifiable
  to E928.8) E929.8
- fall, accidental (accident classifiable to
  E880-E888) E929.3
- fire, accident caused by (accident
  classifiable to E890-E899) E929.4
- homicide, attempt (any means) E969
- injury undetermined whether accidentally
  or purposely inflicted (injury classifiable
  to E980-E988) E989
- legal intervention (injury classifiable to
  E970-E976) E977
- medical or surgical procedure, test or
  therapy
- - as, or resulting in, or from
- - - abnormal or delayed reaction or
  complication - see Reaction,
  abnormal

Late effect of - *continued*
- medical or surgical procedure - *continued*
- - as - *continued*
- - - misadventure - see Misadventure
- motor vehicle accident (accident
  classifiable to E810-E825) E929.0
- natural or environmental factor, accident
  due to (accident classifiable to
  E900-E909) E929.5
- poisoning, accidental (accident
  classifiable to E850-E858, E860-E869)
  E929.2
- suicide, attempt (any means) E959
- transport accident NEC (accident
  classifiable to E800-E807, E826-E838,
  E840-E848) E929.1
- war operations, injury due to (injury
  classifiable to E990-E998) E999
Launching pad accident E845.-
Legal
- execution, any method E978
- intervention (by) (injury from) E976
- - baton E973
- - bayonet E974
- - blow E975
- - blunt object E973
- - cutting or piercing instrument E974
- - dynamite E971
- - execution, any method E978
- - explosive(s) (shell) E971
- - firearm(s) E970
- - gas (asphyxiation) (poisoning) (tear)
  E972
- - grenade E971
- - late effect of E977
- - machine gun E970
- - man-handling E975
- - mortar bomb E971
- - revolver E970
- - rifle E970
- - specified means NEC E975
- - stabbing E974

Legal - *continued*
- intervention - *continued*
- - stave E973
- - truncheon E973
Lifting, injury in E927
Lightning (shock) (stroke) (struck by) E907
Liquid (noncorrosive) in eye E914
- corrosive E924.1
Loss of control
- motor vehicle (on public highway) (without antecedent collision) E816.-
- - not on public highway, nontraffic accident E825.-
- - - with antecedent collision - see Collision, motor vehicle not on public highway
- - with
- - - antecedent collision on public highway - see Collision, motor vehicle
- - - subsequent collision
- - - - involving any object, person or vehicle not on public highway E816.-
- - - - on public highway - see Collision, motor vehicle

Loss of control - *continued*
- off-road type motor vehicle (not on public highway) NEC E821.-
- - on public highway - see Loss of control, motor vehicle
- snow vehicle, motor-driven (not on public highway) E820.-
- - on public highway - see Loss of control, motor vehicle
Lost at sea E832.-
- in war operations E995
- with accident to watercraft E830.-
Low
- pressure, effects - see Effects of air pressure
- temperature, effects - see Cold, exposure to
Lying before train, vehicle or other moving object (unspecified whether accidental or intentional) E988.0
- stated as intentional, purposeful, suicidal (attempt) E958.0
Lynching (see also Assault) E968.9

M

Malfunction, atomic power plant in water transport E838.-
Man-handling (in brawl, fight) E960.0
- legal intervention E975
Mangled (accidentally) NEC E928.9
Manslaughter (nonaccidental) - see also Assault
Marble in nose E912
Mauled by animal E906.8
Medical procedure, complication of
- delayed or as an abnormal reaction without mention of misadventure - see Reaction, abnormal
- due to or as a result of misadventure - see Misadventure
Minamata disease E865.2
Misadventure(s) to patient(s) during surgical or medical care E876.9
- contaminated blood, fluid, drug or biological substance (presence of agents and toxins as listed in E875) E875.9
- - administered (by) NEC E875.9
- - - infusion E875.0

Misadventure(s) to patient(s) - *continued*
- contaminated blood - *continued*
- - administered - *continued*
- - - injection E875.1
- - - specified means NEC E875.2
- - - transfusion E875.0
- - - vaccination E875.1
- cut, cutting, puncture, perforation or hemorrhage (accidental) (inadvertent) (inappropriate) (during) E870.9
- - aspiration of fluid or tissue (by puncture or catheterization, except heart) E870.5
- - biopsy E870.8
- - - needle (aspirating) E870.5
- - blood sampling E870.5
- - catheterization E870.5
- - - heart E870.6
- - dialysis (kidney) E870.2
- - endoscopic examination E870.4
- - enema E870.7
- - infusion E870.1
- - injection E870.3

Misadventure(s) to patient(s) - *continued*
- foreign object left in body - *continued*
- - needle biopsy E871.5
- - paracentesis, abdominal E871.5
- - perfusion E871.2
- - removal of catheter or packing E871.7
- - specified procedure NEC E871.8
- - surgical operation E871.0
- - thoracentesis E871.5
- - transfusion E871.1
- - vaccination E871.3
- hemorrhage - see Misadventure, cut
- inadvertent exposure of patient to radiation (being received for test or therapy) E873.3
- inappropriate
- - operation performed E876.5
- - temperature (too hot or too cold) in local application or packing E873.5
- infusion - see also Misadventure, by specific type, infusion
- - excessive amount of fluid E873.0
- - incorrect dilution of fluid E873.1
- - wrong fluid E876.1
- mismatched blood in transfusion E876.0
- nonadministration of necessary drug or medicament E873.6
- overdose - see also Overdose
- - radiation, in therapy E873.2
- perforation - see Misadventure, cut
- performance of inappropriate operation E876.5
- puncture - see Misadventure, cut
- specified type NEC E876.8
- - failure
- - - suture or ligature during surgical operation E876.2

Misadventure(s) to patient(s) - *continued*
- specified type NEC - *continued*
- - failure - *continued*
- - - to introduce or to remove tube or instrument E876.4
- - - - foreign object left in body E871.9
- - infusion of wrong fluid E876.1
- - performance of inappropriate operation E876.5
- - transfusion of mismatched blood E876.0
- - wrong
- - - fluid in infusion E876.1
- - - placement of endotracheal tube during anesthetic procedure E876.3
- transfusion - see also Misadventure, by specific type, transfusion
- - excessive amount of blood E873.0
- - mismatched blood E876.0
- wrong
- - drug given in error - see Table of drugs and chemicals
- - fluid in infusion E876.1
- - placement of endotracheal tube during anesthetic procedure E876.3
Motion (effects) E903
- sickness E903
Mountain sickness E902.0
Mucus aspiration or inhalation, not of newborn (with asphyxia, obstruction respiratory passage, suffocation) E912
Mudslide of cataclysmic nature E909
Murder (attempt) (see also Assault) E968.9

N

Nail, injury by E920.8
Neglect - see also Privation
- criminal E968.4

Neglect - see also Privation - *continued*
- homicidal intent E968.4
Noise (causing injury) (pollution) E928.1

O

Object

– falling

– – from, in, on, hitting

– – – aircraft E844.-
– – – – due to accident to aircraft - see
     categories E840-E842
– – – machinery - see also Accident,
     machine
– – – – not in operation E916
– – – motor vehicle (in motion) (on public
     highway) E818.-
– – – – not on public highway E825.-
– – – – stationary E916
– – – nonmotor road vehicle NEC
     E829.-
– – – pedal cycle E826.-
– – – person E916
– – – railway rolling stock, train, vehicle
     E806.-
– – – street car E829.-
– – – watercraft E838.-
– – – – due to accident to watercraft
     E831.-

– set in motion by

– – accidental explosion of pressure vessel
     - see category E921

– – firearm - see category E922

– – machine(ry) - see Accident, machine
– – transport vehicle - see categories
     E800-E848

– thrown from, in, on, towards

– – aircraft E844.-
– – cable car (not on rails) E847
– – – on rails E829.-
– – motor vehicle (in motion) (on public
     highway) E818.-
– – – not on public highway E825.-
– – nonmotor road vehicle NEC E829.-
– – pedal cycle E826.-
– – street car E829.-
– – vehicle NEC - see Accident, vehicle
     NEC

Obstruction

– air passages, larynx, respiratory passages

– – by
– – – external means NEC - see
     Suffocation
– – – food, any type (regurgitated)
     (vomited) E911

Obstruction - *continued*

– air passages - *continued*
– – by - *continued*
– – – material or object except food
     E912
– – – mucus E912
– – – phlegm E912
– – – vomitus E911

– digestive tract, except mouth or pharynx
– – by
– – – food, any type E915
– – – foreign body (any) E915

– esophagus
– – food E911
– – foreign body, except food E912
– – without asphyxia or obstruction of
     respiratory passage E915

– mouth or pharynx
– – by
– – – food, any type E911
– – – material or object except food
     E912

– respiration - see Obstruction, air passages

Oil in eye E914

Overdose
– anesthetic (drug) - see Table of drugs and
     chemicals
– drug - see Table of drugs and chemicals

Overexertion (lifting) (pulling) (pushing)
E927

Overexposure (accidental) (to)
– cold - see Cold, exposure to
– – due to manmade conditions E901.1
– heat (see also Heat) E900.9
– radiation - see Radiation
– radioactivity - see Radiation
– sun, except sunburn E900.0
– weather - see Exposure
– wind - see Exposure

Overheated (see also Heat) E900.9

Overlaid E913.0

Overturning (accidental)
– animal-drawn vehicle E827.-
– boat, ship, watercraft
– – causing
– – – drowning, submersion E830.-
– – – injury except drowning,
     submersion E831.-
– machinery - see Accident, machine

Overturning - *continued*
- motor vehicle (see also Loss of control, motor vehicle) E816.-
- - not on public highway, nontraffic accident E825.-
- - - with antecedent collision - see Collision, motor vehicle not on public highway
- - with antecedent collision on public highway - see Collision, motor vehicle

Overturning - *continued*
- nonmotor road vehicle NEC E829.-
- off-road type motor vehicle - see Loss of control, off-road type motor vehicle
- pedal cycle E826.-
- railway rolling stock, train, vehicle (see also Derailment, railway) E802.-
- street car E829.-
- vehicle NEC - see Accident, vehicle NEC

P

Palsy, divers' E902.2
Parachuting (voluntary) (without accident to aircraft) E844.-
- due to accident to aircraft - see categories E840-E842
Paralysis
- divers' E902.2
- lead or saturnine E866.0
- - from pesticide NEC E863.4
Pecked by bird E906.8
Phlegm aspiration or inhalation (with asphyxia, obstruction respiratory passage, suffocation) E912
Piercing (see also Cut) E920.9
Pinched
- between objects (moving) (stationary and moving) E918
- in object E918
Pinned under
- machine(ry) - see Accident, machine
Plumbism E866.0
- from insecticide NEC E863.4
Poisoning (accidental) (by) - see also Table of drugs and chemicals
- carbon monoxide
- - generated by
- - - aircraft in transit E844.-
- - - motor vehicle
- - - - in motion (on public highway) E818.-
- - - - - not on public highway E823.-
- - - watercraft (in transit) (not in transit) E838.-
- caused by injection of poisons or toxins into or through skin by plant thorns, spines or other mechanisms E905.7
- - marine or sea plants E905.6
- fumes or smoke due to
- - conflagration - see Conflagration
- - explosion or fire - see Fire

Poisoning - *continued*
- fumes or smoke due to - *continued*
- - ignition - see Ignition
- gas
- - in legal intervention E972
- - legal execution, by E978
- - on watercraft E838.-
- - used as anesthetic - see Table of drugs and chemicals
- in war operations E997.2
- late effect of - see Late effect
- legal
- - execution E978
- - intervention
- - - by gas E972
Pressure, external, causing asphyxia, suffocation (see also Suffocation) E913.9
Privation E904.9
- food (see also Lack of, food) E904.1
- helpless person, infant, newborn due to abandonment or neglect E904.0
- late effect of NEC E929.5
- resulting from transport accident - see categories E800-E848
- water (see also Lack of, water) E904.2
Projected objects, striking against or struck by - see Striking against, object
Prolonged stay in
- high altitude (causing conditions as listed in E902.0) E902.0
- weightless environment E928.0
Prostration
- heat - see Heat
Pulling, injury in E927
Puncture, puncturing (see also Cut) E920.9
- by
- - plant thorns or spines E920.8
- - - toxic reaction E905.7
- - - - marine or sea plants E905.6

Q

R

Radiation - *continued*
- radioactive isotopes - *continued*
- - misadventure in medical or surgical treatment - see Misadventure, failure, in dosage, radiation
- radiobiologicals - see Radiation, radioactive isotopes
- radiofrequency E926.0
- radiopharmaceuticals - see Radiation, radioactive isotopes
- radium NEC E926.9
- sun E926.2
- - excessive heat from E900.0
- welding arc or torch E926.2
- - excessive heat from E900.1
- x-rays (hard) (soft) E926.3
- - misadventure in medical or surgical treatment - see Misadventure, failure, in dosage, radiation

Rape E960.1

Reaction, abnormal to or following (medical or surgical procedure) E879.9
- amputation (of limbs) E878.5
- anastomosis (arteriovenous) (blood vessel) (gastrojejunal) (skin) (tendon) (natural, artificial material, tissue)
- - external stoma, creation of E878.3
- aspiration (of fluid) E879.4
- - tissue E879.8
- biopsy E879.8
- blood
- - sampling E879.7
- - transfusion
- - - procedure E879.8
- bypass - see Reaction, abnormal, anastomosis
- catheterization
- - cardiac E879.0
- - urinary E879.6
- colostomy E878.3
- cystostomy E878.3
- dialysis (kidney) E879.1
- drugs or biologicals - see Table of drugs and chemicals
- duodenostomy E878.3
- electroshock therapy E879.3
- formation of external stoma E878.3
- gastrostomy E878.3
- graft - see Reaction, abnormal, anastomosis
- hypothermia E879.8
- implant, implantation (of)
- - artificial
- - - internal device (cardiac pacemaker) (electrodes in brain) (heart valve prosthesis) (orthopedic) E878.1

Reaction - *continued*
- implant - *continued*
- - artificial - *continued*
- - - material or tissue (for anastomosis or bypass) E878.2
- - - - with creation of external stoma E878.3
- - natural tissues (for anastomosis or bypass) E878.2
- - - as transplantation - see Reaction, abnormal, transplant
- - - with creation of external stoma E878.3
- infusion
- - procedure E879.8
- injection
- - procedure E879.8
- insertion of gastric or duodenal sound E879.5
- insulin-shock therapy E879.3
- lumbar puncture E879.4
- perfusion E879.1
- procedures other than surgical operation (see also Reaction, abnormal, by specific type of procedure) E879.9
- - specified NEC E879.8
- radiological procedure or therapy E879.2
- removal of organ (partial) (total) NEC E878.6
- sampling
- - blood E879.7
- - fluid NEC E879.4
- - tissue E879.8
- shock therapy E879.3
- surgical operation (see also Reaction, abnormal, by specified type of operation) E878.9
- - restorative NEC E878.4
- - - with
- - - - anastomosis, bypass or graft E878.2
- - - - formation of external stoma E878.3
- - - - implant(ation) - see Reaction, abnormal, implant
- - - - transplant(ation) - see Reaction, abnormal, transplant
- - specified NEC E878.8
- thoracentesis E879.4
- transfusion
- - procedure E879.8
- transplant, transplantation (heart) (kidney) (liver) E878.0
- - partial organ E878.4
- ureterostomy E878.3
- vaccination

S

Shock - *continued*
- anaphylactic - *continued*
- - due to - *continued*
- - - sting - see Sting
- electric (see also Electric shock) E925.9
- from electric appliance or current (see also Electric shock) E925.9
Shooting, shot (accidental(ly)) E922.-

Note – The following fourth-digit subdivisions are for use with categories E922, E955, E965 and E985:

E922	E955	
	E965	
	E985	
.0	.0	*Hand gun* *Pistol* *Revolver (military)*
.1	.1	*Shotgun (automatic)*
.2	.2	*Hunting rifle*
.3	.3	*Military firearm, except hand gun* *Army rifle* *Machine gun*
.8	.4	*Other* *Verey pistol*
.9	.4	*Unspecified.*

Shooting - *continued*
- himself (see also Shooting, self-inflicted) E985.-
- homicide (attempt) E965.-
- in war operations - see War operations, shooting
- inflicted by other person
- - in accidental circumstances E922.-
- - stated as
- - - intentional, homicidal E965.-
- - - undetermined whether accidental or intentional E985.-
- legal
- - execution E978
- - intervention E970
- self-inflicted (unspecified whether accidental or intentional) E985.-
- - accidental E922.-
- - stated as
- - - intentional, purposeful E955.-
- stated as undetermined whether accidental or intentional E985.-
- suicidal (attempt) E955.-
Shoving (accidentally) by other person (see also Pushing by other person) E917.9
Sickness

Sickness - *continued*
- air E903
- alpine E902.0
- car E903
- motion E903
- mountain E902.0
- sea E903
- travel E903
Sinking (accidental)
- boat, ship, watercraft (causing drowning, submersion) E830.-
- - causing injury except drowning, submersion E831.-
Siriasis E900.0
Skydiving E844.-
Slashed wrists (see also Cut, self-inflicted) E986
Slipping (accidental)
- on
- - deck (of boat, ship, watercraft) (icy) (oily) (wet) E835.-
- - ice E885
- - ladder of ship E833.-
- - - due to accident to watercraft E831.-
- - mud E885
- - oil E885
- - snow E885
- - stairs of ship E833.-
- - - due to accident to watercraft E831.-
- - surface
- - - slippery E885
- - - wet E885
Sliver, wood, injury by E920.8
Smothering, smothered (see also Suffocation) E913.9
Solid substance in eye (any part) or adnexa E914
Sound waves (causing injury) E928.1
Splinter, injury by E920.8
Stab, stabbing E966
- accidental - see Cut
Starvation E904.1
- helpless person, infant, newborn - see Lack of food
- homicidal intent E968.4
- late effect of NEC E929.5
- resulting from accident connected with transport - see categories E800-E848
Stepped on
- by
- - animal (not being ridden) E906.8
- - - being ridden (in sport or transport) E828.-
- - crowd E917.1
- - person E917.9

Submersion - *continued*
- in - *continued*
- - sport or recreational activity (without diving equipment) E910.2
- - - water skiing E910.0
- - - with or using diving equipment E910.1
- - swimming pool NEC E910.8
- - war operations E995
- - water transport E832.-
- - - due to accident to boat, ship, watercraft E830.-
- landslide E909
- - overturning boat, ship, watercraft E909
- - sinking boat, ship, watercraft E909
- - submersion boat, ship, watercraft E909
- - tidal wave E909
- - - caused by storm E908
- - torrential rain E908
- late effect of NEC E929.8
- quenching tank E910.8
- self-inflicted (unspecified whether accidental or intentional) E984
- - in accidental circumstances - see category E910
- - stated as intentional, purposeful E954
- stated as undetermined whether accidental or intentional E984
- suicidal (attempted) E954
- while
- - attempting rescue of another person E910.3
- - engaged in
- - - marine salvage E910.3
- - - underwater construction or repairs E910.3
- - fishing, not from boat E910.2
- - hunting, not from boat E910.2
- - ice skating E910.2
- - pearl diving E910.3
- - placing fishing nets E910.3
- - playing in water E910.2
- - scuba diving E910.1
- - - nonrecreational E910.3
- - skin diving E910.1
- - - nonrecreational E910.3
- - snorkel diving E910.2
- - spear fishing underwater E910.1
- - surfboarding E910.2
- - swimming (swimming pool) E910.2
- - wading (in water) E910.2
- - water skiing E910.0
Sucked
- into
- - jet (aircraft) E844.-

Suffocation (accidental) (by external means) (by pressure) (mechanical) E913.9
- caused by other person
- - in accidental circumstances - see category E913
- - stated as
- - - intentional, homicidal E963
- - - undetermined whether accidental or intentional E983.9
- - - - by, in
- - - - - hanging E983.0
- - - - - plastic bag E983.1
- - - - - specified means NEC E983.8
- due to, by
- - avalanche E909
- - bedclothes E913.0
- - bib E913.0
- - blanket E913.0
- - cave-in E913.3
- - - caused by cataclysmic earth surface movement or eruption E909
- - conflagration - see Conflagration
- - explosion - see Explosion
- - falling earth, other substance E913.3
- - fire - see Fire
- - food, any type (ingestion) (inhalation) (regurgitated) (vomited) E911
- - foreign body, except food (ingestion) (inhalation) E912
- - ignition - see Ignition
- - landslide E909
- - machine(ry) - see Accident, machine
- - material, object except food entering by nose or mouth, ingested, inhaled E912
- - mucus (aspiration) (inhalation), not of newborn E912
- - phlegm (aspiration) (inhalation) E912
- - pillow E913.0
- - plastic bag - see Suffocation in plastic bag
- - sheet (plastic) E913.0
- - specified means NEC E913.8
- - vomitus (aspiration) (inhalation) E911
- homicidal (attempt) E963
- in
- - airtight enclosed place E913.2
- - baby carriage E913.0
- - bed E913.0
- - closed place E913.2
- - cot, cradle E913.0
- - perambulator E913.0
- - plastic bag (in accidental circumstances) E913.1

Suffocation - *continued*
- in - *continued*
- - plastic bag - *continued*
- - - homicidal, purposely inflicted by other person E963
- - - self-inflicted (unspecified whether accidental or intentional) E983.1
- - - - in accidental circumstances E913.1
- - - - intentional, suicidal E953.1
- - - stated as undetermined whether accidentally or purposely inflicted E983.1
- - - suicidal, purposely self-inflicted E953.1
- - refrigerator E913.2
- self-inflicted - see also Suffocation stated as undetermined whether accidental or intentional
- - in accidental circumstances - see category E913
- - stated as intentional, purposeful - see Suicide, suffocation
- stated as undetermined whether accidental or intentional E983.9
- - by, in
- - - hanging E983.0
- - - plastic bag E983.1
- - - specified means NEC E983.8
- suicidal - see Suicide, suffocation
Suicide, suicidal (attempted) (by) E958.9
- burning, burns E958.1
- caustic substance E958.7
- - poisoning E950.7
- - swallowed E950.7
- cold, extreme E958.3
- crashing of
- - aircraft E958.6
- - motor vehicle E958.5
- cut (any part of body) E956
- cutting or piercing instrument (classifiable to E920) E956
- drowning E954
- electrocution E958.4
- explosive(s) (classifiable to E923) E955.5
- fire E958.1
- firearm (classifiable to E922) - see Shooting, suicidal
- hanging E953.0

Suicide - *continued*
- jumping
- - before moving object, train, vehicle E958.0
- - from high place - see Jumping from high place stated as suicidal
- knife E956
- late effect of E959
- motor vehicle, crashing of E958.5
- poisoning - see Table of drugs and chemicals
- puncture (any part of body) E956
- scald E958.2
- shooting - see Shooting, suicidal
- specified means NEC E958.8
- stab (any part of body) E956
- strangulation - see Suicide, suffocation
- submersion E954
- suffocation E953.9
- - by, in
- - - hanging E953.0
- - - plastic bag E953.1
- - - specified means NEC E953.8
- wound NEC E958.9
Sunstroke E900.0
Supersonic waves (causing injury) E928.1
Surgical procedure, complication of
- delayed or as an abnormal reaction without mention of misadventure - see Reaction, abnormal
- due to or as a result of misadventure - see Misadventure
Swallowed, swallowing
- foreign body - see Foreign body, alimentary canal
- poison - see Table of drugs and chemicals
- substance
- - caustic - see Table of drugs and chemicals
- - corrosive - see Table of drugs and chemicals
- - poisonous - see Table of drugs and chemicals
Swimmers' cramp (see also Category E910) E910.2
- not in recreation or sport E910.3
Syndrome, battered
- baby or child - see Abuse, child
- wife - see Assault

T

Tackle in sport   E886.0
Thermic fever   E900.9
Thermoplegia   E900.9
Thirst - see also Lack of water
− resulting from accident connected with
   transport - see categories   E800-E848
Thrown (accidentally)
− against object in or part of vehicle
− − by motion of vehicle
− − − aircraft   E844.-
− − − boat, ship, watercraft   E838.-
− − − motor vehicle (on public highway)
      E818.-
− − − − not on public highway   E825.-
− − − − off-road type (not on public
         highway)   E821.-
− − − − − on public highway   E818.-
− − − − − snow vehicle   E820.-
− − − − − − on public highway   E818.-
− − nonmotor road vehicle NEC   E829.-
− − railway rolling stock, train, vehicle
      E806.-
− − street car   E829.-
− from
− − animal (being ridden) (in sport or
      transport)   E828.-
− − high place, homicide (attempt)
      E968.1
− − machinery - see Accident, machine
− − vehicle NEC - see Accident, vehicle
      NEC
− off - see Thrown, from
− overboard (by motion of boat, ship,
   watercraft)   E832.-
− − by accident to boat, ship, watercraft
      E830.-
Thunderbolt NEC   E907
Tidal wave (any injury)   E909
− caused by storm   E908
Took
− overdose of drug - see Table of drugs and
   chemicals

Took - *continued*
− poison - see Table of drugs and chemicals
Tornado (any injury)   E908
Torrential rain (any injury)   E908
Traffic accident NEC   E819.-
Trampled by animal   E906.8
− being ridden (in sport or transport)
   E828.-
Trapped (accidentally)
− between
− − objects (moving) (stationary and
      moving)   E918
− by
− − door of
− − − elevator   E918
− − − motor vehicle (on public highway)
      (while alighting, boarding) - see Fall
      from motor vehicle while alighting
− − − railway train (underground)   E806.-
− − − street car   E829.-
− − − subway train   E806.-
− in object   E918
Travel (effects)   E903
− sickness   E903
Tree
− falling on or hitting   E916
− − motor vehicle (in motion) (on public
      highway)   E818.-
− − − not on public highway   E825.-
− − nonmotor road vehicle NEC   E829.-
− − pedal cycle   E826.-
− − person   E916
− − railway rolling stock, train, vehicle
      E806.-
− − street car   E829.-
Trench foot   E901.0
Tripping over animal, carpet, curb, kerb, rug
   or (small) object (with fall)   E885
− without fall - see Striking against object
Twisting, injury in   E927

U

V

Violence, nonaccidental (see also Assault) E968.9

Volcanic eruption (any injury) E909

Vomitus in air passages (with asphyxia, obstruction or suffocation) E911

W

War operations (during hostilities) (injury) (by) (in) E995

- after cessation of hostilities, injury due to E998
- air blast E993
- aircraft burned, destroyed, exploded, shot down E994
- asphyxia from
- – chemical E997.2
- – fire, conflagration (caused by fire-producing device or conventional weapon) E990.9
- – – from nuclear explosion E996
- – – petrol bomb E990.0
- – fumes E997.2
- – gas E997.2
- battle wound NEC E995
- bayonet E995
- biological warfare agents E997.1
- blast (air) (effects) E993
- – from nuclear explosion E996
- – underwater E992
- bomb (mortar) (explosion) E993
- – after cessation of hostilities E998
- – fragments, injury by E991.9
- – – antipersonnel E991.3
- bullet(s) (from carbine, machine gun, pistol, rifle, shotgun) E991.2
- – rubber E991.0
- burn from
- – chemical E997.2
- – fire, conflagration (caused by fire-producing device or conventional weapon) E990.9
- – – from nuclear explosion E996
- – – petrol bomb E990.0
- – gas E997.2
- burning aircraft E994
- chemical E997.2
- chlorine E997.2
- conventional warfare, specified form NEC E995
- crushing by falling aircraft E994
- depth charge E992
- destruction of aircraft E994

War operations - *continued*
- disability as sequela one year or more after injury due to E999
- drowning E995
- effect (direct) (secondary) nuclear weapon E996
- explosion (artillery shell) (breech block) (cannon shell) E993
- – after cessation of hostilities of bomb, mine placed in war E998
- – aircraft E994
- – bomb (mortar) E993
- – – atom E996
- – – hydrogen E996
- – – injury by fragments from E991.9
- – – – antipersonnel E991.3
- – – nuclear E996
- – depth charge E992
- – injury by fragments from E991.9
- – – antipersonnel E991.3
- – marine weapon E992
- – mine
- – – at sea or in harbor E992
- – – land E993
- – – – injury by fragments from E991.9
- – – marine E992
- – munitions (accidental) (being used in war) (dump) (factory) E993
- – nuclear (weapon) E996
- – own weapons (accidental) E993
- – – injury by fragments from E991.9
- – – – antipersonnel E991.3
- – sea-based artillery shell E992
- – torpedo E992
- exposure to ionizing radiation from nuclear explosion E996
- falling aircraft E994
- fire or fire-producing device E990.9
- – petrol bomb E990.0
- fireball effects from nuclear explosion E996
- fragments from
- – antipersonnel bomb E991.3
- – artillery shell, bomb nec, grenade, guided missile, land mine, rocket, shell, shrapnel E991.9

War operations - *continued*
- fumes E997.2
- gas E997.2
- grenade (explosion) E993
- - fragments, injury by E991.9
- guided missile (explosion) E993
- - fragments, injury by E991.9
- - nuclear E996
- heat from nuclear explosion E996
- injury due to, but occurring after cessation of hostilities E998
- lacrimator (gas) (chemical) E997.2
- land mine (explosion) E993
- - after cessation of hostilities E998
- - fragments, injury by E991.9
- laser(s) E997.0
- late effect of E999
- lewisite E997.2
- lung irritant (chemical) (fumes) (gas) E997.2
- marine mine E992
- mine
- - after cessation of hostilities E998
- - at sea E992
- - in harbor E992
- - land (explosion) E993
- - - fragments, injury by E991.9
- - marine E992
- missile (guided) (explosion) E993
- - fragments, injury by E991.9
- - marine E992
- - nuclear E996
- mortar bomb (explosion) E993
- - fragments, injury by E991.9
- mustard gas E997.2
- nerve gas E997.2
- phosgene E997.2
- poisoning (chemical) (fumes) (gas) E997.2
- radiation, ionizing from nuclear explosion E996
- rocket (explosion) E993
- - fragments, injury by E991.9
- saber, sabre E995
- screening smoke E997.8

War operations - *continued*
- shell (aircraft) (artillery) (cannon) (land-based) (explosion) E993
- - fragments, injury by E991.9
- - sea-based E992
- shooting E991.2
- - after cessation of hostilities E998
- - bullet(s) E991.2
- - - rubber E991.0
- - pellet(s) (rifle) E991.1
- shrapnel E991.9
- submersion E995
- torpedo E992
- unconventional warfare, except by nuclear weapon E997.9
- - biological (warfare) E997.1
- - gas, fumes, chemicals E997.2
- - laser(s) E997.0
- - specified NEC E997.8
- underwater blast E992
- vesicant (chemical) (fumes) (gas) E997.2
- weapon burst E993
Washed
- away by flood - see Flood
- away by tidal wave - see Tidal wave
- off road by storm (transport vehicle) E908
- overboard E832.-
Weather exposure - see also Exposure
- cold E901.0
- hot E900.0
Weightlessness (causing injury) (effects of) (in spacecraft, real or simulated) E928.0
Wound (accidental) NEC (see also Injury) E928.9
- battle (see also War operations) E995
- bayonet E920.3
- - in
- - - legal intervention E974
- - - war operations E995
- gunshot - see Shooting
- incised - see Cut
- saber, sabre E920.3
- - in war operations E995

X   Y   Z

SECTION III

ALPHABETICAL INDEX TO DRUGS AND OTHER CHEMICAL SUBSTANCES
(Table of Drugs and Chemicals)

Section III

ALPHABETICAL INDEX TO DRUGS AND OTHER CHEMICAL SUBSTANCES

(Table of Drugs and Chemicals)

This table gives the code numbers for drugs, medicaments and other chemical substances as the cause of poisoning. The first column provides the code number from Chapter XVII (Injury and Poisoning) in the range 960–989, while the next three columns provide respectively the external cause (E) codes for accidental poisoning (E850–E869, E905), suicidal poisoning (E950–E952) and poisoning undetermined whether accidental or intentional (E980–E982). For drugs and medicaments, a fifth column provides the code numbers for these substances as the cause of adverse effects when properly administered in therapeutic or prophylactic dosage (E930–E949); the adverse effects themselves appear not in this table but in Section I of the Index.

The table contains an extensive but obviously not exhaustive list of drugs, alcohols, petroleum products, industrial solvents, corrosives, metals, gases, noxious foodstuffs, household cleansing agents, pesticides and other chemicals. Although certain substances are indexed with one or more subentries, the great majority are listed in the table according to some one usage or state. It is recognized, however, that many substances can be used in various ways – both in medicine and in industry – and may cause ill effects as solids or liquids and also in terms of their fumes or dusts. In cases in which the reported data indicate clearly a usage or state not shown in the table, or which is plainly different from the one shown, an attempt should be made to classify the substance in the form which more nearly expresses the reported facts. Proprietary names of drugs and medicaments are not listed, since they differ widely from country to country; each country should compile its own list of proprietary names corresponding to the nonproprietary names appearing in the table.

Substance	Poison-ing (Chapter XVII)	External Cause (E Code)			Adverse effect in correct usage
		Poisoning			
		Accident	Suicide (attempt)	Undeter-mined	
Absinthe	980.0	E860.0	E950.9	E980.9	
Acebutolol	971.3	E855.6	E950.4	E980.4	E941.3
Acedapsone	961.8	E857	E950.4	E980.4	E931.8
Acefylline piperazine	975.7	E858.6	E950.4	E980.4	E945.7
Acemorphan	965.0	E850.0	E950.0	E980.0	E935.0
Acenocoumarin	964.2	E858.2	E950.4	E980.4	E934.2
Acepifylline	975.7	E858.6	E950.4	E980.4	E945.7
Acepromazine	969.1	E853.0	E950.3	E980.3	E939.1
Acetal	982.8	E862.4	E950.9	E980.9	
Acetaldehyde (vapor)	987.8	E869.8	E952.8	E982.8	
– liquid	989.8	E866.8	E950.9	E980.9	
Acetaminophen	965.4	E850.2	E950.0	E980.0	E935.2
Acetanilide	965.4	E850.2	E950.0	E980.0	E935.2
Acetarsol	961.1	E857	E950.4	E980.4	E931.1
Acetazolamide	974.2	E858.5	E950.4	E980.4	E944.2
Acetic					
– acid	983.1	E864.1	E950.7	E980.6	
– – medicinal (lotion)	976.2	E858.7	E950.4	E980.4	E946.2
– anhydride	983.1	E864.1	E950.7	E980.6	
– ester	982.8	E862.4	E950.9	E980.9	
– – vapor	987.8	E862.4	E950.9	E980.9	
– ether	982.8	E862.4	E950.9	E980.9	
– – vapor	987.8	E862.4	E950.9	E980.9	
Acetohexamide	962.3	E858.0	E950.4	E980.4	E932.3
Acetomenaphthone	964.3	E858.2	E950.4	E980.4	E934.3
Acetone (oils)	982.8	E862.4	E950.9	E980.9	
– chlorinated	987.5	E869.3	E952.8	E982.8	
– vapor	987.8	E862.4	E950.9	E980.9	
Acetophenazine	969.1	E853.0	E950.3	E980.3	E939.1
Acetophenetedin	965.4	E850.2	E950.0	E980.0	E935.2
Acetophenone	982.8	E862.4	E950.9	E980.9	
Acetrizoic acid	977.8	E858.8	E950.4	E980.4	E947.8
Acetyl					
– bromide	989.8	E866.8	E950.9	E980.9	
– chloride	989.2	E866.8	E950.9	E980.9	
Acetylcholine derivate	971.0	E855.3	E950.4	E980.4	E941.0
Acetylcysteine	975.5	E858.6	E950.4	E980.4	E945.5
Acetyldigitoxin	972.1	E858.3	E950.4	E980.4	E942.1
Acetylene (gas)	987.1	E868.1	E951.8	E981.8	
– dichloride	982.3	E862.4	E950.9	E980.9	
– industrial	987.1	E869.8	E952.8	E982.8	
– tetrachloride	982.3	E862.4	E950.9	E980.9	
– – vapor	987.8	E862.4	E950.9	E980.9	
Acetylsalicylic acid	965.1	E850.1	E950.0	E980.0	E935.1
Acid (corrosive) NEC	983.1	E864.1	E950.7	E980.6	
Acidifying agent NEC	963.2	E858.1	E950.4	E980.4	E933.2
Acridine	983.0	E864.0	E950.7	E980.6	
– vapor	987.8	E869.8	E952.8	E982.8	
Acrolein (gas)	987.8	E869.8	E952.8	E982.8	
– liquid	989.8	E866.8	E950.9	E980.9	
Acrylamide	989.8	E866.8	E950.9	E980.9	

Substance	Poisoning (Chapter XVII)	External Cause (E Code)			Adverse effect in correct usage
		Poisoning			
		Accident	Suicide (attempt)	Undetermined	
Acrylic resin	976.3	E858.7	E950.4	E980.4	E946.3
Acrylonitrile	989.0	E866.8	E950.9	E980.9	
ACTH	962.4	E858.0	E950.4	E980.4	E932.4
Actinomycin(-C)	960.7	E856	E950.4	E980.4	E930.7
Activated charcoal	973.5	E858.4	E950.4	E980.4	E943.5
Adhesive NEC	989.8	E866.6	E950.9	E980.9	
Adicillin	960.5	E856	E950.4	E980.4	E930.5
Adiphenine	975.1	E858.6	E950.4	E980.4	E945.1
Adipiodone	977.8	E858.8	E950.4	E980.4	E947.8
Adrenal steroids NEC	962.0	E858.0	E950.4	E980.4	E932.0
Adrenalin	971.2	E855.5	E950.4	E980.4	E941.2
Adrenergic blocking NEC	971.3	E855.6	E950.4	E980.4	E941.3
— beta, heart	972.0	E858.3	E950.4	E980.4	E942.0
Adrenergic NEC	971.2	E855.5	E950.4	E980.4	E941.2
— specified NEC	971.2	E855.5	E950.4	E980.4	E941.2
Adrenochrome					
— derivative	972.8	E858.3	E950.4	E980.4	E942.8
— semicarbazone	972.8	E858.3	E950.4	E980.4	E942.8
Adrenocorticotrophin	962.4	E858.0	E950.4	E980.4	E932.4
— long-acting	962.4	E858.0	E950.4	E980.4	E932.4
Adriamycin	960.7	E856	E950.4	E980.4	E930.7
Aerosol spray - see Sprays					
Aflatoxin	989.7	E865.9	E950.9	E980.9	
Agar	973.3	E858.4	E950.4	E980.4	E943.3
AHLG	964.6	E858.2	E950.4	E980.4	E934.6
Air contaminant(s), source or type not specified	987.8	E869.9	E925.9	E982.9	
— specified type - see Substance specified					
Ajmaline	972.0	E858.3	E950.4	E980.4	E942.0
Albumin, human serum	964.7	E858.2	E950.4	E980.4	E934.7
Albuterol	975.7	E858.6	E950.4	E980.4	E945.7
Alclofenac	965.6	E850.4	E950.0	E980.0	E935.4
Alcohol	980.9	E860.9	E950.9	E980.9	
— absolute	980.0	E860.1	E950.9	E980.9	
— allyl	980.8	E860.8	E950.9	E980.9	
— amyl	980.3	E860.4	E950.9	E980.9	
— beverage	980.0	E860.0	E950.9	E980.9	
— butyl	980.3	E860.4	E950.9	E980.9	
— dehydrated	980.0	E860.1	E950.9	E980.9	
— — injection	976.4	E858.7	E950.4	E980.4	E946.4
— denatured	980.0	E860.1	E950.9	E980.9	
— deterrent NEC	977.3	E858.8	E950.4	E980.4	E947.3
— ethyl	980.0	E860.1	E950.9	E980.9	
— grain	980.0	E860.1	E950.9	E980.9	
— industrial	980.0	E860.1	E950.9	E980.9	
— isopropyl	980.2	E860.3	E950.9	E980.9	
— methyl	980.1	E860.2	E950.9	E980.9	
— propyl	980.3	E860.4	E950.9	E980.9	
— rubbing	980.2	E860.3	E950.9	E980.9	
— surgical	980.0	E860.1	E950.9	E980.9	
— vapor (from any type of alcohol)	987.8	E869.8	E952.8	E982.8	

Substance	Poisoning (Chapter XVII)	External Cause (E Code)			
		Poisoning			Adverse effect in correct usage
		Accident	Suicide (attempt)	Undetermined	
Alcohol - *continued*					
− wood	980.1	E860.2	E950.9	E980.9	
Alcuronium (chloride)	975.2	E858.6	E950.4	E980.4	E945.2
Aldicarb	989.3	E863.2	E950.6	E980.7	
Aldocorticosterone	962.0	E858.0	E950.4	E980.4	E932.0
Aldosterone	962.0	E858.0	E950.4	E980.4	E932.0
Aldrin (dust)	989.2	E863.0	E950.6	E980.7	
Alkali (caustic)	983.2	E864.2	E950.7	E980.6	
Alkaline aromatic solution	976.6	E858.7	E950.4	E980.4	E946.6
Alkalizing agent NEC	963.3	E858.1	E950.4	E980.4	E933.3
Alkylating drug NEC	963.1	E858.1	E950.4	E980.4	E933.1
− lymphatic	963.1	E858.1	E950.4	E980.4	E933.1
− myeloproliferative	963.1	E858.1	E950.4	E980.4	E933.1
Allantoin	976.4	E858.7	E950.4	E980.4	E946.4
Allethrin	989.4	E863.4	E950.6	E980.7	
Allopurinol	974.7	E858.5	E950.4	E980.4	E944.7
Allyl					
− alcohol	980.8	E860.8	E950.9	E980.9	
− disulfide	972.2	E858.3	E950.4	E980.4	E942.2
Allylestrenol	962.2	E858.0	E950.4	E980.4	E932.2
Aloin	973.1	E858.4	E950.4	E980.4	E943.1
Aloxiprin	965.1	E850.1	E950.0	E980.0	E935.1
Alpha					
− amylase	963.4	E858.1	E950.4	E980.4	E933.4
− prodine	965.0	E850.0	E950.0	E980.0	E935.0
− tocoferol	963.5	E858.1	E950.4	E980.4	E933.5
Alpha-adrenergic blocking drug	971.3	E855.6	E950.4	E980.4	E941.3
Alphadolone	968.3	E855.1	E950.4	E980.4	E938.3
Alphaxolone	968.3	E855.1	E950.4	E980.4	E938.3
Alprenolol	972.0	E858.3	E950.4	E980.4	E942.0
Alseroxylon	972.6	E858.3	E950.4	E980.4	E942.6
Alum (medicinal)	976.4	E858.7	E950.4	E980.4	E946.4
− nonmedicinal (ammonium) (potassium)	983.9	E864.3	E950.7	E980.6	
Aluminum					
− acetate	976.2	E858.7	E950.4	E980.4	E946.2
− carbonate	973.0	E858.4	E950.4	E980.4	E943.0
− glycinate	973.0	E858.4	E950.4	E980.4	E943.0
− hydroxide (gel)	973.0	E858.4	E950.4	E980.4	E943.0
− nicotinate	972.2	E858.3	E950.4	E980.4	E942.2
− phosphate	973.0	E858.4	E950.4	E980.4	E943.0
− sodium silicate	973.0	E858.4	E950.4	E980.4	E943.0
− tannate	973.5	E858.4	E950.4	E980.4	E943.5
Alverine	975.1	E858.6	E950.4	E980.4	E945.1
Amantadine	966.4	E855.0	E950.4	E980.4	E936.4
Ambazone	976.0	E858.7	E950.4	E980.4	E946.0
Ambenonium	971.0	E855.3	E950.4	E980.4	E941.0
Ametazole	977.8	E858.8	E950.4	E980.4	E947.8
Amethocaine	968.5	E855.2	E950.4	E980.4	E938.5
− regional	968.6	E855.2	E950.4	E980.4	E938.6
− spinal	968.7	E855.2	E950.4	E980.4	E938.7
Amfepramone	977.0	E858.8	E950.4	E980.4	E947.0

Substance	Poison-ing (Chapter XVII)	External Cause (E Code)			
		Poisoning			Adverse effect in correct usage
		Accident	Suicide (attempt)	Undeter-mined	
Amylmetacresol	976.6	E858.7	E950.4	E980.4	E946.6
Amylobarbitone	967.0	E851	E950.1	E980.1	E937.0
Amylocaine, regional	968.6	E855.2	E950.4	E980.4	E938.6
Amylopectin	973.5	E858.4	E950.4	E980.4	E943.5
Amyobarbital					
– sodium	967.0	E851	E950.1	E980.1	E937.0
Anabolic steroid	962.1	E858.0	E950.4	E980.4	E932.1
Analeptic NEC	970.0	E854.3	E950.4	E980.4	E940.0
Analgesic NEC	965.9	E850.9	E950.0	E980.0	E935.9
– anti-inflammatory NEC	965.6	E850.4	E950.0	E980.0	E935.4
– – propionic acid derivative	965.6	E850.4	E950.0	E980.0	E935.4
– antirheumatic NEC	965.6	E850.4	E950.0	E980.0	E935.4
– aromatic NEC	965.4	E850.2	E950.0	E980.0	E935.2
– narcotic NEC	965.8	E850.8	E950.0	E980.0	E935.8
– – combination	965.8	E850.8	E950.0	E980.0	E935.8
– – obstetric	965.8	E850.8	E950.0	E980.0	E935.8
– non-narcotic NEC	965.7	E850.5	E950.0	E980.0	E935.5
– – combination	965.7	E850.5	E950.0	E980.0	E935.5
– pyrazole	965.5	E850.3	E950.0	E980.0	E935.3
– specified NEC	965.8	E850.8	E950.0	E980.0	E935.8
Ancrod	964.4	E858.2	E950.4	E980.4	E934.4
Andrenergic NEC	971.2	E855.5	E950.4	E980.4	E941.2
Androgen	962.1	E858.0	E950.4	E980.4	E932.1
Androgen-estrogen mixture	962.1	E858.0	E950.4	E980.4	E932.1
Androstanolone	962.1	E858.0	E950.4	E980.4	E932.1
Anesthesia					
– caudal	968.7	E855.2	E950.4	E980.4	E938.7
– endotracheal	968.2	E855.1	E950.4	E980.4	E938.2
– epidural	968.7	E855.2	E950.4	E980.4	E938.7
– inhalation	968.2	E855.1	E950.4	E980.4	E938.2
– local	968.9	E855.2	E950.4	E980.4	E938.9
– mucosal	968.5	E855.2	E950.4	E980.4	E938.5
– muscle relaxation	975.2	E858.6	E950.4	E980.4	E945.2
– nerve blocking	968.6	E855.2	E950.4	E980.4	E938.6
– plexus blocking	968.6	E855.2	E950.4	E980.4	E938.6
– potentiated	968.4	E855.1	E950.4	E980.4	E938.4
– rectal	968.4	E855.1	E950.4	E980.4	E938.4
– regional	968.6	E855.2	E950.4	E980.4	E938.6
– surface	968.5	E855.2	E950.4	E980.4	E938.5
Anesthetic (see also Anesthesia) NEC	968.9	E855.2	E950.4	E980.4	E938.9
– with muscle relaxant	968.4	E855.1	E950.4	E980.4	E938.4
– gaseous NEC	968.2	E855.1	E950.4	E980.4	E938.2
– – halogenated hydrocarbon	968.2	E855.1	E950.4	E980.4	E938.2
– general NEC	968.4	E855.1	E950.4	E980.4	E938.4
– infiltration NEC	968.5	E855.2	E950.4	E980.4	E938.5
– intravenous NEC	968.3	E855.1	E950.4	E980.4	E938.3
– local NEC	968.9	E855.2	E950.4	E980.4	E938.9
– – acid resistant	973.8	E858.4	E950.4	E980.4	E943.8
– – surface	968.5	E855.2	E950.4	E980.4	E938.5
– rectal	968.4	E855.1	E950.4	E980.4	E938.4
– regional NEC	968.6	E855.2	E950.4	E980.4	E938.6

Substance	Poison-ing (Chapter XVII)	External Cause (E Code)			Adverse effect in correct usage
		Poisoning			
		Accident	Suicide (attempt)	Undeter-mined	
Anesthetic - *continued*					
− spinal NEC	968.7	E855.2	E950.4	E980.4	E938.7
− surface NEC	968.5	E855.2	E950.4	E980.4	E938.5
− thiobarbiturate	968.3	E855.1	E950.4	E980.4	E938.3
Aneurine	963.5	E858.1	E950.4	E980.4	E933.5
Angiotensin	972.8	E858.3	E950.4	E980.4	E942.8
Angiotensinamide	971.2	E855.5	E950.4	E980.4	E941.2
Anileridine	965.0	E850.0	E950.0	E980.0	E935.0
Aniline (dye) (liquid)	983.0	E864.0	E950.7	E980.6	
Anise oil	973.4	E858.4	E950.4	E980.4	E943.4
Anisidine	989.8	E866.8	E950.9	E980.9	
Anisindone	964.2	E858.2	E950.4	E980.4	E934.2
Anisotropine	971.1	E855.4	E950.4	E980.4	E941.1
Anorexiant (central)	977.0	E858.8	E950.4	E980.4	E947.0
Ant poisons - see Insecticide					
Antacid NEC	973.0	E858.4	E950.4	E980.4	E943.0
Antagonist					
− aldosterone	974.4	E858.5	E950.4	E980.4	E944.4
− anticoagulant	964.5	E858.2	E950.4	E980.4	E934.5
− extrapyramidal NEC	971.1	E855.4	E950.4	E980.4	E941.1
− folic acid	963.1	E858.1	E950.4	E980.4	E933.1
− heavy metal	963.8	E858.1	E950.4	E980.4	E933.8
− H-2 receptor	973.0	E858.4	E950.4	E980.4	E943.0
− narcotic analgesic	970.1	E854.3	E950.4	E980.4	E940.1
− opiate	970.1	E854.3	E950.4	E980.4	E940.1
− pyrimidine	963.1	E858.1	E950.4	E980.4	E933.1
− serotonin	972.6	E858.3	E950.4	E980.4	E942.6
Antazoline	963.0	E858.1	E950.4	E980.4	E933.0
Anterior pituitary					
− extract	962.4	E858.0	E950.4	E980.4	E932.4
− hormone NEC	962.4	E858.0	E950.4	E980.4	E932.4
Anthelminthic NEC	961.6	E857	E950.4	E980.4	E931.6
Anthiolimine	961.6	E857	E950.4	E980.4	E931.6
Anthralin	976.4	E858.7	E950.4	E980.4	E946.4
Antiadrenergic NEC	971.3	E855.6	E950.4	E980.4	E941.3
Antiallergic NEC	963.0	E858.1	E950.4	E980.4	E933.0
Anti-amebic drug	961.5	E857	E950.4	E980.4	E931.5
Anti-anemic preparation	964.1	E858.2	E950.4	E980.4	E934.1
Antianxiety drug NEC	969.5	E853.8	E950.3	E980.3	E939.5
Antiarteriosclerotic drug	972.2	E858.3	E950.4	E980.4	E942.2
Antiasthmatic drug NEC	975.7	E858.6	E950.4	E980.4	E945.7
Antibiotic NEC	960.9	E856	E950.4	E980.4	E930.9
− aminoglycide	960.8	E856	E950.4	E980.4	E930.8
− aminoglycoside	960.6	E856	E950.4	E980.4	E930.6
− antifungal	960.1	E856	E950.4	E980.4	E930.1
− antimycobacterial	960.6	E856	E950.4	E980.4	E930.6
− antineoplastic	960.7	E856	E950.4	E980.4	E930.7
− cancer	960.7	E856	E950.4	E980.4	E930.7
− ENT	976.6	E858.7	E950.4	E980.4	E946.6
− eye	976.5	E858.7	E950.4	E980.4	E946.5
− fungicidal (local)	976.0	E858.7	E950.4	E980.4	E946.0

Substance	Poisoning (Chapter XVII)	External Cause (E Code)			Adverse effect in correct usage
		Accident	Suicide (attempt)	Undetermined	
Antibiotic NEC - *continued*					
− intestinal	960.8	E856	E950.4	E980.4	E930.8
− local	976.0	E858.7	E950.4	E980.4	E946.0
− polypeptide	960.8	E856	E950.4	E980.4	E930.8
− specified NEC	960.8	E856	E950.4	E980.4	E930.8
− throat	976.6	E858.7	E950.4	E980.4	E946.6
Anticholesterolemic drug NEC	972.2	E858.3	E950.4	E980.4	E942.2
Anticholinergic NEC	971.1	E855.4	E950.4	E980.4	E941.1
Anticholinesterase	971.0	E855.3	E950.4	E980.4	E941.0
− organophosphorus	971.0	E855.3	E950.4	E980.4	E941.0
Anticoagulant NEC	964.2	E858.2	E950.4	E980.4	E934.2
− antagonists	964.5	E858.2	E950.4	E980.4	E934.5
Anti-common cold drug NEC	975.6	E858.6	E950.4	E980.4	E945.6
Anticonvulsant NEC	966.3	E855.0	E950.4	E980.4	E936.3
− barbiturate	967.0	E851	E950.1	E980.1	E937.0
− combination (with barbiturate)	966.3	E855.0	E950.4	E980.4	E936.3
− hydantoin	966.1	E855.0	E950.4	E980.4	E936.1
− hypnotic	967.8	E852.8	E950.2	E980.2	E937.8
− oxazolidine	966.0	E855.0	E950.4	E980.4	E936.0
− pyrimidine	966.3	E855.0	E950.4	E980.4	E936.3
− succinimide	966.2	E855.0	E950.4	E980.4	E936.2
Antidepressant NEC	969.0	E854.0	E950.3	E980.3	E939.0
− triazolpyridine	969.0	E854.0	E950.3	E980.3	E939.0
− tricyclic	969.0	E854.0	E950.3	E980.3	E939.0
Antidiabetic NEC	962.3	E858.0	E950.4	E980.4	E932.3
− biguanide	962.3	E858.0	E950.4	E980.4	E932.3
− − and sulfonyl combined	962.3	E858.0	E950.4	E980.4	E932.3
− combined	962.3	E858.0	E950.4	E980.4	E932.3
− sulfonylurea	962.3	E858.0	E950.4	E980.4	E932.3
Antidiarrheal drug NEC	973.5	E858.4	E950.4	E980.4	E943.5
− absorbent	973.5	E858.4	E950.4	E980.4	E943.5
Antidiphtheria serum	964.6	E858.2	E950.4	E980.4	E934.6
Antidiuretic hormone	962.5	E858.0	E950.4	E980.4	E932.5
Antidote NEC	977.2	E858.8	E950.4	E980.4	E947.2
− heavy metal	963.8	E858.1	E950.4	E980.4	E933.8
Antiemetic drug	963.0	E858.1	E950.4	E980.4	E933.0
Antifertility pill	962.2	E858.0	E950.4	E980.4	E932.2
Antifibrinolytic drug	964.4	E858.2	E950.4	E980.4	E934.4
Antifilarial drug	961.6	E857	E950.4	E980.4	E931.6
Antiflatulent	973.4	E858.4	E950.4	E980.4	E943.4
Antifreeze	989.8	E866.8	E950.9	E980.9	
− ethylene glycol	982.8	E862.4	E950.9	E980.9	
Antifungal					
− antibiotic (systemic)	960.1	E856	E950.4	E980.4	E930.1
− anti-infective NEC	961.9	E857	E950.4	E980.4	E931.9
− disinfectant	976.0	E858.7	E950.4	E980.4	E946.0
− nonmedicinal (sprays)	989.4	E863.6	E950.6	E980.7	
Anti-gastric-secretion drug NEC	973.0	E858.4	E950.4	E980.4	E943.0
Antihaemoprotozoal drug	961.4	E857	E950.4	E980.4	E931.4
Antihallucinogen	969.5	E853.8	E950.3	E980.3	E939.5
Antihemophilic					

Substance	Poisoning (Chapter XVII)	External Cause (E Code)			
		Poisoning			Adverse effect in correct usage
		Accident	Suicide (attempt)	Undetermined	
Antihemophilic - *continued*					
– factor	964.7	E858.2	E950.4	E980.4	E934.7
– globulin concentrate	964.5	E858.2	E950.4	E980.4	E934.5
– plasma, dried	964.5	E858.2	E950.4	E980.4	E934.5
Antiheparin drug	964.5	E858.2	E950.4	E980.4	E934.5
Antihookworm drug	961.6	E857	E950.4	E980.4	E931.6
Anti-human lymphocytic globulin	964.6	E858.2	E950.4	E980.4	E934.6
Antihypertensive drug NEC	972.6	E858.3	E950.4	E980.4	E942.6
Anti-infective NEC	961.9	E857	E950.4	E980.4	E931.9
– antimony	961.2	E857	E950.4	E980.4	E931.2
– arsenical	961.1	E857	E950.4	E980.4	E931.1
– bismuth					
– – local	976.0	E858.7	E950.4	E980.4	E946.0
– – systemic	961.2	E857	E950.4	E980.4	E931.2
– ENT	976.6	E858.7	E950.4	E980.4	E946.6
– eye NEC	976.5	E858.7	E950.4	E980.4	E946.5
– heavy metal	961.2	E857	E950.4	E980.4	E931.2
– local NEC	976.0	E858.7	E950.4	E980.4	E946.0
– – specified NEC	976.0	E858.7	E950.4	E980.4	E946.0
– mixed	961.9	E857	E950.4	E980.4	E931.9
Anti-inflammatory drug NEC	976.0	E858.7	E950.4	E980.4	E946.0
Antikaluretic	974.5	E858.5	E950.4	E980.4	E944.5
Antiknock (tetraethyl lead)	984.1	E866.6	E950.9	E980.9	
Antilipemic drug NEC	972.2	E858.3	E950.4	E980.4	E942.2
Antimalarial	961.4	E857	E950.4	E980.4	E931.4
– prophylactic NEC	961.4	E857	E950.4	E980.4	E931.4
– pyrimidine derivative	961.4	E857	E950.4	E980.4	E931.4
Antimetabolite	963.1	E858.1	E950.4	E980.4	E933.1
Antimitotic agent	963.1	E858.1	E950.4	E980.4	E933.1
Antimony (compounds) (vapor) NEC	985.4	E866.2	E950.9	E980.9	
– dimercaptosuccinate	961.2	E857	E950.4	E980.4	E931.2
– hydride	985.4	E866.2	E950.9	E980.9	
– pesticides (vapor)	989.4	E863.9	E950.6	E980.7	
Antimuscarinic NEC	971.1	E855.4	E950.4	E980.4	E941.1
Antimycobacterial drug NEC	961.8	E857	E950.4	E980.4	E931.8
– combination	961.8	E857	E950.4	E980.4	E931.8
Antinausea drug	963.0	E858.1	E950.4	E980.4	E933.0
Antinematode drug	961.6	E857	E950.4	E980.4	E931.6
Antineoplastic NEC	963.1	E858.1	E950.4	E980.4	E933.1
– alkaloidal	963.1	E858.1	E950.4	E980.4	E933.1
– combination	963.1	E858.1	E950.4	E980.4	E933.1
– steroid	962.1	E858.0	E950.4	E980.4	E932.1
– – estrogen	962.2	E858.0	E950.4	E980.4	E932.2
Antiparasitic drug	976.0	E858.7	E950.4	E980.4	E946.0
Antiparkinsonism drug NEC	966.4	E855.0	E950.4	E980.4	E936.4
Antiperspirant NEC	971.1	E855.4	E950.4	E980.4	E941.1
Antiphlogistic NEC	965.6	E850.4	E950.0	E980.0	E935.4
Antiplatyhelminthic drug	961.6	E857	E950.4	E980.4	E931.6
Antiprotozoal drug NEC	961.5	E857	E950.4	E980.4	E931.5
– blood protozoa	961.4	E857	E950.4	E980.4	E931.4
– local	976.0	E858.7	E950.4	E980.4	E946.0

Substance	Poisoning (Chapter XVII)	External Cause (E Code)			Adverse effect in correct usage
		Accident	Suicide (attempt)	Undetermined	
Antipruritic drug NEC	976.1	E858.7	E950.4	E980.4	E946.1
Antipsychotic drug NEC	969.3	E853.8	E950.3	E980.3	E939.3
Antipyretic NEC	965.6	E850.4	E950.0	E980.0	E935.4
Antipyrine	965.5	E850.3	E950.0	E980.0	E935.3
Antirabies serum	964.6	E858.2	E950.4	E980.4	E934.6
Antirheumatic NEC	965.6	E850.4	E950.0	E980.0	E935.4
Antirigidity drug NEC	966.4	E855.0	E950.4	E980.4	E936.4
Antischistosomal drug	961.6	E857	E950.4	E980.4	E931.6
Antitapeworm drug	961.6	E857	E950.4	E980.4	E931.6
Antitetanus serum	964.6	E858.2	E950.4	E980.4	E934.6
Antithyroid drug NEC	962.8	E858.0	E950.4	E980.4	E932.8
Antitoxin					
– diphtheria	964.6	E858.2	E950.4	E980.4	E934.6
– gas gangrene	964.6	E858.2	E950.4	E980.4	E934.6
– tetanus	964.6	E858.2	E950.4	E980.4	E934.6
Antitrichomonal drug	961.5	E857	E950.4	E980.4	E931.5
Antitussive NEC	975.4	E858.6	E950.4	E980.4	E945.4
– codeine mixture	965.0	E850.0	E950.0	E980.0	E935.0
– opiate	965.0	E850.0	E950.0	E980.0	E935.0
Antivaricose drug	972.7	E858.3	E950.4	E980.4	E942.7
Antivenin	964.6	E858.2	E950.4	E980.4	E934.6
– crotaline	964.6	E858.2	E950.4	E980.4	E934.6
– spider bite	964.6	E858.2	E950.4	E980.4	E934.6
Antivertigo drug	963.0	E858.1	E950.4	E980.4	E933.0
Antiviral drug NEC	961.7	E857	E950.4	E980.4	E931.7
– eye	976.5	E858.7	E950.4	E980.4	E946.5
Antiwhipworm drug	961.6	E857	E950.4	E980.4	E931.6
ANTU (alpha naphthyl thiourea)	989.4	E863.7	E950.6	E980.7	
APC	965.8	E850.8	E950.0	E980.0	E935.8
– caffeine containing	975.6	E858.6	E950.4	E980.4	E945.6
Apomorphine	973.6	E858.4	E950.4	E980.4	E943.6
Aprindine	972.0	E858.3	E950.4	E980.4	E942.0
Aprobarbital	967.0	E851	E950.1	E980.1	E937.0
Aprotinin	964.4	E858.2	E950.4	E980.4	E934.4
Aqua fortis	983.1	E864.1	E950.7	E980.6	
Arachis oil	972.2	E858.3	E950.4	E980.4	E942.2
Arecoline	971.0	E855.3	E950.4	E980.4	E941.0
Arginine	963.2	E858.1	E950.4	E980.4	E933.2
Aromatics, corrosive	983.0	E864.0	E950.7	E980.6	
Arsenate of lead	985.1	E863.9	E950.6	E980.7	
Arsenic, arsenicals (compounds) (dust) (vapor) NEC	985.1	E866.3	E950.8	E980.8	
– anti-infective	961.1	E857	E950.4	E980.4	E931.1
– – pentavalent	961.1	E857	E950.4	E980.4	E931.1
– hydride	985.1	E866.3	E950.8	E980.8	
– pentavalent	961.1	E857	E950.4	E980.4	E931.1
– pesticide (dust) (fumes)	985.1	E863.9	E950.6	E980.7	
– trioxide	976.7	E858.7	E950.4	E980.4	E946.7
Arsine (gas)	985.1	E866.3	E950.8	E980.8	
Arsthinol	961.1	E857	E950.4	E980.4	E931.1
Asbestos	985.8	E866.4	E950.9	E980.9	

Substance	Poison-ing (Chapter XVII)	External Cause (E Code)			
		Poisoning			Adverse effect in correct usage
		Accident	Suicide (attempt)	Undeter-mined	
Ascaridole	961.6	E857	E950.4	E980.4	E931.6
Ascorbic acid	963.5	E858.1	E950.4	E980.4	E933.5
Asparaginase	963.1	E858.1	E950.4	E980.4	E933.1
Aspidium (oleoresin)	961.6	E857	E950.4	E980.4	E931.6
Aspirin (soluble)	965.1	E850.1	E950.0	E980.0	E935.1
Aspirin-phenacetin-codeine mixture	965.8	E850.8	E950.0	E980.0	E935.8
Astringent (local) NEC	976.2	E858.7	E950.4	E980.4	E946.2
− specified NEC	976.2	E858.7	E950.4	E980.4	E946.2
Ataractic drug NEC	969.5	E853.8	E950.3	E980.3	E939.5
Atropine	971.1	E855.4	E950.4	E980.4	E941.1
− derivatives	971.1	E855.4	E950.4	E980.4	E941.1
− methonitrate	971.1	E855.4	E950.4	E980.4	E941.1
Attapulgite	973.5	E858.4	E950.4	E980.4	E943.5
Auramine	989.8	E866.8	E950.9	E980.9	
Aurothioglucose	965.6	E850.4	E950.0	E980.0	E935.4
Aurothioglycanide	965.6	E850.4	E950.0	E980.0	E935.4
Aurothiolycolanilide	965.6	E850.4	E950.0	E980.0	E935.4
Aurothiomalate sodium	965.6	E850.4	E950.0	E980.0	E935.4
Autonomic nervous system agent NEC	971.9	E855.9	E950.4	E980.4	E941.9
Axerophthol	963.5	E858.1	E950.4	E980.4	E933.5
Azadirachta	989.8	E866.8	E950.9	E980.9	
Azapetine	971.3	E855.6	E950.4	E980.4	E941.3
Azapone	965.5	E850.3	E950.0	E980.0	E935.3
Azapropazone	965.5	E850.3	E950.0	E980.0	E935.3
Azathioprine	963.1	E858.1	E950.4	E980.4	E933.1
Azidocillin	960.8	E856	E950.4	E980.4	E930.8
Azinphos (ethyl) (methyl)	989.3	E863.1	E950.6	E980.7	
Aziridine (chelating)	989.8	E866.8	E950.9	E980.9	
Azobenzene smoke	989.4	E863.4	E950.6	E980.7	
Azocyclonol	969.5	E853.8	E950.3	E980.3	E939.5
Azuresin	977.8	E858.8	E950.4	E980.4	E947.8
Bacillus lactobacillus	973.8	E858.4	E950.4	E980.4	E943.8
Bacitracin zinc	976.0	E858.7	E950.4	E980.4	E946.0
BAL	963.8	E858.1	E950.4	E980.4	E933.8
Bamethan	972.5	E858.3	E950.4	E980.4	E942.5
− sulfate	972.8	E858.3	E950.4	E980.4	E942.8
Bamifylline	975.7	E858.6	E950.4	E980.4	E945.7
Bamipine	963.0	E858.1	E950.4	E980.4	E933.0
Barbital	967.0	E851	E950.1	E980.1	E937.0
− sodium	967.0	E851	E950.1	E980.1	E937.0
Barbital-aminophenazone complex	965.7	E850.5	E950.0	E980.0	E935.5
Barbital-phenacetin complex	965.7	E850.5	E950.0	E980.0	E935.5
Barbitone	967.0	E851	E950.1	E980.1	E937.0
− with amidopyrine	965.5	E850.3	E950.0	E980.0	E935.3
Barbiturate NEC	967.0	E851	E950.1	E980.1	E937.0
− with tranquilizer	967.6	E852.5	E950.2	E980.2	E937.6
Barcetine	965.7	E850.5	E950.0	E980.0	E935.5
Barium (carbonate) (chloride)	985.8	E866.4	E950.9	E980.9	
− pesticide	989.4	E863.9	E950.6	E980.7	
− sulfate (medicinal)	977.8	E858.8	E950.4	E980.4	E947.8
− − nonmedicinal	985.8	E866.4	E950.9	E980.9	

Substance	Poison-ing (Chapter XVII)	External Cause (E Code)			
		Poisoning			Adverse effect in correct usage
		Accident	Suicide (attempt)	Undeter-mined	
Barrier cream	976.3	E858.7	E950.4	E980.4	E946.3
Basic fuchsin	976.0	E858.7	E950.4	E980.4	E946.0
Battery acid or fluid	983.1	E864.1	E950.7	E980.6	
Bay rum	980.8	E860.8	E950.9	E980.9	
BCG (vaccine)	978.0	E858.8	E950.4	E980.4	E948.0
BCNU	963.1	E858.1	E950.4	E980.4	E933.1
Beclamide	966.3	E855.0	E950.4	E980.4	E936.3
Beclometasone	976.0	E858.7	E950.4	E980.4	E946.0
Belladonna leaf	971.1	E855.4	E950.4	E980.4	E941.1
Bemegride	970.0	E854.3	E950.4	E980.4	E940.0
Benactyzine	969.5	E853.8	E950.3	E980.3	E939.5
Benapryzine	971.1	E855.4	E950.4	E980.4	E941.1
Bendrofluazide	974.3	E858.5	E950.4	E980.4	E944.3
Bendroflumethiazide	974.3	E858.5	E950.4	E980.4	E944.3
Benorilate	965.1	E850.1	E950.0	E980.0	E935.1
Benoxinate	968.5	E855.2	E950.4	E980.4	E938.5
Benserazide	966.4	E855.0	E950.4	E980.4	E936.4
Bentonite	976.3	E858.7	E950.4	E980.4	E946.3
Benzalkonium (chloride)	976.0	E858.7	E950.4	E980.4	E946.0
Benzamine	968.5	E855.2	E950.4	E980.4	E938.5
– lactate	976.1	E858.7	E950.4	E980.4	E946.1
Benzene (acetyl) (dimethyl) (methyl) (solvent)	982.0	E862.4	E950.9	E980.9	
– hexachloride (gamma) (insecticide) (vapor)	989.2	E863.0	E950.6	E980.7	
– vapor NEC	987.8	E862.4	E950.9	E980.9	
Benzethonium (chloride)	976.0	E858.7	E950.4	E980.4	E946.0
Benzhexol	971.1	E855.4	E950.4	E980.4	E941.1
Benzhydramine (chloride)	966.4	E855.0	E950.4	E980.4	E936.4
Benzidine	989.8	E866.8	E950.9	E980.9	
Benzilonium bromide	971.1	E855.4	E950.4	E980.4	E941.1
Benzin(e) - see Ligroin					
Benziodarone	974.7	E858.5	E950.4	E980.4	E944.7
Benzocaine	968.5	E855.2	E950.4	E980.4	E938.5
Benzoctamine	969.0	E854.0	E950.3	E980.3	E939.0
Benzoic acid	976.0	E858.7	E950.4	E980.4	E946.0
Benzoin (tincture)	975.6	E858.6	E950.4	E980.4	E945.6
Benzol	982.0	E862.4	E950.9	E980.9	
– vapor	987.8	E862.4	E950.9	E980.9	
Benzonatate	975.4	E858.6	E950.4	E980.4	E945.4
Benzopyrone	972.8	E858.3	E950.4	E980.4	E942.8
Benzoyl peroxide	976.0	E858.7	E950.4	E980.4	E946.0
Benzperidol	969.2	E853.1	E950.3	E980.3	E939.2
Benzphetamine	969.7	E854.2	E950.3	E980.3	E939.7
Benzpyrinium bromide	971.0	E855.3	E950.4	E980.4	E941.0
Benzquinamide	963.0	E858.1	E950.4	E980.4	E933.0
Benzthiazide	974.3	E858.5	E950.4	E980.4	E944.3
Benztropine	971.1	E855.4	E950.4	E980.4	E941.1
Benzydamine	965.8	E850.8	E950.0	E980.0	E935.8
Benzyl					
– acetate	982.8	E862.4	E950.9	E980.9	

Substance	Poison-ing (Chapter XVII)	External Cause (E Code)			
		Poisoning			Adverse effect in correct usage
		Accident	Suicide (attempt)	Undeter-mined	
Bleaching agent	976.4	E858.7	E950.4	E980.4	E946.4
Bleomycin	960.7	E856	E950.4	E980.4	E930.7
Blood					
– dried	989.8	E866.5	E950.9	E980.9	
– drug affecting NEC	964.9	E858.2	E950.4	E980.4	E934.9
– – specified NEC	964.8	E858.2	E950.4	E980.4	E934.8
– expander NEC	964.8	E858.2	E950.4	E980.4	E934.8
– fraction NEC	964.7	E858.2	E950.4	E980.4	E934.7
Bone meal	989.8	E866.5	E950.9	E980.9	
Borate	989.8	E861.3	E950.9	E980.9	
– buffer	977.4	E858.8	E950.4	E980.4	E947.4
– cleanser	989.8	E861.3	E950.9	E980.9	
– sodium	989.8	E861.3	E950.9	E980.9	
Borax (cleanser)	989.8	E861.3	E950.9	E980.9	
Bordeaux mixture	985.8	E863.6	E950.6	E980.7	
Boric acid	976.5	E858.7	E950.4	E980.4	E946.5
Boron	989.8	E866.8	E950.9	E980.9	
– hydride NEC	989.8	E866.8	E950.9	E980.9	
– – fumes or gas	987.8	E869.8	E952.8	E982.8	
– trifluoride	987.8	E869.8	E952.8	E982.8	
Botulinus antitoxin (type A, B)	964.6	E858.2	E950.4	E980.4	E934.6
Bran (wheat)	973.3	E858.4	E950.4	E980.4	E943.3
Brass (fumes)	985.8	E866.4	E950.9	E980.9	
Bretylium (tosilate)	972.5	E858.3	E950.4	E980.4	E942.5
Bromazepam	969.4	E853.2	E950.3	E980.3	E939.4
Brombenzylcyanide	987.5	E869.3	E952.8	E982.8	
Bromelains	963.4	E858.1	E950.4	E980.4	E933.4
Bromhexine	975.5	E858.6	E950.4	E980.4	E945.5
Bromide salts	967.3	E852.2	E950.2	E980.2	E937.3
Bromindione	964.2	E858.2	E950.4	E980.4	E934.2
Bromine	987.8	E869.8	E952.8	E982.8	
– sedative	967.3	E852.2	E950.2	E980.2	E937.3
– vapor	987.8	E869.8	E952.8	E982.8	
Bromisoval	967.3	E852.2	E950.2	E980.2	E937.3
Bromobenzylcyanide	987.5	E869.3	E952.8	E982.8	
Bromocriptine	962.9	E858.0	E950.4	E980.4	E932.9
Bromodiphenhydramine	963.0	E858.1	E950.4	E980.4	E933.0
Brompheniramine	963.0	E858.1	E950.4	E980.4	E933.0
Bromvaletone	967.3	E852.2	E950.2	E980.2	E937.3
Bronchodilator NEC	975.7	E858.6	E950.4	E980.4	E945.7
Broxyquinoline	961.3	E857	E950.4	E980.4	E931.3
Bruceine	975.3	E858.6	E950.4	E980.4	E945.3
Brucine	989.1	E866.6	E950.9	E980.9	
Brunswick green - see Copper					
Buclizine	963.0	E858.1	E950.4	E980.4	E933.0
Buclosamide	976.0	E858.7	E950.4	E980.4	E946.0
Buformin	962.3	E858.0	E950.4	E980.4	E932.3
Bufrolin	975.7	E858.6	E950.4	E980.4	E945.7
Bufylline	975.7	E858.6	E950.4	E980.4	E945.7
Bulk filler	977.0	E858.8	E950.4	E980.4	E947.0
– cathartic	973.3	E858.4	E950.4	E980.4	E943.3

Substance	Poison-ing (Chapter XVII)	External Cause (E Code)			Adverse effect in correct usage
		Poisoning			
		Accident	Suicide (attempt)	Undeter-mined	
Calcium - *continued*					
− ipodate	977.8	E858.8	E950.4	E980.4	E947.8
− lactate	974.6	E858.5	E950.4	E980.4	E944.6
− leucovorin	964.1	E858.2	E950.4	E980.4	E934.1
− oxide	983.2	E864.2	E950.7	E980.6	
− phosphate	974.6	E858.5	E950.4	E980.4	E944.6
− salicylate	965.1	E850.1	E950.0	E980.0	E935.1
− salts	974.6	E858.5	E950.4	E980.4	E944.6
Calculus dissolving drug	977.0	E858.8	E950.4	E980.4	E947.0
Calorific agent	974.5	E858.5	E950.4	E980.4	E944.5
Calusterone	962.2	E858.0	E950.4	E980.4	E932.2
Candicidin	976.0	E858.7	E950.4	E980.4	E946.0
Cannabinol	969.6	E854.1	E950.3	E980.3	E939.6
Cannabis (derivatives)	969.6	E854.1	E950.3	E980.3	E939.6
Capillary-active drug NEC	972.8	E858.3	E950.4	E980.4	E942.8
Capreomycin	960.6	E856	E950.4	E980.4	E930.6
Capsicum	976.4	E858.7	E950.4	E980.4	E946.4
Captan	989.4	E863.6	E950.6	E980.7	
Caramiphen	971.1	E855.4	E950.4	E980.4	E941.1
Carbachol	971.0	E855.3	E950.4	E980.4	E941.0
Carbacrylamine (resin)	974.5	E858.5	E950.4	E980.4	E944.5
Carbamates	989.3	E863.2	E950.6	E980.7	
Carbamazepine	966.3	E855.0	E950.4	E980.4	E936.3
Carbamic esters	967.3	E852.2	E950.2	E980.2	E937.3
Carbamide	974.4	E858.5	E950.4	E980.4	E944.4
Carbarsone	961.1	E857	E950.4	E980.4	E931.1
Carbaryl	989.3	E863.2	E950.6	E980.7	
Carbazochrome	976.4	E858.7	E950.4	E980.4	E946.4
− salicylate	972.8	E858.3	E950.4	E980.4	E942.8
Carbenicillin	960.0	E856	E950.4	E980.4	E930.0
Carbenoxolone	973.8	E858.4	E950.4	E980.4	E943.8
Carbetapentane	975.4	E858.6	E950.4	E980.4	E945.4
Carbethyl salicylate	965.1	E850.1	E950.0	E980.0	E935.1
Carbidopa	966.4	E855.0	E950.4	E980.4	E936.4
Carbimazole	962.8	E858.0	E950.4	E980.4	E932.8
Carbinol	980.1	E860.2	E950.9	E980.9	
Carbinoxamine	963.0	E858.1	E950.4	E980.4	E933.0
Carbitol	982.8	E862.4	E950.9	E980.9	
Carbol fuchsin	976.0	E858.7	E950.4	E980.4	E946.0
Carbolic acid (see also Phenol)	983.0	E864.0	E950.7	E980.6	
Carbolonium (bromide)	975.2	E858.6	E950.4	E980.4	E945.2
Carbon					
− bisulfide (liquid)	982.2	E862.4	E950.9	E980.9	
− − vapor	987.8	E862.4	E950.9	E980.9	
− dioxide					
− − gas					
− − − medicinal	975.8	E858.6	E950.4	E980.4	E945.8
− − − nonmedicinal	987.8	E869.8	E952.8	E982.8	
− − snow	976.4	E858.7	E950.4	E980.4	E946.4
− disulfide (liquid)	982.2	E862.4	E950.9	E980.9	
− − vapor	987.8	E862.4	E950.9	E980.9	

Substance	Poison- ing (Chapter XVII)	External Cause (E Code)			
		Poisoning			Adverse effect in correct usage
		Accident	Suicide (attempt)	Undeter- mined	
Carbon - *continued*					
— monoxide (from incomplete combustion of) (in) NEC	986	E868.9	E952.1	E982.1	
— — blast furnace gas	986	E868.8	E952.1	E982.1	
— — butane (distributed in mobile container)	986	E868.0	E951.1	E981.1	
— — — distributed through pipes	986	E867	E951.0	E981.0	
— — charcoal fumes	986	E868.3	E952.1	E982.1	
— — coal					
— — — gas (piped)	986	E867	E951.0	E981.0	
— — — solid (in domestic stoves, fireplaces)	986	E868.3	E952.1	E982.1	
— — coke (in domestic stoves, fireplaces)	986	E868.3	E952.1	E982.1	
— — exhaust gas (motor) not in transit	986	E868.2	E952.0	E982.0	
— — — combustion engine, any, not in watercraft	986	E868.2	E952.0	E982.0	
— — — farm tractor, not in transit	986	E868.2	E952.0	E982.0	
— — — gas engine	986	E868.2	E952.0	E982.0	
— — — motor pump	986	E868.2	E952.0	E982.0	
— — — motor vehicle, not in transit	986	E868.2	E952.0	E982.0	
— — fuel (in domestic use)	986	E868.3	E952.1	E982.1	
— — — gas (piped)	986	E867	E951.0	E981.0	
— — — — in mobile container	986	E868.0	E951.1	E981.1	
— — — industrial	986	E868.8	E952.1	E982.1	
— — illuminating gas	986	E867	E951.0	E981.0	
— — industrial fuels or gases, any	986	E868.8	E952.1	E982.1	
— — kerosene (in domestic stoves, fireplaces)	986	E868.3	E952.1	E982.1	
— — kiln vapor	986	E868.8	E952.1	E982.1	
— — motor exhaust gas, not in transit	986	E868.2	E952.0	E982.0	
— — paraffin (in domestic stoves, fireplaces)	986	E868.3	E952.1	E982.1	
— — piped gas	986	E867	E951.0	E981.0	
— — producer gas	986	E868.8	E952.1	E982.1	
— — propane (distributed in mobile container)	986	E868.0	E951.1	E981.1	
— — — distributed through pipes	986	E867	E951.0	E981.0	
— — stove gas (piped)	986	E867	E951.0	E981.0	
— — utility gas (piped)	986	E867	E951.0	E981.0	
— — water gas	986	E868.1	E951.8	E981.8	
— — wood (in domestic stoves, fireplaces)	986	E868.3	E952.1	E982.1	
— tetrachloride (vapor) NEC	987.8	E862.4	E950.9	E980.9	
— — liquid (cleansing agent) NEC	982.1	E861.0	E950.9	E980.9	
— — solvent	982.1	E862.4	E950.9	E980.9	
Carbonic acid (gas)	987.8	E869.8	E952.8	E982.8	
— anhydrase inhibitor NEC	974.2	E858.5	E950.4	E980.4	E944.2
Carbophenothion	989.3	E863.1	E950.6	E980.7	
Carbromal	967.3	E852.2	E950.2	E980.2	E937.3
Cardiac rhythm regulator NEC	972.0	E858.3	E950.4	E980.4	E942.0
— specified NEC	972.0	E858.3	E950.4	E980.4	E942.0
Cardiotonic (glycoside) NEC	972.1	E858.3	E950.4	E980.4	E942.1
Cardiovascular drug NEC	972.9	E858.3	E950.4	E980.4	E942.9

Substance	Poison-ing (Chapter XVII)	External Cause (E Code)			Adverse effect in correct usage
		Poisoning			
		Accident	Suicide (attempt)	Undeter-mined	
Carfecillin	960.0	E856	E950.4	E980.4	E930.0
Carisoprodol	968.0	E855.1	E950.4	E980.4	E938.0
Carminative	973.4	E858.4	E950.4	E980.4	E943.4
Carotene	963.5	E858.1	E950.4	E980.4	E933.5
Carphenazine	969.1	E853.0	E950.3	E980.3	E939.1
Carrageenan	973.8	E858.4	E950.4	E980.4	E943.8
Cartecillin	960.8	E856	E950.4	E980.4	E930.8
Cascara (sagrada)	973.1	E858.4	E950.4	E980.4	E943.1
Castor bean	988.2	E865.3	E950.9	E980.9	
Castor oil	973.1	E858.4	E950.4	E980.4	E943.1
Catha (tea)	969.7	E854.2	E950.3	E980.3	E939.7
Cathartic NEC	973.3	E858.4	E950.4	E980.4	E943.3
− anthacene	973.1	E858.4	E950.4	E980.4	E943.1
− bulk	973.3	E858.4	E950.4	E980.4	E943.3
− emollient NEC	973.2	E858.4	E950.4	E980.4	E943.2
− irritant NEC	973.1	E858.4	E950.4	E980.4	E943.1
− mucilage	973.2	E858.4	E950.4	E980.4	E943.2
− vegetable	973.1	E858.4	E950.4	E980.4	E943.1
Cation exchange resin	974.5	E858.5	E950.4	E980.4	E944.5
Caustic(s) NEC	983.9	E864.4	E950.7	E980.6	
− alkali	983.2	E864.2	E950.7	E980.6	
− eye	976.5	E858.7	E950.4	E980.4	E946.5
− hydroxide	983.2	E864.2	E950.7	E980.6	
− potash	983.2	E864.2	E950.7	E980.6	
− soda	983.2	E864.2	E950.7	E980.6	
Cefalexin	960.5	E856	E950.4	E980.4	E930.5
Cefaloglycin	960.5	E856	E950.4	E980.4	E930.5
Cefaloridine	960.5	E856	E950.4	E980.4	E930.5
Cefalosporin	960.5	E856	E950.4	E980.4	E930.5
Cefalotin	960.5	E856	E950.4	E980.4	E930.5
Cefamycin	960.5	E856	E950.4	E980.4	E930.5
Cefapirin	960.5	E856	E950.4	E980.4	E930.5
Cefazolin	960.5	E856	E950.4	E980.4	E930.5
Cefoxitin	960.5	E856	E950.4	E980.4	E930.5
Cefradine	960.5	E856	E950.4	E980.4	E930.5
Cellosolve	982.8	E862.4	E950.9	E980.9	
Cellulose					
− cathartic	973.3	E858.4	E950.4	E980.4	E943.3
− oxidized	976.4	E858.7	E950.4	E980.4	E946.4
Cetalkonium (chloride)	976.0	E858.7	E950.4	E980.4	E946.0
Cetamacrogol	977.4	E858.8	E950.4	E980.4	E947.4
Cetazolin	976.0	E858.7	E950.4	E980.4	E946.0
Cetrimide	976.0	E858.7	E950.4	E980.4	E946.0
Cetrimonium (bromide)	976.0	E858.7	E950.4	E980.4	E946.0
Cetylpyridinium chloride	976.0	E858.7	E950.4	E980.4	E946.0
Cetylpyridium	976.0	E858.7	E950.4	E980.4	E946.0
Ch'an su	972.1	E858.3	E950.4	E980.4	E942.1
Charcoal	973.5	E858.4	E950.4	E980.4	E943.5
− fumes (carbon monoxide)	986	E868.3	E952.1	E982.1	
− − industrial	986	E868.8	E952.1	E982.1	
Chaulmosulfone	961.8	E857	E950.4	E980.4	E931.8

Substance	Poison-ing (Chapter XVII)	External Cause (E Code)			Adverse effect in correct usage
		Poisoning			
		Accident	Suicide (attempt)	Undeter-mined	
Chelating agent NEC	977.2	E858.8	E950.4	E980.4	E947.2
Chemical substance NEC	989.9	E866.9	E950.9	E980.9	
Chenodesoxycholic acid	973.4	E858.4	E950.4	E980.4	E943.4
Chenopodium	961.6	E857	E950.4	E980.4	E931.6
Chiniofon	961.3	E857	E950.4	E980.4	E931.3
Chlophedianol	975.4	E858.6	E950.4	E980.4	E945.4
Chloral	967.1	E852.0	E950.2	E980.2	E937.1
− derivative	967.1	E852.0	E950.2	E980.2	E937.1
− hydrate	967.1	E852.0	E950.2	E980.2	E937.1
Chlorambucil	963.1	E858.1	E950.4	E980.4	E933.1
Chloramine	976.8	E858.7	E950.4	E980.4	E946.8
Chloramphenicol	960.2	E856	E950.4	E980.4	E930.2
Chlorate(s) (potassium) (sodium) NEC	983.9	E864.3	E950.7	E980.6	
− herbicide	989.4	E863.5	E950.6	E980.7	
Chlorbenzene, chlorbenzol	982.0	E862.4	E950.9	E980.9	
Chlorbutol	967.1	E852.0	E950.2	E980.2	E937.1
Chlorcyclizine	963.0	E858.1	E950.4	E980.4	E933.0
Chlordan(e) (dust)	989.2	E863.0	E950.6	E980.7	
Chlordiazepoxide	969.4	E853.2	E950.3	E980.3	E939.4
Chlordiethyl benzamide	976.3	E858.7	E950.4	E980.4	E946.3
Chlorethyl - see Ethyl chloride					
Chlorhexidine	976.0	E858.7	E950.4	E980.4	E946.0
Chloride of lime (bleach)	983.2	E864.2	E950.7	E980.6	
Chlorimipramine	969.0	E854.0	E950.3	E980.3	E939.0
Chlorinated					
− camphene	989.2	E863.0	E950.6	E980.7	
− diphenyl	989.2	E866.8	E950.9	E980.9	
− hydrocarbons NEC	989.2	E863.0	E950.6	E980.7	
− − solvents	982.3	E862.4	E950.9	E980.9	
− lime (bleach)	983.2	E864.2	E950.7	E980.6	
− naphthalene - see Naphthalene					
− pesticides NEC	989.2	E863.0	E950.6	E980.7	
− soda - see Sodium hypochlorite					
Chlorine (fumes) (gas)	987.6	E869.8	E952.8	E982.8	
− bleach	983.9	E864.3	E950.7	E980.6	
− compound NEC	983.9	E864.3	E950.7	E980.6	
− disinfectant	983.9	E861.4	E950.9	E980.9	
− releasing agents NEC	983.9	E861.4	E950.9	E980.9	
Chlorisondamine	972.3	E858.3	E950.4	E980.4	E942.3
Chlormadinone	962.2	E858.0	E950.4	E980.4	E932.2
Chlormerodrin	974.0	E858.5	E950.4	E980.4	E944.0
Chlormethiazole	967.8	E852.8	E950.2	E980.2	E937.8
Chlormethine	963.1	E858.1	E950.4	E980.4	E933.1
Chlormezanone	975.3	E858.6	E950.4	E980.4	E945.3
Chloroacetone	987.5	E869.3	E952.8	E982.8	
Chloroacetophenone	987.5	E869.3	E952.8	E982.8	
Chloroaniline	983.0	E864.0	E950.7	E980.6	
Chlorobenzene, chlorobenzol	982.0	E862.4	E950.9	E980.9	
Chlorobromomethane (fire extinguisher)	989.8	E866.8	E950.9	E980.9	
Chlorobutanol	967.1	E852.0	E950.2	E980.2	E937.1
Chlorodinitrobenzene	983.0	E864.0	E950.7	E980.6	

Substance	Poison-ing (Chapter XVII)	External Cause (E Code)			
		Poisoning			Adverse effect in correct usage
		Accident	Suicide (attempt)	Undeter-mined	
Chlorodinitrobenzene - *continued*					
– dust or vapor	987.8	E869.8	E952.8	E982.8	
Chlorodiphenyl	989.8	E866.8	E950.9	E980.9	
Chloroethane - see Ethyl chloride					
Chloroethylene	987.8	E869.8	E952.8	E982.8	
Chloroform (fumes) (vapor)	987.8	E862.4	E950.9	E980.9	
– anesthetic	968.2	E855.1	E950.4	E980.4	E938.2
– solvent	982.8	E862.4	E950.9	E980.9	
Chloroguanide	961.4	E857	E950.4	E980.4	E931.4
Chloromycine	960.1	E856	E950.4	E980.4	E930.1
Chloronitrobenzene	983.0	E864.0	E950.7	E980.6	
– dust or vapor	987.8	E869.8	E952.8	E982.8	
Chlorophenol	983.0	E864.0	E950.7	E980.6	
Chlorophenothane	989.2	E863.0	E950.6	E980.7	
Chlorophyll	977.4	E858.8	E950.4	E980.4	E947.4
Chloropicrin (fumes)	987.8	E869.8	E952.8	E982.8	
– pesticide (fumes)	989.4	E863.9	E950.6	E980.7	
Chloroprocaine, spinal	968.7	E855.2	E950.4	E980.4	E938.7
Chloropurine	963.1	E858.1	E950.4	E980.4	E933.1
Chloropyrilene	963.0	E858.1	E950.4	E980.4	E933.0
Chloroquine	961.4	E857	E950.4	E980.4	E931.4
Chlorothiazide	974.3	E858.5	E950.4	E980.4	E944.3
Chlorothymol	976.4	E858.7	E950.4	E980.4	E946.4
Chlorotrianisene	962.2	E858.0	E950.4	E980.4	E932.2
Chlorovinyldichloroarsine, not in war	985.1	E866.3	E950.8	E980.8	
Chloroxylenol	976.0	E858.7	E950.4	E980.4	E946.0
Chlorphenamine	963.0	E858.1	E950.4	E980.4	E933.0
Chlorphenesin	976.0	E858.7	E950.4	E980.4	E946.0
– carbamate	968.0	E855.1	E950.4	E980.4	E938.0
Chlorphenisate	972.2	E858.3	E950.4	E980.4	E942.2
Chlorphenoxamine	966.4	E855.0	E950.4	E980.4	E936.4
Chlorphentermine	977.0	E858.8	E950.4	E980.4	E947.0
Chlorpromazine	969.1	E853.0	E950.3	E980.3	E939.1
Chlorpropamide	962.3	E858.0	E950.4	E980.4	E932.3
Chlorprothixene	969.5	E853.8	E950.3	E980.3	E939.5
Chlorquinaldol	961.3	E857	E950.4	E980.4	E931.3
Chlortalidone	974.3	E858.5	E950.4	E980.4	E944.3
Chlortetracycline	960.4	E856	E950.4	E980.4	E930.4
Chlorthenoxazin	965.7	E850.5	E950.0	E980.0	E935.5
Chlorthion	989.3	E863.1	E950.6	E980.7	
Chlorzoxazone	968.0	E855.1	E950.4	E980.4	E938.0
Choke damp	987.8	E869.8	E952.8	E982.8	
Cholagogues	973.4	E858.4	E950.4	E980.4	E943.4
Cholecalciferol	963.5	E858.1	E950.4	E980.4	E933.5
Cholecystokinin	973.4	E858.4	E950.4	E980.4	E943.4
Cholera vaccine	978.2	E858.8	E950.4	E980.4	E948.2
Choleretic	973.4	E858.4	E950.4	E980.4	E943.4
Cholestyramine (resin)	972.2	E858.3	E950.4	E980.4	E942.2
Cholic acid	973.4	E858.4	E950.4	E980.4	E943.4
Choline	975.7	E858.6	E950.4	E980.4	E945.7
– dihydrogen citrate	977.1	E858.8	E950.4	E980.4	E947.1

Substance	Poisoning (Chapter XVII)	External Cause (E Code)			
		Poisoning			Adverse effect in correct usage
		Accident	Suicide (attempt)	Undetermined	
Clorprenaline	975.7	E858.6	E950.4	E980.4	E945.7
Clortermine	977.0	E858.8	E950.4	E980.4	E947.0
Clotrimazole	961.9	E857	E950.4	E980.4	E931.9
Cloxacillin	960.0	E856	E950.4	E980.4	E930.0
CMF (cyclophosphamide, methotrexate, fluorouracil)	963.1	E858.1	E950.4	E980.4	E933.1
Coagulant NEC	964.5	E858.2	E950.4	E980.4	E934.5
Coal (carbon monoxide from) - see Carbon monoxide, coal					
− oil - see Kerosene					
− tar	976.1	E858.7	E950.4	E980.4	E946.1
− − fumes	987.8	E869.8	E952.8	E982.8	
− − naphtha (solvent)	982.0	E862.4	E950.9	E980.9	
− − nonmedicinal	983.0	E864.0	E950.7	E980.6	
Cobalamine	963.5	E858.1	E950.4	E980.4	E933.5
Cobalt					
− medicinal (trace) (chloride)	964.1	E858.2	E950.4	E980.4	E934.1
− nonmedicinal (fumes) (industrial)	985.8	E866.4	E950.9	E980.9	
Cocaine	968.5	E855.2	E950.4	E980.4	E938.5
Coccidiodin	977.8	E858.8	E950.4	E980.4	E947.8
Cochineal	989.8	E866.8	E950.9	E980.9	
Cocillana	975.5	E858.6	E950.4	E980.4	E945.5
Cod liver oil	963.5	E858.1	E950.4	E980.4	E933.5
Codeine	965.0	E850.4	E950.0	E980.0	E935.0
Co-enzymes	963.4	E858.1	E950.4	E980.4	E933.4
Coffee	988.2	E865.3	E950.9	E980.9	
Coke fumes or gas (carbon monoxide)	986	E868.3	E952.1	E982.1	
− industrial use	986	E868.8	E952.1	E982.1	
Colchicine	974.7	E858.5	E950.4	E980.4	E944.7
Colistimethate	960.8	E856	E950.4	E980.4	E930.8
Colistin	960.8	E856	E950.4	E980.4	E930.8
Collagenase	976.4	E858.7	E950.4	E980.4	E946.4
Collodion	976.3	E858.7	E950.4	E980.4	E946.3
Colocynth	973.1	E858.4	E950.4	E980.4	E943.1
Colophony adhesive	976.3	E858.7	E950.4	E980.4	E946.3
Colorant	977.4	E858.8	E950.4	E980.4	E947.4
Colymicin	960.8	E856	E950.4	E980.4	E930.8
Combustion gas - see Carbon monoxide					
Compound					
− F	962.0	E858.0	E950.4	E980.4	E932.0
− 1080 (sodium fluoroacetate)	989.4	E863.7	E950.6	E980.7	
− 269 (endrin)	989.2	E863.0	E950.6	E980.7	
− 3422 (parathion)	989.3	E863.1	E950.6	E980.7	
− 3911 (phorate)	989.3	E863.1	E950.6	E980.7	
− 3956 (toxaphene)	989.2	E863.0	E950.6	E980.7	
− 4049 (malathion)	989.3	E863.1	E950.6	E980.7	
− 4124 (dicapthon)	989.3	E863.1	E950.6	E980.7	
− 42 (warfarin)	989.4	E863.7	E950.6	E980.7	
− 497 (dieldrin)	989.2	E863.0	E950.6	E980.7	
Conjugated estrogenic substances	962.2	E858.0	E950.4	E980.4	E932.2
Contraceptive (pill)	962.2	E858.0	E950.4	E980.4	E932.2

| Substance | Poison-ing (Chapter XVII) | External Cause (E Code) | | | Adverse effect in correct usage |
| | | Poisoning | | | |
		Accident	Suicide (attempt)	Undeter-mined	
Crude oil	981	E862.9	E950.9	E980.9	
Cryolite	983.9	E864.3	E950.7	E980.6	
− insecticide (vapour)	989.4	E863.4	E950.6	E980.7	
− vapor NEC	987.8	E869.8	E952.8	E982.8	
Cryptenamine	972.6	E858.3	E950.4	E980.4	E942.6
Crystal violet	976.0	E858.7	E950.4	E980.4	E946.0
Cyanacetyl hydrazide	961.8	E857	E950.4	E980.4	E931.8
Cyanic acid (gas)	989.8	E869.8	E952.8	E982.8	
Cyanide(s) (compounds) (hydrogen) (potassium) (sodium) NEC	989.0	E866.8	E950.9	E980.9	
− dust (inhalation) or gas NEC	987.8	E869.8	E952.8	E982.8	
− mercuric - see Mercury					
− pesticide (dust) (fumes)	989.0	E863.8	E950.6	E980.7	
Cyanoacrylate adhesive	976.3	E858.7	E950.4	E980.4	E946.3
Cyanocobalamin	963.5	E858.1	E950.4	E980.4	E933.5
Cyanogen (chloride) (gas) NEC	987.8	E869.8	E952.8	E982.8	
Cyanopsis tetragonoloba	972.2	E858.3	E950.4	E980.4	E942.2
Cyclacillin	960.8	E856	E950.4	E980.4	E930.8
Cyclamate	977.4	E858.8	E950.4	E980.4	E947.4
Cyclandelate	972.5	E858.3	E950.4	E980.4	E942.5
Cyclazocine	970.1	E854.3	E950.4	E980.4	E940.1
Cyclizine	963.0	E858.1	E950.4	E980.4	E933.0
Cyclobarbital	968.3	E855.1	E950.4	E980.4	E938.3
Cycloguanil (embonate)	961.4	E857	E950.4	E980.4	E931.4
Cycloheptadiene	969.0	E854.0	E950.3	E980.3	E939.0
Cyclohexane	982.8	E862.4	E950.9	E980.9	
Cyclohexanol	980.8	E860.8	E950.9	E980.9	
Cyclohexanone	982.8	E862.4	E950.9	E980.9	
Cycloheximide	989.4	E863.6	E950.6	E980.7	
Cyclohexyl acetate	982.8	E862.4	E950.9	E980.9	
Cyclomethycaine	968.5	E855.2	E950.4	E980.4	E938.5
Cyclopenthiazide	974.3	E858.5	E950.4	E980.4	E944.3
Cyclopentolate	976.5	E858.7	E950.4	E980.4	E946.5
Cyclophosphamide	963.1	E858.1	E950.4	E980.4	E933.1
Cycloplegic drug	976.5	E858.7	E950.4	E980.4	E946.5
Cyclopropane	968.2	E855.1	E950.4	E980.4	E938.2
Cyclopyrabital	965.7	E850.5	E950.0	E980.0	E935.5
Cycloserine	960.6	E856	E950.4	E980.4	E930.6
Cyclothiazide	974.3	E858.5	E950.4	E980.4	E944.3
Cycrimine	971.1	E855.4	E950.4	E980.4	E941.1
Cyproheptadine	977.0	E858.8	E950.4	E980.4	E947.0
Cyproterone	962.2	E858.0	E950.4	E980.4	E932.2
Cysteamine	977.1	E858.8	E950.4	E980.4	E947.1
Cytarabine	963.1	E858.1	E950.4	E980.4	E933.1
Cytosine arabinoside	963.1	E858.1	E950.4	E980.4	E933.1
Cytozyme	964.5	E858.2	E950.4	E980.4	E934.5
Dacarbazine	963.1	E858.1	E950.4	E980.4	E933.1
Dactinomycin	960.7	E856	E950.4	E980.4	E930.7
DADPS	961.8	E857	E950.4	E980.4	E931.8
Dalapon	989.2	E863.5	E950.6	E980.7	
Danthron	973.1	E858.4	E950.4	E980.4	E943.1

Substance	Poisoning (Chapter XVII)	External Cause (E Code)			
		Poisoning			Adverse effect in correct usage
		Accident	Suicide (attempt)	Undetermined	
Dantrolene	975.2	E858.6	E950.4	E980.4	E945.2
Dapsone	961.8	E857	E950.4	E980.4	E931.8
Daunomycin	960.7	E856	E950.4	E980.4	E930.7
Daunorubicin	960.7	E856	E950.4	E980.4	E930.7
D-CON (rodenticide)	989.4	E863.7	E950.6	E980.7	
D-D (vapor)	989.2	E863.0	E950.6	E980.7	
DDAVP	962.5	E858.0	E950.4	E980.4	E932.5
DDE	989.2	E863.0	E950.6	E980.7	
DDT (dust)	989.2	E863.0	E950.6	E980.7	
Deadly nightshade	988.2	E865.4	E950.9	E980.9	
Deanol (aceglumate)	970.8	E854.3	E950.4	E980.4	E940.8
Debrisoquine	972.6	E858.3	E950.4	E980.4	E942.6
Decaborane	989.8	E866.8	E950.9	E980.9	
− fumes	987.8	E869.8	E952.8	E982.8	
Decahydronaphthalene	982.0	E862.4	E950.9	E980.9	
Decalin	982.0	E862.4	E950.9	E980.9	
Decamethonium (bromide)	975.2	E858.6	E950.4	E980.4	E945.2
Decongestant, nasal (mucosa)	975.6	E858.6	E950.4	E980.4	E945.6
− combination	975.6	E858.6	E950.4	E980.4	E945.6
Deet	989.4	E863.4	E950.6	E980.7	
Deferoxamine	963.8	E858.1	E950.4	E980.4	E933.8
Deglycyrrhinised liquorice	973.8	E858.4	E950.4	E980.4	E943.8
Dehydrocholic acid	973.4	E858.4	E950.4	E980.4	E943.4
Dehydroemetine	961.6	E857	E950.4	E980.4	E931.6
Dekalin	982.0	E862.4	E950.9	E980.9	
Demecarium (bromide)	976.5	E858.7	E950.4	E980.4	E946.5
Demeclocycline	960.4	E856	E950.4	E980.4	E930.4
Demecolcine	974.7	E858.5	E950.4	E980.4	E944.7
Demethylchlortetracycline	960.4	E856	E950.4	E980.4	E930.4
Demeton	989.3	E863.1	E950.6	E980.7	
Demulcent (external) NEC	976.3	E858.7	E950.4	E980.4	E946.3
− specified NEC	976.3	E858.7	E950.4	E980.4	E946.3
Denatured alcohol	980.0	E860.1	E950.9	E980.9	
Dental drug, topical application NEC	976.7	E858.7	E950.4	E980.4	E946.7
Dentifrice	976.7	E858.7	E950.4	E980.4	E946.7
Deoxycortone	962.0	E858.0	E950.4	E980.4	E932.0
Deoxyfluoruridine	963.1	E858.1	E950.4	E980.4	E933.1
Deoxyribonuclease	976.4	E858.7	E950.4	E980.4	E946.4
Depilatory	976.4	E858.7	E950.4	E980.4	E946.4
Deprenil	966.4	E855.0	E950.4	E980.4	E936.4
Depressant					
− appetite	977.0	E858.8	E950.4	E980.4	E947.0
− central nervous system	968.9	E855.2	E950.4	E980.4	E938.9
Deptropine	975.7	E858.6	E950.4	E980.4	E945.7
Dequalinium (chloride)	976.0	E858.7	E950.4	E980.4	E946.0
Derris	989.4	E863.4	E950.6	E980.7	
Desamino-d-arginine vasopressin	962.5	E858.0	E950.4	E980.4	E932.5
Deserpidine	972.6	E858.3	E950.4	E980.4	E942.6
Desferrioxamine	963.8	E858.1	E950.4	E980.4	E933.8
Desipramine	969.0	E854.0	E950.3	E980.3	E939.0
Deslanoside	972.1	E858.3	E950.4	E980.4	E942.1

Substance	Poison-ing (Chapter XVII)	External Cause (E Code)			Adverse effect in correct usage
		Poisoning			
		Accident	Suicide (attempt)	Undeter-mined	
Desloughing agent	976.4	E858.7	E950.4	E980.4	E946.4
Desmopressin	962.5	E858.0	E950.4	E980.4	E932.5
Desonide	976.0	E858.7	E950.4	E980.4	E946.0
Desoxycorticosteroid	962.0	E858.0	E950.4	E980.4	E932.0
Desoxycortone	962.0	E858.0	E950.4	E980.4	E932.0
Desoxyephedrine	969.7	E854.2	E950.3	E980.3	E939.7
Detergent (local) (medicinal) NEC	976.2	E858.7	E950.4	E980.4	E946.2
− nonmedicinal	989.6	E861.0	E950.9	E980.9	
− specified NEC	976.2	E858.7	E950.4	E980.4	E946.2
Detoxifying agent	977.2	E858.8	E950.4	E980.4	E947.2
Dexamethasone	962.0	E858.0	E950.4	E980.4	E932.0
Dexamphetamine	969.7	E854.2	E950.3	E980.3	E939.7
Dexbrompheniramine	963.0	E858.1	E950.4	E980.4	E933.0
Dexchlorpheniramine	963.0	E858.1	E950.4	E980.4	E933.0
Dextran	964.8	E858.2	E950.4	E980.4	E934.8
Dextromethorphan	975.4	E858.6	E950.4	E980.4	E945.4
Dextromoramide	965.0	E850.0	E950.0	E980.0	E935.0
Dextropropoxyphene	965.7	E850.5	E950.0	E980.0	E935.5
Dextrose	974.5	E858.5	E950.4	E980.4	E944.5
− concentrated solution, intravenous	972.7	E858.3	E950.4	E980.4	E942.7
Dextrothyroxine sodium	962.7	E858.0	E950.4	E980.4	E932.7
DFP	971.0	E855.3	E950.4	E980.4	E941.0
DHE-45	972.6	E858.3	E950.4	E980.4	E942.6
Diacetone alcohol	982.8	E862.4	E950.9	E980.9	
Diacetylmorphine	965.0	E850.0	E950.0	E980.0	E935.0
Diachylon plaster	976.4	E858.7	E950.4	E980.4	E946.4
Diagnostic agent NEC	977.8	E858.8	E950.4	E980.4	E947.8
Di-alkyl carbonate	982.8	E862.4	E950.9	E980.9	
Dialysis solution	974.5	E858.5	E950.4	E980.4	E944.5
Diaminodiphenylsulphone	961.8	E857	E950.4	E980.4	E931.8
Diamorphine	965.0	E850.0	E950.0	E980.0	E935.0
Diamthazole	976.0	E858.7	E950.4	E980.4	E946.0
Diastase	963.4	E858.1	E950.4	E980.4	E933.4
Diatol	982.8	E862.4	E950.9	E980.9	
Diatrizoate	977.8	E858.8	E950.4	E980.4	E947.8
Diazepam	969.4	E853.2	E950.3	E980.3	E939.4
Diazinon	989.3	E863.1	E950.6	E980.7	
Diazomethane (gas)	987.8	E869.8	E952.8	E982.8	
Diazoxide	972.5	E858.3	E950.4	E980.4	E942.5
Diborane (gas)	987.8	E869.8	E952.8	E982.8	
Dibromoethane	989.8	E866.8	E950.9	E980.9	
Dibromopropamidine isethionate	976.0	E858.7	E950.4	E980.4	E946.0
Dibucaine	968.5	E855.2	E950.4	E980.4	E938.5
Dibutoline	971.1	E855.4	E950.4	E980.4	E941.1
Dibutyryl	977.1	E858.8	E950.4	E980.4	E947.1
Dicamba	989.4	E863.5	E950.6	E980.7	
Dicapthon	989.3	E863.1	E950.6	E980.7	
Dichloral phenazone	967.6	E852.5	E950.2	E980.2	E937.6
Dichlorbenzene	989.2	E863.0	E950.6	E980.7	
Dichlorbenzidine	989.2	E866.8	E950.9	E980.9	
Dichlorhydrin, dichlorohydrin	982.3	E862.4	E950.9	E980.9	

Substance	Poison-ing (Chapter XVII)	External Cause (E Code)			
		Poisoning			Adverse effect in correct usage
		Accident	Suicide (attempt)	Undeter-mined	
Dichlorhydroxyquinoline	961.3	E857	E950.4	E980.4	E931.3
Dichlorodifluoromethane	987.4	E869.2	E952.8	E982.8	
Dichloroethane	982.3	E862.4	E950.9	E980.9	
Dichloroethyl sulfide, not in war	987.8	E869.8	E952.8	E982.8	
Dichloroethylene	982.3	E862.4	E950.9	E980.9	
Dichloroformoxine, not in war	989.8	E866.8	E950.9	E980.9	
Dichlorohydrin	982.3	E862.4	E950.9	E980.9	
Dichloromethane (solvent)	982.3	E862.4	E950.9	E980.9	
− vapor	987.8	E862.4	E950.9	E980.9	
Dichloronaphthoquinone	989.2	E863.0	E950.6	E980.7	
Dichlorophen	961.6	E857	E950.4	E980.4	E931.6
Dichloropropionic acid	989.2	E863.5	E950.6	E980.7	
Dichlorvos	989.3	E863.1	E950.6	E980.7	
Diclofenamide	974.2	E858.5	E950.4	E980.4	E944.2
Dicloxacillin	960.0	E856	E950.4	E980.4	E930.0
Dicophane	976.0	E858.7	E950.4	E980.4	E946.0
Dicoumarol, dicoumarin, dicumarol	964.2	E858.2	E950.4	E980.4	E934.2
Dicyanogen (gas)	987.8	E869.8	E952.8	E982.8	
Dicyclomine	971.1	E855.4	E950.4	E980.4	E941.1
Dieldrin (vapor)	989.2	E863.0	E950.6	E980.7	
Dielene	982.8	E862.4	E950.9	E980.9	
Dienestrol	962.2	E858.0	E950.4	E980.4	E932.2
Dietetic drug NEC	977.0	E858.8	E950.4	E980.4	E947.0
Diethazine	966.4	E855.0	E950.4	E980.4	E936.4
Diethyl					
− carbinol	980.3	E860.4	E950.9	E980.9	
− carbonate	982.8	E862.4	E950.9	E980.9	
− ether (vapor) (see also Ether(s))	987.8	E869.8	E952.8	E982.8	
− oxide	982.8	E862.4	E950.9	E980.9	
− toluamide (nonmedicinal)	989.4	E863.4	E950.6	E980.7	
− − medicinal	976.3	E858.7	E950.4	E980.4	E946.3
Diethylamine acetarsol	961.1	E857	E950.4	E980.4	E931.1
Diethylcarbamazine	961.6	E857	E950.4	E980.4	E931.6
Diethylene					
− dioxide	982.8	E862.4	E950.9	E980.9	
− glycol (monoacetate) (monoethyl ether) .	982.8	E862.4	E950.9	E980.9	
Diethylpropion	977.0	E858.8	E950.4	E980.4	E947.0
Diethylstilbestrol	962.2	E858.0	E950.4	E980.4	E932.2
Diethylstilboestrol	962.2	E858.0	E950.4	E980.4	E932.2
Difebuzol	965.5	E850.3	E950.0	E980.0	E935.3
Difenoxin	973.5	E858.4	E950.4	E980.4	E943.5
Diflucortolone	976.0	E858.7	E950.4	E980.4	E946.0
Digestant NEC	973.4	E858.4	E950.4	E980.4	E943.4
Digitalis	972.1	E858.3	E950.4	E980.4	E942.1
− glycoside NEC	972.1	E858.3	E950.4	E980.4	E942.1
− lanata (leaf) (glycoside)	972.1	E858.3	E950.4	E980.4	E942.1
− leaf	972.1	E858.3	E950.4	E980.4	E942.1
− purpurea (leaf) (glycoside)	972.1	E858.3	E950.4	E980.4	E942.1
Digitoxin	972.1	E858.3	E950.4	E980.4	E942.1
Digitoxose	972.1	E858.3	E950.4	E980.4	E942.1
Digoxin	972.1	E858.3	E950.4	E980.4	E942.1

Substance	Poisoning (Chapter XVII)	External Cause (E Code)			Adverse effect in correct usage
		Poisoning			
		Accident	Suicide (attempt)	Undeter-mined	
Dihydralazine	972.6	E858.3	E950.4	E980.4	E942.6
Dihydrazine	972.6	E858.3	E950.4	E980.4	E942.6
Dihydrocodeinone	965.0	E850.0	E950.0	E980.0	E935.0
Dihydroergocornine	972.5	E858.3	E950.4	E980.4	E942.5
Dihydroergocristine	972.5	E858.3	E950.4	E980.4	E942.5
Dihydroergokryptine	972.5	E858.3	E950.4	E980.4	E942.5
Dihydroergotamine	972.6	E858.3	E950.4	E980.4	E942.6
Dihydrohydroxycodeinone	965.0	E850.0	E950.0	E980.0	E935.0
Dihydromorphinone	965.0	E850.0	E950.0	E980.0	E935.0
Dihydrostreptomycin	960.6	E856	E950.4	E980.4	E930.6
Dihydrotachysterol	962.9	E858.0	E950.4	E980.4	E932.9
Dihydroxyaluminium aminoacetate	973.0	E858.4	E950.4	E980.4	E943.0
Dihydroxyanthraquinone	973.1	E858.4	E950.4	E980.4	E943.1
Dihydroxypropyl theophylline	974.1	E858.5	E950.4	E980.4	E944.1
Diiodohydroxyquinoline	976.0	E858.7	E950.4	E980.4	E946.0
Diisopropylfluorophosphonate	971.0	E855.3	E950.4	E980.4	E941.0
Dill	973.4	E858.4	E950.4	E980.4	E943.4
Dimazole	976.0	E858.7	E950.4	E980.4	E946.0
Dimefox	989.3	E863.1	E950.6	E980.7	
Dimenhydrinate	963.0	E858.1	E950.4	E980.4	E933.0
Dimercaprol (British anti-lewisite)	963.8	E858.1	E950.4	E980.4	E933.8
Dimethicone	973.0	E858.4	E950.4	E980.4	E943.0
Dimethindene	963.0	E858.1	E950.4	E980.4	E933.0
Dimethisoquin	976.1	E858.7	E950.4	E980.4	E946.1
Dimethisterone	962.2	E858.0	E950.4	E980.4	E932.2
Dimethoxanate	975.4	E858.6	E950.4	E980.4	E945.4
Dimethyl					
− arsine, arsinic acid - see Arsenic					
− carbinol	980.2	E860.3	E950.9	E980.9	
− carbonate	982.8	E862.4	E950.9	E980.9	
− ketone	982.8	E862.4	E950.9	E980.9	
− − vapor	987.8	E862.4	E950.9	E980.9	
− phthlate	976.3	E858.7	E950.4	E980.4	E946.3
− sulfate (fumes)	987.8	E869.8	E952.8	E982.8	
− − liquid	983.9	E864.3	E950.7	E980.6	
− sulfoxide (nonmedicinal)	982.8	E862.4	E950.9	E980.9	
− − medicinal	977.4	E858.8	E950.4	E980.4	E947.4
Dimethylamine sulfate	976.4	E858.7	E950.4	E980.4	E946.4
Dimethyltubocurarine	975.2	E858.6	E950.4	E980.4	E945.2
Dimetilan	989.3	E863.2	E950.6	E980.7	
Dimetindene	976.1	E858.7	E950.4	E980.4	E946.1
Dinitro(-ortho-)cresol (pesticide) (spray)	989.4	E863.4	E950.6	E980.7	
Dinitrobenzene	983.0	E864.0	E950.7	E980.6	
− vapor	987.8	E869.8	E952.8	E982.8	
Dinitrobenzol	983.0	E864.0	E950.7	E980.6	
− vapor	987.8	E869.8	E952.8	E982.8	
Dinitrobutylphenol	989.4	E863.4	E950.6	E980.7	
Dinitrocyclohexylphenol	989.4	E863.9	E950.6	E980.7	
Dinitrophenol	989.8	E866.8	E950.9	E980.9	
Dinoprostone	975.0	E858.6	E950.4	E980.4	E945.0
Dinoseb (DNBP)	989.4	E863.4	E950.6	E980.7	

Substance	Poisoning (Chapter XVII)	External Cause (E Code)			Adverse effect in correct usage
		Poisoning			
		Accident	Suicide (attempt)	Undetermined	
Diodone	977.8	E858.8	E950.4	E980.4	E947.8
Dionine	965.0	E850.0	E950.0	E980.0	E935.0
Dioxane	982.8	E862.4	E950.9	E980.9	
Dioxathion	989.3	E863.1	E950.6	E980.7	
Dioxin	989.2	E866.8	E950.9	E980.9	
Dioxyline	972.4	E858.3	E950.4	E980.4	E942.4
Dipentene	982.8	E862.4	E950.9	E980.9	
Diperodon	968.5	E855.2	E950.4	E980.4	E938.5
Diphacinone	989.4	E863.7	E950.6	E980.7	
Diphenadione	964.2	E858.2	E950.4	E980.4	E934.2
Diphenamil	971.1	E855.4	E950.4	E980.4	E941.1
Diphenhydramine	963.0	E858.1	E950.4	E980.4	E933.0
Diphenidol	963.0	E858.1	E950.4	E980.4	E933.0
Diphenoxylate	973.5	E858.4	E950.4	E980.4	E943.5
Diphenylamine	989.8	E866.8	E950.9	E980.9	
Diphenylbutazone	965.5	E850.3	E950.0	E980.0	E935.3
Diphenylchloroarsine, not in war	985.1	E866.3	E950.8	E980.8	
Diphenylmethane dye	989.8	E866.8	E950.9	E980.9	
Diphenylpyraline	963.0	E858.1	E950.4	E980.4	E933.0
Diphtheria toxoid or vaccine	978.5	E858.8	E950.4	E980.4	E948.5
Dipipanone	965.0	E850.0	E950.0	E980.0	E935.0
Diprophylline	974.1	E858.5	E950.4	E980.4	E944.1
Dipropyline	975.1	E858.6	E950.4	E980.4	E945.1
Dipropyridine	967.8	E852.8	E950.2	E980.2	E937.8
Dipyridamole	972.4	E858.3	E950.4	E980.4	E942.4
Diquat (salt)	989.4	E863.5	E950.6	E980.7	
Disinfectant	983.9	E861.4	E950.9	E980.9	
− alkaline	983.2	E861.4	E950.9	E980.9	
− aromatic	983.0	E861.4	E950.9	E980.9	
− intestinal	961.9	E857	E950.4	E980.4	E931.9
Disodium edetate	977.2	E858.8	E950.4	E980.4	E947.2
Disopyramide	972.0	E858.3	E950.4	E980.4	E942.0
Distigmine	971.0	E855.3	E950.4	E980.4	E941.0
Disulfamide	974.3	E858.5	E950.4	E980.4	E944.3
Disulfiram	977.3	E858.8	E950.4	E980.4	E947.3
Disulfoton	989.3	E863.1	E950.6	E980.7	
Dithranol	976.4	E858.7	E950.4	E980.4	E946.4
Diuretic NEC	974.4	E858.5	E950.4	E980.4	E944.4
− benzothiadiazine	974.3	E858.5	E950.4	E980.4	E944.3
− furfuryl NEC	974.3	E858.5	E950.4	E980.4	E944.3
− mercurial NEC	974.0	E858.5	E950.4	E980.4	E944.0
− osmotic	974.3	E858.5	E950.4	E980.4	E944.3
− purine NEC	974.1	E858.5	E950.4	E980.4	E944.1
− saluretic NEC	974.3	E858.5	E950.4	E980.4	E944.3
− sulphonamide	974.4	E858.5	E950.4	E980.4	E944.4
− thiazide NEC	974.3	E858.5	E950.4	E980.4	E944.3
− xanthine	974.1	E858.5	E950.4	E980.4	E944.1
Dizoxide	972.5	E858.3	E950.4	E980.4	E942.5
DMSO	982.8	E862.4	E950.9	E980.9	
DNOC	989.4	E863.4	E950.6	E980.7	
Dobutamine	975.7	E858.6	E950.4	E980.4	E945.7

Substance	Poisoning (Chapter XVII)	External Cause (E Code)			Adverse effect in correct usage
		Poisoning			
		Accident	Suicide (attempt)	Undeter-mined	
DOCA	962.0	E858.0	E950.4	E980.4	E932.0
Domestic gas - see Gas, utility					
Domestos	983.2	E864.2	E950.7	E980.6	
Domiphen (bromide)	976.0	E858.7	E950.4	E980.4	E946.0
Dopa	971.2	E855.5	E950.4	E980.4	E941.2
Dopamine	971.2	E855.5	E950.4	E980.4	E941.2
Dornase	975.5	E858.6	E950.4	E980.4	E945.5
Dothiepin	969.0	E854.0	E950.3	E980.3	E939.0
Doxantrazole	975.7	E858.6	E950.4	E980.4	E945.7
Doxapram	970.0	E854.3	E950.4	E980.4	E940.0
Doxepin	969.0	E854.0	E950.3	E980.3	E939.0
Doxorubicin	960.7	E856	E950.4	E980.4	E930.7
Doxycycline	960.4	E856	E950.4	E980.4	E930.4
Doxylamine	963.0	E858.1	E950.4	E980.4	E933.0
Dressing, live pulp	976.7	E858.7	E950.4	E980.4	E946.7
Droperidol	969.2	E853.1	E950.3	E980.3	E939.2
Drostanolone	962.1	E858.0	E950.4	E980.4	E932.1
Drug NEC	977.9	E858.9	E950.5	E980.5	E947.9
− specified NEC	977.8	E858.8	E950.4	E980.4	E947.8
DTIC	963.1	E858.1	E950.4	E980.4	E933.1
Dursban	989.3	E863.1	E950.6	E980.7	
Dybenal	976.0	E858.7	E950.4	E980.4	E946.0
Dyclonine	976.1	E858.7	E950.4	E980.4	E946.1
Dydrogesterone	962.2	E858.0	E950.4	E980.4	E932.2
Dye(s) NEC	989.8	E866.8	E950.9	E980.9	
− antiseptic	976.0	E858.7	E950.4	E980.4	E946.0
Dyflos	971.0	E855.3	E950.4	E980.4	E941.0
Dynamite	989.8	E866.8	E950.9	E980.9	
− fumes	987.8	E869.8	E952.8	E982.8	
Dynaphylline	975.7	E858.6	E950.4	E980.4	E945.7
Ear drug NEC	976.6	E858.7	E950.4	E980.4	E946.6
Ecothiopate iodide	971.0	E855.3	E950.4	E980.4	E941.0
Ectylurea	969.5	E853.8	E950.3	E980.3	E939.5
Edrophonium	971.0	E855.3	E950.4	E980.4	E941.0
EDTA	977.2	E858.8	E950.4	E980.4	E947.2
Elatine	975.2	E858.6	E950.4	E980.4	E945.2
Electrolyte balance drug	974.5	E858.5	E950.4	E980.4	E944.5
Elemental diet	977.0	E858.8	E950.4	E980.4	E947.0
Embramine	963.0	E858.1	E950.4	E980.4	E933.0
Emepronium	971.1	E855.4	E950.4	E980.4	E941.1
Emetic NEC	973.6	E858.4	E950.4	E980.4	E943.6
Emetine	961.5	E857	E950.4	E980.4	E931.5
Emollient NEC	976.3	E858.7	E950.4	E980.4	E946.3
Emylcamate	968.0	E855.1	E950.4	E980.4	E938.0
Endosulfan	989.4	E863.4	E950.6	E980.7	
Endothal	989.4	E863.5	E950.6	E980.7	
Endrin	989.2	E863.0	E950.6	E980.7	
Enflurane	968.2	E855.1	E950.4	E980.4	E938.2
Enzyme NEC	963.4	E858.1	E950.4	E980.4	E933.4
− depolymerizing	976.8	E858.7	E950.4	E980.4	E946.8
− fibrolytic	963.4	E858.1	E950.4	E980.4	E933.4

Substance	Poisoning (Chapter XVII)	External Cause (E Code)			Adverse effect in correct usage
		Poisoning			
		Accident	Suicide (attempt)	Undetermined	
Enzyme NEC - *continued*					
– gastric	963.4	E858.1	E950.4	E980.4	E933.4
– intestinal	973.4	E858.4	E950.4	E980.4	E943.4
– local action	976.4	E858.7	E950.4	E980.4	E946.4
– proteolytic	976.4	E858.7	E950.4	E980.4	E946.4
– thrombolytic	963.4	E858.1	E950.4	E980.4	E933.4
Ephedra	971.2	E855.5	E950.4	E980.4	E941.2
Ephedrine	971.2	E855.5	E950.4	E980.4	E941.2
Epicillin	960.8	E856	E950.4	E980.4	E930.8
Epinephrine	971.2	E855.5	E950.4	E980.4	E941.2
Epipodophyllotoxin	963.1	E858.1	E950.4	E980.4	E933.1
EPN	989.3	E863.1	E950.6	E980.7	
Epoxy resin	989.8	E866.8	E950.9	E980.9	
Epsilon aminocaproic acid	964.4	E858.2	E950.4	E980.4	E934.4
Ergobasine	975.0	E858.6	E950.4	E980.4	E945.0
Ergocalciferol	963.5	E858.1	E950.4	E980.4	E933.5
Ergometrine	975.0	E858.6	E950.4	E980.4	E945.0
Ergonovine	975.0	E858.6	E950.4	E980.4	E945.0
Ergot NEC	988.2	E865.4	E950.9	E980.9	
– derivative	975.0	E858.6	E950.4	E980.4	E945.0
Ergotamine	972.6	E858.3	E950.4	E980.4	E942.6
Ergotocine	975.0	E858.6	E950.4	E980.4	E945.0
Erythrityl tetranitrate	972.4	E858.3	E950.4	E980.4	E942.4
Erythrol tetranitrate	972.4	E858.3	E950.4	E980.4	E942.4
Erythromycin (salts)	960.3	E856	E950.4	E980.4	E930.3
Eserine	971.0	E855.3	E950.4	E980.4	E941.0
ESTD (ether soluble tar distillate)	976.1	E858.7	E950.4	E980.4	E946.1
Estradiol	962.2	E858.0	E950.4	E980.4	E932.2
– with testosterone	962.1	E858.0	E950.4	E980.4	E932.1
Estriol	962.2	E858.0	E950.4	E980.4	E932.2
Estrogen	962.2	E858.0	E950.4	E980.4	E932.2
– with progesterone	962.2	E858.0	E950.4	E980.4	E932.2
Estrone	962.2	E858.0	E950.4	E980.4	E932.2
Etacrynic acid	974.4	E858.5	E950.4	E980.4	E944.4
Etafedrine	975.7	E858.6	E950.4	E980.4	E945.7
Etamidate	968.3	E855.1	E950.4	E980.4	E938.3
Etamiphyllin	975.7	E858.6	E950.4	E980.4	E945.7
Ethacrynic acid	974.4	E858.5	E950.4	E980.4	E944.4
Ethambutol	961.8	E857	E950.4	E980.4	E931.8
Ethamivan	970.0	E854.3	E950.4	E980.4	E940.0
Ethamsylate	964.5	E858.2	E950.4	E980.4	E934.5
Ethanol	980.0	E860.1	E950.9	E980.9	
Ethanolamine oleate	972.7	E858.3	E950.4	E980.4	E942.7
Ethchlorvynol	967.8	E852.8	E950.2	E980.2	E937.8
Ether(s) (vapor)	987.8	E862.4	E950.9	E980.9	
– divinyl	968.2	E855.1	E950.4	E980.4	E938.2
– ethyl (medicinal)	968.2	E855.1	E950.4	E980.4	E938.2
– – nonmedicinal	987.8	E862.4	E950.9	E980.9	
– petroleum - see Ligroin					
– solvent	982.8	E862.4	E950.9	E980.9	
Ethidine chloride (vapor)	987.8	E862.4	E950.9	E980.9	

Substance	Poison-ing (Chapter XVII)	External Cause (E Code)			Adverse effect in correct usage
		Poisoning			
		Accident	Suicide (attempt)	Undeter-mined	
Ethidine chloride - *continued*					
− liquid (solvent)	982.8	E862.4	E950.9	E980.9	
Ethinamate	967.8	E852.8	E950.2	E980.2	E937.8
Ethinylestradiol	962.2	E858.0	E950.4	E980.4	E932.2
Ethion	989.3	E863.1	E950.6	E980.7	
Ethionamide	961.8	E857	E950.4	E980.4	E931.8
Ethisterone	962.2	E858.0	E950.4	E980.4	E932.2
Ethoheptazine	965.7	E850.5	E950.0	E980.0	E935.5
Ethopropazine	966.4	E855.0	E950.4	E980.4	E936.4
Ethosuximide	966.2	E855.0	E950.4	E980.4	E936.2
Ethotoin	966.1	E855.0	E950.4	E980.4	E936.1
Ethoxzolamide	974.2	E858.5	E950.4	E980.4	E944.2
Ethyl					
− acetate	982.8	E862.4	E950.9	E980.9	
− − vapor	987.8	E862.4	E950.9	E980.9	
− alcohol	980.0	E860.1	E950.9	E980.9	
− aldehyde (vapor)	987.8	E869.8	E952.8	E982.8	
− − liquid	989.8	E866.8	E950.9	E980.9	
− aminobenzoate	968.5	E855.2	E950.4	E980.4	E938.5
− benzoate	982.8	E862.4	E950.9	E980.9	
− biscoumacetate	964.2	E858.2	E950.4	E980.4	E934.2
− carbamate	963.1	E858.1	E950.4	E980.4	E933.1
− carbinol	980.2	E860.3	E950.9	E980.9	
− chaulmoograte	961.8	E857	E950.4	E980.4	E931.8
− chloride (anesthetic)	968.2	E855.1	E950.4	E980.4	E938.2
− − local	976.4	E858.7	E950.4	E980.4	E946.4
− − solvent	982.3	E862.4	E950.9	E980.9	
− dibunate	975.4	E858.6	E950.4	E980.4	E945.4
− dichloroarsine (vapor)	985.1	E866.3	E950.8	E980.8	
− ether (see also Ether(s))	987.8	E862.4	E950.9	E980.9	
− formate NEC (solvent)	982.8	E862.4	E950.9	E980.9	
− hydroxyisobutyrate NEC (solvent)	982.8	E862.4	E950.9	E980.9	
− iodoacetate	987.5	E869.3	E952.8	E982.8	
− lactate NEC (solvent)	982.8	E862.4	E950.9	E980.9	
− mercuric chloride	985.0	E863.6	E950.6	E980.7	
− noradrenaline	975.7	E858.6	E950.4	E980.4	E945.7
− oxybutyrate NEC (solvent)	982.8	E862.4	E950.9	E980.9	
Ethylamino					
− benzoate	968.5	E855.2	E950.4	E980.4	E938.5
− phenothiazine	969.1	E853.0	E950.3	E980.3	E939.1
Ethylene (gas)	987.1	E869.8	E952.8	E982.8	
− chlorohydrin	982.3	E862.4	E950.9	E980.9	
− − vapor	987.8	E862.4	E950.9	E980.9	
− dichloride	982.3	E862.4	E950.9	E980.9	
− − vapor	987.8	E862.4	E950.9	E980.9	
− dinitrate	982.4	E862.4	E950.9	E980.9	
− glycol(s) (any)	982.8	E862.4	E950.9	E980.9	
− − dinitrate	982.4	E862.4	E950.9	E980.9	
− − vapor	987.8	E862.4	E950.9	E980.9	
− oxide (fumigant) (nonmedicinal)	987.8	E863.8	E950.6	E980.7	
− − medicinal	976.0	E858.7	E950.4	E980.4	E946.0

Substance	Poison-ing (Chapter XVII)	External Cause (E Code)			Adverse effect in correct usage
		Accident	Suicide (attempt)	Undeter-mined	
Ethylenediamine teophylline	975.7	E858.6	E950.4	E980.4	E945.7
Ethylenediaminetetraacetic acid	977.2	E858.8	E950.4	E980.4	E947.2
Ethylenedinitrilotetraacetate	977.2	E858.8	E950.4	E980.4	E947.2
Ethyleneimine	989.8	E866.8	E950.9	E980.9	
Ethylestrenol	962.1	E858.0	E950.4	E980.4	E932.1
Ethylidene					
− chloride NEC	982.3	E862.4	E950.9	E980.9	
− diethyl ether	982.8	E862.4	E950.9	E980.9	
Ethylmorphine	965.0	E850.0	E950.0	E980.0	E935.0
Ethylparachlorophenoxyisobutyrate	972.2	E858.3	E950.4	E980.4	E942.2
Ethynodiol	962.2	E858.0	E950.4	E980.4	E932.2
Etoglucide	963.1	E858.1	E950.4	E980.4	E933.1
Eucaine	968.5	E855.2	E950.4	E980.4	E938.5
Eucalyptus oil	976.7	E858.7	E950.4	E980.4	E946.7
Eucatropine	971.1	E855.4	E950.4	E980.4	E941.1
Eusolvan	982.8	E862.4	E950.9	E980.9	
Evans blue	977.8	E858.8	E950.4	E980.4	E947.8
Exhaust gas - see Carbon monoxide, exhaust gas					
Expectorant NEC	975.5	E858.6	E950.4	E980.4	E945.5
Extended insulin zinc suspension	962.3	E858.0	E950.4	E980.4	E932.3
Extrapyramidal antagonist NEC	971.1	E855.4	E950.4	E980.4	E941.1
Eye drug NEC	976.5	E858.7	E950.4	E980.4	E946.5
FAC (fluorouracil, adriamycin, cyclophosphamide)	963.1	E858.1	E950.4	E980.4	E933.1
Factor IX complex	964.5	E858.2	E950.4	E980.4	E934.5
Fat suspension, intravenous	977.0	E858.8	E950.4	E980.4	E947.0
Fecal softener	973.2	E858.4	E950.4	E980.4	E943.2
Felypressin	972.8	E858.3	E950.4	E980.4	E942.8
Fenbutrazate	977.0	E858.8	E950.4	E980.4	E947.0
Fenfluramine	977.0	E858.8	E950.4	E980.4	E947.0
Fenoprofen	965.6	E850.4	E950.0	E980.0	E935.4
Fentanyl	965.0	E850.0	E950.0	E980.0	E935.0
Fenthion	989.3	E863.1	E950.6	E980.7	
Fenticlor	976.0	E858.7	E950.4	E980.4	E946.0
Ferric - see Iron					
Ferrocholinate	964.0	E858.2	E950.4	E980.4	E934.0
Ferrous - see Iron					
Ferrovanadium (fumes)	985.8	E866.4	E950.9	E980.9	
Ferrum - see Iron					
Fertilizers NEC	989.8	E866.5	E950.9	E980.9	
Fibrinogen (human)	964.7	E858.2	E950.4	E980.4	E934.7
Fibrinolysin	964.4	E858.2	E950.4	E980.4	E934.4
− inhibitor NEC	964.4	E858.2	E950.4	E980.4	E934.4
Fibrinolysis affecting drug	964.4	E858.2	E950.4	E980.4	E934.4
Fibrinolytic drug	964.4	E858.2	E950.4	E980.4	E934.4
Fibrolysin, human	963.4	E858.1	E950.4	E980.4	E933.4
Filix mas	961.6	E857	E950.4	E980.4	E931.6
Filtering cream	976.3	E858.7	E950.4	E980.4	E946.3
Fire damp	987.1	E869.8	E952.8	E982.8	
Fish, nonbacterial or noxious	988.0	E865.2	E950.9	E980.9	

Substance	Poison-ing (Chapter XVII)	External Cause (E Code)			Adverse effect in correct usage
		Poisoning			
		Accident	Suicide (attempt)	Undeter-mined	
Fish - *continued*					
- shell	988.0	E865.1	E950.9	E980.9	
Flavoxate	975.1	E858.6	E950.4	E980.4	E945.1
Floxuridine	963.1	E858.1	E950.4	E980.4	E933.1
Fluandrenolone	976.0	E858.7	E950.4	E980.4	E946.0
Flucloxacillin	960.0	E856	E950.4	E980.4	E930.0
Flucytosine	961.9	E857	E950.4	E980.4	E931.9
Fludrocortisone	962.0	E858.0	E950.4	E980.4	E932.0
Flufenamic acid	965.6	E850.4	E950.0	E980.0	E935.4
Flumetasone	976.0	E858.7	E950.4	E980.4	E946.0
Flunitrazepam	969.4	E853.2	E950.3	E980.3	E939.4
Fluocinolone	976.0	E858.7	E950.4	E980.4	E946.0
Fluocortolone	976.0	E858.7	E950.4	E980.4	E946.0
Fluometholone	976.0	E858.7	E950.4	E980.4	E946.0
Fluopromazine	969.1	E853.0	E950.3	E980.3	E939.1
Fluoride(s) (nonmedicinal) (pesticides) (sodium) NEC	989.4	E863.9	E950.6	E980.7	
- hydrogen - see Hydrofluoric acid					
- medicinal NEC	974.6	E858.5	E950.4	E980.4	E944.6
- - dental use	976.7	E858.7	E950.4	E980.4	E946.7
- not pesticides NEC	983.9	E864.3	E950.7	E980.6	
Fluorine (gas)	987.8	E869.8	E952.8	E982.8	
- salt - see Fluoride(s)					
Fluoroacetate	989.4	E863.7	E950.6	E980.7	
Fluorocarbon monomer	987.4	E869.2	E952.8	E982.8	
Fluorohydrocortisone	962.0	E858.0	E950.4	E980.4	E932.0
Fluorophosphate	989.4	E863.6	E950.6	E980.7	
Fluorouracil	963.1	E858.1	E950.4	E980.4	E933.1
Fluorphenylalanine	976.5	E858.7	E950.4	E980.4	E946.5
Fluoxymesterone	962.1	E858.0	E950.4	E980.4	E932.1
Flupenthixol	969.5	E853.8	E950.3	E980.3	E939.5
Fluphenazine	969.1	E853.0	E950.3	E980.3	E939.1
Fluprednisolone	962.0	E858.0	E950.4	E980.4	E932.0
Flurazepam	969.4	E853.2	E950.3	E980.3	E939.4
Flurothyl	970.8	E854.3	E950.4	E980.4	E940.8
Fluroxene	968.2	E855.1	E950.4	E980.4	E938.2
Fluspirilene	969.2	E853.1	E950.3	E980.3	E939.2
Folic acid	964.1	E858.2	E950.4	E980.4	E934.1
- antagonist	963.1	E858.1	E950.4	E980.4	E933.1
Folinic acid	964.1	E858.2	E950.4	E980.4	E934.1
Folpet	989.2	E863.0	E950.6	E980.7	
Food, foodstuffs, nonbacterial or noxious NEC	988.8	E865.8	E950.9	E980.9	
Formaldehyde (solution)	989.8	E861.4	E950.9	E980.9	
- gas or vapor	987.8	E869.8	E952.8	E982.8	
Formalin	989.8	E861.4	E950.9	E980.9	
- vapor	987.8	E869.8	E952.8	E982.8	
Formic acid	983.1	E864.1	E950.7	E980.6	
- vapor	987.8	E869.8	E952.8	E982.8	
Foxglove	988.2	E865.4	E950.9	E980.9	
Framycetin	960.8	E856	E950.4	E980.4	E930.8

Substance	Poison-ing (Chapter XVII)	External Cause (E Code)			Adverse effect in correct usage
		Poisoning			
		Accident	Suicide (attempt)	Undeter-mined	
Frangula	973.1	E858.4	E950.4	E980.4	E943.1
Frei antigen	977.8	E858.8	E950.4	E980.4	E947.8
Freon	987.4	E869.2	E952.8	E982.8	
Fructose	974.5	E858.5	E950.4	E980.4	E944.5
Frusemide	974.3	E858.5	E950.4	E980.4	E944.3
FSH (follicle stimulating hormone)	962.4	E858.0	E950.4	E980.4	E932.4
Fuel					
– automobile	981	E862.1	E950.9	E980.9	
– – exhaust gas, not in transit	986	E868.2	E952.0	E982.0	
– – vapor NEC	987.1	E862.4	E950.9	E980.9	
– gas (domestic use) - see Carbon monoxide, fuel					
– industrial, incomplete combustion	986	E868.8	E952.1	E982.1	
Fulminate of mercury	985.0	E866.1	E950.9	E980.9	
Fumagillin	960.8	E856	E950.4	E980.4	E930.8
Fumes (from)	987.9	E869.9	E925.9	E982.9	
– carbon monoxide - see Carbon monoxide					
– charcoal (domestic use)	986	E868.3	E952.1	E982.1	
– coke (in domestic stoves, fireplaces)	986	E868.3	E952.1	E982.1	
– corrosive NEC	987.9	E869.8	E952.8	E982.8	
– ether - see Ether(s)					
– lead - see Lead					
– metals - see Metals, or the specified metal					
– specified source NEC	987.9	E869.8	E952.8	E982.8	
Fumigant	989.4	E863.8	E950.6	E980.7	
Fungi, noxious, used as food	988.1	E865.5	E950.9	E980.9	
Fungicide	989.4	E863.6	E950.6	E980.7	
Furazolidone	961.9	E857	E950.4	E980.4	E931.9
Furfural	982.8	E862.4	E950.9	E980.9	
Furnace (coal burning) (domestic), gas from industrial	986	E868.8	E952.1	E982.1	
Furniture polish	989.8	E861.2	E950.9	E980.9	
Furosemide	974.3	E858.5	E950.4	E980.4	E944.3
Fusel oil (any) (amyl) (butyl) (propyl)	980.3	E860.4	E950.9	E980.9	
– vapor	987.8	E869.8	E952.8	E982.8	
Fusidate (sodium) (ethanolamine)	960.8	E856	E950.4	E980.4	E930.8
Fusidic acid	960.8	E856	E950.4	E980.4	E930.8
Gaba	969.8	E855.8	E950.3	E980.3	E939.8
Galactose	974.5	E858.5	E950.4	E980.4	E944.5
Gallamine (triethiodide)	975.2	E858.6	E950.4	E980.4	E945.2
Gamma globulin NEC	964.6	E858.2	E950.4	E980.4	E934.6
Gamma-aminobutyric acid	969.8	E855.8	E950.3	E980.3	E939.8
Gamma-benzene hexachloride (medicinal)	976.0	E858.7	E950.4	E980.4	E946.0
– nonmedicinal (vapor)	989.2	E863.0	E950.6	E980.7	
Ganglionic blocking drug NEC	972.3	E858.3	E950.4	E980.4	E942.3
– specified NEC	972.3	E858.3	E950.4	E980.4	E942.3
Ganja	969.6	E854.1	E950.3	E980.3	E939.6
Gas	987.9	E869.9	E925.9	E982.9	
– acetylene	987.1	E868.1	E951.8	E981.8	

Substance	Poison-ing (Chapter XVII)	External Cause (E Code)			Adverse effect in correct usage
		Poisoning			
		Accident	Suicide (attempt)	Undeter-mined	
Gas - *continued*					
– air contaminants, source or type not specified	987.8	E869.9	E925.9	E982.9	
– anesthetic	968.2	E855.1	E950.4	E980.4	
– blast furnace	986	E868.8	E952.1	E982.1	
– butane - see Butane					
– carbon monoxide - see Carbon monoxide					
– chlorine	987.6	E869.8	E952.8	E982.8	
– coal - see Carbon monoxide, coal					
– cyanide	987.7	E869.8	E952.8	E982.8	
– dicyanogen	987.8	E869.8	E952.8	E982.8	
– domestic - see Gas, utility					
– exhaust - see Carbon monoxide, exhaust gas					
– from wood- or coal-burning stove or fireplace	986	E868.3	E952.1	E982.1	
– fuel (domestic use) - see also Carbon monoxide, fuel					
– – industrial use	986	E868.8	E952.1	E982.1	
– garage	986	E868.2	E952.0	E982.0	
– hydrocarbon NEC	987.1	E869.8	E952.8	E982.8	
– – liquefied - see Butane					
– hydrocyanic acid	987.7	E869.8	E952.8	E982.8	
– illuminating - see Gas, utility					
– incomplete combustion, any - see Carbon monoxide					
– kiln	986	E868.8	E952.1	E982.1	
– lacrimogenic	987.5	E869.3	E952.8	E982.8	
– – liquefied petroleum - see Butane					
– marsh	987.1	E869.8	E952.8	E982.8	
– motor exhaust, not in transit	986	E868.2	E952.0	E982.0	
– mustard, not in war	987.8	E869.8	E952.8	E982.8	
– natural	987.1	E867	E951.0	E981.0	
– nerve, not in war	987.9	E869.8	E952.8	E982.8	
– oil	981	E862.1	E950.9	E980.9	
– producer	986	E868.8	E952.1	E982.1	
– propane - see Propane					
– refrigerant (freon)	987.4	E869.2	E952.8	E982.8	
– – not freon	987.8	E869.8	E952.8	E982.8	
– sewer	987.8	E869.8	E952.8	E982.8	
– specified source NEC	987.9	E869.8	E952.8	E982.8	
– stove - see Gas, utility					
– utility (for cooking, eating, or lighting) NEC	986	E868.1	E951.8	E981.8	
– – in mobile container	987.0	E868.0	E951.1	E981.1	
– – natural	987.1	E867	E951.0	E981.0	
– – piped	986	E867	E951.0	E981.0	
– – specified type NEC	986	E868.1	E951.8	E981.8	
– water	986	E868.1	E951.8	E981.8	
Gaseous substance - see Gas					

Substance	Poison-ing (Chapter XVII)	External Cause (E Code)			
		Poisoning			Adverse effect in correct usage
		Accident	Suicide (attempt)	Undeter-mined	
Griseofulvin	960.1	E856	E950.4	E980.4	E930.1
Guaiacol derivative	975.5	E858.6	E950.4	E980.4	E945.5
Guaifenesin	975.5	E858.6	E950.4	E980.4	E945.5
Guanacline	972.6	E858.3	E950.4	E980.4	E942.6
Guanethidine	972.6	E858.3	E950.4	E980.4	E942.6
Guano	989.8	E866.5	E950.9	E980.9	
Guanochlor	972.6	E858.3	E950.4	E980.4	E942.6
Guanoxan	972.6	E858.3	E950.4	E980.4	E942.6
Guar gum	972.2	E858.3	E950.4	E980.4	E942.2
Hachimycin	960.1	E856	E950.4	E980.4	E930.1
Hag	973.0	E858.4	E950.4	E980.4	E943.0
Hair					
− dye	976.4	E858.7	E950.4	E980.4	E946.4
− preparation NEC	976.4	E858.7	E950.4	E980.4	E946.4
Halcinolone	976.0	E858.7	E950.4	E980.4	E946.0
Hallucinogen NEC	969.6	E854.1	E950.3	E980.3	E939.6
Halofenate	972.2	E858.3	E950.4	E980.4	E942.2
Haloperidol	969.2	E853.1	E950.3	E980.3	E939.2
Haloprogin	976.0	E858.7	E950.4	E980.4	E946.0
Haloquinol	961.3	E857	E950.4	E980.4	E931.3
Halothane	968.1	E855.1	E950.4	E980.4	E938.1
Hamamelis	976.2	E858.7	E950.4	E980.4	E946.2
Hartmann's solution	977.4	E858.8	E950.4	E980.4	E947.4
Hashish	969.6	E854.1	E950.3	E980.3	E939.6
HCH	989.2	E863.0	E950.6	E980.7	
HCN	989.0	E866.8	E950.9	E980.9	
Headache remedy	965.7	E850.5	E950.0	E980.0	E935.5
Health salts	973.3	E858.4	E950.4	E980.4	E943.3
Heavy metal antidote	963.8	E858.1	E950.4	E980.4	E933.8
Helium	975.8	E858.6	E950.4	E980.4	E945.8
Hematinic preparation	964.1	E858.2	E950.4	E980.4	E934.1
Hemlock	988.2	E865.4	E950.9	E980.9	
Hemostatic	976.4	E858.7	E950.4	E980.4	E946.4
− drug, systemic	964.5	E858.2	E950.4	E980.4	E934.5
Hemostyptic	976.4	E858.7	E950.4	E980.4	E946.4
Heparin (sodium)	964.2	E858.2	E950.4	E980.4	E934.2
− action reverser	964.5	E858.2	E950.4	E980.4	E934.5
Heparinoid	963.4	E858.1	E950.4	E980.4	E933.4
Hepatic secretion stimulant	973.8	E858.4	E950.4	E980.4	E943.8
Heptachlor	989.2	E863.0	E950.6	E980.7	
Heptaminol	972.4	E858.3	E950.4	E980.4	E942.4
Herbicide	989.4	E863.5	E950.6	E980.7	
Heroin	965.0	E850.0	E950.0	E980.0	E935.0
Hesperidin	963.5	E858.1	E950.4	E980.4	E933.5
Hetacillin	960.0	E856	E950.4	E980.4	E930.0
Hetastarch	974.5	E858.5	E950.4	E980.4	E944.5
HETP	989.3	E863.1	E950.6	E980.7	
Hexachlorobenzene (vapor)	989.2	E863.0	E950.6	E980.7	
Hexachlorocyclohexane	989.2	E863.0	E950.6	E980.7	
Hexachlorophene	976.0	E858.7	E950.4	E980.4	E946.0
Hexadylamine	972.4	E858.3	E950.4	E980.4	E942.4

Substance	Poison-ing (Chapter XVII)	External Cause (E Code)			Adverse effect in correct usage
		Poisoning			
		Accident	Suicide (attempt)	Undeter-mined	
Hexaethyl tetraphosphate	989.3	E863.1	E950.6	E980.7	
Hexafluorenium (bromide)	975.2	E858.6	E950.4	E980.4	E945.2
Hexafluorodiethyl ether	968.2	E855.1	E950.4	E980.4	E938.2
Hexahydrobenzol	982.8	E862.4	E950.9	E980.9	
Hexahydrocresol	980.8	E860.8	E950.9	E980.9	
− arsenide	985.1	E866.3	E950.8	E980.8	
− arseniuretted	985.1	E866.3	E950.8	E980.8	
− cyanide	989.0	E866.8	E950.9	E980.9	
− − gas	987.8	E869.8	E952.8	E982.8	
− fluoride (liquid)	983.1	E864.1	E950.7	E980.6	
− − vapor	987.8	E869.8	E952.8	E982.8	
− phosphuretted	987.8	E869.8	E952.8	E982.8	
− sulfate	983.1	E864.1	E950.7	E980.6	
− sulfide (gas)	987.8	E869.8	E952.8	E982.8	
− − arseniuretted	985.1	E866.3	E950.8	E980.8	
− sulfuretted	987.8	E869.8	E952.8	E982.8	
Hexahydrophenol	980.8	E860.8	E950.9	E980.9	
Hexamethonium bromide	972.3	E858.3	E950.4	E980.4	E942.3
Hexamethylene	982.8	E862.4	E950.9	E980.9	
Hexamine (mandelate)	961.9	E857	E950.4	E980.4	E931.9
Hexanone	982.8	E862.4	E950.9	E980.9	
Hexcarbacholine bromide	975.2	E858.6	E950.4	E980.4	E945.2
Hexestrol	962.2	E858.0	E950.4	E980.4	E932.2
Hexetidine	961.8	E857	E950.4	E980.4	E931.8
Hexobarbital	967.0	E851	E950.1	E980.1	E937.0
− rectal	968.4	E855.1	E950.4	E980.4	E938.4
− sodium	968.3	E855.1	E950.4	E980.4	E938.3
Hexocyclium	971.1	E855.4	E950.4	E980.4	E941.1
Hexone	982.8	E862.4	E950.9	E980.9	
Hexylcaine	968.5	E855.2	E950.4	E980.4	E938.5
Hexylresorcinol	983.0	E864.0	E950.7	E980.6	
HGH (human growth hormone)	962.4	E858.0	E950.4	E980.4	E932.4
Histamine (phosphate)	977.8	E858.8	E950.4	E980.4	E947.8
Histoplasmin	977.8	E858.8	E950.4	E980.4	E947.8
Homatropine	971.1	E855.4	E950.4	E980.4	E941.1
Hormone NEC	962.9	E858.0	E950.4	E980.4	E932.9
− androgenic	962.1	E858.0	E950.4	E980.4	E932.1
− anterior pituitary NEC	962.4	E858.0	E950.4	E980.4	E932.4
− antidiuretic	962.5	E858.0	E950.4	E980.4	E932.5
− cancer therapy	962.9	E858.0	E950.4	E980.4	E932.9
− luteinizing	962.4	E858.0	E950.4	E980.4	E932.4
− ovarian	962.2	E858.0	E950.4	E980.4	E932.2
− oxytocic	975.0	E858.6	E950.4	E980.4	E945.0
− pituitary (posterior) NEC	962.5	E858.0	E950.4	E980.4	E932.5
− thyroid	962.7	E858.0	E950.4	E980.4	E932.7
Horse anti-human lymphocytic serum	964.6	E858.2	E950.4	E980.4	E934.6
Human immune serum	964.6	E858.2	E950.4	E980.4	E934.6
Hyaluronidase	976.8	E858.7	E950.4	E980.4	E946.8
Hydantoin derivative NEC	966.1	E855.0	E950.4	E980.4	E936.1
Hydralazine	972.6	E858.3	E950.4	E980.4	E942.6
Hydrargaphen	976.0	E858.7	E950.4	E980.4	E946.0

Substance	Poisoning (Chapter XVII)	External Cause (E Code)			Adverse effect in correct usage
		Poisoning			
		Accident	Suicide (attempt)	Undetermined	
Hydrastine	975.3	E858.6	E950.4	E980.4	E945.3
Hydrazine	983.9	E864.3	E950.7	E980.6	
– monoamine oxidase inhibitors	969.0	E854.0	E950.3	E980.3	E939.0
Hydrazoic acid, azides	989.8	E866.8	E950.9	E980.9	
Hydriodic acid	975.5	E858.6	E950.4	E980.4	E945.5
Hydrochloric acid (liquid)	983.1	E864.1	E950.7	E980.6	
– medicinal (digestant)	973.4	E858.4	E950.4	E980.4	E943.4
– vapor	987.8	E869.8	E952.8	E982.8	
Hydrochlorothiazide	974.3	E858.5	E950.4	E980.4	E944.3
Hydrocodone	965.0	E850.0	E950.0	E980.0	E935.0
Hydrocortisone	962.0	E858.0	E950.4	E980.4	E932.0
Hydrocyanic acid (liquid)	989.0	E866.8	E950.9	E980.9	
– gas	987.7	E869.8	E952.8	E982.8	
Hydroflumethiazide	974.3	E858.5	E950.4	E980.4	E944.3
Hydrofluoric acid (liquid)	983.1	E864.1	E950.7	E980.6	
– vapor	987.8	E869.8	E952.8	E982.8	
Hydrogen	987.8	E869.8	E952.8	E982.8	
– chloride	983.1	E864.1	E950.7	E980.6	
– cyanide	989.0	E866.8	E950.9	E980.9	
– – gas	987.7	E869.8	E952.8	E982.8	
– peroxide	976.0	E858.7	E950.4	E980.4	E946.0
Hydromorphone	965.0	E850.0	E950.0	E980.0	E935.0
Hydrophilic salt	973.3	E858.4	E950.4	E980.4	E943.3
Hydroquinone	983.0	E864.0	E950.7	E980.6	
– vapor	987.8	E869.8	E952.8	E982.8	
Hydrosulfuric acid (gas)	987.8	E869.8	E952.8	E982.8	
Hydrous wool fat	976.3	E858.7	E950.4	E980.4	E946.3
Hydroxide of aluminum gel	973.0	E858.4	E950.4	E980.4	E943.0
Hydroxide, caustic	983.2	E864.2	E950.7	E980.6	
Hydroxyamphetamine	976.5	E858.7	E950.4	E980.4	E946.5
Hydroxymethylpentanone	982.8	E862.4	E950.9	E980.9	
Hydroxyprogesterone	962.2	E858.0	E950.4	E980.4	E932.2
Hydroxyquinoline (derivatives) NEC	961.3	E857	E950.4	E980.4	E931.3
Hydroxystilbamide	961.2	E857	E950.4	E980.4	E931.2
Hydroxystilbamidine	961.2	E857	E950.4	E980.4	E931.2
Hydroxytoluene	983.0	E861.4	E950.9	E980.9	
Hydroxyurea	963.1	E858.1	E950.4	E980.4	E933.1
Hydroxyzine	969.5	E853.8	E950.3	E980.3	E939.5
Hyoscine	971.1	E855.4	E950.4	E980.4	E941.1
Hyoscyamus, hyoscyamine	971.1	E855.4	E950.4	E980.4	E941.1
Hypnotic NEC	967.9	E852.9	E950.2	E980.2	E937.9
– anticonvulsant	967.8	E852.8	E950.2	E980.2	E937.8
– specified NEC	967.8	E852.8	E950.2	E980.2	E937.8
Hypochlorite	976.0	E858.7	E950.4	E980.4	E946.0
Hypotensive NEC	972.6	E858.3	E950.4	E980.4	E942.6
Hypromellose	976.5	E858.7	E950.4	E980.4	E946.5
Ibufenac	965.6	E850.4	E950.0	E980.0	E935.4
Ibuprofen	965.6	E850.4	E950.0	E980.0	E935.4
Ibuterol	975.7	E858.6	E950.4	E980.4	E945.7
Ichthammol	976.4	E858.7	E950.4	E980.4	E946.4
Idoxuridine	976.5	E858.7	E950.4	E980.4	E946.5

Substance	Poison-ing (Chapter XVII)	External Cause (E Code)			Adverse effect in correct usage
		Poisoning			
		Accident	Suicide (attempt)	Undeter-mined	
Illuminating gas - see Gas, utility					
Imipramine	969.0	E854.0	E950.3	E980.3	E939.0
Immune					
– globulin	964.6	E858.2	E950.4	E980.4	E934.6
– serum globulin	964.6	E858.2	E950.4	E980.4	E934.6
Immunoglobin					
– human	964.6	E858.2	E950.4	E980.4	E934.6
Immunosuppressive drug	963.1	E858.1	E950.4	E980.4	E933.1
Indandione (derivatives)	964.2	E858.2	E950.4	E980.4	E934.2
Indian hemp	969.6	E854.1	E950.3	E980.3	E939.6
Indigo carmine	977.8	E858.8	E950.4	E980.4	E947.8
Indometacin	965.6	E850.4	E950.0	E980.0	E935.4
Indoramin	971.3	E855.6	E950.4	E980.4	E941.3
Ingested substances NEC	989.9	E866.9	E950.9	E980.9	
INH	961.8	E857	E950.4	E980.4	E931.8
Inhalation medicaments	975.6	E858.6	E950.4	E980.4	E945.6
Inhibitor					
– fibrinolysis	964.4	E858.2	E950.4	E980.4	E934.4
– monoamine oxidase NEC	969.0	E854.0	E950.3	E980.3	E939.0
– – hydrazine	969.0	E854.0	E950.3	E980.3	E939.0
– postsynaptic	969.8	E855.8	E950.3	E980.3	E939.8
– protease	964.4	E858.2	E950.4	E980.4	E934.4
– prothrombin synthesis	964.2	E858.2	E950.4	E980.4	E934.2
– steroid synthesis	962.9	E858.0	E950.4	E980.4	E932.9
Inoleic acid	972.2	E858.3	E950.4	E980.4	E942.2
Inositol	977.1	E858.8	E950.4	E980.4	E947.1
– nicotinate	972.2	E858.3	E950.4	E980.4	E942.2
Insect (sting), venomous	989.5	E905.	E950.9	E980.9	
Insecticide NEC	989.4	E863.4	E950.6	E980.7	
– carbamates	989.3	E863.2	E950.6	E980.7	
– mixed	989.4	E863.3	E950.6	E980.7	
– organochlorine	989.2	E863.0	E950.6	E980.7	
– organophosphorus	989.3	E863.1	E950.6	E980.7	
Insular tissue extract	962.3	E858.0	E950.4	E980.4	E932.3
Insulin NEC	962.3	E858.0	E950.4	E980.4	E932.3
– protamine zinc	962.3	E858.0	E950.4	E980.4	E932.3
– slow acting	962.3	E858.0	E950.4	E980.4	E932.3
– zinc suspension (amorphous)	962.3	E858.0	E950.4	E980.4	E932.3
Interferon	979.9	E858.8	E950.4	E980.4	E949.9
Intestinal motility control drug	973.5	E858.4	E950.4	E980.4	E943.5
– biological	973.8	E858.4	E950.4	E980.4	E943.8
Intravenous					
– aminoacids	977.0	E858.8	E950.4	E980.4	E947.0
– fat suspension	977.0	E858.8	E950.4	E980.4	E947.0
Invert sugar	974.5	E858.5	E950.4	E980.4	E944.5
Iobenzamic acid	977.8	E858.8	E950.4	E980.4	E947.8
Iocetamic acid	977.8	E858.8	E950.4	E980.4	E947.8
Iodide NEC	975.5	E858.6	E950.4	E980.4	E945.5
Iodinated contrast medium	977.8	E858.8	E950.4	E980.4	E947.8
Iodine (antiseptic, external) (tincture) NEC	976.0	E858.7	E950.4	E980.4	E946.0
– vapor	987.8	E869.8	E952.8	E982.8	

Substance	Poison-ing (Chapter XVII)	External Cause (E Code)			
		Poisoning			Adverse effect in correct usage
		Accident	Suicide (attempt)	Undeter-mined	
Iodipamide	977.8	E858.8	E950.4	E980.4	E947.8
Iodized (poppy seed) oil	977.8	E858.8	E950.4	E980.4	E947.8
Iodochlorhydroxyquinoline	961.3	E857	E950.4	E980.4	E931.3
Iodoform	976.0	E858.7	E950.4	E980.4	E946.0
Iodohippuric acid	977.8	E858.8	E950.4	E980.4	E947.8
Iodophthalein	977.8	E858.8	E950.4	E980.4	E947.8
Iodopyracet	977.8	E858.8	E950.4	E980.4	E947.8
Iodoquinolin	961.3	E857	E950.4	E980.4	E931.3
Iofendylate	977.8	E858.8	E950.4	E980.4	E947.8
Ioglycamic acid	977.8	E858.8	E950.4	E980.4	E947.8
Ion exchange resin					
− anion	973.8	E858.4	E950.4	E980.4	E943.8
− cation	974.5	E858.5	E950.4	E980.4	E944.5
− cholestyramine	972.2	E858.3	E950.4	E980.4	E942.2
− intestinal	973.8	E858.4	E950.4	E980.4	E943.8
Iopanoic acid	977.8	E858.8	E950.4	E980.4	E947.8
Iophendyte	977.8	E858.8	E950.4	E980.4	E947.8
Iophenoic acid	977.8	E858.8	E950.4	E980.4	E947.8
Iopydol	977.8	E858.8	E950.4	E980.4	E947.8
Iotalamic acid	977.8	E858.8	E950.4	E980.4	E947.8
Ipecacuanha, ipecac	975.5	E858.6	E950.4	E980.4	E945.5
Ipodate (sodium)	977.8	E858.8	E950.4	E980.4	E947.8
Ipratropium (bromide)	975.7	E858.6	E950.4	E980.4	E945.7
Iprindole	969.0	E854.0	E950.3	E980.3	E939.0
Iproniazid	969.0	E854.0	E950.3	E980.3	E939.0
Iproveratril	972.0	E858.3	E950.4	E980.4	E942.0
Iron (compounds) (medicinal) NEC	964.0	E858.2	E950.4	E980.4	E934.0
− and ammonium citrate	964.0	E858.2	E950.4	E980.4	E934.0
− dextran injection	964.0	E858.2	E950.4	E980.4	E934.0
− nonmedicinal (fumes) (dust) NEC	985.8	E866.4	E950.9	E980.9	
− sorbital citric acid complex	964.0	E858.2	E950.4	E980.4	E934.0
− sorbitex	964.0	E858.2	E950.4	E980.4	E934.0
Irrigating fluid	976.8	E858.7	E950.4	E980.4	E946.8
− eye	976.5	E858.7	E950.4	E980.4	E946.5
Isoamanile (citrate)	975.4	E858.6	E950.4	E980.4	E945.4
Isobenzan	989.4	E863.4	E950.6	E980.7	
Isobutyl acetate	982.8	E862.4	E950.9	E980.9	
Isocarboxazid	969.0	E854.0	E950.3	E980.3	E939.0
Isoetarine	975.7	E858.6	E950.4	E980.4	E945.7
Isoethadione	966.0	E855.0	E950.4	E980.4	E936.0
Isoflurophate	971.0	E855.3	E950.4	E980.4	E941.0
Isometheptene	971.2	E855.5	E950.4	E980.4	E941.2
Isoniazid	961.8	E857	E950.4	E980.4	E931.8
Isonicotinic acid hydrazide	961.8	E857	E950.4	E980.4	E931.8
Isonipecaine	965.0	E850.0	E950.0	E980.0	E935.0
Isophorone	989.8	E866.8	E950.9	E980.9	
Isoprenaline	975.7	E858.6	E950.4	E980.4	E945.7
Isopropamide	971.1	E855.4	E950.4	E980.4	E941.1
Isopropanol	980.2	E860.3	E950.9	E980.9	
Isopropyl					
− acetate	982.8	E862.4	E950.9	E980.9	

Substance	Poison-ing (Chapter XVII)	External Cause (E Code)			Adverse effect in correct usage
		Poisoning			
		Accident	Suicide (attempt)	Undeter-mined	
Isopropyl - *continued*					
– alcohol	980.2	E860.3	E950.9	E980.9	
– – medicinal	976.4	E858.7	E950.4	E980.4	E946.4
– ether	982.8	E862.4	E950.9	E980.9	
Isoproterenol	975.7	E858.6	E950.4	E980.4	E945.7
Isosorbide dinitrate	972.4	E858.3	E950.4	E980.4	E942.4
Isothipendyl	963.0	E858.1	E950.4	E980.4	E933.0
Isoxsuprine	972.5	E858.3	E950.4	E980.4	E942.5
Ispaghula	973.3	E858.4	E950.4	E980.4	E943.3
Izal (disinfectant)	983.0	E861.4	E950.9	E980.9	
Jalap	973.1	E858.4	E950.4	E980.4	E943.1
Jamaica ginger	989.8	E866.8	E950.9	E980.9	
Jimson weed	988.2	E865.4	E950.9	E980.9	
Juniper tar	976.1	E858.7	E950.4	E980.4	E946.1
Kallikrein	972.5	E858.3	E950.4	E980.4	E942.5
Kanamycin	960.6	E856	E950.4	E980.4	E930.6
Kaolin	973.5	E858.4	E950.4	E980.4	E943.5
Keratolytic drug NEC	976.4	E858.7	E950.4	E980.4	E946.4
– anthracene	976.4	E858.7	E950.4	E980.4	E946.4
Keratoplastic NEC	976.4	E858.7	E950.4	E980.4	E946.4
Kerosene, kerosine (fuel) (solvent) NEC	981	E862.1	E950.9	E980.9	
– insecticide	981	E863.4	E950.6	E980.7	
– vapor	987.1	E862.1	E950.9	E980.9	
Ketamine	968.3	E855.1	E950.4	E980.4	E938.3
Ketobemidone	965.0	E850.0	E950.0	E980.0	E935.0
Ketols	982.8	E862.4	E950.9	E980.9	
Ketone oils	982.8	E862.4	E950.9	E980.9	
Ketoprofen	965.6	E850.4	E950.0	E980.0	E935.4
Khat	969.7	E854.2	E950.3	E980.3	E939.7
Khelline	972.4	E858.3	E950.4	E980.4	E942.4
Kiln gas or vapor (carbon monoxide)	986	E868.8	E952.1	E982.1	
Kwell (insecticide)	989.2	E863.0	E950.6	E980.7	
Labetalol	972.6	E858.3	E950.4	E980.4	E942.6
Laburnum (seeds)	988.2	E865.3	E950.9	E980.9	
Lachesine	976.5	E858.7	E950.4	E980.4	E946.5
Lacquers	989.8	E861.6	E950.9	E980.9	
Lactated potassic saline	974.6	E858.5	E950.4	E980.4	E944.6
Lactic acid	976.8	E858.7	E950.4	E980.4	E946.8
Lactobacillus acidophilus	973.8	E858.4	E950.4	E980.4	E943.8
Lactulose	973.3	E858.4	E950.4	E980.4	E943.3
Laevo - see Levo-					
Lanatoside-C	972.1	E858.3	E950.4	E980.4	E942.1
Lanoline	976.3	E858.7	E950.4	E980.4	E946.3
Lassar's paste	976.4	E858.7	E950.4	E980.4	E946.4
Lauryl sulfoacetate	976.2	E858.7	E950.4	E980.4	E946.2
Lead (dust) (fumes) (vapor) NEC	984.9	E866.0	E950.9	E980.9	
– acetate	976.2	E858.7	E950.4	E980.4	E946.2
– alkyl (fuel additive)	984.1	E862.1	E950.9	E980.9	
– arsenate, arsenite (dust) (herbicide) (insecticide) (vapor)	985.1	E863.9	E950.6	E980.7	
– inorganic	984.0	E866.0	E950.9	E980.9	

Substance	Poison-ing (Chapter XVII)	External Cause (E Code)			Adverse effect in correct usage
		Poisoning			
		Accident	Suicide (attempt)	Undeter-mined	
Lead - *continued*					
− organic	984.1	E866.0	E950.9	E980.9	
Leptazol	970.0	E854.3	E950.4	E980.4	E940.0
Leucovorin (factor)	964.1	E858.2	E950.4	E980.4	E934.1
Levallorphan	970.1	E854.3	E950.4	E980.4	E940.1
Levarterenol	971.2	E855.5	E950.4	E980.4	E941.2
Levodopa	966.4	E855.0	E950.4	E980.4	E936.4
Levomepromazine	969.3	E853.8	E950.3	E980.3	E939.3
Levopropoxyphene	975.4	E858.6	E950.4	E980.4	E945.4
Levoproxyphylline	975.1	E858.6	E950.4	E980.4	E945.1
Levorphanol	965.0	E850.0	E950.0	E980.0	E935.0
Levothyroxine	962.7	E858.0	E950.4	E980.4	E932.7
Levulose	974.5	E858.5	E950.4	E980.4	E944.5
Lewisite (gas), not in war	985.1	E866.3	E950.8	E980.8	
Lidocaine	968.5	E855.2	E950.4	E980.4	E938.5
− regional	968.6	E855.2	E950.4	E980.4	E938.6
− spinal	968.7	E855.2	E950.4	E980.4	E938.7
Lighter fluid	981	E862.1	E950.9	E980.9	
Lignin hemicellulose	973.5	E858.4	E950.4	E980.4	E943.5
Lignocaine	968.5	E855.2	E950.4	E980.4	E938.5
− regional	968.6	E855.2	E950.4	E980.4	E938.6
− spinal	968.7	E855.2	E950.4	E980.4	E938.7
Ligroin(e) (solvent)	981	E862.0	E950.9	E980.9	
− vapor	987.1	E862.0	E950.9	E980.9	
Lime (chloride)	983.2	E864.2	E950.7	E980.6	
Limonene	982.8	E862.4	E950.9	E980.9	
Lincomycin	960.3	E856	E950.4	E980.4	E930.3
Lindane (insecticide) (nonmedicinal) (vapor)	989.2	E863.0	E950.6	E980.7	
− medicinal	976.0	E858.7	E950.4	E980.4	E946.0
Linolenic acid	972.2	E858.3	E950.4	E980.4	E942.2
Linseed	976.3	E858.7	E950.4	E980.4	E946.3
Liothyronine	962.7	E858.0	E950.4	E980.4	E932.7
Liotrix	962.7	E858.0	E950.4	E980.4	E932.7
Lipotropic drug NEC	977.1	E858.8	E950.4	E980.4	E947.1
Liquid paraffin	973.2	E858.4	E950.4	E980.4	E943.2
Liquid substance NEC	989.9	E866.9	E950.9	E980.9	
Liquor creosolis compositus	983.0	E861.4	E950.9	E980.9	
Liquorice extract	973.8	E858.4	E950.4	E980.4	E943.8
Lithium	985.8	E866.4	E950.9	E980.9	
− salts	969.8	E855.8	E950.3	E980.3	E939.8
Liver extract	964.1	E858.2	E950.4	E980.4	E934.1
Lobeline	970.0	E854.3	E950.4	E980.4	E940.0
Local action drug NEC	976.9	E858.7	E950.4	E980.4	E946.9
− specified NEC	976.8	E858.7	E950.4	E980.4	E946.8
Loperamide	973.5	E858.4	E950.4	E980.4	E943.5
Lorazepam	969.4	E853.2	E950.3	E980.3	E939.4
LSD	969.6	E854.1	E950.3	E980.3	E939.6
L-tryptophan	969.0	E854.0	E950.3	E980.3	E939.0
Lubricant, eye	976.5	E858.7	E950.4	E980.4	E946.5
Lubricating oil NEC	981	E862.2	E950.9	E980.9	

Substance	Poisoning (Chapter XVII)	External Cause (E Code)			Adverse effect in correct usage
		Poisoning			
		Accident	Suicide (attempt)	Undetermined	
Lucanthone	961.6	E857	E950.4	E980.4	E931.6
Lung irritant (gas) NEC	987.8	E869.8	E952.8	E982.8	
Lung tissue extract	964.5	E858.2	E950.4	E980.4	E934.5
Luteinizing hormone	962.4	E858.0	E950.4	E980.4	E932.4
Lututrin	975.1	E858.6	E950.4	E980.4	E945.1
Lye (concentrated)	983.2	E864.2	E950.7	E980.6	
Lymecycline	960.4	E856	E950.4	E980.4	E930.4
Lymphogranuloma venereum antigen	977.8	E858.8	E950.4	E980.4	E947.8
Lynestrenol	962.2	E858.0	E950.4	E980.4	E932.2
Lypressin	962.5	E858.0	E950.4	E980.4	E932.5
Lysergic acid diethylamide	969.6	E854.1	E950.3	E980.3	E939.6
Lysergide	969.6	E854.1	E950.3	E980.3	E939.6
Lysol	983.0	E861.4	E950.9	E980.9	
Lytic cocktail	965.8	E850.8	E950.0	E980.0	E935.8
Macrisalb	977.4	E858.8	E950.4	E980.4	E947.4
Macrogol	977.4	E858.8	E950.4	E980.4	E947.4
Macrolide NEC	964.8	E858.2	E950.4	E980.4	E934.8
− antibiotic	960.3	E856	E950.4	E980.4	E930.3
Mafenide	976.0	E858.7	E950.4	E980.4	E946.0
Magaldrate	973.0	E858.4	E950.4	E980.4	E943.0
Magnesia magma	973.0	E858.4	E950.4	E980.4	E943.0
Magnesium NEC	985.8	E866.4	E950.9	E980.9	
− carbonate	973.0	E858.4	E950.4	E980.4	E943.0
− choline	977.0	E858.8	E950.4	E980.4	E947.0
− citrate	973.3	E858.4	E950.4	E980.4	E943.3
− fumes	987.8	E869.8	E952.8	E982.8	
− hydroxide	973.0	E858.4	E950.4	E980.4	E943.0
− silicofluoride	974.6	E858.5	E950.4	E980.4	E944.6
− sodium citrate	977.0	E858.8	E950.4	E980.4	E947.0
− sulfate	973.3	E858.4	E950.4	E980.4	E943.3
− thiosulfate	963.0	E858.1	E950.4	E980.4	E933.0
− trisilicate	973.0	E858.4	E950.4	E980.4	E943.0
Majoon	969.6	E854.1	E950.3	E980.3	E939.6
Malathion (medicinal)	976.0	E858.7	E950.4	E980.4	E946.0
− insecticide	989.3	E863.1	E950.6	E980.7	
Male fern extract	961.6	E857	E950.4	E980.4	E931.6
Mandelic acid	961.9	E857	E950.4	E980.4	E931.9
Manganese (dioxide) (nonmedicinal)	985.2	E866.4	E950.9	E980.9	
− medicinal (trace)	964.1	E858.2	E950.4	E980.4	E934.1
Mannitol	974.4	E858.5	E950.4	E980.4	E944.4
− hexanitrate	972.4	E858.3	E950.4	E980.4	E942.4
Mannomustine	963.1	E858.1	E950.4	E980.4	E933.1
Maphenide	976.0	E858.7	E950.4	E980.4	E946.0
Marihuana	969.6	E854.1	E950.3	E980.3	E939.6
Marsh gas	987.1	E869.8	E952.8	E982.8	
Mazindol	977.0	E858.8	E950.4	E980.4	E947.0
MCPA	989.2	E863.5	E950.6	E980.7	
Measles virus vaccine (attenuated)	979.4	E858.8	E950.4	E980.4	E949.4
Meat, noxious	988.8	E865.0	E950.9	E980.9	
Mebanazine	969.0	E854.0	E950.3	E980.3	E939.0
Mebendazole	961.6	E857	E950.4	E980.4	E931.6

Substance	Poison-ing (Chapter XVII)	External Cause (E Code)			
		Poisoning			Adverse effect in correct usage
		Accident	Suicide (attempt)	Undeter-mined	
Mebeverine	975.1	E858.6	E950.4	E980.4	E945.1
Mebhydrolin	963.0	E858.1	E950.4	E980.4	E933.0
Mebutamate	972.6	E858.3	E950.4	E980.4	E942.6
Mecamine	972.3	E858.3	E950.4	E980.4	E942.3
Mecamylamine	972.3	E858.3	E950.4	E980.4	E942.3
Mechlorethamine	963.1	E858.1	E950.4	E980.4	E933.1
Mecillinam	960.8	E856	E950.4	E980.4	E930.8
Meclizine	963.0	E858.1	E950.4	E980.4	E933.0
Meclofenoxate	969.7	E854.2	E950.3	E980.3	E939.7
Meclozine	963.0	E858.1	E950.4	E980.4	E933.0
Mecoprop	989.2	E863.5	E950.6	E980.7	
Medazepam	969.4	E853.2	E950.3	E980.3	E939.4
Medicament NEC	977.9	E858.9	E950.5	E980.5	E947.9
− local NEC	976.4	E858.7	E950.4	E980.4	E946.4
− specified NEC	977.8	E858.8	E950.4	E980.4	E947.8
Medroxyprogesterone	962.2	E858.0	E950.4	E980.4	E932.2
Medrysone	976.0	E858.7	E950.4	E980.4	E946.0
Mefenamic acid	965.6	E850.4	E950.0	E980.0	E935.4
Mefruside	974.3	E858.5	E950.4	E980.4	E944.3
Megestrol	962.2	E858.0	E950.4	E980.4	E932.2
Meglumine					
− antilmoniate	961.2	E857	E950.4	E980.4	E931.2
− diatrizoate	977.8	E858.8	E950.4	E980.4	E947.8
− iodipamide	977.8	E858.8	E950.4	E980.4	E947.8
MEK	982.8	E862.4	E950.9	E980.9	
Melarsonyl	961.1	E857	E950.4	E980.4	E931.1
Melarsoprol	961.1	E857	E950.4	E980.4	E931.1
Melphalan	963.1	E858.1	E950.4	E980.4	E933.1
Menadiol	964.3	E858.2	E950.4	E980.4	E934.3
Menadione	964.3	E858.2	E950.4	E980.4	E934.3
Menaphtone	964.3	E858.2	E950.4	E980.4	E934.3
Menaquinone	964.3	E858.2	E950.4	E980.4	E934.3
Menthol	975.6	E858.6	E950.4	E980.4	E945.6
Mepacrine	961.4	E857	E950.4	E980.4	E931.4
Meparfynol	967.8	E852.8	E950.2	E980.2	E937.8
Mepenzolate	971.1	E855.4	E950.4	E980.4	E941.1
Meperidine	965.0	E850.0	E950.0	E980.0	E935.0
Mephenamine	971.1	E855.4	E950.4	E980.4	E941.1
Mephenesin	968.0	E855.1	E950.4	E980.4	E938.0
Mephenoxalone	969.5	E853.8	E950.3	E980.3	E939.5
Mephentermine	971.2	E855.5	E950.4	E980.4	E941.2
Mephenytoin	966.1	E855.0	E950.4	E980.4	E936.1
− with phenobarbital	966.3	E855.0	E950.4	E980.4	E936.3
Mephobarbital	967.0	E851	E950.1	E980.1	E937.0
Mepivacaine, epidural	968.7	E855.2	E950.4	E980.4	E938.7
Meprednisone	962.9	E858.0	E950.4	E980.4	E932.9
Meprobamate	969.5	E853.8	E950.3	E980.3	E939.5
Meprophenhydramine	963.0	E858.1	E950.4	E980.4	E933.0
Meprylcaine	968.5	E855.2	E950.4	E980.4	E938.5
Mepyramine	963.0	E858.1	E950.4	E980.4	E933.0
Meralluride	974.0	E858.5	E950.4	E980.4	E944.0

Substance	Poisoning (Chapter XVII)	External Cause (E Code)			
		Poisoning			Adverse effect in correct usage
		Accident	Suicide (attempt)	Undetermined	
Merbromin	976.0	E858.7	E950.4	E980.4	E946.0
Mercaptomerin	974.0	E858.5	E950.4	E980.4	E944.0
Mercaptopurine	963.1	E858.1	E950.4	E980.4	E933.1
Mercuramide	974.0	E858.5	E950.4	E980.4	E944.0
Mercurophylline	974.0	E858.5	E950.4	E980.4	E944.0
Mercury, mercurial, mercuric, mercurous (compounds) (cyanide) (fumes) (nonmedicinal) (vapor) NEC	985.0	E866.1	E950.9	E980.9	
– anti-infective					
– – local	976.0	E858.7	E950.4	E980.4	E946.0
– – systemic	961.2	E857	E950.4	E980.4	E931.2
– bichloride	985.0	E863.6	E950.6	E980.7	
– diuretic NEC	974.0	E858.5	E950.4	E980.4	E944.0
– insecticide (vapor)	989.4	E863.4	E950.6	E980.7	
– organic (fungicide) (seed dressing)	989.4	E863.6	E950.6	E980.7	
Mersalyl	974.0	E858.5	E950.4	E980.4	E944.0
Merthiolate	976.0	E858.7	E950.4	E980.4	E946.0
Mescaline	969.6	E854.1	E950.3	E980.3	E939.6
Mesoridazine	969.1	E853.0	E950.3	E980.3	E939.1
Mestanolone	962.1	E858.0	E950.4	E980.4	E932.1
Mestranol	962.2	E858.0	E950.4	E980.4	E932.2
Mesuximide	966.2	E855.0	E950.4	E980.4	E936.2
Metabutethamine	968.5	E855.2	E950.4	E980.4	E938.5
Metacresylate	976.6	E858.7	E950.4	E980.4	E946.6
Metacycline	960.4	E856	E950.4	E980.4	E930.4
Metaldehyde (snail killer) NEC	989.4	E863.9	E950.6	E980.7	
Metals (heavy) (nonmedicinal) NEC	985.9	E866.4	E950.9	E980.9	
– anti-infective	961.2	E857	E950.4	E980.4	E931.2
– dust, fumes, or vapor NEC	985.9	E866.4	E950.9	E980.9	
– light NEC	985.8	E866.4	E950.9	E980.9	
– – dust, fumes or vapor NEC	987.8	E869.8	E952.8	E982.8	
– pesticides (dust) (vapor)	989.4	E863.9	E950.6	E980.7	
Metamizole	965.5	E850.3	E950.0	E980.0	E935.3
Metaproterenol	975.1	E858.6	E950.4	E980.4	E945.1
Metaraminol	972.8	E858.3	E950.4	E980.4	E942.8
Metaxalone	968.0	E855.1	E950.4	E980.4	E938.0
Metergoline	966.4	E855.0	E950.4	E980.4	E936.4
Metformin	962.3	E858.0	E950.4	E980.4	E932.3
Methacholine	971.0	E855.3	E950.4	E980.4	E941.0
Methadone	965.0	E850.0	E950.0	E980.0	E935.0
Methallenestril	962.2	E858.0	E950.4	E980.4	E932.2
Methallenoestril	962.2	E858.0	E950.4	E980.4	E932.2
Methamphetamine	969.7	E854.2	E950.3	E980.3	E939.7
Methampyrone	965.5	E850.3	E950.0	E980.0	E935.3
Methandienone	962.1	E858.0	E950.4	E980.4	E932.1
Methandrostanolone	962.1	E858.0	E950.4	E980.4	E932.1
Methane	987.1	E869.8	E952.8	E982.8	
Methanethiol	987.8	E869.8	E952.8	E982.8	
Methanol	980.1	E860.2	E950.9	E980.9	
– vapor	987.8	E869.8	E952.8	E982.8	
Methantheline	971.1	E855.4	E950.4	E980.4	E941.1

Substance	Poisoning (Chapter XVII)	External Cause (E Code)			Adverse effect in correct usage
		Poisoning			
		Accident	Suicide (attempt)	Undetermined	
Methapyrilene	963.0	E858.1	E950.4	E980.4	E933.0
Methaqualone (compound)	967.4	E852.3	E950.2	E980.2	E937.4
Metharbital	967.0	E851	E950.1	E980.1	E937.0
Methazolamide	974.2	E858.5	E950.4	E980.4	E944.2
Methdilazine	969.1	E853.0	E950.3	E980.3	E939.1
Methenamine	961.9	E857	E950.4	E980.4	E931.9
Methenolone	962.1	E858.0	E950.4	E980.4	E932.1
Methimazole	962.8	E858.0	E950.4	E980.4	E932.8
Methionine	977.1	E858.8	E950.4	E980.4	E947.1
Methixene	971.1	E855.4	E950.4	E980.4	E941.1
Methocarbamol	968.0	E855.1	E950.4	E980.4	E938.0
– smooth muscle relaxant	975.2	E858.6	E950.4	E980.4	E945.2
Methohexital	968.3	E855.1	E950.4	E980.4	E938.3
Methohexitone	968.3	E855.1	E950.4	E980.4	E938.3
Methoin	966.1	E855.0	E950.4	E980.4	E936.1
Methoserpidine	972.6	E858.3	E950.4	E980.4	E942.6
Methotrexate	963.1	E858.1	E950.4	E980.4	E933.1
Methotrimeprazine	969.3	E853.8	E950.3	E980.3	E939.3
Methoxamine	971.2	E855.5	E950.4	E980.4	E941.2
Methoxsalen	976.3	E858.7	E950.4	E980.4	E946.3
Methoxyaniline	989.8	E866.8	E950.9	E980.9	
Methoxychlor	989.2	E863.0	E950.6	E980.7	
Methoxy-DDT	989.2	E863.0	E950.6	E980.7	
Methoxyflurane	968.2	E855.1	E950.4	E980.4	E938.2
Methoxyphenamine	975.7	E858.6	E950.4	E980.4	E945.7
Methscopolamine	971.1	E855.4	E950.4	E980.4	E941.1
Methsuximide	966.2	E855.0	E950.4	E980.4	E936.2
Methyclothiazide	974.3	E858.5	E950.4	E980.4	E944.3
Methyl					
– acetate	982.8	E862.4	E950.9	E980.9	
– acetone	982.8	E862.4	E950.9	E980.9	
– acrylate	989.8	E866.8	E950.9	E980.9	
– alcohol	980.1	E860.2	E950.9	E980.9	
– aminophenol	989.8	E866.8	E950.9	E980.9	
– benzene	982.0	E862.4	E950.9	E980.9	
– benzoate	982.8	E862.4	E950.9	E980.9	
– benzol	982.0	E862.4	E950.9	E980.9	
– bromide (gas)	987.8	E869.8	E952.8	E982.8	
– – fumigant	987.8	E863.8	E950.6	E980.7	
– butanol	980.3	E860.4	E950.9	E980.9	
– cellosolve	982.8	E862.4	E950.9	E980.9	
– chloride (gas)	987.8	E869.8	E952.8	E982.8	
– chloroformate	987.5	E869.3	E952.8	E982.8	
– cyclohexane	982.8	E862.4	E950.9	E980.9	
– cyclohexanol	980.8	E860.8	E950.9	E980.9	
– cyclohexanone	982.8	E862.4	E950.9	E980.9	
– cyclohexyl acetate	982.8	E862.4	E950.9	E980.9	
– demeton	989.3	E863.1	E950.6	E980.7	
– ethyl ketone	982.8	E862.4	E950.9	E980.9	
– glucamine antimonate	961.2	E857	E950.4	E980.4	E931.2
– hydrazine	983.9	E864.3	E950.7	E980.6	

Substance	Poisoning (Chapter XVII)	External Cause (E Code)			Adverse effect in correct usage
		Poisoning			
		Accident	Suicide (attempt)	Undetermined	
Methyl - *continued*					
– isobutyl ketone	982.8	E862.4	E950.9	E980.9	
– mercaptan	987.8	E869.8	E952.8	E982.8	
– paraben	976.0	E858.7	E950.4	E980.4	E946.0
– parathion	989.3	E863.1	E950.6	E980.7	
– propylcarbinol	980.3	E860.4	E950.9	E980.9	
– salicylate	976.2	E858.7	E950.4	E980.4	E946.2
– sulfate (fumes)	987.8	E869.8	E952.8	E982.8	
– – liquid	983.9	E864.3	E950.7	E980.6	
Methylamphetamine	969.7	E854.2	E950.3	E980.3	E939.7
Methylated spirit	980.1	E860.2	E950.9	E980.9	
Methylatropine	971.1	E855.4	E950.4	E980.4	E941.1
Methylcellulose					
– laxative	973.3	E858.4	E950.4	E980.4	E943.3
Methylchlorophenoxyacetic acid	989.2	E863.5	E950.6	E980.7	
Methyldopa	972.6	E858.3	E950.4	E980.4	E942.6
Methylene					
– blue	961.9	E857	E950.4	E980.4	E931.9
– chloride or dichloride (solvent) NEC	982.3	E862.4	E950.9	E980.9	
– – vapor NEC	987.8	E862.4	E950.9	E980.9	
Methylergometrine	975.0	E858.6	E950.4	E980.4	E945.0
Methylergonovine	975.0	E858.6	E950.4	E980.4	E945.0
Methylethyl cellulose	977.4	E858.8	E950.4	E980.4	E947.4
Methylmeprobamate	969.5	E853.8	E950.3	E980.3	E939.5
Methylmorphine	965.0	E850.0	E950.0	E980.0	E935.0
Methylnicotinate	976.4	E858.7	E950.4	E980.4	E946.4
Methylparafynol	967.8	E852.8	E950.2	E980.2	E937.8
Methylphenidate	969.7	E854.2	E950.3	E980.3	E939.7
Methylphenobarbital	967.0	E851	E950.1	E980.1	E937.0
Methylpolysiloxane	973.0	E858.4	E950.4	E980.4	E943.0
Methylprednisolone	962.0	E858.0	E950.4	E980.4	E932.0
Methylrosaniline	976.0	E858.7	E950.4	E980.4	E946.0
Methylrosanilinium chloride	976.0	E858.7	E950.4	E980.4	E946.0
Methyltestosterone	962.1	E858.0	E950.4	E980.4	E932.1
Methylthionine chloride	961.9	E857	E950.4	E980.4	E931.9
Methylthiouracil	962.8	E858.0	E950.4	E980.4	E932.8
Methyprylon	967.8	E852.8	E950.2	E980.2	E937.8
Methysergide	972.6	E858.3	E950.4	E980.4	E942.6
Metiamide	973.0	E858.4	E950.4	E980.4	E943.0
Meticillin	960.0	E856	E950.4	E980.4	E930.0
Metisazone	961.7	E857	E950.4	E980.4	E931.7
Metixene	975.1	E858.6	E950.4	E980.4	E945.1
Metizoline	975.6	E858.6	E950.4	E980.4	E945.6
Metoclopramide	963.0	E858.1	E950.4	E980.4	E933.0
Metolazine	972.6	E858.3	E950.4	E980.4	E942.6
Metoprolol	972.0	E858.3	E950.4	E980.4	E942.0
Metrizoic acid	977.8	E858.8	E950.4	E980.4	E947.8
Metronidazole	976.0	E858.7	E950.4	E980.4	E946.0
Metyrapone	962.9	E858.0	E950.4	E980.4	E932.9
Mexenone	976.3	E858.7	E950.4	E980.4	E946.3
Mexiletine	972.0	E858.3	E950.4	E980.4	E942.0

Substance	Poisoning (Chapter XVII)	External Cause (E Code)			Adverse effect in correct usage
		Accident	Suicide (attempt)	Undetermined	
Mianserin	969.0	E854.0	E950.3	E980.3	E939.0
Miconazole	976.0	E858.7	E950.4	E980.4	E946.0
Milk of magnesia	973.0	E858.4	E950.4	E980.4	E943.0
Mineral					
– oil (laxative) (medicinal)	973.2	E858.4	E950.4	E980.4	E943.2
– – nonmedicinal	981	E862.2	E950.9	E980.9	
– salt NEC	974.6	E858.5	E950.4	E980.4	E944.6
Mineralocorticosteroid	962.0	E858.0	E950.4	E980.4	E932.0
Minocycline	960.4	E856	E950.4	E980.4	E930.4
Minoxidil	972.8	E858.3	E950.4	E980.4	E942.8
Miotic drug	976.5	E858.7	E950.4	E980.4	E946.5
Mipafox	971.0	E855.3	E950.4	E980.4	E941.0
Mirex	989.2	E863.0	E950.6	E980.7	
Mithramycin	960.7	E856	E950.4	E980.4	E930.7
Mitobronitol	963.1	E858.1	E950.4	E980.4	E933.1
Mitomycin	960.7	E856	E950.4	E980.4	E930.7
Mitotane	963.1	E858.1	E950.4	E980.4	E933.1
Mofebutazone	965.5	E850.3	E950.0	E980.0	E935.3
Molindone	969.5	E853.8	E950.3	E980.3	E939.5
Monoamine oxidase inhibitor NEC	969.0	E854.0	E950.3	E980.3	E939.0
– hydrazine	969.0	E854.0	E950.3	E980.3	E939.0
Monobenzone	976.4	E858.7	E950.4	E980.4	E946.4
Monochlorobenzene	982.0	E862.4	E950.9	E980.9	
Monoethanolamine	972.7	E858.3	E950.4	E980.4	E942.7
Monophenylbutazone	965.5	E850.3	E950.0	E980.0	E935.3
Monosulfiram	976.0	E858.7	E950.4	E980.4	E946.0
Monoxide, carbon - see Carbon monoxide					
Monuron	989.4	E863.5	E950.6	E980.7	
MOPP (mustard, vincristine, prednisone, procarbazine)	963.1	E858.1	E950.4	E980.4	E933.1
Morinamide	961.8	E857	E950.4	E980.4	E931.8
Morphazinamide	961.8	E857	E950.4	E980.4	E931.8
Morphine	965.0	E850.0	E950.0	E980.0	E935.0
– antagonist	970.1	E854.3	E950.4	E980.4	E940.1
Moth balls	989.4	E863.4	E950.6	E980.7	
Motor exhaust gas - see Carbon monoxide, exhaust gas					
Mouth wash (antiseptic) (zinc chloride)	976.6	E858.7	E950.4	E980.4	E946.6
Moxisylyste	971.3	E855.6	E950.4	E980.4	E941.3
Mucilage, plant	973.2	E858.4	E950.4	E980.4	E943.2
Mucolytic drug	975.5	E858.6	E950.4	E980.4	E945.5
Muriatic acid - see Hydrochloric acid					
Muscle relaxant - see Relaxant, muscle					
Muscle-tone depressant					
– central NEC	968.0	E855.1	E950.4	E980.4	E938.0
– – specified NEC	968.0	E855.1	E950.4	E980.4	E938.0
Muscle-action drug NEC	975.3	E858.6	E950.4	E980.4	E945.3
Mushroom, noxious	988.1	E865.5	E950.9	E980.9	
Mussel, noxious	988.0	E865.1	E950.9	E980.9	
Mustard (emetic)	973.6	E858.4	E950.4	E980.4	E943.6
– black	973.6	E858.4	E950.4	E980.4	E943.6

| Substance | Poison-ing (Chapter XVII) | External Cause (E Code) | | | Adverse effect in correct usage |
| | | Poisoning | | | |
		Accident	Suicide (attempt)	Undeter-mined	
Mustard - *continued*					
– gas, not in war	987.9	E869.8	E952.8	E982.8	
Mustine	963.1	E858.1	E950.4	E980.4	E933.1
Mycotoxins	989.7	E865.9	E950.9	E980.9	
Mydriatic drug	976.5	E858.7	E950.4	E980.4	E946.5
Myralact	976.0	E858.7	E950.4	E980.4	E946.0
Nafcillin (sodium)	960.0	E856	E950.4	E980.4	E930.0
Nafoxidine	962.9	E858.0	E950.4	E980.4	E932.9
Naftidrofuryl (oxalate)	972.5	E858.3	E950.4	E980.4	E942.5
Naled	989.3	E863.1	E950.6	E980.7	
Nalidixic acid	961.9	E857	E950.4	E980.4	E931.9
Nalorphine	970.1	E854.3	E950.4	E980.4	E940.1
Naloxone	970.1	E854.3	E950.4	E980.4	E940.1
Nandrolone	962.1	E858.0	E950.4	E980.4	E932.1
Naphazoline	975.6	E858.6	E950.4	E980.4	E945.6
Naphtha (painters') (petroleum)	981	E862.0	E950.9	E980.9	
– solvent	982.0	E862.4	E950.9	E980.9	
– vapor	987.1	E862.0	E950.9	E980.9	
Naphthalene (chlorinated)	983.0	E864.0	E950.7	E980.6	
– insecticide or moth repellant	983.0	E863.4	E950.6	E980.7	
– vapor	987.8	E869.8	E952.8	E982.8	
Naphthol	983.0	E864.0	E950.7	E980.6	
Naphthylamine	983.0	E864.0	E950.7	E980.6	
Naphthylthiourea	989.4	E863.7	E950.6	E980.7	
Naproxen	965.6	E850.4	E950.0	E980.0	E935.4
Narcotic NEC	965.8	E850.8	E950.0	E980.0	E935.8
– opiate NEC	965.0	E850.0	E950.0	E980.0	E935.0
Nasal drug NEC	976.6	E858.7	E950.4	E980.4	E946.6
Natamycin	960.1	E856	E950.4	E980.4	E930.1
Natural gas	987.1	E867	E951.0	E981.0	
– incomplete combustion	986	E867	E951.0	E981.0	
Nealbarbital	967.0	E851	E950.1	E980.1	E937.0
Neoarsphenamine	961.1	E857	E950.4	E980.4	E931.1
Neomycin	976.0	E858.7	E950.4	E980.4	E946.0
Neostigmine bromide	971.0	E855.3	E950.4	E980.4	E941.0
Nerium oleander	988.2	E865.4	E950.9	E980.9	
Nerve gases, not in war	987.9	E869.8	E952.8	E982.8	
Neuroleptic drug NEC	969.3	E853.8	E950.3	E980.3	E939.3
Neuromuscular blocking brug	975.2	E858.6	E950.4	E980.4	E945.2
Niacin	972.2	E858.3	E950.4	E980.4	E942.2
Nialamide	969.0	E854.0	E950.3	E980.3	E939.0
Nickel (carbonyl) (tetracarbonyl) (fumes) (vapor)	985.8	E866.4	E950.9	E980.9	
Nickelocene	985.8	E866.4	E950.9	E980.9	
Niclosamide	961.6	E857	E950.4	E980.4	E931.6
Nicotinamide	963.5	E858.1	E950.4	E980.4	E933.5
Nicotine (insecticide) (spray) (sulfate) NEC	989.4	E863.4	E950.6	E980.7	
– not insecticide	989.8	E866.8	E950.9	E980.9	
Nicotinic acid	972.2	E858.3	E950.4	E980.4	E942.2
Nicotinyl alcohol	972.5	E858.3	E950.4	E980.4	E942.5
Nicoumalone	964.2	E858.2	E950.4	E980.4	E934.2

Substance	Poisoning (Chapter XVII)	External Cause (E Code)			
		Poisoning			Adverse effect in correct usage
		Accident	Suicide (attempt)	Undetermined	
Nifenazone	965.5	E850.3	E950.0	E980.0	E935.3
Nifuratel	961.9	E857	E950.4	E980.4	E931.9
Nightshade, deadly	988.2	E865.4	E950.9	E980.9	
Nikethamide	970.0	E854.3	E950.4	E980.4	E940.0
Nimorazole	961.5	E857	E950.4	E980.4	E931.5
Niridazole	961.6	E857	E950.4	E980.4	E931.6
Nitrate, organic	972.4	E858.3	E950.4	E980.4	E942.4
Nitrazepam	969.4	E853.2	E950.3	E980.3	E939.4
Nitric					
— acid (liquid)	983.1	E864.1	E950.7	E980.6	
— — vapor	987.8	E869.8	E952.8	E982.8	
— oxide (gas)	987.8	E869.8	E952.8	E982.8	
Nitroaniline	983.0	E864.0	E950.7	E980.6	
— vapor	987.8	E869.8	E952.8	E982.8	
Nitrobenzene, nitrobenzol	983.0	E864.0	E950.7	E980.6	
— vapor	987.8	E869.8	E952.8	E982.8	
Nitrocellulose	989.8	E866.8	E950.9	E980.9	
— lacquer	989.8	E861.6	E950.9	E980.9	
Nitrodiphenyl	989.8	E866.8	E950.9	E980.9	
Nitrofural	961.9	E857	E950.4	E980.4	E931.9
Nitrofurantoin	961.9	E857	E950.4	E980.4	E931.9
Nitrofurazone	961.9	E857	E950.4	E980.4	E931.9
Nitrogen (dioxide) (oxide) (gas)	987.2	E869.0	E952.8	E982.8	
— mustard	963.1	E858.1	E950.4	E980.4	E933.1
Nitroglycerin, nitroglycerol (medicinal)	972.4	E858.3	E950.4	E980.4	E942.4
— nonmedicinal	989.8	E866.8	E950.9	E980.9	
— — fumes	987.8	E869.8	E952.8	E982.8	
Nitroglycol	982.4	E862.4	E950.9	E980.9	
Nitrohydrochloric acid	983.1	E864.1	E950.7	E980.6	
Nitronaphthalene	983.0	E864.0	E950.7	E980.6	
Nitrophenol	983.0	E864.0	E950.7	E980.6	
Nitroprusside	972.5	E858.3	E950.4	E980.4	E942.5
Nitrosodimethylamine	989.8	E866.8	E950.9	E980.9	
Nitrosourea	963.1	E858.1	E950.4	E980.4	E933.1
Nitrotoluene, nitrotoluol	983.0	E864.0	E950.7	E980.6	
— vapor	987.8	E869.8	E952.8	E982.8	
Nitrous					
— acid (liquid)	983.1	E864.1	E950.7	E980.6	
— — fumes	987.8	E869.8	E952.8	E982.8	
— oxide	968.2	E855.1	E950.4	E980.4	E938.2
Nonionic acid	976.0	E858.7	E950.4	E980.4	E946.0
Nonylphenoxy (polyethoxyethanol)	976.8	E858.7	E950.4	E980.4	E946.8
Noradrenalin	971.2	E855.5	E950.4	E980.4	E941.2
Noramidopyridine	965.5	E850.3	E950.0	E980.0	E935.3
Norbormide	989.4	E863.7	E950.6	E980.7	
Norepinephrine	971.2	E855.5	E950.4	E980.4	E941.2
Norethandrolone	962.1	E858.0	E950.4	E980.4	E932.1
Norethindrone	962.2	E858.0	E950.4	E980.4	E932.2
Norethisterone	962.2	E858.0	E950.4	E980.4	E932.2
Norethynodrel	962.2	E858.0	E950.4	E980.4	E932.2
Norgestrel	962.2	E858.0	E950.4	E980.4	E932.2

Substance	Poison-ing (Chapter XVII)	External Cause (E Code)			
		Poisoning			Adverse effect in correct usage
		Accident	Suicide (attempt)	Undeter-mined	
Norpseudoephedrine	977.0	E858.8	E950.4	E980.4	E947.0
Nortriptyline	969.0	E854.0	E950.3	E980.3	E939.0
Noscapine	965.0	E850.0	E950.0	E980.0	E935.0
Novobiocin	960.8	E856	E950.4	E980.4	E930.8
Noxious foodstuffs NEC	988.9	E865.9	E950.9	E980.9	
– specified NEC	988.8	E865.8	E950.9	E980.9	
Nutmeg	975.1	E858.6	E950.4	E980.4	E945.1
Nutritional supplement	977.0	E858.8	E950.4	E980.4	E947.0
Nylidrin	971.2	E855.5	E950.4	E980.4	E941.2
Nystatin	960.1	E856	E950.4	E980.4	E930.1
Octafonium (chloride)	976.3	E858.7	E950.4	E980.4	E946.3
Octamethyl pyrophosphoramide	989.3	E863.1	E950.6	E980.7	
Oestradiol	962.2	E858.0	E950.4	E980.4	E932.2
Oestriol	962.2	E858.0	E950.4	E980.4	E932.2
Oestrogen	962.2	E858.0	E950.4	E980.4	E932.2
Oestrone	962.2	E858.0	E950.4	E980.4	E932.2
Oil (of) NEC	989.8	E866.8	E950.9	E980.9	
– bitter almond	989.0	E866.8	E950.9	E980.9	
– cloves	976.7	E858.7	E950.4	E980.4	E946.7
– colors	989.8	E861.6	E950.9	E980.9	
– fumes	987.8	E869.8	E952.8	E982.8	
– lubricating	981	E862.2	E950.9	E980.9	
– niobe	982.8	E862.4	E950.9	E980.9	
– vitriol (liquid)	983.1	E864.1	E950.7	E980.6	
– – fumes	987.8	E869.8	E952.8	E982.8	
Oily preparation (for skin)	976.3	E858.7	E950.4	E980.4	E946.3
Ointment NEC	976.3	E858.7	E950.4	E980.4	E946.3
Oleander	988.2	E865.4	E950.9	E980.9	
Oleandomycin	960.3	E856	E950.4	E980.4	E930.3
Oleic acid	972.2	E858.3	E950.4	E980.4	E942.2
Oleovitamin	963.5	E858.1	E950.4	E980.4	E933.5
Oleum ricini	973.1	E858.4	E950.4	E980.4	E943.1
OMPA	989.3	E863.1	E950.6	E980.7	
Opiate NEC	965.0	E850.0	E950.0	E980.0	E935.0
Opipramol	969.0	E854.0	E950.3	E980.3	E939.0
Opium alkaloids	965.0	E850.0	E950.0	E980.0	E935.0
Orciprenaline	975.1	E858.6	E950.4	E980.4	E945.1
Organonitrate NEC	972.4	E858.3	E950.4	E980.4	E942.4
Organophosphates	989.3	E863.1	E950.6	E980.7	
Orphenadrine	971.1	E855.4	E950.4	E980.4	E941.1
Orthodichloro-ethane	982.3	E862.4	E950.9	E980.9	
Osmic acid (liquid)	983.1	E864.1	E950.7	E980.6	
– fumes	987.8	E869.8	E952.8	E982.8	
Ouabaine	972.1	E858.3	E950.4	E980.4	E942.1
Ovarian					
– hormone	962.2	E858.0	E950.4	E980.4	E932.2
– stimulant	962.2	E858.0	E950.4	E980.4	E932.2
Ox bile extract	973.4	E858.4	E950.4	E980.4	E943.4
Oxacillin	960.0	E856	E950.4	E980.4	E930.0
Oxalic acid	983.1	E864.1	E950.7	E980.6	
Oxandrolone	962.1	E858.0	E950.4	E980.4	E932.1

Substance	Poisoning (Chapter XVII)	External Cause (E Code)			Adverse effect in correct usage
		Poisoning			
		Accident	Suicide (attempt)	Undetermined	
Oxantel	961.6	E857	E950.4	E980.4	E931.6
Oxazepam	969.4	E853.2	E950.3	E980.3	E939.4
Oxazimedrine	977.0	E858.8	E950.4	E980.4	E947.0
Oxazolidine derivative NEC	966.0	E855.0	E950.4	E980.4	E936.0
Oxedrine	971.2	E855.5	E950.4	E980.4	E941.2
Oxeladin (citrate)	975.4	E858.6	E950.4	E980.4	E945.4
Oxethacaine	973.8	E858.4	E950.4	E980.4	E943.8
Oxidizing agents NEC	983.9	E864.3	E950.7	E980.6	
Oxophenarsine	961.1	E857	E950.4	E980.4	E931.1
Oxprenolol	972.0	E858.3	E950.4	E980.4	E942.0
Oxtocic drug NEC	975.0	E858.6	E950.4	E980.4	E945.0
Oxtriphylline	975.7	E858.6	E950.4	E980.4	E945.7
Oxybuprocaine	968.5	E855.2	E950.4	E980.4	E938.5
Oxycodone	965.0	E850.0	E950.0	E980.0	E935.0
Oxygen	975.8	E858.6	E950.4	E980.4	E945.8
Oxymesterone	962.1	E858.0	E950.4	E980.4	E932.1
Oxymetazoline	975.6	E858.6	E950.4	E980.4	E945.6
Oxymetholone	962.1	E858.0	E950.4	E980.4	E932.1
Oxymorphone	965.0	E850.0	E950.0	E980.0	E935.0
Oxyphenbutazone	965.5	E850.3	E950.0	E980.0	E935.3
Oxyphencyclimine	971.1	E855.4	E950.4	E980.4	E941.1
Oxyphenisatine	973.1	E858.4	E950.4	E980.4	E943.1
Oxyphenonium bromide	971.1	E855.4	E950.4	E980.4	E941.1
Oxytetracycline	960.4	E856	E950.4	E980.4	E930.4
Oxytocin (synthetic)	975.0	E858.6	E950.4	E980.4	E945.0
Ozone	987.8	E869.8	E952.8	E982.8	
Paint NEC	989.8	E861.6	E950.9	E980.9	
– cleaner	982.8	E862.4	E950.9	E980.9	
– fumes NEC	987.8	E869.8	E952.8	E982.8	
– lead (fumes)	984.0	E861.5	E950.9	E980.9	
– solvent NEC	982.8	E862.4	E950.9	E980.9	
– stripper	982.8	E862.4	E950.9	E980.9	
Palm kernel oil	977.4	E858.8	E950.4	E980.4	E947.4
Palmitamide	965.8	E850.8	E950.0	E980.0	E935.8
PAM	971.0	E855.3	E950.4	E980.4	E941.0
Pancreatic					
– digestive secretion stimulant	973.8	E858.4	E950.4	E980.4	E943.8
– dornase	973.4	E858.4	E950.4	E980.4	E943.4
Pancreatin	973.4	E858.4	E950.4	E980.4	E943.4
Pancuronium (bromide)	975.2	E858.6	E950.4	E980.4	E945.2
Pantothenic acid	963.5	E858.1	E950.4	E980.4	E933.5
Papain	963.4	E858.1	E950.4	E980.4	E933.4
– digestant	973.4	E858.4	E950.4	E980.4	E943.4
Papaveretum	965.0	E850.0	E950.0	E980.0	E935.0
Papaverine	972.5	E858.3	E950.4	E980.4	E942.5
Para-acetamidophenol	965.4	E850.2	E950.0	E980.0	E935.2
Para-aminobenzoic acid	976.3	E858.7	E950.4	E980.4	E946.3
Para-aminosalicylic acid	961.8	E857	E950.4	E980.4	E931.8
Paracetaldehyde	967.2	E852.1	E950.2	E980.2	E937.2
Paracetamol	965.4	E850.2	E950.0	E980.0	E935.2
Paraffin(s) (wax)	981	E862.3	E950.9	E980.9	

Substance	Poison-ing (Chapter XVII)	External Cause (E Code)			Adverse effect in correct usage
		Poisoning			
		Accident	Suicide (attempt)	Undeter-mined	
Paraffin(s) - *continued*					
− liquid (medicinal)	973.2	E858.4	E950.4	E980.4	E943.2
− − nonmedicinal	981	E862.1	E950.9	E980.9	
Paraformaldehyde	989.4	E863.6	E950.6	E980.7	
Paraldehyde	967.2	E852.1	E950.2	E980.2	E937.2
Paramethadione	966.0	E855.0	E950.4	E980.4	E936.0
Paramethasone	962.0	E858.0	E950.4	E980.4	E932.0
− acetate	976.0	E858.7	E950.4	E980.4	E946.0
Paraoxon	989.3	E863.1	E950.6	E980.7	
Paraquat	989.4	E863.5	E950.6	E980.7	
Parasympatholytic NEC	971.1	E855.4	E950.4	E980.4	E941.1
Parasympathomimetic drug NEC	971.0	E855.3	E950.4	E980.4	E941.0
Parathion	989.3	E863.1	E950.6	E980.7	
Parathyroid extract	962.6	E858.0	E950.4	E980.4	E932.6
Parazolidin	965.7	E850.5	E950.0	E980.0	E935.5
Pargyline	969.0	E854.0	E950.3	E980.3	E939.0
Paris green	985.1	E866.3	E950.8	E980.8	
− insecticide	985.1	E863.4	E950.6	E980.7	
Paromomycin	960.8	E856	E950.4	E980.4	E930.8
PAS	961.8	E857	E950.4	E980.4	E931.8
Pasiniazid	961.8	E857	E950.4	E980.4	E931.8
PCB	989.8	E866.8	E950.9	E980.9	
PCP	989.4	E863.6	E950.6	E980.7	
Pectin	973.5	E858.4	E950.4	E980.4	E943.5
Pelletierine tannate	961.6	E857	E950.4	E980.4	E931.6
Pemoline	969.7	E854.2	E950.3	E980.3	E939.7
Pempidine	972.3	E858.3	E950.4	E980.4	E942.3
Penamecillin	960.0	E856	E950.4	E980.4	E930.0
Penfluridol	969.2	E853.1	E950.3	E980.3	E939.2
Penicillamine	963.8	E858.1	E950.4	E980.4	E933.8
Penicillin (any)	960.0	E856	E950.4	E980.4	E930.0
Penicillinase	963.4	E858.1	E950.4	E980.4	E933.4
Pent	972.4	E858.3	E950.4	E980.4	E942.4
Pentachloronaphthalene	989.2	E866.8	E950.9	E980.9	
Pentachlorophenol (pesticide)	989.4	E863.6	E950.6	E980.7	
Pentaerithrityl tetranitrate	972.4	E858.3	E950.4	E980.4	E942.4
Pentagastrin	977.8	E858.8	E950.4	E980.4	E947.8
Pentalin	982.8	E862.4	E950.9	E980.9	
Pentamethonium bromide	972.3	E858.3	E950.4	E980.4	E942.3
Pentamidine	961.5	E857	E950.4	E980.4	E931.5
Pentanol	980.3	E860.4	E950.9	E980.9	
Pentapyrrolidinium	972.3	E858.3	E950.4	E980.4	E942.3
Pentaquine	961.4	E857	E950.4	E980.4	E931.4
Pentazocine	965.8	E850.8	E950.0	E980.0	E935.8
Penthienate	971.1	E855.4	E950.4	E980.4	E941.1
Pentobarbital	967.0	E851	E950.1	E980.1	E937.0
− sodium	967.0	E851	E950.1	E980.1	E937.0
Pentolonium (tartrate)	972.3	E858.3	E950.4	E980.4	E942.3
Pentoxyverine	975.4	E858.6	E950.4	E980.4	E945.4
Pentylenetetral	970.0	E854.3	E950.4	E980.4	E940.0
Pentylenetetrazol	970.0	E854.3	E950.4	E980.4	E940.0

Substance	Poison-ing (Chapter XVII)	External Cause (E Code)			
		Poisoning			Adverse effect in correct usage
		Accident	Suicide (attempt)	Undeter-mined	
Peppermint (oil)	973.4	E858.4	E950.4	E980.4	E943.4
Pepsin	963.4	E858.1	E950.4	E980.4	E933.4
– digestant	973.4	E858.4	E950.4	E980.4	E943.4
Peptide, non-antigenic	962.4	E858.0	E950.4	E980.4	E932.4
Perchloroethylene	982.3	E862.4	E950.9	E980.9	
– vapor	987.8	E862.4	E950.9	E980.9	
Perhexilene	972.4	E858.3	E950.4	E980.4	E942.4
Periciazine	969.1	E853.0	E950.3	E980.3	E939.1
Peritoneal dialysis solution	974.5	E858.5	E950.4	E980.4	E944.5
Permanganates	983.9	E864.3	E950.7	E980.6	
Perphenazine	969.1	E853.0	E950.3	E980.3	E939.1
Pertussis vaccine	978.6	E858.8	E950.4	E980.4	E948.6
Pesticides (dust) (fumes) (vapor) NEC	989.4	E863.9	E950.6	E980.7	
– chlorinated	989.2	E863.0	E950.6	E980.7	
Pethidine	965.0	E850.0	E950.0	E980.0	E935.0
Petrol	981	E862.1	E950.9	E980.9	
– vapor	987.1	E862.1	E950.9	E980.9	
Petrolatum	973.2	E858.4	E950.4	E980.4	E943.2
– nonmedicinal	981	E862.3	E950.9	E980.9	
– red veterinary	976.3	E858.7	E950.4	E980.4	E946.3
– white	976.3	E858.7	E950.4	E980.4	E946.3
Petroleum (products) NEC	981	E862.9	E950.9	E980.9	
– benzin(e) - see Ligroin					
– ether - see Ligroin					
– jelly - see Petrolatum					
– naphtha - see Ligroin					
– pesticide	989.4	E863.9	E950.6	E980.7	
– vapor	987.1	E862.9	E950.9	E980.9	
Peyote	969.6	E854.1	E950.3	E980.3	E939.6
Pharmaceutical					
– adjunct NEC	977.4	E858.8	E950.4	E980.4	E947.4
– excipient NEC	977.4	E858.8	E950.4	E980.4	E947.4
– sweetener	977.4	E858.8	E950.4	E980.4	E947.4
– viscous agent	977.4	E858.8	E950.4	E980.4	E947.4
Phenacemide	966.3	E855.0	E950.4	E980.4	E936.3
Phenacetin	965.4	E850.2	E950.0	E980.0	E935.2
Phenaglycodol	969.5	E853.8	E950.3	E980.3	E939.5
Phenantoin	966.1	E855.0	E950.4	E980.4	E936.1
Phenazocine	965.8	E850.8	E950.0	E980.0	E935.8
Phenazone	965.5	E850.3	E950.0	E980.0	E935.3
Phenazopyridine	961.9	E857	E950.4	E980.4	E931.9
Phenbutrazate	977.0	E858.8	E950.4	E980.4	E947.0
Phendimetrazine	977.0	E858.8	E950.4	E980.4	E947.0
Phenelzine	969.0	E854.0	E950.3	E980.3	E939.0
Pheneticillin	960.0	E856	E950.4	E980.4	E930.0
Pheneturide	966.3	E855.0	E950.4	E980.4	E936.3
Phenformin	962.3	E858.0	E950.4	E980.4	E932.3
Phenglutarimide	971.1	E855.4	E950.4	E980.4	E941.1
Phenindamine	963.0	E858.1	E950.4	E980.4	E933.0
Phenindione	964.2	E858.2	E950.4	E980.4	E934.2
Pheniprazine	969.0	E854.0	E950.3	E980.3	E939.0

Substance	Poison-ing (Chapter XVII)	External Cause (E Code)			
		Poisoning			Adverse effect in correct usage
		Accident	Suicide (attempt)	Undeter-mined	
Pheniramine	963.0	E858.1	E950.4	E980.4	E933.0
Phenmetrazine	977.0	E858.8	E950.4	E980.4	E947.0
Phenobarbital	967.0	E851	E950.1	E980.1	E937.0
– with					
– – mephenytoin	966.3	E855.0	E950.4	E980.4	E936.3
– – phenytoin	966.3	E855.0	E950.4	E980.4	E936.3
– sodium	967.0	E851	E950.1	E980.1	E937.0
Phenobutiodol	977.8	E858.8	E950.4	E980.4	E947.8
Phenol					
– disinfectant	983.0	E861.4	E950.9	E980.9	
– in oil injection	972.7	E858.3	E950.4	E980.4	E942.7
– medicinal	976.1	E858.7	E950.4	E980.4	E946.1
– nonmedicinal NEC	983.0	E864.0	E950.7	E980.6	
– pesticide	989.4	E863.9	E950.6	E980.7	
– red	977.8	E858.8	E950.4	E980.4	E947.8
Phenolic preparation	976.1	E858.7	E950.4	E980.4	E946.1
Phenolphthalein	973.1	E858.4	E950.4	E980.4	E943.1
Phenolsulfonphthalein	977.8	E858.8	E950.4	E980.4	E947.8
Phenoperidine	965.0	E850.0	E950.0	E980.0	E935.0
Phenopyrazone	972.8	E858.3	E950.4	E980.4	E942.8
Phenoquin	974.7	E858.5	E950.4	E980.4	E944.7
Phenothiazine (tranquilizer) NEC	969.1	E853.0	E950.3	E980.3	E939.1
– insecticide	989.4	E863.4	E950.6	E980.7	
Phenoxybenzamine	971.3	E855.6	E950.4	E980.4	E941.3
Phenoxyethanol	976.6	E858.7	E950.4	E980.4	E946.6
Phenoxymethylpenicillin	960.0	E856	E950.4	E980.4	E930.0
Phenprocoumon	964.2	E858.2	E950.4	E980.4	E934.2
Phensuximide	966.2	E855.0	E950.4	E980.4	E936.2
Phentermine	977.0	E858.8	E950.4	E980.4	E947.0
Phentolamine	971.3	E855.6	E950.4	E980.4	E941.3
Phenyl					
– enediamine	983.0	E864.0	E950.7	E980.6	
– hydrazine	983.0	E864.0	E950.7	E980.6	
– mercuric compounds - see Mercury					
Phenylalanine mustard	963.1	E858.1	E950.4	E980.4	E933.1
Phenylbutazone	965.5	E850.3	E950.0	E980.0	E935.3
Phenylenediamin	989.8	E866.8	E950.9	E980.9	
Phenylephrine	971.2	E855.5	E950.4	E980.4	E941.2
Phenylmercuric nitrate	976.0	E858.7	E950.4	E980.4	E946.0
Phenylmethylbarbitone	967.0	E851	E950.1	E980.1	E937.0
Phenylpropanol	973.4	E858.4	E950.4	E980.4	E943.4
Phenylpropanolamine	977.0	E858.8	E950.4	E980.4	E947.0
Phenylpropylamine	975.6	E858.6	E950.4	E980.4	E945.6
Phenylstibamic acid	961.2	E857	E950.4	E980.4	E931.2
Phenylsulphthion	989.3	E863.1	E950.6	E980.7	
Phenyltoloxamine	963.0	E858.1	E950.4	E980.4	E933.0
Phenytoin	966.1	E855.0	E950.4	E980.4	E936.1
– with phenobarbital	966.3	E855.0	E950.4	E980.4	E936.3
Pholcodine	965.0	E850.0	E950.0	E980.0	E935.0
Pholedrin	972.8	E858.3	E950.4	E980.4	E942.8
Phorate	989.3	E863.1	E950.6	E980.7	

Substance	Poisoning (Chapter XVII)	External Cause (E Code)			
		Poisoning			Adverse effect in correct usage
		Accident	Suicide (attempt)	Undetermined	
Phosdrin	989.3	E863.1	E950.6	E980.7	
Phosgene (gas)	987.8	E869.8	E952.8	E982.8	
Phosphamidon	989.3	E863.1	E950.6	E980.7	
Phosphate					
— laxative	973.3	E858.4	E950.4	E980.4	E943.3
— tricresyl	982.8	E862.4	E950.9	E980.9	
Phosphine	987.9	E863.8	E950.6	E980.7	
Phosphoric acid	983.1	E864.1	E950.7	E980.6	
Phosphorus (compounds) NEC	983.9	E864.3	E950.7	E980.6	
— pesticides	989.3	E863.1	E950.6	E980.7	
Phthalic anhydride	989.8	E866.8	E950.9	E980.9	
Phthalylsulfathiazole	961.0	E857	E950.4	E980.4	E931.0
Phylloquinone	964.3	E858.2	E950.4	E980.4	E934.3
Physostigmine	971.0	E855.3	E950.4	E980.4	E941.0
Phytomenadione	964.3	E858.2	E950.4	E980.4	E934.3
Picosulfate (sodium)	973.1	E858.4	E950.4	E980.4	E943.1
Picric (acid)	983.0	E864.0	E950.7	E980.6	
Picrotoxin	970.0	E854.3	E950.4	E980.4	E940.0
Pilocarpine	971.0	E855.3	E950.4	E980.4	E941.0
Pimelic ketone	982.8	E862.4	E950.9	E980.9	
Pimozide	969.8	E855.8	E950.3	E980.3	E939.8
Pindone	989.4	E863.4	E950.6	E980.7	
Pine oil, pinesol (disinfectant)	983.9	E861.4	E950.9	E980.9	
Pipamazine	963.0	E858.1	E950.4	E980.4	E933.0
Pipazetate	975.4	E858.6	E950.4	E980.4	E945.4
Pipenzolate	971.1	E855.4	E950.4	E980.4	E941.1
Piperacetazine	969.1	E853.0	E950.3	E980.3	E939.1
Piperazine	961.6	E857	E950.4	E980.4	E931.6
Piperidolate	971.1	E855.4	E950.4	E980.4	E941.1
Piperocaine	976.6	E858.7	E950.4	E980.4	E946.6
Piperonyl butoxide	989.4	E863.4	E950.6	E980.7	
Pipobroman	963.1	E858.1	E950.4	E980.4	E933.1
Pipradrol	969.7	E854.2	E950.3	E980.3	E939.7
Pitch	983.0	E864.0	E950.7	E980.6	
Placental extract	962.9	E858.0	E950.4	E980.4	E932.9
Plague vaccine	978.3	E858.8	E950.4	E980.4	E948.3
Plant foods or fertilizers NEC	989.8	E866.5	E950.9	E980.9	
— containing herbicide	989.4	E863.5	E950.6	E980.7	
Plants, noxious, used as food	988.2	E865.4	E950.9	E980.9	
Plasma expander NEC	964.8	E858.2	E950.4	E980.4	E934.8
Plasma protein fraction	964.7	E858.2	E950.4	E980.4	E934.7
Plasmin(-ogen)	964.4	E858.2	E950.4	E980.4	E934.4
Plaster dressing	976.3	E858.7	E950.4	E980.4	E946.3
Plastic dressing	976.3	E858.7	E950.4	E980.4	E946.3
Podophyllum	976.4	E858.7	E950.4	E980.4	E946.4
Poison NEC	989.9	E866.9	E950.9	E980.9	
Pokeweed (any part)	988.2	E865.4	E950.9	E980.9	
Poldine	971.1	E855.4	E950.4	E980.4	E941.1
Polidexide	972.2	E858.3	E950.4	E980.4	E942.2
Poliomyelitis vaccine	979.5	E858.8	E950.4	E980.4	E949.5

Substance	Poison-ing (Chapter XVII)	External Cause (E Code)			
		Poisoning			Adverse effect in correct usage
		Accident	Suicide (attempt)	Undeter-mined	
Polish (car) (floor) (furniture) (metal) (porcelain) (silver)	989.8	E861.2	E950.9	E980.9	
Poloxalkol	973.2	E858.4	E950.4	E980.4	E943.2
Polychlorinated biphenyl	989.8	E866.8	E950.9	E980.9	
Polyester fumes	987.8	E869.8	E952.8	E982.8	
Polyestradiol (phosphate)	962.2	E858.0	E950.4	E980.4	E932.2
Polyethanolamine alkyl sulfate	976.2	E858.7	E950.4	E980.4	E946.2
Polyethylene adhesive	976.3	E858.7	E950.4	E980.4	E946.3
Polymyxin					
– eye	976.5	E858.7	E950.4	E980.4	E946.5
– systemic	960.8	E856	E950.4	E980.4	E930.8
Polynoxylin	976.0	E858.7	E950.4	E980.4	E946.0
Polyoestradiol (phosphate)	962.2	E858.0	E950.4	E980.4	E932.2
Polytetrafluoroethylene (inhaled)	987.8	E869.8	E952.8	E982.8	
Polythiazide	974.3	E858.5	E950.4	E980.4	E944.3
Polyvidone	964.8	E858.2	E950.4	E980.4	E934.8
Polyvinylpyrrolidine	964.8	E858.2	E950.4	E980.4	E934.8
Posterior pituitary					
– extract	962.5	E858.0	E950.4	E980.4	E932.5
– hormone NEC	962.5	E858.0	E950.4	E980.4	E932.5
Potash (caustic)	983.2	E864.2	E950.7	E980.6	
Potassium (salts) NEC	974.6	E858.5	E950.4	E980.4	E944.6
– aminobenzoate	963.8	E858.1	E950.4	E980.4	E933.8
– aminosalicilate	961.8	E857	E950.4	E980.4	E931.8
– antimony tartrate	961.2	E857	E950.4	E980.4	E931.2
– bichromate	983.9	E864.3	E950.7	E980.6	
– bisulfate	983.9	E864.3	E950.7	E980.6	
– bromide	967.3	E852.2	E950.2	E980.2	E937.3
– carbonate	983.2	E864.2	E950.7	E980.6	
– chlorate NEC	983.9	E864.3	E950.7	E980.6	
– chloride	974.6	E858.5	E950.4	E980.4	E944.6
– citrate	963.3	E858.1	E950.4	E980.4	E933.3
– citratobismuthate	961.2	E857	E950.4	E980.4	E931.2
– cyanide (see also Cyanide)	989.0	E866.8	E950.9	E980.9	
– fluoride	974.6	E858.5	E950.4	E980.4	E944.6
– hydroxide	983.2	E864.2	E950.7	E980.6	
– iodide	975.5	E858.6	E950.4	E980.4	E945.5
– nitrate	989.8	E866.8	E950.9	E980.9	
– oxalate	983.9	E864.3	E950.7	E980.6	
– perchlorate (nonmedicinal) NEC	983.9	E864.3	E950.7	E980.6	
– – medicinal	962.8	E858.0	E950.4	E980.4	E932.8
– permanganate (nonmedicinal)	983.9	E864.3	E950.7	E980.6	
– – medicinal	976.0	E858.7	E950.4	E980.4	E946.0
Potassium-removing resin	974.5	E858.5	E950.4	E980.4	E944.5
Potassium-retaining drug	974.5	E858.5	E950.4	E980.4	E944.5
Povidone					
– iodine	976.0	E858.7	E950.4	E980.4	E946.0
– PVP	964.8	E858.2	E950.4	E980.4	E934.8
Practolol	972.0	E858.3	E950.4	E980.4	E942.0
Pralidoxime	971.0	E855.3	E950.4	E980.4	E941.0
Pramocaine	976.1	E858.7	E950.4	E980.4	E946.1

Substance	Poison-ing (Chapter XVII)	External Cause (E Code)			
		Poisoning			Adverse effect in correct usage
		Accident	Suicide (attempt)	Undeter-mined	
Pramoxine	976.1	E858.7	E950.4	E980.4	E946.1
Prazosin	972.6	E858.3	E950.4	E980.4	E942.6
Precursor for synthesis	963.5	E858.1	E950.4	E980.4	E933.5
Prednisolone	962.0	E858.0	E950.4	E980.4	E932.0
Prednisone	962.0	E858.0	E950.4	E980.4	E932.0
Premedication anesthetic	968.4	E855.1	E950.4	E980.4	E938.4
Prenylamine	972.4	E858.3	E950.4	E980.4	E942.4
Preparation, local	976.4	E858.7	E950.4	E980.4	E946.4
Preservatives (nonmedicinal)	989.8	E866.8	E950.9	E980.9	
− medicinal	977.4	E858.8	E950.4	E980.4	E947.4
Prethcamide	970.0	E854.3	E950.4	E980.4	E940.0
Prilocaine, regional	968.6	E855.2	E950.4	E980.4	E938.6
Primaquine	961.4	E857	E950.4	E980.4	E931.4
Primidone	966.3	E855.0	E950.4	E980.4	E936.3
Pristinamycin	960.8	E856	E950.4	E980.4	E930.8
Probenecid	974.7	E858.5	E950.4	E980.4	E944.7
Procainamide	972.0	E858.3	E950.4	E980.4	E942.0
Procaine (infiltration)	968.5	E855.2	E950.4	E980.4	E938.5
− penicillin	960.0	E856	E950.4	E980.4	E930.0
− regional	968.6	E855.2	E950.4	E980.4	E938.6
− spinal	968.7	E855.2	E950.4	E980.4	E938.7
Procarbazine	963.1	E858.1	E950.4	E980.4	E933.1
Prochlorperazine	969.1	E853.0	E950.3	E980.3	E939.1
Procyclidine	971.1	E855.4	E950.4	E980.4	E941.1
Producer gas	986	E868.8	E952.1	E982.1	
Profenamine	966.4	E855.0	E950.4	E980.4	E936.4
Progesterone	962.2	E858.0	E950.4	E980.4	E932.2
Progestogen NEC	962.2	E858.0	E950.4	E980.4	E932.2
Proguanil	961.4	E857	E950.4	E980.4	E931.4
Prolintane	969.7	E854.2	E950.3	E980.3	E939.7
Promazine	969.1	E853.0	E950.3	E980.3	E939.1
Promethazine	969.1	E853.0	E950.3	E980.3	E939.1
Propafenon	972.0	E858.3	E950.4	E980.4	E942.0
Propamidine	976.0	E858.7	E950.4	E980.4	E946.0
Propane (distributed in mobile container)	987.0	E868.0	E951.1	E981.1	
− distributed through pipes	987.0	E867	E951.0	E981.0	
− incomplete combustion - see Carbon monoxide, propane					
Propanidid	968.3	E855.1	E950.4	E980.4	E938.3
Propanol	980.2	E860.3	E950.9	E980.9	
Propantheline	971.1	E855.4	E950.4	E980.4	E941.1
Proparacaine	968.5	E855.2	E950.4	E980.4	E938.5
Propicillin	960.0	E856	E950.4	E980.4	E930.0
Propiolactone	976.0	E858.7	E950.4	E980.4	E946.0
Propiomazine	969.1	E853.0	E950.3	E980.3	E939.1
Propionate (sodium) (calcium)	976.0	E858.7	E950.4	E980.4	E946.0
Propoxur	989.3	E863.2	E950.6	E980.7	
Propoxycaine	968.5	E855.2	E950.4	E980.4	E938.5
Propoxyphene	965.7	E850.5	E950.0	E980.0	E935.5
Propranolol	972.0	E858.3	E950.4	E980.4	E942.0
Propylaminophenothiazine	969.1	E853.0	E950.3	E980.3	E939.1

Substance	Poisoning (Chapter XVII)	External Cause (E Code)			Adverse effect in correct usage
		Accident	Suicide (attempt)	Undetermined	
Propylene	987.1	E869.8	E952.8	E982.8	
Propylhexedrine	975.6	E858.6	E950.4	E980.4	E945.6
Propyliodone	977.8	E858.8	E950.4	E980.4	E947.8
Propylthiouracil	962.8	E858.0	E950.4	E980.4	E932.8
Proscillaridin	972.1	E858.3	E950.4	E980.4	E942.1
Prostaglandin	975.0	E858.6	E950.4	E980.4	E945.0
Protamine sulfate	964.5	E858.2	E950.4	E980.4	E934.5
Protectant, skin NEC	976.3	E858.7	E950.4	E980.4	E946.3
– specified NEC	976.3	E858.7	E950.4	E980.4	E946.3
Protein hydrolysate	977.0	E858.8	E950.4	E980.4	E947.0
Prothionamide	961.8	E857	E950.4	E980.4	E931.8
Prothrombin					
– activator	964.5	E858.2	E950.4	E980.4	E934.5
– synthesis inhibitor	964.2	E858.2	E950.4	E980.4	E934.2
Protokylol	975.7	E858.6	E950.4	E980.4	E945.7
Protoveratrine	972.6	E858.3	E950.4	E980.4	E942.6
Protriptyline	969.0	E854.0	E950.3	E980.3	E939.0
Proxymetacaine	968.5	E855.2	E950.4	E980.4	E938.5
Proxyphylline	975.1	E858.6	E950.4	E980.4	E945.1
Prussic acid	989.0	E866.8	E950.9	E980.9	
– vapor	987.7	E869.8	E952.8	E982.8	
Pseudoephedrine	975.6	E858.6	E950.4	E980.4	E945.6
Psilocin	969.6	E854.1	E950.3	E980.3	E939.6
Psilocybine	969.6	E854.1	E950.3	E980.3	E939.6
Psychodysleptic drug NEC	969.6	E854.1	E950.3	E980.3	E939.6
Psychostimulant NEC	969.7	E854.2	E950.3	E980.3	E939.7
Psychotherapeutic drug NEC	969.9	E855.9	E950.3	E980.3	E939.9
Psychotropic drug NEC	969.9	E855.9	E950.3	E980.3	E939.9
– specified NEC	969.8	E855.8	E950.3	E980.3	E939.8
Pteroylglutamic acid	964.1	E858.2	E950.4	E980.4	E934.1
PTFE	987.8	E869.8	E952.8	E982.8	
Pulp					
– devitalizing paste	976.7	E858.7	E950.4	E980.4	E946.7
– dressing	976.7	E858.7	E950.4	E980.4	E946.7
Pumpkin seed extract	961.6	E857	E950.4	E980.4	E931.6
Purgative (see also Cathartic) NEC	973.3	E858.4	E950.4	E980.4	E943.3
Purine analogues	963.1	E858.1	E950.4	E980.4	E933.1
Pyrabital	965.7	E850.5	E950.0	E980.0	E935.5
Pyramidon	965.5	E850.3	E950.0	E980.0	E935.3
Pyrantel	961.6	E857	E950.4	E980.4	E931.6
Pyrazinamide	961.8	E857	E950.4	E980.4	E931.8
Pyrazole analgesic NEC	965.5	E850.3	E950.0	E980.0	E935.3
Pyrazolone analgesic NEC	965.5	E850.3	E950.0	E980.0	E935.3
Pyrethrins, pyrethrum	989.4	E863.4	E950.6	E980.7	
Pyridine (liquid)	982.0	E862.4	E950.9	E980.9	
– aldoxime methiodide	971.0	E855.3	E950.4	E980.4	E941.0
– vapor	987.8	E862.4	E950.9	E980.9	
Pyridostigmine bromide	971.0	E855.3	E950.4	E980.4	E941.0
Pyridoxine	963.5	E858.1	E950.4	E980.4	E933.5
Pyrilamine	963.0	E858.1	E950.4	E980.4	E933.0
Pyrimethamine	961.4	E857	E950.4	E980.4	E931.4

Substance	Poisoning (Chapter XVII)	External Cause (E Code)			
		Poisoning			Adverse effect in correct usage
		Accident	Suicide (attempt)	Undetermined	
Pyrimidine antagonist	963.1	E858.1	E950.4	E980.4	E933.1
Pyrogallic acid	983.0	E864.0	E950.7	E980.6	
Pyroxylin	976.3	E858.7	E950.4	E980.4	E946.3
Pyrrobutamine	963.0	E858.1	E950.4	E980.4	E933.0
Pyrvinium chloride	961.6	E857	E950.4	E980.4	E931.6
Quaternary ammonium					
− anti-infective	976.0	E858.7	E950.4	E980.4	E946.0
− ganglion blocking	972.3	E858.3	E950.4	E980.4	E942.3
− parasympatholytic	971.1	E855.4	E950.4	E980.4	E941.1
Quicklime	983.2	E864.2	E950.7	E980.6	
Quinacrine	961.4	E857	E950.4	E980.4	E931.4
Quinalbarbital	967.0	E851	E950.1	E980.1	E937.0
Quinaldol	976.0	E858.7	E950.4	E980.4	E946.0
Quinazolinone	974.4	E858.5	E950.4	E980.4	E944.4
Quinethazone	974.4	E858.5	E950.4	E980.4	E944.4
Quinidine	972.0	E858.3	E950.4	E980.4	E942.0
Quinine	961.4	E857	E950.4	E980.4	E931.4
Quinisocaine	976.1	E858.7	E950.4	E980.4	E946.1
Quinocide	961.4	E857	E950.4	E980.4	E931.4
Quinoline (derivatives) NEC	961.3	E857	E950.4	E980.4	E931.3
Rabies					
− immune globulin (human)	964.6	E858.2	E950.4	E980.4	E934.6
− vaccine	979.1	E858.8	E950.4	E980.4	E949.1
Radioactive drug NEC	977.8	E858.8	E950.4	E980.4	E947.8
Rat poison	989.4	E863.7	E950.6	E980.7	
Rauwolfia (alkaloids)	972.6	E858.3	E950.4	E980.4	E942.6
Razoxane	976.4	E858.7	E950.4	E980.4	E946.4
Red blood cells, packed	964.7	E858.2	E950.4	E980.4	E934.7
Reducing agents, industrial NEC	983.9	E864.3	E950.7	E980.6	
Refrigerant gas (freon)	987.4	E869.2	E952.8	E982.8	
− not freon	987.8	E869.8	E952.8	E982.8	
Relaxant					
− muscle					
− − anesthetic	975.2	E858.6	E950.4	E980.4	E945.2
− − skeletal NEC	975.2	E858.6	E950.4	E980.4	E945.2
− − smooth NEC	975.1	E858.6	E950.4	E980.4	E945.1
Replacement solution	974.5	E858.5	E950.4	E980.4	E944.5
Rescinnamine	972.6	E858.3	E950.4	E980.4	E942.6
Reserpine	972.6	E858.3	E950.4	E980.4	E942.6
Resorcin, resorcinol (nonmedicinal)	983.0	E864.0	E950.7	E980.6	
− medicinal	976.4	E858.7	E950.4	E980.4	E946.4
Respiratory drug NEC	975.8	E858.6	E950.4	E980.4	E945.8
− antiasthmatic NEC	975.7	E858.6	E950.4	E980.4	E945.7
− anti-common cold NEC	975.6	E858.6	E950.4	E980.4	E945.6
− expectorant NEC	975.5	E858.6	E950.4	E980.4	E945.5
− stimulant	975.8	E858.6	E950.4	E980.4	E945.8
Retabolil	975.3	E858.6	E950.4	E980.4	E945.3
Riboflavine	963.5	E858.1	E950.4	E980.4	E933.5
Ricin	989.8	E866.8	E950.9	E980.9	
Rickettsial vaccine NEC	979.6	E858.8	E950.4	E980.4	E949.6
Rifamide	960.6	E856	E950.4	E980.4	E930.6

Substance	Poison-ing (Chapter XVII)	External Cause (E Code)			Adverse effect in correct usage
		Poisoning			
		Accident	Suicide (attempt)	Undeter-mined	
Rifampicin	960.6	E856	E950.4	E980.4	E930.6
Rifamycin	960.6	E856	E950.4	E980.4	E930.6
Ringer (lactate) solution	974.5	E858.5	E950.4	E980.4	E944.5
Ristocetin	960.8	E856	E950.4	E980.4	E930.8
Ritodrine	971.2	E855.5	E950.4	E980.4	E941.2
Roach killers - see Insecticide					
Roburite	989.8	E866.8	E950.9	E980.9	
Rodenticide	989.4	E863.7	E950.6	E980.7	
Rolitetracycline	960.4	E856	E950.4	E980.4	E930.4
Rotenone	989.4	E863.4	E950.6	E980.7	
Rotoxamine	963.0	E858.1	E950.4	E980.4	E933.0
Rubbing alcohol	980.2	E860.3	E950.9	E980.9	
Rubefacient	976.4	E858.7	E950.4	E980.4	E946.4
Rubidomycin	960.7	E856	E950.4	E980.4	E930.7
Rue	988.2	E865.4	E950.9	E980.9	
Russel's viper venin	964.5	E858.2	E950.4	E980.4	E934.5
Saccharin	977.4	E858.8	E950.4	E980.4	E947.4
Safflower oil	972.2	E858.3	E950.4	E980.4	E942.2
Salazosulfapyridine	961.0	E857	E950.4	E980.4	E931.0
Salbutamol	975.7	E858.6	E950.4	E980.4	E945.7
Salicylamide	965.4	E850.2	E950.0	E980.0	E935.2
Salicylate NEC	965.1	E850.1	E950.0	E980.0	E935.1
Salicylazosulfapyridine	961.0	E857	E950.4	E980.4	E931.0
Salicylic acid	976.4	E858.7	E950.4	E980.4	E946.4
- derivative	965.1	E850.1	E950.0	E980.0	E935.1
Salsalate	965.1	E850.1	E950.0	E980.0	E935.1
Salt substitute	977.0	E858.8	E950.4	E980.4	E947.0
Salt-replacing drug	977.0	E858.8	E950.4	E980.4	E947.0
Salt-retaining mineralcorticoid	962.0	E858.0	E950.4	E980.4	E932.0
Saluretic NEC	974.3	E858.5	E950.4	E980.4	E944.3
Santonin	961.6	E857	E950.4	E980.4	E931.6
Saralasin	972.6	E858.3	E950.4	E980.4	E942.6
Sarcolysin	963.1	E858.1	E950.4	E980.4	E933.1
Saturnine - see Lead					
S-carboxymethyl cysteine	975.5	E858.6	E950.4	E980.4	E945.5
Scheele's green	985.1	E866.3	E950.8	E980.8	
- insecticide	985.1	E863.4	E950.6	E980.7	
Schradan	989.3	E863.1	E950.6	E980.7	
Schweinfurth green	985.1	E866.3	E950.8	E980.8	
- insecticide	985.1	E863.4	E950.6	E980.7	
Scilla, rat poison	989.4	E863.7	E950.6	E980.7	
Sclerosing agent	972.7	E858.3	E950.4	E980.4	E942.7
Scopolamine	971.1	E855.4	E950.4	E980.4	E941.1
Secobarbital	967.0	E851	E950.1	E980.1	E937.0
Secretin	973.4	E858.4	E950.4	E980.4	E943.4
Secretion suppressant NEC	971.1	E855.4	E950.4	E980.4	E941.1
Sedative NEC	967.9	E852.9	E950.2	E980.2	E937.9
- mixed NEC	967.6	E852.5	E950.2	E980.2	E937.6
- specified NEC	967.8	E852.8	E950.2	E980.2	E937.8
Seed disinfectant or dressing	989.4	E863.6	E950.6	E980.7	
Seeds, poisonous	988.2	E865.3	E950.9	E980.9	

Substance	Poison-ing (Chapter XVII)	External Cause (E Code)			Adverse effect in correct usage
		Poisoning			
		Accident	Suicide (attempt)	Undeter-mined	
Selenium NEC	989.8	E866.8	E950.9	E980.9	
− fumes	987.8	E869.8	E952.8	E982.8	
− sulfide	976.4	E858.7	E950.4	E980.4	E946.4
Senna	973.1	E858.4	E950.4	E980.4	E943.1
Serum					
− antibotulinus	964.6	E858.2	E950.4	E980.4	E934.6
− anticytotoxic	964.6	E858.2	E950.4	E980.4	E934.6
− antidiphtheria	964.6	E858.2	E950.4	E980.4	E934.6
− antimeningococcus	964.6	E858.2	E950.4	E980.4	E934.6
− anti-Rh	964.6	E858.2	E950.4	E980.4	E934.6
− antisnake bite	964.6	E858.2	E950.4	E980.4	E934.6
− antitetanic	964.6	E858.2	E950.4	E980.4	E934.6
− antitoxic	964.6	E858.2	E950.4	E980.4	E934.6
− complement (inhibitor)	964.7	E858.2	E950.4	E980.4	E934.7
− convalescent	964.6	E858.2	E950.4	E980.4	E934.6
− haemolytic complement	964.7	E858.2	E950.4	E980.4	E934.7
− immune (human)	964.6	E858.2	E950.4	E980.4	E934.6
− protective NEC	964.6	E858.2	E950.4	E980.4	E934.6
Sewer gas	987.8	E869.8	E952.8	E982.8	
Shampoo	989.8	E861.0	E950.9	E980.9	
Shellfish, nonbacterial or noxious	988.0	E865.1	E950.9	E980.9	
Silicones NEC	989.8	E866.8	E950.9	E980.9	
− medicinal	976.3	E858.7	E950.4	E980.4	E946.3
Silver					
− nitrate	976.0	E858.7	E950.4	E980.4	E946.0
− nonmedicinal (dust)	985.8	E866.4	E950.9	E980.9	
− protein	976.5	E858.7	E950.4	E980.4	E946.5
Simazine	989.4	E863.5	E950.6	E980.7	
Simethicone	973.4	E858.4	E950.4	E980.4	E943.4
Sisomicin	960.8	E856	E950.4	E980.4	E930.8
Sitosterol	972.2	E858.3	E950.4	E980.4	E942.2
Sleeping draught, pill	967.9	E852.9	E950.2	E980.2	E937.9
Smallpox vaccine	979.0	E858.8	E950.4	E980.4	E949.0
Smelter fumes NEC	985.9	E866.4	E950.9	E980.9	
Smog	987.3	E869.1	E952.8	E982.8	
Smoke NEC	987.8	E869.8	E952.8	E982.8	
Snail killer	989.4	E863.9	E950.6	E980.7	
Snake venom or bite	989.5	E905.0	E950.9	E980.9	
− defibrinating	964.4	E858.2	E950.4	E980.4	E934.4
− hemocoagulase	964.5	E858.2	E950.4	E980.4	E934.5
Snuff	989.8	E866.8	E950.9	E980.9	
Soap (powder) (product)	989.6	E861.1	E950.9	E980.9	
− superfatted	976.2	E858.7	E950.4	E980.4	E946.2
Soda (caustic)	983.2	E864.2	E950.7	E980.6	
Sodium					
− acetosulfone	961.8	E857	E950.4	E980.4	E931.8
− amidotrizoate	977.8	E858.8	E950.4	E980.4	E947.8
− aminopterin	963.1	E858.1	E950.4	E980.4	E933.1
− antimony gluconate	961.2	E857	E950.4	E980.4	E931.2
− arsenate - see Arsenic					
− aurothiomalate	965.6	E850.4	E950.0	E980.0	E935.4

Substance	Poison- ing (Chapter XVII)	External Cause (E Code)			
		Poisoning			Adverse effect in correct usage
		Accident	Suicide (attempt)	Undeter- mined	
Sodium - *continued*					
– barbiturate	967.0	E851	E950.1	E980.1	E937.0
– basic phosphate	973.3	E858.4	E950.4	E980.4	E943.3
– benzoate	977.8	E858.8	E950.4	E980.4	E947.8
– bicarbonate	963.3	E858.1	E950.4	E980.4	E933.3
– bichromate	983.9	E864.3	E950.7	E980.6	
– biphosphate	963.2	E858.1	E950.4	E980.4	E933.2
– bisulfate	983.9	E864.3	E950.7	E980.6	
– borate (cleanser)	989.8	E861.3	E950.9	E980.9	
– – eye	976.5	E858.7	E950.4	E980.4	E946.5
– bromide	967.3	E852.2	E950.2	E980.2	E937.3
– calcium ededate	963.8	E858.1	E950.4	E980.4	E933.8
– carbonate NEC	983.2	E864.2	E950.7	E980.6	
– chlorate NEC	983.9	E864.3	E950.7	E980.6	
– chromate	983.9	E864.3	E950.7	E980.6	
– citrate	963.3	E858.1	E950.4	E980.4	E933.3
– cromoglicate	975.7	E858.6	E950.4	E980.4	E945.7
– cyanide - see Cyanide(s)					
– dehydrocholate	977.8	E858.8	E950.4	E980.4	E947.8
– dibunate	975.4	E858.6	E950.4	E980.4	E945.4
– dioctyl sulfosuccinate	973.2	E858.4	E950.4	E980.4	E943.2
– etacrynate	974.4	E858.5	E950.4	E980.4	E944.4
– feredetate	964.0	E858.2	E950.4	E980.4	E934.0
– fluoride - see Fluoride(s)					
– fluoroacetate (dust) (pesticide)	989.4	E863.7	E950.6	E980.7	
– fusidate	960.8	E856	E950.4	E980.4	E930.8
– glucosulfone	961.8	E857	E950.4	E980.4	E931.8
– glutamate	963.2	E858.1	E950.4	E980.4	E933.2
– hydroxide	983.2	E864.2	E950.7	E980.6	
– hypochlorite (bleach) NEC	983.9	E864.3	E950.7	E980.6	
– – vapor	987.8	E869.8	E952.8	E982.8	
– indigotindisulfonate	977.8	E858.8	E950.4	E980.4	E947.8
– iopodate	977.8	E858.8	E950.4	E980.4	E947.8
– lactate	963.3	E858.1	E950.4	E980.4	E933.3
– lauryl sulphate	976.2	E858.7	E950.4	E980.4	E946.2
– L-triiodothyronine	962.7	E858.0	E950.4	E980.4	E932.7
– magnesium citrate	977.0	E858.8	E950.4	E980.4	E947.0
– mersalate	974.0	E858.5	E950.4	E980.4	E944.0
– monofluoroacetate (dust) (pesticide)	989.4	E863.7	E950.6	E980.7	
– morrhuate	972.7	E858.3	E950.4	E980.4	E942.7
– nitrate (oxidizing agent)	983.9	E864.3	E950.7	E980.6	
– nitrite	977.2	E858.8	E950.4	E980.4	E947.2
– oxalate	989.8	E866.8	E950.9	E980.9	
– perborate (nonmedicinal) NEC	989.8	E866.8	E950.9	E980.9	
– – medicinal	976.0	E858.7	E950.4	E980.4	E946.0
– phytate	977.2	E858.8	E950.4	E980.4	E947.2
– polyhydroxyaluminium monocarbonate	973.0	E858.4	E950.4	E980.4	E943.0
– polystyrene sulfonate	974.5	E858.5	E950.4	E980.4	E944.5
– propyl hydroxybenzoate	977.4	E858.8	E950.4	E980.4	E947.4
– salicylate	965.1	E850.1	E950.0	E980.0	E935.1
– salt NEC	974.6	E858.5	E950.4	E980.4	E944.6

Substance	Poison-ing (Chapter XVII)	External Cause (E Code)			Adverse effect in correct usage
		Poisoning			
		Accident	Suicide (attempt)	Undeter-mined	
Sodium - *continued*					
— selenate	989.4	E863.4	E950.6	E980.7	
— sulfate	973.3	E858.4	E950.4	E980.4	E943.3
— sulfoxone	961.8	E857	E950.4	E980.4	E931.8
— thiosulfate	977.2	E858.8	E950.4	E980.4	E947.2
— tolbutamide	962.3	E858.0	E950.4	E980.4	E932.3
— versenate	977.2	E858.8	E950.4	E980.4	E947.2
Sodium-free salt	977.0	E858.8	E950.4	E980.4	E947.0
Sodium-removing resin	974.5	E858.5	E950.4	E980.4	E944.5
Soframycin	960.8	E856	E950.4	E980.4	E930.8
Solactol	982.8	E862.4	E950.9	E980.9	
Solapsone	961.8	E857	E950.4	E980.4	E931.8
Solar lotion	976.3	E858.7	E950.4	E980.4	E946.3
Soldering fluid	983.1	E864.1	E950.7	E980.6	
Solid substance NEC	989.9	E866.9	E950.9	E980.9	
Solvents, industrial NEC	982.8	E862.4	E950.9	E980.9	
Solvulose	982.8	E862.4	E950.9	E980.9	
Somatotropin	962.4	E858.0	E950.4	E980.4	E932.4
Soporific	967.9	E852.9	E950.2	E980.2	E937.9
Sorbide nitrate	972.4	E858.3	E950.4	E980.4	E942.4
Sorbitol	977.4	E858.8	E950.4	E980.4	E947.4
Sotalol	972.0	E858.3	E950.4	E980.4	E942.0
Sparteine	975.0	E858.6	E950.4	E980.4	E945.0
Spasmolytic					
— autonomic	971.1	E855.4	E950.4	E980.4	E941.1
— bronchial NEC	975.7	E858.6	E950.4	E980.4	E945.7
— quaternary ammonium	971.1	E855.4	E950.4	E980.4	E941.1
— skeletal muscle NEC	975.2	E858.6	E950.4	E980.4	E945.2
Spectinomycin	960.6	E856	E950.4	E980.4	E930.6
Spermicide	976.8	E858.7	E950.4	E980.4	E946.8
Spindle inactivators	974.7	E858.5	E950.4	E980.4	E944.7
Spiperone	969.2	E853.1	E950.3	E980.3	E939.2
Spiramycin	960.3	E856	E950.4	E980.4	E930.3
Spirit(s) (neutral) NEC	980.0	E860.1	E950.9	E980.9	
— industrial	980.0	E860.1	E950.9	E980.9	
— of salt - see Hydrochloric acid					
— surgical	980.0	E860.1	E950.9	E980.9	
Spironolactone	974.4	E858.5	E950.4	E980.4	E944.4
Spiroperidol	969.2	E853.1	E950.3	E980.3	E939.2
Sprays (aerosol)	989.8	E866.8	E950.9	E980.9	
— cosmetic	989.8	E866.7	E950.9	E980.9	
— specified content - see Substance specified					
Spreading factor	976.8	E858.7	E950.4	E980.4	E946.8
Sputum viscosity lowering drug	975.5	E858.6	E950.4	E980.4	E945.5
Squill, rat poison	989.3	E863.7	E950.6	E980.7	
Stains	989.8	E866.8	E950.9	E980.9	
Stannous					
— fluoride	974.6	E858.5	E950.4	E980.4	E944.6
— oxide	961.2	E857	E950.4	E980.4	E931.2
Stanolone	962.1	E858.0	E950.4	E980.4	E932.1

Substance	Poison-ing (Chapter XVII)	External Cause (E Code)			
		Poisoning			Adverse effect in correct usage
		Accident	Suicide (attempt)	Undeter-mined	
Stanozolol	962.1	E858.0	E950.4	E980.4	E932.1
Sterculia	973.3	E858.4	E950.4	E980.4	E943.3
Sternutator gas	987.8	E869.8	E952.8	E982.8	
Steroid					
– adrenal cortical	962.0	E858.0	E950.4	E980.4	E932.0
– anabolic	962.1	E858.0	E950.4	E980.4	E932.1
– androgenic	962.1	E858.0	E950.4	E980.4	E932.1
– antineoplastic	962.1	E858.0	E950.4	E980.4	E932.1
– – estrogen	962.2	E858.0	E950.4	E980.4	E932.2
Stibine	985.4	E866.2	E950.9	E980.9	
Stibogluconate	961.2	E857	E950.4	E980.4	E931.2
Stibophen	961.2	E857	E950.4	E980.4	E931.2
Stilbamide	961.2	E857	E950.4	E980.4	E931.2
Stilbestrol	962.2	E858.0	E950.4	E980.4	E932.2
Stimulant					
– central nervous system	970.9	E854.3	E950.4	E980.4	E940.9
– – specified NEC	970.8	E854.3	E950.4	E980.4	E940.8
– respiratory	970.0	E854.3	E950.4	E980.4	E940.0
Stone dissolving drug	977.0	E858.8	E950.4	E980.4	E947.0
Storage batteries (cells) (acid)	983.1	E864.1	E950.7	E980.6	
Stove gas - see Gas, utility					
Stramonium	975.7	E858.6	E950.4	E980.4	E945.7
Streptodornase	964.4	E858.2	E950.4	E980.4	E934.4
Streptoduocin	960.6	E856	E950.4	E980.4	E930.6
Streptokinase	963.4	E858.1	E950.4	E980.4	E933.4
Streptomycin	960.6	E856	E950.4	E980.4	E930.6
Streptonivicin	960.8	E856	E950.4	E980.4	E930.8
Stripper (paint) (solvent)	982.8	E862.4	E950.9	E980.9	
Strobane	989.2	E863.0	E950.6	E980.7	
Strophanthin-G	972.1	E858.3	E950.4	E980.4	E942.1
Strophanthus	972.1	E858.3	E950.4	E980.4	E942.1
Strophantin	972.1	E858.3	E950.4	E980.4	E942.1
Strychnine (nonmedicinal) (pesticide) (salts)	989.1	E863.9	E950.6	E980.7	
– medicinal	975.3	E858.6	E950.4	E980.4	E945.3
Styramate	968.0	E855.1	E950.4	E980.4	E938.0
Styrene	983.0	E864.0	E950.7	E980.6	
Succinimides	966.2	E855.0	E950.4	E980.4	E936.2
Succinylcholine	975.2	E858.6	E950.4	E980.4	E945.2
Succinylsulfathiazole	961.0	E857	E950.4	E980.4	E931.0
Sucrose	974.5	E858.5	E950.4	E980.4	E944.5
Sulfacetamide	976.5	E858.7	E950.4	E980.4	E946.5
Sulfachlorpyridazine	961.0	E857	E950.4	E980.4	E931.0
Sulfadiazine	961.0	E857	E950.4	E980.4	E931.0
Sulfadimethoxine	961.0	E857	E950.4	E980.4	E931.0
Sulfadimidine	961.0	E857	E950.4	E980.4	E931.0
Sulfafurazole	961.0	E857	E950.4	E980.4	E931.0
Sulfaguanidine	961.0	E857	E950.4	E980.4	E931.0
Sulfaloxate	961.0	E857	E950.4	E980.4	E931.0
Sulfaloxic acid	961.0	E857	E950.4	E980.4	E931.0
Sulfamerazine	961.0	E857	E950.4	E980.4	E931.0

Substance	Poisoning (Chapter XVII)	External Cause (E Code)			Adverse effect in correct usage
		Poisoning			
		Accident	Suicide (attempt)	Undetermined	
Sulfameter	961.0	E857	E950.4	E980.4	E931.0
Sulfamethizole	961.0	E857	E950.4	E980.4	E931.0
Sulfamethoxazole	961.0	E857	E950.4	E980.4	E931.0
Sulfamethoxydiazine	961.0	E857	E950.4	E980.4	E931.0
Sulfamethoxypyridazine	961.0	E857	E950.4	E980.4	E931.0
Sulfamyxin	960.8	E856	E950.4	E980.4	E930.8
Sulfanilamide	961.0	E857	E950.4	E980.4	E931.0
Sulfaphenazole	961.0	E857	E950.4	E980.4	E931.0
Sulfaproxyline	961.0	E857	E950.4	E980.4	E931.0
Sulfapyridine	961.0	E857	E950.4	E980.4	E931.0
Sulfasalazine	961.0	E857	E950.4	E980.4	E931.0
Sulfated amylopectin	973.8	E858.4	E950.4	E980.4	E943.8
Sulfathiazole	961.0	E857	E950.4	E980.4	E931.0
Sulfatostearate	976.2	E858.7	E950.4	E980.4	E946.2
Sulfinpyrazone	974.7	E858.5	E950.4	E980.4	E944.7
Sulfisomidine	961.0	E857	E950.4	E980.4	E931.0
Sulfisoxazole	961.0	E857	E950.4	E980.4	E931.0
Sulfobromophthalein sodium	977.8	E858.8	E950.4	E980.4	E947.8
Sulfomyxin (sodium)	976.6	E858.7	E950.4	E980.4	E946.6
Sulfonamide NEC	961.0	E857	E950.4	E980.4	E931.0
− eye	976.5	E858.7	E950.4	E980.4	E946.5
Sulfone	961.8	E857	E950.4	E980.4	E931.8
Sulfur, sulfuretted, sulfuric, sulfurous, sulfuryl (compounds) NEC	989.8	E866.8	E950.9	E980.9	
− acid	983.1	E864.1	E950.7	E980.6	
− dioxide (gas)	987.3	E869.1	E952.8	E982.8	
− ether − see Ether(s)					
− hydrogen	987.8	E869.8	E952.8	E982.8	
− lime	976.4	E858.7	E950.4	E980.4	E946.4
− medicinal (ointment) NEC	976.4	E858.7	E950.4	E980.4	E946.4
− pesticide (vapor)	989.4	E863.9	E950.6	E980.7	
− vapor NEC	987.8	E869.8	E952.8	E982.8	
Sulindac	965.8	E850.8	E950.0	E980.0	E935.8
Sulph − see Sulf-					
Sulphapyrimidine glymidine	962.3	E858.0	E950.4	E980.4	E932.3
Sulpiride	969.5	E853.8	E950.3	E980.3	E939.5
Sulthiame, sultiame	966.3	E855.0	E950.4	E980.4	E936.3
Sunflower seed oil	972.2	E858.3	E950.4	E980.4	E942.2
Suramin (sodium)	961.6	E857	E950.4	E980.4	E931.6
Suxamethonium (chloride)	975.2	E858.6	E950.4	E980.4	E945.2
Sweetener	977.4	E858.8	E950.4	E980.4	E947.4
Sym-dichloroethyl ether	982.3	E862.4	E950.9	E980.9	
Sympatholytic NEC	971.3	E855.6	E950.4	E980.4	E941.3
− haloalkylamine	971.3	E855.6	E950.4	E980.4	E941.3
Sympathomimetic NEC	971.2	E855.5	E950.4	E980.4	E941.2
− anti-common-cold	975.6	E858.6	E950.4	E980.4	E945.6
− bronchodilator	975.7	E858.6	E950.4	E980.4	E945.7
− specified NEC	971.2	E855.5	E950.4	E980.4	E941.2
Syrosingopine	972.6	E858.3	E950.4	E980.4	E942.6
Systemic drug	963.9	E858.1	E950.4	E980.4	E933.9
− specified NEC	963.8	E858.1	E950.4	E980.4	E933.8

Substance	Poison-ing (Chapter XVII)	External Cause (E Code)			Adverse effect in correct usage
		Poisoning			
		Accident	Suicide (attempt)	Undeter-mined	
Tacrine	970.0	E854.3	E950.4	E980.4	E940.0
Talampicillin	960.0	E856	E950.4	E980.4	E930.0
Talbutal	967.0	E851	E950.1	E980.1	E937.0
Talc powder	976.3	E858.7	E950.4	E980.4	E946.3
Tamoxifen	962.9	E858.0	E950.4	E980.4	E932.9
Tannic acid	976.2	E858.7	E950.4	E980.4	E946.2
Tar NEC	983.0	E864.0	E950.7	E980.6	
− camphor - see Naphthalene					
− distillate	976.1	E858.7	E950.4	E980.4	E946.1
− fumes	987.8	E869.8	E952.8	E982.8	
− medicinal	976.1	E858.7	E950.4	E980.4	E946.1
− ointment	976.1	E858.7	E950.4	E980.4	E946.1
Tartar emetic	961.2	E857	E950.4	E980.4	E931.2
Tartaric acid	983.1	E864.1	E950.7	E980.6	
Tartrate, laxative	973.3	E858.4	E950.4	E980.4	E943.3
TCA	983.1	E864.1	E950.7	E980.6	
TCDD	989.2	E866.8	E950.9	E980.9	
TDI	983.0	E864.0	E950.7	E980.6	
− vapor	987.8	E869.8	E952.8	E982.8	
Tear gas	987.5	E869.3	E952.8	E982.8	
Tear solution	976.5	E858.7	E950.4	E980.4	E946.5
Teclothiazide	974.3	E858.5	E950.4	E980.4	E944.3
Tellurium	989.8	E866.8	E950.9	E980.9	
− fumes	987.8	E869.8	E952.8	E982.8	
Tepa	963.1	E858.1	E950.4	E980.4	E933.1
Tepp	989.3	E863.1	E950.6	E980.7	
Teprotide	972.6	E858.3	E950.4	E980.4	E942.6
Terbutaline	975.7	E858.6	E950.4	E980.4	E945.7
Terpin hydrate	975.5	E858.6	E950.4	E980.4	E945.5
Testolactone	962.1	E858.0	E950.4	E980.4	E932.1
Testosterone	962.1	E858.0	E950.4	E980.4	E932.1
Tetanus toxoid or vaccine	978.4	E858.8	E950.4	E980.4	E948.4
Tetrabenazine	967.8	E852.8	E950.2	E980.2	E937.8
Tetracaine	968.5	E855.2	E950.4	E980.4	E938.5
− regional	968.6	E855.2	E950.4	E980.4	E938.6
− spinal	968.7	E855.2	E950.4	E980.4	E938.7
Tetrachlorethylene - see Tetrachloroethylene					
Tetrachloroethane	982.3	E862.4	E950.9	E980.9	
− vapor	987.8	E862.4	E950.9	E980.9	
Tetrachloroethylene (liquid)	982.3	E862.4	E950.9	E980.9	
− medicinal	961.6	E857	E950.4	E980.4	E931.6
− vapor	987.8	E862.4	E950.9	E980.9	
Tetrachloromethane - see Carbon tetrachloride					
Tetracosactide	962.4	E858.0	E950.4	E980.4	E932.4
Tetracycline	960.4	E856	E950.4	E980.4	E930.4
Tetraethyl					
− lead	984.1	E866.0	E950.9	E980.9	
− pyrophosphate	989.3	E863.1	E950.6	E980.7	
Tetrahydrofuran	982.8	E862.4	E950.9	E980.9	

Substance	Poison- ing (Chapter XVII)	External Cause (E Code)			
		Poisoning			Adverse effect in correct usage
		Accident	Suicide (attempt)	Undeter- mined	
Tetrahydronaphthalene	982.0	E862.4	E950.9	E980.9	
Tetrahydrozoline	976.5	E858.7	E950.4	E980.4	E946.5
Tetralin(e)	982.0	E862.4	E950.9	E980.9	
Tetramethylthiuram (disulfide) NEC	989.4	E863.9	E950.6	E980.7	
Tetranicotinoyl fructose	972.5	E858.3	E950.4	E980.4	E942.5
Tetranitromethylaniline	983.0	E864.0	E950.7	E980.6	
Tetryl	983.0	E864.0	E950.7	E980.6	
Tetrylammonium chloride	972.3	E858.3	E950.4	E980.4	E942.3
Tetryzoline	976.5	E858.7	E950.4	E980.4	E946.5
Thalidomide	963.1	E858.1	E950.4	E980.4	E933.1
Thallium (compounds) (dust) NEC	985.8	E866.4	E950.9	E980.9	
– pesticide	985.8	E863.7	E950.6	E980.7	
THAM	963.3	E858.1	E950.4	E980.4	E933.3
Thenyldiamine	963.0	E858.1	E950.4	E980.4	E933.0
Theobromine (calcium salicylate)	974.1	E858.5	E950.4	E980.4	E944.1
Theophylline	974.1	E858.5	E950.4	E980.4	E944.1
Thiacetazone	961.8	E857	E950.4	E980.4	E931.8
Thialbarbital	968.3	E855.1	E950.4	E980.4	E938.3
Thiamazole	962.8	E858.0	E950.4	E980.4	E932.8
Thiambutozine	961.8	E857	E950.4	E980.4	E931.8
Thiamine	963.5	E858.1	E950.4	E980.4	E933.5
Thiamphenicol	960.2	E856	E950.4	E980.4	E930.2
Thiamylal	967.0	E851	E950.1	E980.1	E937.0
– sodium	968.3	E855.1	E950.4	E980.4	E938.3
Thiethylperazine	969.1	E853.0	E950.3	E980.3	E939.1
Thiobarbital sodium	968.3	E855.1	E950.4	E980.4	E938.3
Thiobarbiturate anesthetic	968.3	E855.1	E950.4	E980.4	E938.3
Thioglycolate	976.4	E858.7	E950.4	E980.4	E946.4
Thioglycolic acid	989.8	E866.7	E950.9	E980.9	
Thioguanine	963.1	E858.1	E950.4	E980.4	E933.1
Thiomersal	976.0	E858.7	E950.4	E980.4	E946.0
Thionazin	989.4	E863.9	E950.6	E980.7	
Thiopental (sodium)	968.3	E855.1	E950.4	E980.4	E938.3
Thiopentone (sodium)	968.3	E855.1	E950.4	E980.4	E938.3
Thiopropazate	969.3	E853.8	E950.3	E980.3	E939.3
Thioproperazine	969.1	E853.0	E950.3	E980.3	E939.1
Thioridazine	969.1	E853.0	E950.3	E980.3	E939.1
Thiosinamine	976.4	E858.7	E950.4	E980.4	E946.4
Thiotepa	963.1	E858.1	E950.4	E980.4	E933.1
Thiphenamil	971.1	E855.4	E950.4	E980.4	E941.1
Thiram NEC	989.4	E863.9	E950.6	E980.7	
Thonzylamine (systemic)	963.0	E858.1	E950.4	E980.4	E933.0
– mucosal decongestant	975.6	E858.6	E950.4	E980.4	E945.6
Throat drug NEC	976.6	E858.7	E950.4	E980.4	E946.6
Thromboplastin	964.5	E858.2	E950.4	E980.4	E934.5
Thurfyl nicotinate	976.4	E858.7	E950.4	E980.4	E946.4
Thymol	983.0	E864.0	E950.7	E980.6	
Thymoxamine	971.3	E855.6	E950.4	E980.4	E941.3
Thymus extract	962.9	E858.0	E950.4	E980.4	E932.9
Thyroglobulin	962.7	E858.0	E950.4	E980.4	E932.7
Thyroid extract	962.7	E858.0	E950.4	E980.4	E932.7

Substance	Poison-ing (Chapter XVII)	External Cause (E Code)			Adverse effect in correct usage
		Poisoning			
		Accident	Suicide (attempt)	Undeter-mined	
Thyrotrophic hormone	962.4	E858.0	E950.4	E980.4	E932.4
Thyrotrophine	962.4	E858.0	E950.4	E980.4	E932.4
Thyroxine	962.7	E858.0	E950.4	E980.4	E932.7
Tiabendazole	961.6	E857	E950.4	E980.4	E931.6
Tiemonium	971.1	E855.4	E950.4	E980.4	E941.1
Timolol	971.3	E855.6	E950.4	E980.4	E941.3
Tin (chloride) (dust) (oxide) NEC	985.8	E866.4	E950.9	E980.9	
– anti-infective	961.2	E857	E950.4	E980.4	E931.2
Tincture, iodine - see Iodine					
Tiotixene	969.5	E853.8	E950.3	E980.3	E939.5
Tioxolone	976.4	E858.7	E950.4	E980.4	E946.4
Titanium (compounds) (vapor)	985.8	E866.4	E950.9	E980.9	
– dioxide	976.3	E858.7	E950.4	E980.4	E946.3
– oxide	976.3	E858.7	E950.4	E980.4	E946.3
– tetrachloride	985.8	E866.4	E950.9	E980.9	
Titanocene	985.8	E866.4	E950.9	E980.9	
TMTD	989.4	E863.9	E950.6	E980.7	
TNT	989.8	E866.8	E950.9	E980.9	
– fumes	987.8	E869.8	E952.8	E982.8	
Toadstool	988.1	E865.5	E950.9	E980.9	
Tobacco NEC	989.8	E866.8	E950.9	E980.9	
Tobramycin	960.8	E856	E950.4	E980.4	E930.8
Tocoferol	963.5	E858.1	E950.4	E980.4	E933.5
Todralazine	972.6	E858.3	E950.4	E980.4	E942.6
Toilet deodorizer	989.8	E866.8	E950.9	E980.9	
Tolamolol	972.0	E858.3	E950.4	E980.4	E942.0
Tolazamide	962.3	E858.0	E950.4	E980.4	E932.3
Tolazoline (hydrochloride)	971.3	E855.6	E950.4	E980.4	E941.3
Tolbutamide	962.3	E858.0	E950.4	E980.4	E932.3
Tolmetin	965.8	E850.8	E950.0	E980.0	E935.8
Tolnaftate	976.0	E858.7	E950.4	E980.4	E946.0
Toluene (liquid)	982.0	E862.4	E950.9	E980.9	
– diisocyanate	983.0	E864.0	E950.7	E980.6	
– vapor	987.8	E862.4	E950.9	E980.9	
Toluidine	983.0	E864.0	E950.7	E980.6	
– vapor	987.8	E869.8	E952.8	E982.8	
Toluol (liquid)	982.0	E862.4	E950.9	E980.9	
– vapor	987.8	E862.4	E950.9	E980.9	
Toluylenediamine	983.9	E864.3	E950.7	E980.6	
Tolylene-2, 4-diisocyanate	983.0	E864.0	E950.7	E980.6	
Tonic NEC	977.0	E858.8	E950.4	E980.4	E947.0
Topical action drug NEC	976.9	E858.7	E950.4	E980.4	E946.9
– ear, nose or throat	976.6	E858.7	E950.4	E980.4	E946.6
– eye	976.5	E858.7	E950.4	E980.4	E946.5
– skin	976.4	E858.7	E950.4	E980.4	E946.4
– specified NEC	976.8	E858.7	E950.4	E980.4	E946.8
Tosylchloramide sodium	976.8	E858.7	E950.4	E980.4	E946.8
Totaquin	961.4	E857	E950.4	E980.4	E931.4
Toxaphene (dust) (spray)	989.2	E863.0	E950.6	E980.7	
Toxin, diphtheria (schick test)	977.8	E858.8	E950.4	E980.4	E947.8
Toxoid					

Substance	Poisoning (Chapter XVII)	External Cause (E Code)			Adverse effect in correct usage
		Poisoning			
		Accident	Suicide (attempt)	Undetermined	
Toxoid - *continued*					
– combined	978.9	E858.8	E950.4	E980.4	E948.9
– diphtheria	978.5	E858.8	E950.4	E980.4	E948.5
– tetanus	978.4	E858.8	E950.4	E980.4	E948.4
Trace element NEC	964.1	E858.2	E950.4	E980.4	E934.1
Tractor fuel NEC	981	E862.1	E950.9	E980.9	
Tragacanth	977.4	E858.8	E950.4	E980.4	E947.4
Tramazoline	975.6	E858.6	E950.4	E980.4	E945.6
Tranexamic acid	964.4	E858.2	E950.4	E980.4	E934.4
Tranquilizer NEC	969.5	E853.8	E950.3	E980.3	E939.5
– with hypnotic or sedative	967.6	E852.5	E950.2	E980.2	E937.6
– benzodiazepine NEC	969.4	E853.2	E950.3	E980.3	E939.4
– butyrophenone NEC	969.2	E853.1	E950.3	E980.3	E939.2
– carbamate	969.5	E853.8	E950.3	E980.3	E939.5
– dimethylamine	969.1	E853.0	E950.3	E980.3	E939.1
– ethylamino	969.1	E853.0	E950.3	E980.3	E939.1
– hydroxyzine	969.5	E853.8	E950.3	E980.3	E939.5
– major NEC	969.3	E853.8	E950.3	E980.3	E939.3
– phenothiazine NEC	969.1	E853.0	E950.3	E980.3	E939.1
– piperazine	969.1	E853.0	E950.3	E980.3	E939.1
– piperidine	969.1	E853.0	E950.3	E980.3	E939.1
– propylamine	969.1	E853.0	E950.3	E980.3	E939.1
– thioxanthine NEC	969.5	E853.8	E950.3	E980.3	E939.5
Tranylcypromine	969.0	E854.0	E950.3	E980.3	E939.0
Trazadone	969.0	E854.0	E950.3	E980.3	E939.0
Tretamine	963.1	E858.1	E950.4	E980.4	E933.1
Triacetin	976.0	E858.7	E950.4	E980.4	E946.0
Triacetoxyanthracene	976.4	E858.7	E950.4	E980.4	E946.4
Triacetyloleandomycin	960.3	E856	E950.4	E980.4	E930.3
Triamcinolone	962.0	E858.0	E950.4	E980.4	E932.0
Triamterene	974.5	E858.5	E950.4	E980.4	E944.5
Triaziquone	963.1	E858.1	E950.4	E980.4	E933.1
Tribromethanol, rectal	968.4	E855.1	E950.4	E980.4	E938.4
Trichloethylene	968.2	E855.1	E950.4	E980.4	E938.2
Trichloracetic acid	976.4	E858.7	E950.4	E980.4	E946.4
Trichlorfon	989.2	E863.0	E950.6	E980.7	
Trichlormethiazide	974.3	E858.5	E950.4	E980.4	E944.3
Trichloroacetic acid	983.1	E864.1	E950.7	E980.6	
– medicinal	976.4	E858.7	E950.4	E980.4	E946.4
Trichloroethane	982.3	E862.4	E950.9	E980.9	
Trichloroethylene	982.3	E862.4	E950.9	E980.9	
– vapor NEC	987.8	E862.4	E950.9	E980.9	
Trichlorofluoromethane NEC	987.4	E869.2	E952.8	E982.8	
Trichloropropane	982.3	E862.4	E950.9	E980.9	
Trichomycin	960.1	E856	E950.4	E980.4	E930.1
Tricresyl phosphate	989.8	E866.8	E950.9	E980.9	
Tricyclamol	971.1	E855.4	E950.4	E980.4	E941.1
Tridihexethyl	971.1	E855.4	E950.4	E980.4	E941.1
Triethanolamine NEC	983.2	E864.2	E950.7	E980.6	
– detergent	983.2	E861.0	E950.9	E980.9	
– trinitrate biphosphate	972.4	E858.3	E950.4	E980.4	E942.4

Substance	Poison- ing (Chapter XVII)	External Cause (E Code)			Adverse effect in correct usage
		Poisoning			
		Accident	Suicide (attempt)	Undeter- mined	
Triethanomelamine	963.1	E858.1	E950.4	E980.4	E933.1
Triethylenethiophosphoramide	963.1	E858.1	E950.4	E980.4	E933.1
Trifluoperazine	969.1	E853.0	E950.3	E980.3	E939.1
Trifluoroethyl vinyl ether	968.2	E855.1	E950.4	E980.4	E938.2
Trifluperidol	969.2	E853.1	E950.3	E980.3	E939.2
Triflupromazine	969.1	E853.0	E950.3	E980.3	E939.1
Trihexyphenidyl	971.1	E855.4	E950.4	E980.4	E941.1
Trilene - see Trichloroethylene					
Trimeprazine	969.1	E853.0	E950.3	E980.3	E939.1
Trimetazidine	972.4	E858.3	E950.4	E980.4	E942.4
Trimethadione	966.0	E855.0	E950.4	E980.4	E936.0
Trimethaphan	972.3	E858.3	E950.4	E980.4	E942.3
Trimethidium	972.3	E858.3	E950.4	E980.4	E942.3
Trimethobenzamide	963.0	E858.1	E950.4	E980.4	E933.0
Trimethoprim	961.4	E857	E950.4	E980.4	E931.4
Trimethylcarbinol	980.3	E860.4	E950.9	E980.9	
Trimipramine	969.0	E854.0	E950.3	E980.3	E939.0
Trinitrin	972.4	E858.3	E950.4	E980.4	E942.4
Trinitrobenzol	983.0	E864.0	E950.7	E980.6	
Trinitrophenol	983.0	E864.0	E950.7	E980.6	
Trinitrotoluene	989.8	E866.8	E950.9	E980.9	
— fumes	987.8	E869.8	E952.8	E982.8	
Triorthocresyl phosphate	989.8	E866.8	E950.9	E980.9	
Trioxide of arsenic - see Arsenic					
Tripelennamine	963.0	E858.1	E950.4	E980.4	E933.0
Triperidol	969.2	E853.1	E950.3	E980.3	E939.2
Triphenylphosphate	989.8	E866.8	E950.9	E980.9	
Triple					
— bromides	967.3	E852.2	E950.2	E980.2	E937.3
— carbonate	973.0	E858.4	E950.4	E980.4	E943.0
— vaccine, including pertussis	978.6	E858.8	E950.4	E980.4	E948.6
Triprolidine	963.0	E858.1	E950.4	E980.4	E933.0
Trisodium hydrogen edetate	977.2	E858.8	E950.4	E980.4	E947.2
Trisulfapyrimidines	961.0	E857	E950.4	E980.4	E931.0
Troleandomycin	960.3	E856	E950.4	E980.4	E930.3
Trometamol	963.3	E858.1	E950.4	E980.4	E933.3
Tromethamine	963.3	E858.1	E950.4	E980.4	E933.3
Tropicamide	971.1	E855.4	E950.4	E980.4	E941.1
Troxidone	966.0	E855.0	E950.4	E980.4	E936.0
Tryparsamide	961.1	E857	E950.4	E980.4	E931.1
Trypsin	973.4	E858.4	E950.4	E980.4	E943.4
TSH	962.4	E858.0	E950.4	E980.4	E932.4
Tuaminoheptane	975.6	E858.6	E950.4	E980.4	E945.6
Tubocurarine (chloride)	975.2	E858.6	E950.4	E980.4	E945.2
Turpentine (spirits of)	982.8	E862.4	E950.9	E980.9	
— vapor	987.8	E862.4	E950.9	E980.9	
Twilight sleep	969.5	E853.8	E950.3	E980.3	E939.5
Tybamate	969.5	E853.8	E950.3	E980.3	E939.5
Tyloxapol	975.5	E858.6	E950.4	E980.4	E945.5
Tymazoline	975.6	E858.6	E950.4	E980.4	E945.6
Typhoid-paratyphoid vaccine	978.1	E858.8	E950.4	E980.4	E948.1

Substance	Poison-ing (Chapter XVII)	External Cause (E Code)			
		Poisoning			Adverse effect in correct usage
		Accident	Suicide (attempt)	Undeter-mined	
Typhus vaccine	979.2	E858.8	E950.4	E980.4	E949.2
Tyrothricin	976.6	E858.7	E950.4	E980.4	E946.6
Ultraviolet light protectant	976.3	E858.7	E950.4	E980.4	E946.3
Undecenoic acid	976.0	E858.7	E950.4	E980.4	E946.0
Undecylenic acid	976.0	E858.7	E950.4	E980.4	E946.0
Unsaturated fatty acid	972.2	E858.3	E950.4	E980.4	E942.2
Upas	989.8	E866.8	E950.9	E980.9	
Uracil mustard	963.1	E858.1	E950.4	E980.4	E933.1
Uramustine	963.1	E858.1	E950.4	E980.4	E933.1
Urea	974.4	E858.5	E950.4	E980.4	E944.4
– peroxide	976.0	E858.7	E950.4	E980.4	E946.0
– stabamine	961.2	E857	E950.4	E980.4	E931.2
Urethane	963.1	E858.1	E950.4	E980.4	E933.1
Uric acid metabolism drug NEC	974.7	E858.5	E950.4	E980.4	E944.7
Uricosuric	974.7	E858.5	E950.4	E980.4	E944.7
Urinary anti-infective	961.9	E857	E950.4	E980.4	E931.9
Urokinase	964.4	E858.2	E950.4	E980.4	E934.4
Ursodeoxycholic acid	977.0	E858.8	E950.4	E980.4	E947.0
Uterine relaxing factor	962.2	E858.0	E950.4	E980.4	E932.2
Utility gas - see Gas, utility					
Vaccine NEC	979.9	E858.8	E950.4	E980.4	E949.9
– antineoplastic	979.9	E858.8	E950.4	E980.4	E949.9
– bacterial NEC	978.8	E858.8	E950.4	E980.4	E948.8
– – mixed NEC	978.9	E858.8	E950.4	E980.4	E948.9
– BCG	978.0	E858.8	E950.4	E980.4	E948.0
– cholera	978.2	E858.8	E950.4	E980.4	E948.2
– diphtheria	978.5	E858.8	E950.4	E980.4	E948.5
– influenza	979.6	E858.8	E950.4	E980.4	E949.6
– measles	979.4	E858.8	E950.4	E980.4	E949.4
– mixed, viral-rickettsial(-bacterial)	979.7	E858.8	E950.4	E980.4	E949.7
– mumps	979.6	E858.8	E950.4	E980.4	E949.6
– pertussis	978.6	E858.8	E950.4	E980.4	E948.6
– – with diphtheria	978.6	E858.8	E950.4	E980.4	E948.6
– – – and tetanus	978.6	E858.8	E950.4	E980.4	E948.6
– plague	978.3	E858.8	E950.4	E980.4	E948.3
– poliomyelitis	979.5	E858.8	E950.4	E980.4	E949.5
– rabies	979.1	E858.8	E950.4	E980.4	E949.1
– rickettsial NEC	979.6	E858.8	E950.4	E980.4	E949.6
– rocky mountain spotted fever	979.6	E858.8	E950.4	E980.4	E949.6
– rubella	979.6	E858.8	E950.4	E980.4	E949.6
– smallpox	979.0	E858.8	E950.4	E980.4	E949.0
– TAB	978.1	E858.8	E950.4	E980.4	E948.1
– tetanus	978.4	E858.8	E950.4	E980.4	E948.4
– typhoid	978.1	E858.8	E950.4	E980.4	E948.1
– typhus	979.2	E858.8	E950.4	E980.4	E949.2
– viral NEC	979.6	E858.8	E950.4	E980.4	E949.6
– yellow fever	979.3	E858.8	E950.4	E980.4	E949.3
Vaccinia immune globulin	964.6	E858.2	E950.4	E980.4	E934.6
Valethamate	971.1	E855.4	E950.4	E980.4	E941.1
Valproate (sodium)	966.3	E855.0	E950.4	E980.4	E936.3
Vanadium	985.8	E866.4	E950.9	E980.9	

Substance	Poison-ing (Chapter XVII)	External Cause (E Code)			Adverse effect in correct usage
		Poisoning			
		Accident	Suicide (attempt)	Undeter-mined	
Vancomycin	960.8	E856	E950.4	E980.4	E930.8
Vapor (see also Gas)	987.8	E869.9	E925.9	E982.9	
– kiln (carbon monoxide)	986	E868.8	E952.1	E982.1	
– lead - see Lead					
– specified source NEC	987.9	E869.8	E952.8	E982.8	
Varicose reduction drug	972.7	E858.3	E950.4	E980.4	E942.7
Varnish	989.8	E861.6	E950.9	E980.9	
– cleaner	982.8	E862.4	E950.9	E980.9	
Vasoconstrictor, local	972.8	E858.3	E950.4	E980.4	E942.8
Vasodilator					
– coronary NEC	972.4	E858.3	E950.4	E980.4	E942.4
– peripheral NEC	972.5	E858.3	E950.4	E980.4	E942.5
Vasopressin (injection)	962.5	E858.0	E950.4	E980.4	E932.5
Vasopressor drug NEC	962.5	E858.0	E950.4	E980.4	E932.5
Vegetable extract, astringent	976.2	E858.7	E950.4	E980.4	E946.2
Venom (centipede) (insect) (reptile) (snake) (spider)	989.5	E905.	E950.9	E980.9	
Venous sclerosing drug NEC	972.7	E858.3	E950.4	E980.4	E942.7
Verapamil	972.0	E858.3	E950.4	E980.4	E942.0
Veratrum alkaloid, veratrine	972.6	E858.3	E950.4	E980.4	E942.6
Verdigris (see also Copper)	985.8	E866.4	E950.9	E980.9	
Versenate	977.2	E858.8	E950.4	E980.4	E947.2
Vienna					
– green	985.1	E866.3	E950.8	E980.8	
– – insecticide	985.1	E863.4	E950.6	E980.7	
– red	989.8	E866.8	E950.9	E980.9	
Viloxazine	969.0	E854.0	E950.3	E980.3	E939.0
Vinblastine	963.1	E858.1	E950.4	E980.4	E933.1
Vincristine	963.1	E858.1	E950.4	E980.4	E933.1
Vinyl					
– bromide	987.8	E869.8	E952.8	E982.8	
– chloride	987.8	E869.8	E952.8	E982.8	
– ether	968.2	E855.1	E950.4	E980.4	E938.2
Viomycin	960.6	E856	E950.4	E980.4	E930.6
Viprynium	961.6	E857	E950.4	E980.4	E931.6
Viral vaccine NEC	979.6	E858.8	E950.4	E980.4	E949.6
Viscous agent	977.4	E858.8	E950.4	E980.4	E947.4
Vitamin NEC	963.5	E858.1	E950.4	E980.4	E933.5
– A	963.5	E858.1	E950.4	E980.4	E933.5
– B NEC	963.5	E858.1	E950.4	E980.4	E933.5
– – nicotinic acid	972.2	E858.3	E950.4	E980.4	E942.2
– B-1	963.5	E858.1	E950.4	E980.4	E933.5
– B-12	963.5	E858.1	E950.4	E980.4	E933.5
– C	963.5	E858.1	E950.4	E980.4	E933.5
– D	963.5	E858.1	E950.4	E980.4	E933.5
– E	963.5	E858.1	E950.4	E980.4	E933.5
– K NEC	964.3	E858.2	E950.4	E980.4	E934.3
Warfarin	964.2	E858.2	E950.4	E980.4	E934.2
– rodenticide	989.4	E863.7	E950.6	E980.7	
Water					
– balance drug	974.5	E858.5	E950.4	E980.4	E944.5

Substance	Poisoning (Chapter XVII)	External Cause (E Code)			
		Poisoning			Adverse effect in correct usage
		Accident	Suicide (attempt)	Undetermined	
Water - *continued*					
– distilled	974.5	E858.5	E950.4	E980.4	E944.5
– gas	986	E868.1	E951.8	E981.8	
– purified	974.5	E858.5	E950.4	E980.4	E944.5
Wax (paraffin) (petroleum)	981	E862.3	E950.9	E980.9	
– automobile	989.8	E861.2	E950.9	E980.9	
Weedkiller	989.4	E863.5	E950.6	E980.7	
White					
– arsenic - see Arsenic					
– spirit	981	E862.0	E950.9	E980.9	
Whitewashes	989.8	E861.6	E950.9	E980.9	
Whole blood (human)	964.7	E858.2	E950.4	E980.4	E934.7
Window cleaning fluid	989.8	E861.3	E950.9	E980.9	
Wood					
– alcohol	980.1	E860.2	E950.9	E980.9	
– spirit	980.1	E860.2	E950.9	E980.9	
Wormseed, american	961.6	E857	E950.4	E980.4	E931.6
Xanthinol nicotinate	972.5	E858.3	E950.4	E980.4	E942.5
Xantocillin	976.0	E858.7	E950.4	E980.4	E946.0
Xenysalate	976.4	E858.7	E950.4	E980.4	E946.4
Xylene	982.0	E862.4	E950.9	E980.9	
– vapor	987.8	E862.4	E950.9	E980.9	
Xylol	982.0	E862.4	E950.9	E980.9	
– vapor	987.8	E862.4	E950.9	E980.9	
Xylometazoline	975.6	E858.6	E950.4	E980.4	E945.6
Yeast	963.5	E858.1	E950.4	E980.4	E933.5
Yellow fever vaccine	979.3	E858.8	E950.4	E980.4	E949.3
Yew	988.2	E865.4	E950.9	E980.9	
Zinc (compounds) (fumes) (vapor) NEC	985.8	E866.4	E950.9	E980.9	
– chloride, mouth wash	976.6	E858.7	E950.4	E980.4	E946.6
– chromate	985.8	E861.6	E950.9	E980.9	
– intravenous	972.7	E858.3	E950.4	E980.4	E942.7
– oxide	976.3	E858.7	E950.4	E980.4	E946.3
– – plaster	976.3	E858.7	E950.4	E980.4	E946.3
– peroxide	976.0	E858.7	E950.4	E980.4	E946.0
– phosphide	985.8	E863.7	E950.6	E980.7	
– stearate	976.3	E858.7	E950.4	E980.4	E946.3
– sulfate	976.5	E858.7	E950.4	E980.4	E946.5
Zineb	989.3	E863.2	E950.6	E980.7	
2,3,7,8-tetrachlorodibenzo-P-dioxin	989.2	E866.8	E950.9	E980.9	
2,4,5-T	989.2	E863.5	E950.6	E980.7	
2,4D	989.4	E863.5	E950.6	E980.7	
2,4-toluene diisocyanate	983.0	E864.0	E950.7	E980.6	
8-aminoquinoline drugs	961.4	E857	E950.4	E980.4	E931.4

CORRIGENDA, VOLUME 1

Page

137	228.0	Delete "NOS" and "vascular" under "Naevus:"
143	238.7	Amend exclusion code "298.8" to "289.8"
144	239.2	Amend exclusion code "239.8" to "239.0"
204	307.8	Amend exclusion code "784.5" to "724.5"
238	365.0	Align "Anatomical narrow angle Ocular hypertension Steroid responder"
260	393	Amend exclusion code "423.9" to "423.–"
281	457.1	Amend exclusion code "628.4" to "624.8"
308	528.4	Delete "Palatal papilla cyst"
347	620.7 } 620.8	Transfer "Haematosalpinx" from 620.7 to 620.8
363	648.6	Amend inclusion term to: "Conditions in 390–398, 410–429, 435, 440 to 459" Amend first exclusion term to: "cerebrovascular disorders in the puerperium (674.0)"
412	736.2	"clubbing of fingers (781.5)" is part of the exclusion note
418	742.4	Delete "Lissencephaly"
419	743.8	Add " †" after "270.2"
423	747.6	Amend exclusion code "743.8" to "743.5"
	747.8	Amend exclusion code "743.8" to "743.5"
428	752	Amend exclusion code "251.8" to "257.8"
429	752.7	Amend exclusion code "257.9" to "257.8"
435	757.3	Delete "Harlequin foetus"
436	758.7	Amend inclusion term to: "XXY syndrome"
457	781.2	Amend exclusion code "094.2" to "094.0"
466	790.6	Delete "hyperglycaemia NOS (250.9)" in exclusion note
530	980–989	Add exclusion term: "localized toxic effects indexed elsewhere (001 to 799)"
543	997.5	Amend exclusion code "539.3" to "593.3"
563	.1	Amend exclusion code ".3" to ".4"
578	E864.0 } E864.1	Transfer "Carbolic acid or phenol" from E864.1 to E864.0
635	Para. 1, line 2.	Amend "000–999" to "001–999"
638	V10–V19	Amend exclusion code "V50" to "V51"
639	V10.7	Delete "and 209"
649	V45.0	Amend exclusion code "V52.3" to "V53.3"
659	V70–V82	Amend "790–795" to "790–796" in Note

659

667	Table	Amend "M8000–M8002" to "M8000–M8004"
673		Amend code for "Mucoepidermoid tumour" to "M8430/1"
704	Example 12	Amend "example 52" to "example 59"
741	Rule MB3	Amend code "188.4" to "236.7"
748	182	Hyperlipoproteinaemia Amend codes to "272.0–272.4"
749	217	Amend "malnutrition" to "malfunction"
758	350	Nephritis, etc. Amend "500–589" to "580–589"

WHO publications may be obtained, direct or through booksellers, from:

ALGERIA: Société Nationale d'Edition et de Diffusion, 3 bd Zirout Youcef, ALGIERS

ARGENTINA: Carlos Hirsch SRL, Florida 165, Galerias Güemes, Escritorio 453/465, BUENOS AIRES

AUSTRALIA: Mail Order Sales: Australian Government Publishing Service, P.O. Box 84, CANBERRA A.C.T. 2600; or over the counter from Australian Government Publishing Service Bookshops at: 70 Alinga Street, CANBERRA CITY A.C.T. 2600; 294 Adelaide Street, BRISBANE, Queensland 4000; 347 Swanston Street, MELBOURNE, VIC 3000; 309 Pitt Street, SYDNEY, N.S.W. 2000; Mt Newman House, 200 St. George's Terrace, PERTH, WA 6000; Industry House, 12 Pirie Street, ADELAIDE, SA 5000; 156–162 Macquarie Street. HOBART, TAS 7000 — Hunter Publications, 58A Gipps Street, COLLINGWOOD, VIC 3066 — R. Hill & Son Ltd, 608 St. Kilda Road, MELBOURNE, VIC 3004; Lawson House, 10–12 Clark Street, CROW'S NEST, NSW 2065

AUSTRIA: Gerold & Co., Graben 31, 1011 VIENNA I

BANGLADESH: The WHO Programme Coordinator, G.P.O. Box 250, DACCA 5 — The Association of Voluntary Agencies, P.O. Box 5045, DACCA 5

BELGIUM: Office international de Librairie, 30 avenue Marnix, 1050 BRUSSELS — Subscriptions to World Health only: Jean de Lannoy, 202 avenue du Roi, 1060 BRUSSELS

BRAZIL: Biblioteca Regional de Medicina OMS/OPS, Unidade de Venda de Publicações, Caixa Postal 20.381, Vila Clementino, 04023 SÃO PAULO, S.P.

BURMA: see India, WHO Regional Office

CANADA: Single and bulk copies of individual publications (not subscriptions): Canadian Public Health Association, 1335 Carling Avenue, Suite 210, OTTAWA, Ont. K1Z 8N8. Subscriptions: Subscription orders, accompanied by cheque made out to the Royal Bank of Canada, OTTAWA, Account World Health Organization, should be sent to the World Health Organization, P.O. Box 1800, Postal Station B, OTTAWA, Ont. K1P 5R5. Correspondence concerning subscriptions should be addressed to the World Health Organization, Distribution and Sales, 1211 GENEVA 27, Switzerland

CHINA: China National Publications Import Corporation, P.O. Box 88, BEIJING (PEKING)

COLOMBIA: Distrilibros Ltd, Pio Alfonso Garcia, Carrera 4a, Nos 36–119, CARTAGENA

CYPRUS: Publishers' Distributors Cyprus, 30 Democratias Ave Ayios Dhometious, P.O. Box 4165, NICOSIA

CZECHOSLOVAKIA: Artia, Ve Smeckach 30, 11127 PRAGUE I

DENMARK: Munksgaard Export and Subscription Service, Nørre Søgade 35, 1370 COPENHAGEN K

ECUADOR: Libreria Cientifica S.A., P.O. Box 362, Luque 223, GUAYAQUIL

EGYPT: Osiris Office for Books and Reviews, 50 Kasr El Nil Street, CAIRO

EL SALVADOR: Libreria Estudiantil, Edificio Comercial B No 3, Avenida Libertad, SAN SALVADOR

FIJI: The WHO Programme Coordinator, P.O. Box 113, SUVA

FINLAND: Akateeminen Kirjakauppa, Keskuskatu 2, 00101 HELSINKI 10

FRANCE: Librairie Arnette, 2 rue Casimir-Delavigne, 75006 PARIS

GERMAN DEMOCRATIC REPUBLIC: Buchhaus Leipzig, Postfach 140, 701 LEIPZIG

GERMANY, FEDERAL REPUBLIC OF: Govi-Verlag GmbH, Ginnheimerstrasse 20, Postfach 5360, 6236 ESCHBORN — W. E. Saarbach, Postfach 101610, Follerstrasse 2, 5000 KÖLN 1 — Alex. Horn, Spiegelgasse 9, Postfach 3340, 6200 WIESBADEN

GHANA: Fides Enterprises, P.O. Box 1628, ACCRA

GREECE: G. C. Eleftheroudakis S.A., Librairie internationale, rue Nikis 4, ATHENS (T. 126)

HAITI: Max Bouchereau, Librairie "A la Caravelle", Boîte postale 111-B, PORT-AU-PRINCE

HONG KONG: Hong Kong Government Information Services, Beaconsfield House, 6th Floor, Queen's Road, Central, VICTORIA

HUNGARY: Kultura, P.O.B. 149, BUDAPEST 62 — Akadémiai Könyvesbolt, Váci utca 22, BUDAPEST V

ICELAND: Snaebjørn Jonsson & Co., P.O. Box 1131, Hafnarstraeti 9, REYKJAVIK

INDIA: WHO Regional Office for South-East Asia, World Health House, Indraprastha Estate, Ring Road, NEW DELHI 110002 — Oxford Book & Stationery Co., Scindia House, NEW DELHI 110001; 17 Park Street, CALCUTTA 700016 (Sub-agent)

INDONESIA: M/s Kalman Book Service Ltd. Kwitang Raya No. 11, P.O. Box 3105/Jkt., JAKARTA

IRAN: Iranian Amalgamated Distribution Agency, 151 Khiaban Soraya, TEHERAN

IRAQ: Ministry of Information, National House for Publishing, Distributing and Advertising, BAGHDAD

IRELAND: The Stationery Office, DUBLIN 4

ISRAEL: Heiliger & Co., 3 Nathan Strauss Street, JERUSALEM

ITALY: Edizioni Minerva Medica, Corso Bramante 83–85, 10126 TURIN; Via Lamarmora 3, 20100 MILAN

JAPAN: Maruzen Co. Ltd, P.O. Box 5050, TOKYO International, 100–31

KOREA, REPUBLIC OF: The WHO Programme Coordinator, Central P.O. Box 540, SEOUL

KUWAIT: The Kuwait Bookshops Co. Ltd, Thunayan Al-Ghanem Bldg, P.O. Box 2942, KUWAIT

LAO PEOPLE'S DEMOCRATIC REPUBLIC: The WHO Programme Coordinator, P.O. Box 343, VIENTIANE

LEBANON: The Levant Distributors Co. S.A.R.L., Box 1181, Makdassi Street, Hanna Bldg, BEIRUT

LUXEMBOURG: Librairie du Centre, 49 bd Royal, LUXEMBOURG

MALAWI: Malawi Book Service, P.O. Box 30044, Chichiti, BLANTYRE 3

MALAYSIA: The WHO Programme Coordinator, Room 1004, Fitzpatrick Building, Jalan Raja Chulan, KUALA LUMPUR 05–02 — Jubilee (Book) Store Ltd, 97 Jalan Tuanku Abdul Rahman, P.O. Box 629, KUALA LUMPUR 01–08 — Parry's Book Center, K. L. Hilton Hotel, Jln. Treacher, P.O. Box 960, KUALA LUMPUR

MEXICO: La Prensa Médica Mexicana, Ediciones Cientificas, Paseo de las Facultades 26, Apt. Postal 20–413, MEXICO CITY 20, D.F.

MONGOLIA: see India, WHO Regional Office

MOROCCO: Editions La Porte, 281 avenue Mohammed V, RABAT

MOZAMBIQUE: INLD, Caixa Postal 4030, MAPUTO

NEPAL: see India, WHO Regional Office

NETHERLANDS: Medical Books Europe BV, Noorderwal 38, 7241 BL LOCHEM

NEW ZEALAND: Government Printing Office, Publications Section, Mulgrave Street, Private Bag, WELLINGTON 1; Walter Street, WELLINGTON; World Trade Building, Cubacade, Cuba Street, WELLINGTON. Government Bookshops at: Hannaford Burton Building, Rutland Street, Private Bag, AUCKLAND; 159 Hereford Street, Private Bag, CHRISTCHURCH; Alexandra Street, P.O. Box 857, HAMILTON; T & G Building, Princes Street, P.O. Box 1104, DUNEDIN — R. Hill & Son, Ltd, Ideal House, Cnr Gillies Avenue & Eden St., Newmarket, AUCKLAND 1

NIGERIA: University Bookshop Nigeria Ltd, University of Ibadan, IBADAN

NORWAY: J. G. Tanum A/S, P.O. Box 1177 Sentrum, OSLO 1

PAKISTAN: Mirza Book Agency, 65 Shahrah-E-Quaid-E-Azam, P.O. Box 729, LAHORE 3

PAPUA NEW GUINEA: The WHO Programme Coordinator, P.O. Box 5896, BOROKO

PHILIPPINES: World Health Organization, Regional Office for the Western Pacific, P.O. Box 2932, MANILA — The Modern Book Company Inc., P.O. Box 632, 922 Rizal Avenue, MANILA 2800

POLAND: Składnica Księgarska, ul Mazowiecka 9, 00052 WARSAW (except periodicals) — BKWZ Ruch, ul Wronia 23, 00840 WARSAW (periodicals only)

PORTUGAL: Livraria Rodrigues, 186 Rua do Ouro, LISBON 2

SIERRA LEONE: Njala University College Bookshop (University of Sierra Leone), Private Mail Bag, FREETOWN

SINGAPORE: The WHO Programme Coordinator, 144 Moulmein Road, G.P.O. Box 3457, SINGAPORE 1 — Select Books (Pte) Ltd, 215 Tanglin Shopping Centre, 2/F, 19 Tanglin Road, SINGAPORE 10

SOUTH AFRICA: Van Schaik's Bookstore (Pty) Ltd, P.O. Box 724, 268 Church Street, PRETORIA 0001

SPAIN: Comercial Atheneum S.A., Consejo de Ciento 130–136, BARCELONA 15; General Moscardó 29, MADRID 20 — Libreria Díaz de Santos, Lagasca 95 y Maldonado 6, MADRID 6; Balmes 417 y 419, BARCELONA 22

SRI LANKA: see India, WHO Regional Office

SWEDEN: Aktiebolaget C. E. Fritzes Kungl. Hovbokhandel, Regeringsgatan 12, 10327 STOCKHOLM

SWITZERLAND: Medizinischer Verlag Hans Huber, Länggass Strasse 76, 3012 BERN 9

SYRIAN ARAB REPUBLIC: M. Farras Kekhia, P.O. Box No. 5221, ALEPPO

THAILAND: see India, WHO Regional Office

TUNISIA: Société Tunisienne de Diffusion, 5 avenue de Carthage, TUNIS

TURKEY: Haset Kitapevi, 469 Istiklal Caddesi, Beyoglu, ISTANBUL

UNITED KINGDOM: H.M. Stationery Office: 49 High Holborn, LONDON WC1V 6HB; 13a Castle Street, EDINBURGH EH2 3AR; 41 The Hayes, CARDIFF CF1 1JW; 80 Chichester Street, BELFAST BT1 4JY; Brazennose Street, MANCHESTER M60 8AS; 258 Broad Street, BIRMINGHAM B1 2HE; Southey House, Wine Street, BRISTOL BS1 2BQ. All mail orders should be sent to P.O. Box 569, LONDON SE1 9NH

UNITED STATES OF AMERICA: Single and bulk copies of individual publications (not subscriptions): WHO Publications Centre USA, 49 Sheridan Avenue, ALBANY, N.Y. 12210. Subscriptions: Subscription orders, accompanied by check made out to the Chemical Bank, New York, Account World Health Organization, should be sent to the World Health Organization, P.O. Box 5284, Church Street Station, NEW YORK, N.Y. 10249. Correspondence concerning subscriptions should be addressed to the World Health Organization, Distribution and Sales, 1211 GENEVA 27, Switzerland. Publications are also available from the United Nations Bookshop, NEW YORK, N.Y. 10017 (retail only)

USSR: For readers in the USSR requiring Russian editions: Komsomolskij prospekt 18, Medicinskaja Kniga, MOSCOW — For readers outside the USSR requiring Russian editions: Kuzneckij most 18, Meždunarodnaja Kniga, MOSCOW G-200

VENEZUELA: Editorial Interamericana de Venezuela C.A., Apartado 50.785, CARACAS 105 — Libreria del Este, Apartado 60.337, CARACAS 106 — Libreria Médica Paris, Apartado 60.681, CARACAS 106

YUGOSLAVIA: Jugoslovenska Knjiga, Terazije 27/II, 11000 BELGRADE

ZAIRE: Librairie universitaire, avenue de la Paix Nº 167, B.P. 1682, KINSHASA I

Special terms for developing countries are obtainable on application to the WHO Programme Coordinators or WHO Regional Offices listed above or to the World Health Organization, Distribution and Sales Service, 1211 Geneva 27, Switzerland. Orders from countries where sales agents have not yet been appointed may also be sent to the Geneva address, but must be paid for in pounds sterling, US dollars, or Swiss francs.

Price: Sw. fr. 30.—   Prices are subject to change without notice.   C/1/81